GYNECOLOGIC SURGERY
Errors, Safeguards, and Salvage

CONTRIBUTORS

Howard W. Jones, Jr., M.D., Professor of Gynecology and Obstetrics, The Johns Hopkins University School of Medicine, Baltimore, MD.
> *In collaboration with*
>> **Mason C. Andrews, M.D.,** Professor and Chairman, Department of Obstetrics and Gynecology, Eastern Virginia Medical School, Norfolk, VA.

George W. Mitchell, Jr., M.D., Professor and Chairman, Department of Obstetrics and Gynecology, Tufts University School of Medicine; Gynecologist-in-Chief, New England Medical Center Hospital; Boston, MA.

John L. Moore, Jr., LL.B., Attorney at Law; B.Litt. Oxon 1953 (Rhodes Scholar); LL.B. Harvard 1956; formerly Lecturer in Law and Medicine, Emory University School of Law; formerly Lecturer in Forensic Psychiatry, Emory University School of Medicine; Atlanta, GA.

John H. Ridley, M.D., Chairman, Department of Gynecology and Obstetrics, Piedmont Hospital; Clinical Professor, Department of Gynecology and Obstetrics, Emory University School of Medicine; Atlanta, GA.

Felix N. Rutledge, M.D., Professor of Gynecology, University of Texas Medical School; Chief, Department of Gynecology, University of Texas M.D. Anderson Hospital; Houston, TX.

Lawrence R. Wharton, Jr., M.D., Assistant Professor of Gynecology and Obstetrics, The Johns Hopkins School of Medicine, Baltimore, MD.

Tiffany J. Williams, M.D., Associate Professor of Obstetrics and Gynecology, Mayo Medical School; Division of Gynecologic Surgery, Mayo Clinic; Rochester, MN.

J. Donald Woodruff, M.D., Professor of Gynecology and Obstetrics; Associate Professor of Pathology; The Johns Hopkins University School of Medicine, Baltimore, MD.
> *In collaboration with*
>> **Conrad G. Julian, M.D.,** Associate Professor of Gynecology and Obstetrics; Assistant Professor of Radiology; The Johns Hopkins University School of Medicine, Baltimore, MD.

GYNECOLOGIC SURGERY
Errors, Safeguards, and Salvage

authored and edited by
JOHN H. RIDLEY, M.D.

foreword by
RICHARD W. TE LINDE, M.D.

The Williams & Wilkins Co. / Baltimore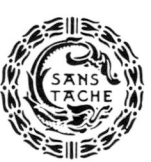

Made in the United States of America

Library of Congress Cataloging in Publication Data

Ridley, John H   1914–
    Gynecologic surgery.

    1. Gynecology, Operative. I. Title.
DNLM: 1. Gynecologic diseases—Surgery.
WP660 R545g 1974
RG104.R53   618.1   73-17408
ISBN 0-683-07276-5

Composed and printed at the
Waverly Press, Inc.
Mt. Royal and Guilford Aves.
Baltimore, Md. 21202, U.S.A.

Dedicated to
RICHARD W. TE LINDE, M.D.
Surgeon, Teacher, Friend

FOREWORD

It is with great pleasure and a feeling of satisfaction that I write the foreword to this volume. All of the surgical contributors to this work have had residency training at the Johns Hopkins Hospital. I believe that after reading this volume the reader will agree with me that it is the work of master pelvic surgeons.

The surgeon who has never committed an error has never done an appreciable amount of surgery. Every honest operator will admit to his errors and hopefully profit by them. To avoid errors in judgment or technic is the aim of all, but since surgeons are made of the same material as the rest of mankind, they naturally make their share of mistakes.

The greatest factor in the development of surgical judgment and technic is adequate training. The long term residency training program was conceived at the Johns Hopkins Hospital by Welch, Osler, Kelly and Halsted. Perhaps it was a contrivance on the part of these professors to lessen the burden of their work. In the last year of a five-year residency, with each year of increasing responsibility, the resident can naturally assume much of the professors' burden of teaching and performing surgery. Regardless of the motive of the professors, the creation of the long term residency training program has been the greatest factor in surgical training in the country in the past 75 years. All of the surgical authors of this work have had the advantage of this type of training.

In spite of the best of training and the greatest care by the most conscientious surgeon, things do happen in surgery which are unavoidable. Sometimes, legal action results. The jury may feel sorry for the patient who has really suffered, even though the surgeon may be completely innocent. A verdict against the surgeon is not uncommon under such circumstances. Many examples may be cited. An operator may close all abdominal incisions in the same manner. Ninety-nine of a hundred patients will heal perfectly with a strong abdominal wall. The hundredth patient may develop a hernia. Tissues vary in their healing qualities in different individuals but unfortunately, this cannot be determined pre-operatively by any known test. Then there are deviations in anatomy in different individuals. There may, for example, be a duplication of ureters or a deviation in the course of the ureter. In spite of meticulous care, the ureter may be injured under such circumstances. Vesicovaginal fistulas, especially those resulting from irradiation, may be practically incurable due to scarring and poor blood supply. The experienced surgeon is cognizant of the difficulties but because of compassion for the patient, he may undertake the job of curing the patient surgically. A failure of cure naturally results in great disappointment to the patient and the occasional resentful one may bring legal action.

When errors are committed at the operating table, they can often be corrected.

I have witnessed surgeons making technical errors become tremendously upset and loose their ordinarily good judgment. Often, some improvised procedure can be done on the spot to correct or alleviate the error but much can be accomplished by anticipating the possibility pre-operatively and carefully considering the method of correction. The means of avoiding or correcting such errors is what this book is about. I believe the wise counsel contained herein will be of value to all pelvic surgeons.

RICHARD W. TE LINDE, M.D.

PREFACE

The art and science of gynecologic surgery has kept well apace with the great advancements and responsibilities that have benefitted the practice of medicine and surgery in recent years. Our particular specialty has responded to the increasing demands of surgery of malignant and benign disease and of congenital deformities in the female pelvis. We are caring for these problems in a bolder and more comprehensive manner than ever before. Although this task has been made much easier by the modern, well-trained anesthesiologist and the internist, nevertheless the increased skill and confidence of the gynecologic surgeon is the main ingredient which gives the newer dimensions of effectiveness to his efforts.

Errors in the practice of gynecologic surgery are inevitable. This is true of any surgical specialty. These errors can occur in three areas: technique, surgical judgment, and the patient care, whether this be preoperative or postoperative. The main theme of this volume is the recognition of the possibility of these errors, with suggestions as to how these may be avoided by proper safeguards of alertness and skill, and with advice on what to do in an effort to salvage the failure or the less-than-satisfactory end result. Regardless of the maturity of the pelvic surgeon, he will remember the errors he has made or be confronted with errors he is making. With his broadening surgical experience, however, and with his knowledge of the numerous pitfalls that are possible, he will be less likely to make these errors, be more likely to employ safeguards against errors, and be more able to salvage a failure

The first milestone of the maturing surgeon is his frankness to admit that he has made an error or that his operative procedure is wrong to any varying degree. This important milestone may occur while the surgeon is yet a tyro; or may never occur at all. This latter intransigence may be influenced by a basic ignorance, which is forgiven if the surgeon learns more and broadens his skills. Or, intractability may be based upon stupidity, which is usually irreversible and should be the reason for dismissal from surgical practice. If, on the other hand, false pride is predominant, the trait is unforgivable and invites just criticism to himself and to the standard of his profession.

Even the most skilled and mature surgeon will inevitably make errors. There are such variations in human anatomy that no amount of previous experience and knowledge will prevent this from being a factor in contributing to errors. Also, there are individual responses of tissue healing and strength that are completely unpredictable. Further, there are problems of patient behavior which are beyond the control of the most conscientious surgeon. The presence of one or all of these factors in a given surgical problem may contribute to the failure or to the less-than-satisfactory end result of the operation. Thus the surgeon must be forewarned of the unexpected or uncontrollable factors in the care of his patient.

In addition, the iatrogenic pitfalls are possibly the most disturbing because of direct reflection upon the skill and judgment of the surgeon—productive of a sense of frustration, guilt and disappointment. Not in the least, iatrogenic casualties promote invitations for litigation in malpractice suits. In the past two decades this has been increasingly true, to a point where the surgeon must frequently compromise his better judgment of technique and patient care. In summary, the fact that an error has been made in surgical management is not usually *ipse res loquitur* of negligence, inexperience or indifference, but most frequently is related to these many variable factors in conscientious and skilled surgical care that are beyond the control of the operator.

The majority of textbooks of surgical technique deal with the "how to" of various operations. However, the purpose of this textbook is to point out the various possible errors that may occur, how errors can be avoided by modifying certain procedures, and, finally, how to salvage a failure if possible.

The basic approach of this textbook, then, is to suggest a general philosophy of operating with anticipation of possible errors, not operating fearfully but operating without hesitation, knowing that if such errors are committed, which in a career will be at times inevitable, that the surgeon will know how to recognize the error and take immediate appropriate action to correct this. Such anticipation can avoid a disastrous loss of composure and clear thinking which would impede a successful correction of the error and salvage of the case.

The contributors to *Gynecologic Surgery: Errors, Safeguards, and Salvage* have a background in common; their basic residency training was in the tradition of Howard A. Kelly, Thomas S. Cullen, and Richard W. Te Linde. To this training program has been added a considerable number of years of teaching, writing, and practicing of all phases of gynecologic surgery. In this time these men have been in the positions to judge not only themselves but have been called upon to teach others, to aid the erring surgeon, and to persistently demand perfection rather than mediocrity in gynecologic surgery.

This volume has another objective. By explaining that some errors are predictably possible and therefore are not matters of individual negligence, the book offers some refuge to gynecologic surgeons who have committed such errors. It is hoped that the defendant and defense attorney will find aid and reassurance within this volume, for we attempt to show that even men of broad surgical experience cannot always control the potential hazards of surgery and the capriciousness of anatomy and tissue behavior. A legal point of view is given by a competent lawyer who has had many years of experience in dealing with threatened and actual malpractice suits.

Although any one contributor to this volume could write comprehensively about the broad selection of subjects, it was nevertheless decided that particular sections would be done by the individual surgeon who through his years of experience and personal interest more or less specialized in his assigned field of writing for this volume.

Besides the work of the contributors, the various artists selected by these surgeons have done an outstanding job, uniform in fine quality, in their task of depicting graphically the thoughts of the surgeons.

Appreciation is expressed to the staffs of the Piedmont Hospital and of the Grady Memorial Hospital (Emory University School of Medicine) of Atlanta for the help given in the operating room, on the wards, and in the reference libraries. Dr. Lorna Beldia has given unselfishly much of her time and advice in helping to compose this volume. Consultations and suggestions by Dr. Mark P. Pentecost, Jr. have been most helpful.

Without adequate and competent secretarial help, no such volume would have been possible. My staff, selected and supervised by Mrs. Fabie Lasseter, has contributed immeasurably toward properly typing and helping to complete this textbook.

Mr. Dick Hoover, Editor-in-Chief of The Williams & Wilkins Company, has made most valuable practical suggestions toward finally publishing this volume. The job has been made much easier by his patience and cooperation.

Finally, mention must be made of the encouragement, tolerance, and patience on the part of my family during the preparation for final delivery of this volume.

JOHN H. RIDLEY, M.D.

CONTENTS

CHAPTER ONE

TIFFANY J. WILLIAMS, M.D.

ABDOMINAL HYSTERECTOMY, MYOMECTOMY, AND PRESACRAL NEURECTOMY: WITH MANAGEMENT OF BLADDER INJURY AND ATTENTION TO THROMBOEMBOLIC DISEASE

Any surgical procedure performed on the female pelvic organs subjects the patient to the risks of general anesthesia and general surgery. The surgeon is wise who recalls that the preoperative evaluation must be as complete as possible, even in emergency situations. Short-cuts taken for convenience or for socio-economic reasons are condemned as inadequate and incompetent medical care. This holds true regardless of whether they are taken before operation, during the surgical procedure, or after the operation and during convalescence.

Three abdominal procedures will be considered in separate sections of this chapter. Particular attention will be directed to vesical injury occurring during abdominal procedures and to thromboembolic disease. The other complications and problems that are common to each procedure will be discussed together. The indications and expected results for each procedure will be considered separately.

Preliminary Preparation

General Considerations

Certain general considerations apply to all gynecologic surgical procedures and particularly to those requiring abdominal incision. These factors apply before, during, and after the operation.

The preoperative period may be divided into two separate categories: before hospitalization and before surgical treatment. Evaluation before hospitalization is carried out in an office or clinic; nearly all preliminary study is best accomplished and evaluated during this period for several important reasons. Primarily, it allows for complete work-up and full discussion of the problem, including indications, complications, and anticipated results. It also allows time for the patient to recall other events or problems that may have been forgotten or ignored during the first interview. Particularly, it allows the patient and her family to consider and adjust to the psychologic ramifications of female pelvic surgery. Also of importance are the facts that hospital beds are not occupied unnecessarily and the high expense of hospitalization is avoided.

History. Taking the history is an intellectual exercise that cannot be overstressed. The history of any patient contemplating major surgery must include information about all organ systems. Questionnaires are helpful, but they are no substitute for personal confrontation, which assures understanding, insofar as possible, by both the patient and the physician.

The general history should include the cardiac as well as the respiratory status. Particular attention should be directed to any gastrointestinal and urologic problems that might be related to or might complicate the gynecologic condition. Allergies or hypersensitive conditions are particularly important in patients who may be exposed to additional drugs or transfusion.

Inquiry about medications that have been used in the past or present is imperative. Identification of unknown drugs is necessary, because many patients are unable to tell what their medication is or why they are using it. This may provide a significant clue to a condition or disease otherwise unknown to the patient. Patients who have been on long term medications are likely to ignore certain drugs unless specifically questioned on this point.

Three specific categories of drugs will be mentioned: endocrine, cardiovascular, and antibiotic. In the endocrine category, thyroid, estrogens, and cortisone must be mentioned specifically; insulin for diabetes is seldom forgotten since it is given by injection. Cardiovascular medications, such as the antihypertensive drugs and diuretics, are often ignored as may be even digitalis preparations and anticoagulants. Antibiotics used in the past may be of significance in future infection, and if allergic or hypersensitive reactions have occurred, these must be known and recorded.

Medications that need documentation may be categorized in three groups. Group 1 includes those medications that may affect the anesthesia or the surgical procedure itself. Diuretics, antihypertensive medication, cortisone, thyroid, insulin, and anticoagulants are examples. It may be necessary to discontinue some of these medications, or with drugs such as cortisone, preliminary preparation may be satisfactory.

Group 2 includes medications that would be required by the patient regardless of any surgical procedure such as cardiac glycosides, thyroid, insulin, estrogens, anticoagulants, antacids, anticonvulsants, and antihypertensive preparations. It is important to remember that when the patient's routine medications are taken away on admission to the hospital, oftentimes she forgets about them subsequently because she has placed herself in the care of the surgeon. Necessary orders must be written concerning these medications, but this may be overlooked by the busy surgeon concentrating on his surgical specialty if the patient has failed to mention them when asked about her medications.

Group 3 includes drugs related to the surgical procedure or to the hospitalization. Analgesics for postoperative pain are probably the most necessary of this group, and it should be stressed that such medications are best used in their therapeutic doses. Sedation for sleep and cathartics are commonly required for patient satisfaction. Antibiotics are indicated prophylactically with cardiac valvular disease but otherwise should be reserved for therapeutic use. Sensitivity or adverse reaction to such medication should be recorded as part of the preliminary evaluation.

On completion of the general history, more detailed attention is turned to the specific gynecologic complaint. A complete menstrual history should be followed by the obstetric history. Pelvic conditions or disease diagnosed or treated in the past must be recorded and may be relevant to the present problem. Of particular importance are all previous surgical procedures, especially those in the pelvis. The operative report should be obtained, and the histologic and cytologic findings should be reviewed to confirm previous diagnoses. All information should be obtained because any decision to take shortcuts to save time during this preliminary preparation may result in unnecessary surgical procedures.

Physical Examination. On completion of the general and specific gynecologic history, attention is directed to the physical examination. The compulsive intellectual discipline required in obtaining the history applies to the physical examination as well. When major pelvic surgery is anticipated, the cardiovascular and respiratory systems are of particular importance because of the anesthesia required, the status of surgery, and the subsequent convalescence. Cardiac enlargement, hypertension, arrhythmia, and arteriosclerosis are warning signs and require evaluation and consultation prior to consideration of surgery. Such abnormal conditions increase the risk of anesthesia and operation. Varicose veins are of special importance in pelvic surgery, and appropriate management is necessary to minimize significant postoperative complications.

Respiratory conditions such as asthma or emphysema may present problems not only with proper anesthesia but also with the postoperative respiratory toilet. Chronic bronchitis may require a period of respiratory preparation prior to surgical treatment. The chronic smoker must be encouraged to decrease her use of cigarettes. Anesthesia and surgery are contraindicated in the presence of an acute upper respiratory infection except in the most dire emergency. Appropriate treatment and convalescence are required to minimize risks of postoperative pneumonia.

Gastrointestinal symptoms may be of significance when considering gynecologic surgery. Signs of intestinal obstruction may reveal the true condition or may be evidence of more extensive disease. Similarly, evidence of extensive colitis or diverticulitis may lead to the conclusion that the intestinal disease is primary and gynecologic symptoms are secondary. Malignancy of both gynecologic and intestinal origin must be considered. Anticipation and preparation will minimize the risks of otherwise unexpected complications.

Urologic examination is particularly significant because of the close embryologic and anatomic relationship of the urinary and genital tracts. Anomaly in one tract is often associated with anomaly in the other, and preliminary evaluation is necessary. Similarly, infection in one system is often associated with infection in another. Indeed, the symptom in one system may be due to disease in another system.

The specific physical examination of most importance is that area at risk: the lower part of the abdomen and the pelvis. Adequate examination must include the entire abdomen, but particularly the hypogastrium and even the inguinal areas.

Pelvic examination is the *sine qua non*. No surgeon should operate on someone with whom he has not talked personally or whom he has not examined. Attention must be paid to all of the pelvic organs: the vulva and its parts, the vagina and its support (both anatomic and hormonal), the cervix, the uterus, and the adnexa. The position, size, and consistency of these organs are important.

No pelvic examination is complete without a rectal component; a combined rectovagino-abdominal bimanual examination is the single most useful clinical gynecologic examination. This examination should be confirmatory of previous examination and compatible with the history. In particular, the possibility of pregnancy must always be considered when dealing with the functioning female pelvis.

Laboratory Studies, Special Examinations, and Tests. Although certain laboratory studies are mandatory prior to any surgical procedure, more intelligent selection of necessary tests may be made on completion of the history and physical examination. These tests may be broken down into several categories.

Some tests are considered to be general in nature as they supply pertinent information relative to the patient undergoing any major surgical procedure. Among these tests are those that give information on blood status—*e.g.,* the hematocrit reading and hemoglobin. It is

important to remember that if these tests are performed when the patient is in the fasting or dehydrated state, they may give values that are somewhat misleading; clinical information and impressions should always be given due consideration. This holds true for all laboratory tests and diagnostic aids. Older individuals, in particular, are likely to present under such conditions. If prolonged anesthesia and surgical procedure are anticipated with the possibility of major blood loss and replacement, blood volume determinations may be useful. Baseline levels will be necessary in order to interpret subsequent values.

Renal status in general may be evaluated by routine urinalysis, which should include tests for sugar, protein, specific gravity, and acidity, and microscopic study for bacteria and cellular elements. When such study reveals normal findings, further laboratory study of the urinary tract is unnecessary unless abnormalities are reported in the history or found on physical examination. In such instances, treatment and/or blood urea nitrogen (BUN) may be required in addition to cystoscopy, cultures, and excretory urograms.

X-ray examination of the chest is also mandatory before use of any general anesthetic and major operation. Abnormal configuration of the cardiovascular tree dictates further evaluation, as does abnormality of the pulmonary fields. The findings of tuberculosis, emphysema, bronchiectasis, atelectasis, or metastatic disease could significantly alter the therapeutic plans. If chronic lung disease is present, preoperative pulmonary preparation is often useful in minimizing subsequent complications.

An electrocardiogram should be available for all patients more than 50 years of age even in the absence of a history of cardiovascular problems. It is a useful baseline for every patient but is mandatory if the patient has a family history or personal history of cardiac disease. In patients who have hypertension, evaluation of sodium and potassium are necessary.

Multiple other tests may be required because of abnormal findings in the history, physical examination, or laboratory studies. Any abnormality should be fully evaluated prior to major operation so that the surgeon can avoid being trapped by a significant complication during or soon after the operation. Conversely, there is no justification for ordering a meaningless battery of tests for the sole purpose of filling in blank spaces in the record.

In the event of significant gastrointestinal symptoms or findings, radiologic and endoscopic studies of this system are helpful. Occasionally, esophagoscopy, gastroscopy, and a gastrointestinal series are indicated, but with pelvic problems, the large bowel is more likely to be significant. Proctoscopy and roentgenograms of the colon are often useful adjuncts in ruling out intestinal disease or in pointing to the probability of complications in the bowel.

More important in pelvic surgery is the urinary tract, and some surgeons have gone so far as to recommend that cystoscopy and excretory urography be performed on all patients who are to undergo major gynecologic operations. Once again, such studies are considered necessary if there is a history of urologic disease or if the physical or laboratory examinations suggest involvement of or association with the urinary tract.

Specific tests relative to the pelvic organs also must be carried out. A cervicovaginal cytology study is mandatory in any pelvic examination or preoperative work-up. Similarly, if any visible or palpable abnormalities are amenable to biopsy, this should be performed. The same is true if there is a cervical lesion even in the presence of a negative smear.

Pregnancy is always a possibility in any female during the reproductive years. The marital status and the menstrual and gynecologic history may have no bearing on this possibility. Laboratory tests are likewise subject to error and, in general, the clinical impression of pregnancy takes precedence over the history and laboratory reports. Entirely aside from the moral question concerning abortion is the hard cold fact of increased risk in surgery performed on the pregnant woman.

If any significant abnormality has been determined by the preceding evaluation, then specialty consultation is in order. Cardiovascular problems are the most frequent. A history of infarction, cardiac failure, arrhythmia, hypertension, embolism, and the like may not be contraindications to surgical treatment but each requires close monitoring and followup during the surgical stress and recovery.

Metabolic problems such as diabetes and thyroid disease frequently are encountered and are deserving of knowledgeable and competent evaluation and treatment. Emphysema, chronic bronchitis, bronchiectasis, asthma, and similar respiratory problems may require preoperative preparation and recommendation concerning subsequent care. Such information and planning are far better outlined prior to the operation than later.

Diagnosis and Related Problems. On completion of the preoperative and prehospital evaluation, all information, reports, and tests should be gathered together and studied. It is then that the most significant part of the preoperative consultation takes place; a diagnosis is formulated and the condition or disease is explained to the patient. It is important that thorough discussion be carried out with the patient and, if possible, with the husband or relatives involved. A simple explanation of the disease or condition is in order.

The indications for surgery and its risks must be discussed. It is wise to mention the alternatives as well as to give the logical reasons for the selected treatment. The aims and results to be accomplished by operation are outlined. It is important to mention the significant risks and side-effects as well as the complications that may occur. There is a fine line between causing undue alarm because of certain problems and giving no information at all. The surgeon must tailor his discussion, which varies more in its presentation than in its content, to the personality of the patient and her family.

Of particular importance are the childbearing status and wishes of the woman. The patient must be aware of the possibilities that may eventuate from the surgery. It is a wise policy to make no guarantees concerning the surgical procedure to be performed or the results. It is not reasonable to accept the risks of major surgery when the surgeon is confined to performance of only a specific procedure or prohibited from carrying out an indicated operation. Most people understand such problems and if their faith and trust in the surgeon cannot surmount preconceived desires, then they should seek care elsewhere.

Many patients will raise the question of sexual performance or changes with aging relative to the operation. Whatever reassurance is possible should be offered concerning these factors. The discussion should contain comment concerning anesthesia, hospitalization, and convalescence. Financial arrangements are legitimate points for question and should be discussed. It is also important to point out the negative as well as the positive effects to be expected from the indicated operation. If these are ignored, many patients will assume that all of their problems will be solved by the operative procedure and will be dissatisfied when their wishes are not fulfilled.

Time should be available for questions from the patient and her husband and these should be given serious and honest answers. If all parties are in agreement and surgical treatment is elected, hospital and surgical arrangements are made. Further questions often will arise or need reiteration and can be answered in the hospital.

The situations arising relative to the operative procedures may be divided into three rather general categories: presurgical, surgical, and postsurgical. The presurgical period covers the time from hospital admittance to surgical incision. The surgical component covers the time between the incision and the patient's exit from the operating room. The postsurgical period covers the time between the patient's leaving the operating room and her return to her hospital bed. These three periods are common to whichever operation is to be done.

Presurgical Period

The time between the patient's admittance to the hospital and the performance of the surgical procedure allows for completion of any additional consultations or tests that may have been indicated. It is, likewise, a time when any additional questions may be answered and discussed or any additional complications or problems evaluated.

Admission to Hospital. When the patient is admitted, her chart should be reviewed for completeness and she should be questioned concerning any changes that may have arisen relative to her general health or specific gynecologic problems since she was last seen by the surgeon. Any necessary consultations should be obtained and the laboratory studies checked. The routine vital signs, pulse, respiration, temperature, and blood pressure are obtained and recorded. Reconfirmation of a

normal cardiorespiratory system is indicated and pelvic examination should confirm the previous findings. Abnormalities or changes require further evaluations and possibly additional treatment before the patient undergoes the risk of anesthesia and surgery.

The usual hospital routines require confiscation of the patient's own medications so that harmful duplication will be avoided. It is imperative, however, to remember that these medications are important to the patient's health, and it is the surgeon's responsibility to see that such necessary medications are continued and not ignored simply because they are not of gynecologic significance. Specific allergic reactions and sensitivities to medications should be recorded on the hospital chart and such information prominently attached to the patient, by means of a wrist band or some method that will not permit easy detachment, so that it is immediately available in the event of catastrophe or when the patient may be unconscious. Special emergency situations may arise in patients with heart disease, diabetes, or problems of similar severity. It is important that the nursing staff be aware of any such complications and alert to recognition of significant changes and symptoms.

Preparatory Cleansing. Certain routine preparations are indicated for the patient who is to undergo a major pelvic operation. Most important is cleansing of the involved area. Shaving and cleansing may be done the night before operation to permit time for more relaxation and more efficiency on the day of operation. Additional cleansing may be repeated the day of operation to minimize chances for infection. In abdominal procedures this includes the abdomen and the vagina, and if the possibility of combined procedures exists, the vulva and the perineum as well.

Scrubbing the skin with hexachlorophene (pHisoHex) is advantageous after excess bacteria-bearing hair has been shaved. The vagina is prepared in all instances and a cleansing douche may be followed by use of an antibiotic cream or suppository to minimize vaginal wall infection. Evacuation and cleansing of the bowel will lessen the chances of contamination of the operative field by fecal material whether from injury or muscular activity. The bladder is emptied to avoid trauma to it by distortion of the anatomy and to avoid distention from the fluids given during the procedure.

Certain other special preparations also are often required in pelvic surgery. Any organ or part of an organ situated in the pelvis should be given additional care because it may become involved during the operation. Most significant is the bowel. If there is known or suspected gastrointestinal complication, such as tumor, malignancy, adhesions, endometriosis, or diverticulitis, which may necessitate operation on the bowel, not only mechanical cleansing but also antibiotic cleansing is of value. An example is 15 ml of neothalidine every 4 hours for four doses and then every 6 hours until operation.

Care for Special Problems. Treatment for any infection of the bladder should be started promptly on diagnosis. Unless surgical treatment of the bladder or the urinary tract itself is contemplated, it is not necessary to delay operation, provided the patient is afebrile and responding to therapy. It is also important to complete the therapeutic course during the convalescence.

Varicose veins, also a special problem, frequently are present in women requiring major pelvic surgery. Because of the inactivity and stasis resulting from the anesthesia and the operation, as well as the immediate postoperative period, clotting is a likely complication. Thrombophlebitis and embolization may occur subsequently, and it is important to minimize these significant and conceivably lethal complications. If possible, surgical therapy for the varicose veins should precede major pelvic surgery, thereby decreasing the likelihood of these complications. Many times this is not feasible and supportive measures are required. Wrapping of the calf and thigh to collapse the veins will minimize stasis. Some routinely recommend antiembolic support of the calf, and if any emboli can be prevented thereby, it is a valuable addition to the program of treatment.

Medications. Two groups of medications are used: (1) those used for anesthetic and operative reasons and (2) special medications, some of which are reused for anesthetic and operative reasons and some of which are required for the patient's medical condition or complications. Two specific types are used routinely—the antianxiety variety and the antisecretory group.

The antianxiety group includes tranquilizers, narcotics, sedatives, and analgesics; the aim in using them is exactly as stated—to obtain relaxation and cooperation in a patient facing the stress of major surgery. Unless pain is a significant part of the problem, there is no real rationale for the use of analgesics or narcotics. Mild sedatives or tranquilizers are more likely to provide the desired result without potentiating or undesirable side-effects.

The antisecretory group is primarily for anesthetic benefit. The aim is to diminish respiratory, oral, and bronchial secretions and to avoid obstruction with diminished aeration and oxygenation. This group includes atropine and scopolamine. It must be remembered that there are contraindications to all medications. Similarly, the dosages of the medications must be tailored to the patient considering the size, weight, age, and medical condition. There is no such thing as a routine dose suitable for all patients.

Transfer to Operating Room. Medications are often given prior to transfer of the patient from her room to the operating room. It must be remembered that such premedicated patients are not in full control of their facilities and may be unduly sedated or even hyperexcited. Transfer should be well controlled and is best done with the patient supine on a stretcher under constant supervision. At no time should a patient in a wheelchair or on a stretcher be left unattended after medications have been given. Restraining straps should be used on stretchers to avoid an unexpected jolt, turn, or fall. The patient may be taken to a preanesthetic waiting room where intravenous injection of fluids may be started or she may be taken directly to the operating room. It is unwise to start anesthesia in one room and then remove a completely anesthetized patient to another operating room and table.

When the patient arrives at the operating room, she is moved from the transportation stretcher to the operating table; if she has received appropriate premedication, she may be aroused enough so that she may help move herself to the operating table. It is necessary, however, to have adequate personnel for proper control of the patient in the event that she is too sedated to be aware or helpful.

Positioning of Patient. Proper positioning of the patient on the table from the beginning is essential so that further movement is not required. Since many women have problems or complaints referable to the back, care must be taken to avoid undue extension or flexion of this region. Many of these patients are older women, and hip problems also are likely to be encountered and require special attention. It is wise to place the patient in position prior to anesthesia to avoid undue stress, particularly if the lithotomy position is required. In all situations it is important to move the legs, thighs, and hips together and with gentleness to avoid trauma. When the patient is anesthetized, there is no protective action of the skeletal muscles, and fracture may occur.

Pressure points on the legs, calves, and feet are to be avoided even in short procedures. Only slight additional trauma to a dilated blood vessel may result in thrombophlebitis. Restraints and supports should be well padded wherever they are in contact with the patient.

Since the Trendelenburg position is useful in many gynecologic procedures, care must be taken to avoid pressure points with the positional change. A particularly important area is the calf of the leg at the lower break in the operating table. Pressure here or laterally may cause foot drop from nerve damage, which may be transient and inconvenient or permanent and incapacitating. Also to be avoided are shoulder braces that support the patient's entire weight. Extensive and permanent damage to the brachial plexus may result. Hyperextension of the arms may place undue tension on the nerves and eventuate in paralysis. The arms are best placed by the patient's side in a natural position and further protected from the pressure of the surgeons, nurses, and assistants leaning on them. An additional point to be remembered is that the possibility of intracranial lesions contraindicates the use of the Trendelenburg position when castrating procedures are performed for metastatic carcinoma of the breast.

Discussion of anesthesia is beyond the scope of this work. Competent specialist consultation should be available as well as the equipment for any desired or required anesthetic. Adequate monitoring equipment and facilities for emergency resuscitation are necessary. During the induction of anesthesia, it is important that the patient have the full opportunity to reach the desired depth of anesthesia without extraneous stimulation. Examination under anesthesia is mandatory in all patients to confirm and re-evaluate the previous findings. Adequate

muscular relaxation may show the pelvis to be within normal limits and physiologic masses may resolve without surgery.

Completion of Cleansing and Preparation. On completion of the confirming examination, cleansing and preparation are completed. Antiseptic and drying solutions are commonly utilized and entirely satisfactory in conjunction with mechanical cleansing provided subsequent pressure on wet areas is avoided. Antibacterial solutions have gained some favor, but none seems to have advantage over another. Materials to which the patient may be hypersensitive should be avoided. The mercurial compounds are the most frequent offenders and may cause severe reactions.

Compulsive attention must be paid to the details of the cleansing. All areas that may be violated by the scalpel must be prepared, and contamination from unprepared areas must be avoided. Extension of incisions must be considered and the trunk must be cleansed between the breasts and thighs. It is important that the patient be dried thoroughly because moisture and pressure may combine to cause a mechanical or chemical burn that presents a more annoying problem than the surgery itself. Dragging or pulling of the drapes should be avoided, as this too may cause significant damage to the tissues.

When electrocoagulation or cautery is anticipated during the procedure, placement of the contact pad is best done under full vision to be sure that good contact is made. This is far easier when done prior to draping of the patient rather than subsequently by fumbling blindly beneath drapes and contaminating the area.

Of particular importance in abdominal surgery of the pelvic organs is the empty bladder. Even though the patient is instructed to void prior to coming to the surgical suite, delays are unavoidable and intravenous fluids may rapidly fill the bladder. Adequate pelvic examination is impossible with a distended bladder and after the urethral cleansing and catheterization, the bladder should be emptied and the pelvis examined without waste of time. It must be stressed that a pelvic examination with the patient under anesthesia and adequately relaxed is mandatory before any surgical procedure. This must be done to confirm the previous findings and to become aware of any changes that may have occurred since the last examination. Bimanual compression of the bladder is often required to provide adequate emptying, without which trauma is likely.

Choice of Incision. Although the incision itself initiates the surgical procedure, the selection of the incision must precede the draping of the patient. The intent of the draping is to exclude all other areas from the surgical field. Extension of the incision must be considered, however, and the draping should allow for this. In order to accomplish the proper draping, the selection of the incision is best made while the entire abdomen is exposed.

Several factors need consideration in selection of the incision. General considerations involve first the exposure that the incision will allow. Next in importance is the relative strength of various types of incisions and the subsequent healing processes, followed by the ease with which the incision and its repair may be accomplished, and then the complications or difficulties to be anticipated. Also to be considered is the pain related to the incision itself and, lastly, the cosmetic result.

Two factors may modify the selection of the incision. One is the presence of a previous scar and the other is the need for exposure. If there has been previous surgery, there will be compromise of the blood supply and, hence, compromise of healing in that area. It is better to excise a previous scar than to place an incision near it. Crossing or angling of incisions should be avoided, even though such an incision would otherwise be preferable.

Exposure in the event of large tumors or some intestinal complications may require extension of the incision into the upper part of the abdomen. In these instances a paramedian or low midline incision is best. Such incisions are likely to be somewhat easier and quicker to perform and perhaps they cause somewhat less postoperative discomfort; however, because of the blood and nerve supply, they are likely to be weaker incisions. The strongest incisions are transverse, and when they are placed lower in the abdomen they will be more cosmetic, because they follow the skin lines. Somewhat more discomfort may be experienced after the operation, however, and they require more time to make and to repair. Adequate exposure of the pelvic organs can generally be obtained by cutting the muscles, but if upper abdominal

procedures are required or anticipated, an additional incision may be necessary.

Because of the multiplicity of problems that may be encountered in the female pelvis, buttonhole incisions or small gridiron incisions, which cannot be extended if necessary, should be avoided. It is foolish to persist in making a surgical procedure more difficult than necessary because of poor exposure; to do so increases the risks and compromises the aims and results of the operation.

Once the patient has been anesthetized, cleansed, and draped, the time for the surgical procedure has arrived. Adequate anesthesia coverage and competent surgical and nursing assistance are of utmost importance. Surgical procedures are an exercise in teamwork and efficiency, and all members of the team, from the surgeon and the assistants to the scrub nurses, circulating nurses, and aides, must be aware of their responsibilities and duties during the operation. All preparations, instruments, and equipment should be available and ready prior to the start of the operation. The duration of the operation and of the anesthesia is related directly to the morbidity and complications. Speed *per se* is not of value, but the entire knowledge, understanding, and competence of the surgical team will promote the desired efficiency and so serve to minimize morbidity.

The Surgical Procedure

The one component of the surgical procedure that is common to all operations under consideration is the incision itself. Regardless of what procedure is required, the selection of the incision, the surgical techniques used, and the subsequent repair are identical.

The Incision. Whatever type of incision is selected, basic precepts will apply. Some of these, such as excision of the old scar, have been mentioned. Absence of occult herniation, which might damage other structures, must be assured. Incision is made on either side of the scar and joined beneath so that a wedge of scar and subcutaneous fat is removed. The incision is then carried deeper into the tissues and is identical with a primary incision, with the exception that adhesions and incorporation of bowel or bladder into the scar are possible. Even in the absence of previous surgical procedures, diastasis and herniation with adhesions may be present; therefore, equal care is required in all instances. At any time that the surgeon is unsure of the anatomy or tissue location, particular care must be taken to avoid unnecessary trauma to unexpected tissues.

As the incision is extended beneath the skin, vessels will be cut and will bleed. Some will be immediately beneath the dermis and these should be controlled by hemostats while the dissection is continued through the subcutaneous fat. Occasionally large bleeding vessels will be incised and will require control. Most vessels, however, will be small and will provide their own hemostasis by contracture of their walls.

Avoidance of trauma to fatty tissue is important because, in general, blood supply is poor and healing is retarded. Because of this trauma, necrosis and liquefaction may occur with subsequent infection and compromise of wound healing. Midline incisions usually have less bleeding inasmuch as the vessels come into the area laterally and terminate in the midline. However, large vessels, if present, will require ligation at the lower end of the incision; if such vessels have not been encountered, it is likely that the lower end of the incision has not gained full exposure.

The convenient way of controlling bleeding in subcutaneous tissues is by hemostats left in place until the procedure is completed. When they are removed just prior to closure, constriction and clotting usually render ligature unnecessary. If bleeding points must be ligated, the tie should be placed from the opposite side of the incision, so that the knot, and thus the bulk of the suture, is deeper in the tissues and less likely to form "stitch" abscess and "spit." Fine chromic or plain catgut suffices for such ligature.

A frequent fault is cleansing the adjacent overlying fat from the fascia. The excuse may be given that this allows better approximation of tissue; in fact, however, such "stripping" serves only to create dead space for the collection of serum, blood, or pus and should be avoided. In addition, a slip at this point could serve only to "buttonhole" and to weaken the fascia further and unnecessarily.

As the scalpel reaches the fascia, the dissection should be carried down through this layer in a definitive manner. Small sweeping strokes which do not incise the full thickness of the fascia serve only to attenuate and weaken this important tissue. Once the fascia has been incised, tension on both sides will allow extension of the incision upward toward the umbilicus and downward toward the pubis.

The position of the musculus pyramidalis will point toward the actual midline, and blunt finger dissection will separate the underlying properitoneal fat. Care must be taken that the tension is exactly in the midline so that the forceps do not hook beneath the belly of the muscle and affect its blood supply or cause unnecessary bleeding.

The foregoing comments apply particularly to the low midline incision. To summarize, such incisions are easier to perform, less vascular, less painful, may be easily extended to the upper part of the abdomen, and are weaker and more likely to herniate, particularly if there is obesity or infection. The transverse incision with or without muscle cutting will supply adequate exposure but is more vascular, more tender, stronger, and more cosmetic but will not allow adequate exposure or extension to the upper portion of the abdomen if this is required.

The most logical transverse incision would appear to be the Pfannenstiel, whereby the fascia is incised transversely. Longitudinal fascial incision in the midline causes development of a dead space between the fat and fascia that is subject to formation of seroma or infection and should be avoided. If transverse incision is carried widely, ligature of the inferior hypogastric vessels will be required; if these vessels are not reached, exposure is likely to be inadequate. Separation of the muscles in the midline would seem more logical and less traumatic than cutting of the muscles unless additional exposure is required. Care must be taken, however, to avoid cutting or weakening of the fascia when the peritoneum is freed.

If exposure requires cutting of the muscles, the use of scissors will often cause occlusion of small vessels that otherwise cause annoying bleeding. Significant bleeding vessels will require control, but trauma to the muscle itself is to be avoided.

The properitoneal fat should be separated from the region in which the peritoneum is to be incised. This may be done by sharp or blunt dissection. The position of entry into the peritoneal cavity is critical. The safest area is in the upper portion of the incision. The tissue of the posterior rectus sheath and peritoneum is grasped on either side and incised. Almost no bleeding should accompany this step, and the tissue itself has a distinctive appearance. Picking up small portions of tissue will increase the chances of recognizing problems and minimize the possibility of bowel damage. Bleeding, oozing, or red muscular tissue are evidence of a problem and require close attention to be sure that neither bowel nor bladder is involved. Although the most important points referable to damage of the bladder or bowel are prompt recognition and appropriate repair, it is far more satisfactory to avoid the complication entirely. More time and morbidity will result from slashing, hurried incisions, and repairs than will result from meticulous, careful dissection and avoidance of damage and trauma to other organs.

If the patient is adequately anesthetized and relaxed, there will be an inrush of air as the vented peritoneum is entered and the abdominal contents drop away. Extension of the peritoneal incision is done best with scissors, being sure that no bowel will be included in the cut. Proper use of the dissecting scissors is as two opposed cutting blades rather than the closing of the handles in a shearing action. Such closing will sever whatever is between the jaws of the scissors, whereas, when the scissors are properly utilized, resistance will be encountered as a warning that different tissue may be present. This is particularly important when there has been previous surgery and bowel adhesions may be encountered.

The bladder is always a problem at the lower end of the incision. Proper surgical technique will alert one to the presence of bladder muscularis. Not only the consistency but also the vascularity of the muscularis is different and will alert the surgeon to the presence of adjacent structures. When in doubt, slow down and be sure of the exact anatomic position. There is little cause for incising the bladder, but no excuse for failure to recognize the problem. If damage has occurred, recognition and appropriate repair provide satisfactory results without increasing the morbidity. Incision may be made into the bladder or the bowel and this may be entirely unavoidable because of pre-senting conditions; however, this never occurs without adequate warning so that proper recognition and repair can be carried out.

If the bladder has been elevated or is high so that it compromises the lower extension of the incision, then lateral incision downward along the side will allow adequate exposure. This will minimize the possibility of trauma to the bladder and bleeding from its highly vascular tissues.

The first step on opening the peritoneal cavity is thorough and complete exploration of the abdominal contents. Only in the presence of pelvic infection should upper abdominal exploration and contamination be avoided. It is best, first, to confirm the pelvic diagnosis when intra-abdominal hemorrhage and/or infection are complicating factors. Attention may then be turned to the other abdominal organs.

Exploration. Exploration should be systematic. The liver is a good starting place. Its size, shape, and consistency should be noted. Metastatic disease or nodules may be recorded if present. Similarly, the gallbladder should be palpated for stones, and if present their size should be noted. Both kidneys should be checked for presence, size, and consistency. The spleen, pancreas, and stomach should be checked and the diaphragm as well to note the possibility of herniation. The intestine should be checked from the standpoint of Meckel's diverticulum and the appendix. However, if there are no other gastrointestinal problems requiring manipulation of the bowel, handling should be kept to a minimum to avoid postoperative ileus.

The pelvic organs should be carefully evaluated to confirm the preoperative diagnosis and to determine the appropriate operative procedure. It is best to avail oneself of all possible information about the pelvic organs before starting on a definitive procedure. If there are adhesions, they should be freed prior to committing oneself to a specific operation. In this way, all tissues may be visualized, palpated, and evaluated in order to avoid unnecessary procedures or unwanted surprises.

The bowel and any adhesions should be freed and removed from the field of operation. If trauma or bleeding occurs, repair and hemostasis should be performed promptly so that there is no unnecessary loss of blood or contamination.

Also, such dissection will remove any adherent intestine from the area of retraction which could cause additional trauma to the bowel.

Proper anesthesia and relaxation will simplify handling and manipulation of the intestines, and if a mild Trendelenburg position is used, no manipulation whatsoever may be required. It is wise, however, to pack the bowels away from the operative field to facilitate the procedure. This should be done gently with moist packs blocking the gutters laterally as well as the region between them. If relaxation is poor, it is best to wait until adequate anesthesia has been attained rather than to proceed with forceful manipulation of the intestines.

The bladder, also, may present a problem, even though catheterization has been carried out. As mentioned previously, if a distended bladder obscures the field of surgery, it should be emptied before the operation is continued. Pressure may accomplish this, or needle aspiration may be required to evacuate the urine so that exposure is adequate. This may be done extraperitoneally with an 18- to 20-gauge needle and a 30- to 50-ml syringe. Both the bladder and bowel should be freed from any adhesions to the pelvic organs. Similarly, they should be extracted from the field of exposure so that neither the bladder nor the bowels will unexpectedly obstruct the vision in the surgical field at a critical time.

As was mentioned earlier, the pelvic organs themselves should be adequately visualized for confirmation of the diagnosis. Complicating factors such as diverticulitis, endometriosis, tumors, and malignant lesions may distort the anatomy. More time may be required for dissection to determine the proper diagnosis and surgical treatment. The appropriate plan of attack is best organized at this time, rather than when partially through a difficult operative procedure.

Specific procedures will now be considered. The diagnosis has been confirmed and the procedure to be carried out will be determined. Hysterectomy, myomectomy, and presacral neurectomy will be considered in sequence up to the time of the completion of the specific technique.

Abdominal Hysterectomy

The general and specific history, physical examination, and laboratory tests have been discussed earlier. Some mention, however, needs to be made concerning the indications for abdominal hysterectomy. Abdominal hysterectomy refers to the removal of the entire uterus, cervix, and fundus through an abdominal incision.

Seldom is there cause to remove only the fundus of the uterus and leave behind a troublesome cervix. Extenuating circumstances, however, do arise, and the technique of a rapid subtotal or supracervical hysterectomy should be known by all pelvic surgeons. The flat statement made by some individuals that there "is no place for the subtotal hysterectomy" is an absurd one. Generally there is no indication for planning such a procedure, but the operative findings and the patient's condition may dictate a course of discretion. In the event of anesthetic or surgical problems, it is better to have a live patient with a cervical stump than a dead patient without one.

The indications for abdominal hysterectomy are confined to two broad categories: benign and malignant disease involving the pelvic organs. A basic consideration is whether the patient herself has any symptoms or problems from the condition. A second consideration is whether, even if asymptomatic, the condition presents a risk to the patient.

For Benign Conditions

The benign conditions include tumors, inflammatory disease, and endometriosis. Although fibroid tumors of the uterus are the most commonly encountered, benign pelvic tumors may require exploration and removal. The presence of fibroids *per se* is not alone an indication for hysterectomy. In all instances it is important that the question of future childbearing be settled and that the wishes of the patient be respected if they are within the limits of good surgical practice. The surgeon must not be restricted, however, in choosing the required procedure. In general, when laparotomy has been undertaken and the risks of general anesthesia and major surgery have been accepted, it is unwise not to perform complete and adequate surgery. All diseased organs should be removed. Leaving damaged tissue behind only subjects the patient to the risk of subsequent surgery and morbidity.

The adnexa are discussed elsewhere, but they should be mentioned briefly. If castrating surgery or sterilizing surgery is required because of adnexal disease, then the uterus should be removed. There is no reason to leave behind an organ whose only subsequent function is loss of blood or growth of tumor.

Infection requiring hysterectomy is related to the adnexa in most instances, although on occasion uterine abscess and pelvic abscess may occur requiring removal of the diseased tissue. When this much infection is present, there is no way whereby the uterus and childbearing capability can be preserved; removal of these organs is indicated to permit adequate rehabilitation of the patient.

Endometriosis is another condition that involves the pelvic organs and may require hysterectomy. If the family is complete and endometriosis is symptomatic, total abdominal hysterectomy and bilateral salpingo-oophorectomy are the procedures of choice. When children are desired, conservative surgery is justified as a calculated risk with acceptance of the fact that additional surgery may be required. Numerous studies have demonstrated a pregnancy rate of about 30% as opposed to a reoperation rate of 10 to 15%. On occasion, laparotomy is necessary because of a pelvic mass that subsequently proves to be endometriosis even in the absence of symptoms. In such instances, preliminary discussion will have enabled the surgeon to know the patient's wishes and will allow him to perform the required surgery.

The other uterine disease leading to abdominal hysterectomy is benign fibroid tumors. These cases present two broad indications for surgery: symptoms or disability secondary to fibroids and changes found on examination. Pain discomfort, pressure, a mass, and bleeding are the symptoms that alert the patient to the presence of tumors. Removal of the uterus is indicated if tumors are responsible for these symptoms.

Fibroid tumors gradually grow during active menstrual life, and if unstimulated by hormones, they often regress after the estrogen depletion of the menopause. If there is a rapid change in the size of the tumors, malignant degeneration must be suspected and hysterectomy is advised. Hemorrhage and secondary anemia are likewise indications that may require abdominal hysterectomy. Size alone is a valid indication for hysterectomy when the tumors have grown to such an extent that the pelvic organs cannot be delineated and ovarian neoplasm or malignancy cannot be ruled out.

There are variations in technique for abdominal hysterectomy when performed for benign and malignant disease and mention of the variations will be made at the specific points in the technical progress of the operation.

For Malignant Disease

Malignant disease of the cervix, uterus, tubes, and ovaries is also an indication for abdominal hysterectomy. Invasive cervical cancer, which is considered elsewhere in this book, may be amenable to radical hysterectomy. Preinvasive carcinoma of the cervix may be treated by simple extrafascial hysterectomy removing a wide vaginal cuff. This is more easily performed by the vaginal than the abdominal route unless other problems require the latter approach.

Carcinoma of the endometrium is treated by extrafascial hysterectomy with bilateral salpingo-oophorectomy. Preliminary suture of the cervix (Fig. 1.1) and ligation of the tubes or clamping the cervical ends of the tubes immediately on opening the abdomen prevent dissemination of malignant cells by those avenues (Fig. 1.2). These steps should precede manipulation of the pelvic organs. Radiation before or after operation and with or without chemotherapy completes the therapy for endometrial malignancy. Preoperative catheterization and a sponge saturated with 95% alcohol placed in the vagina are of value.

Procedures for treatment of carcinoma of the tubes and ovaries are laparotomy and total abdominal hysterectomy with bilateral salpingo-oophorectomy and omentectomy. Even when the disease is extensive, it is felt that the bulk of the tumor should be removed if possible. However, hysterectomy should be avoided if it means leaving a large malignant crater where the cervix used to be.

It is of paramount importance that all gynecologic symptoms be evaluated before starting the operation, to minimize the chances of removing an undiagnosed carcinoma by an inadequate operation, which would significantly jeopardize the patient's chances for survival. Smears are required before beginning

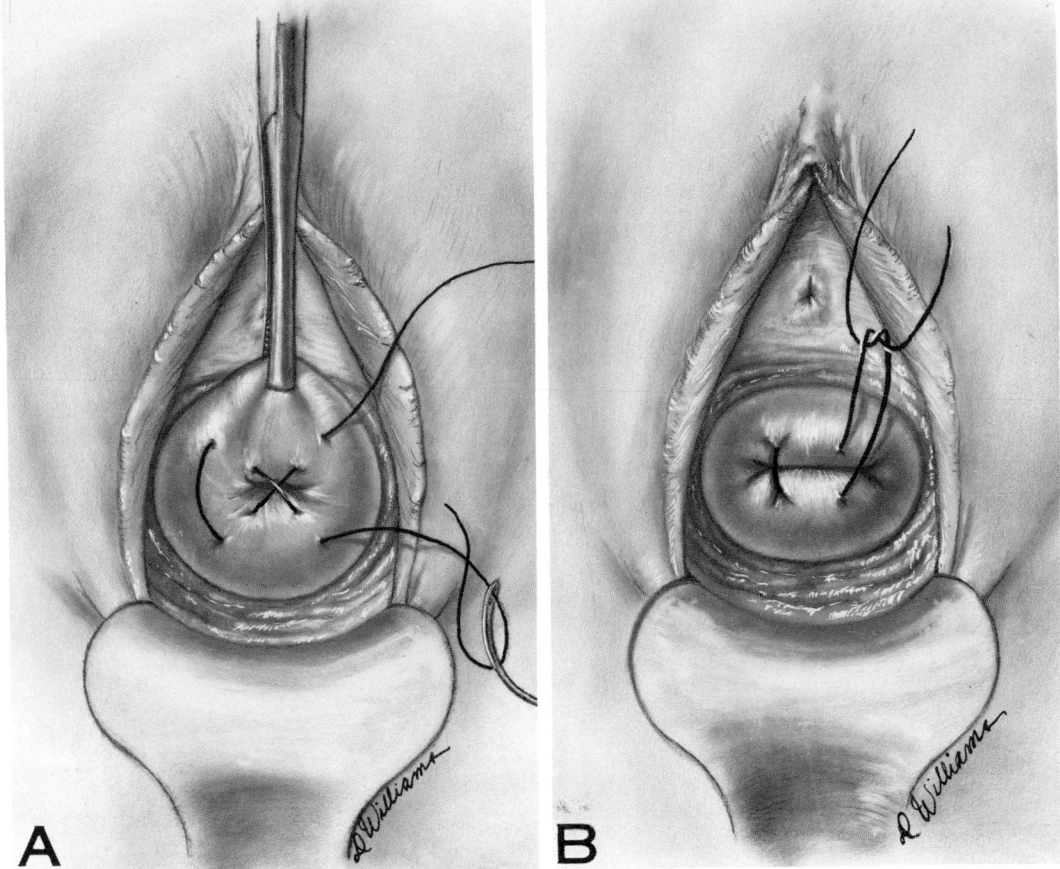

Fig. 1.1. A, Placement of figure-of-eight suture to close cervix. B, Closure of cervix by suture to prevent spill of malignant cells.

any procedure as is cervical biopsy or endometrial curettage if symptoms of a lesion or of bleeding are noted. Because of the dissemination mode of tubal, ovarian, and endometrial carcinoma, radical operation generally is not of value and is contraindicated.

Technique

After the abdomen has been opened by an appropriate incision and its contents have been explored, attention may be turned to the pelvic surgery. The judgment should be made as to whether hysterectomy is indicated; if it is, one should proceed with the operation.

Subsequent to freeing adhesions, if they are present, the first step is to isolate the round ligament by clamping it (Fig. 1.3), then tying and cutting it to enter the retroperitoneal space at the top of the broad ligament. Often a small

blood vessel lies beneath the round ligament and this should be included in the clamp and ligature. Leaving a clamp on the uterine remnant of the ligament allows a means of traction to improve exposure.

Chromic catgut (1-0) is a reasonable ligature and suture size. It is strong enough to tighten against large ligamentous and vascular pedicles and does not tend to cut through soft or edematous tissues. Newer collagen suture material and Dexon are satisfactory and are likely to be used more commonly in the future. It is best to use the smallest size of surgical gut that is of adequate strength and the smallest amount that is required and can be handled comfortably. Atraumatic sutures seem more logical from the standpoint of tearing and damage to the tissues, but interrupted ones work satisfactorily. Because of the difficulty in adequately cleansing the vagina and the proximity of the ligatures to

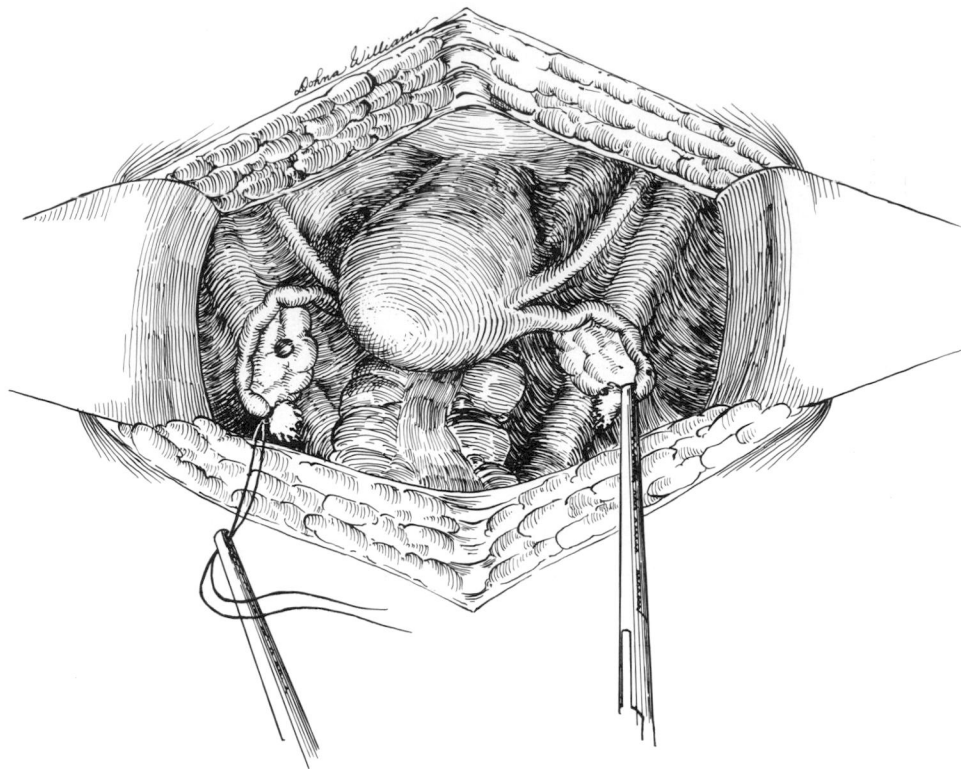

Fig. 1.2. Ligation of distal ends of tube to prevent intraperitoneal spread during hysterectomy for carcinoma of endometrium.

a potentially infected vaginal vault, permanent sutures are usually avoided in favor of the catgut.

If pelvic varices are present, they should be avoided and the procedure tailored or modified so as to avoid the error of unnecessary trauma and troublesome bleeding. These vessels are often encountered in the infundibulopelvic and broad ligaments and extend down laterally to the cervix and vagina beneath the bladder. When present, it is wise to have clamps or ligatures on both sides of the incisions. If heavy bleeding obscures the field, it is better to turn all attention to the bleeding and its control, rather than to operate blindly in a pool of blood, even if one is positive about the anatomic structures involved. Figure 1.3 demonstrates the relative positions and courses of the uterine, ovarian, and iliac vessels as well as the ureter and bladder.

After the round ligament is cared for, the uterus is held laterally and anteriorly so that the infundibulopelvic or utero-ovarian ligament can be isolated (Fig. 1.3). The posterior parietal peritoneum is entered either by sharp or blunt dissection through the avascular space so that the pedicle bearing the blood vessels is isolated. It is wise to check the ureter (Fig. 1.3) to confirm that it has not been included along with the blood vessels. Before clamping, either visualization or palpation of the ureter is required as a safeguard against including it in the clamps along with the ovarian vessels.

If space permits, three clamps with similar jaws (Fig. 1.4) are utilized, cutting between them so that the double clamps are left distally and the single clamp is on the uterine side to control back-bleeding and to serve for traction. The double clamps minimize the chances of tissue pulling out before ligation or retracting during the process. Use of a free tie just behind the distal clamp will control the blood supply, and a transfixion suture may be placed behind the remaining clamp without fear of vessel perforation with bleeding or formation of a hematoma.

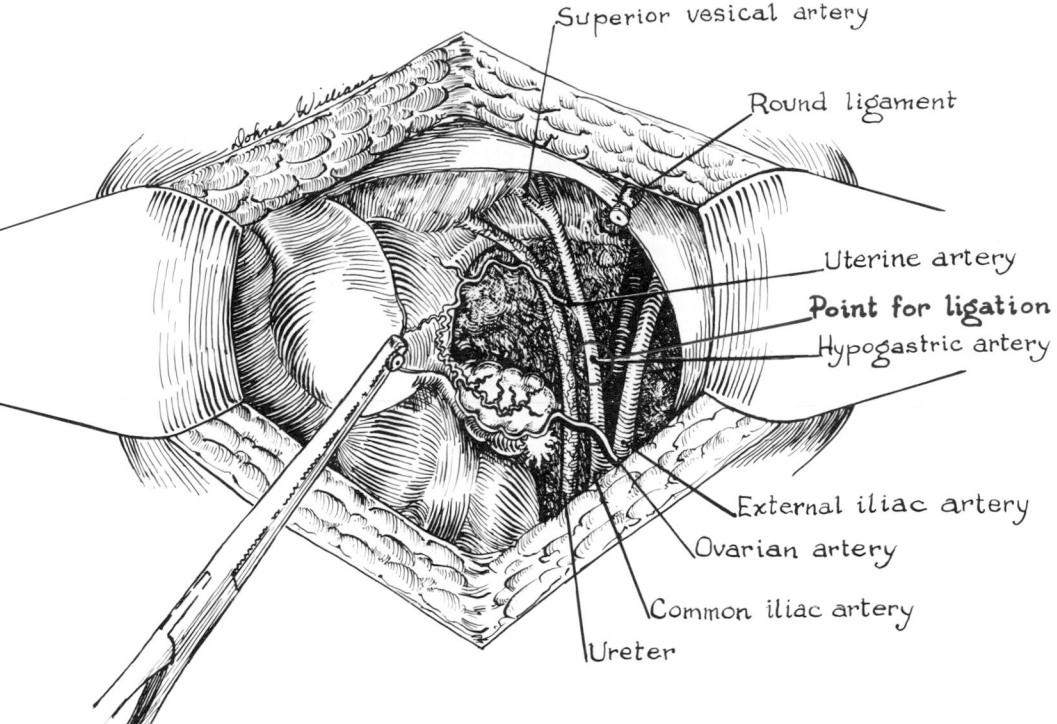

Fig. 1.3. Retroperitoneal anatomy with blood vessels and ureter.

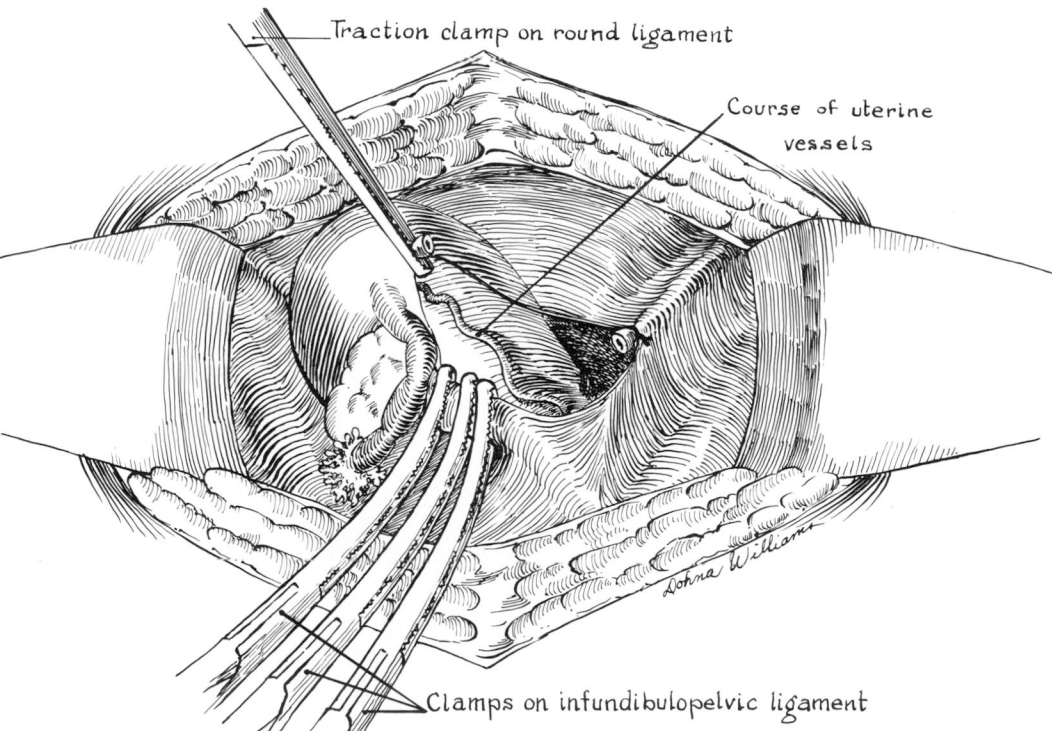

Fig. 1.4. Triple clamping of infundibulopelvic ligament when tube and ovary are to be removed.

If the artery does retract and a hematoma forms, the bleeding should be controlled immediately. Delay only allows increase in the size and extent of the hematoma and makes eventual control of the bleeding vessel more hazardous. As soon as a hematoma is noted, incision is made into the retroperitoneal space of the hematoma and the vessel is controlled under direct vision. If a tie is required for control higher up on the whole pedicle, care must be taken to re-evaluate the position of the ureter in relation to the tie so that it will not be traumatized, tied, or kinked by the ligature.

Particular care must be taken in searching for the ureter if there are complicating factors such as diverticulitis, ovarian mass, endometriosis, or infection. Combined visualization and palpation are best. Although the ureter has a distinctive feel and "snap" when rolled between the fingers, large veins also may present similar sensations. Peristalsis and the characteristic wavy blood vessel on the ureteral surface are not duplicated by any other structure (Fig. 1.3).

The opposite side of the pelvis is managed similarly, and bilateral control of the ovarian vessels will decrease some of the blood supply to the uterus, diminishing subsequent blood loss and improving visualization.

The third step involves freeing the bladder from its attachment to the anterior surface of the uterus. Tension and traction on the peritoneal edges from the round ligament area enable one to stay within the loose areolar tissue and to dissect this toward the symphysis. Bleeding is minimal when dissection is in the proper plane of cleavage. A common error is to make the peritoneal incision too close to the uterus; dissection will then be more difficult and bloody. Conversely, however, when there has been previous surgery, particularly cesarean section or uterine suspension, one may find that the bladder has been advanced to the top of the fundus. In such cases it is important to utilize the proper plane and to be sure that part of the bladder is not left attached to the uterus and subsequently traumatized. Inflammatory conditions and adhesions may also affect the bladder position by distorting its anatomy and changing the nature and character of the tissues. An additional safeguard would be to leave myometrium on the bladder rather than the bladder on the uterus.

When the bladder itself is approached, the tissue is entirely different. Vascularity is encountered with bleeding from multiple small vessels. The vesical muscularis has soft, meaty red fibers. Progression of dissection will lead to the mucosa through which fluid may be seen, and when the mucosa is incised, the urine itself will escape. If the bladder has been opened, the urine itself may not be noted but the indwelling catheter may be both seen and palpated. If the dissection is difficult and exposure is poor, it is best to check the position of the catheter frequently to avoid incising the bladder. Repair will be discussed in a subsequent section.

When dissecting the bladder flap, the safest use of dissecting scissors is to push them against the peritoneum with the tips slightly apart and with the blades serving as opposing cutting edges. Change in the tissue character will be noted immediately. However, if scissors are used with an opening and closing "guillotine" action, it may be too late to avoid damage to the encountered tissue. The back of the bladder may be dissected from the anterior surface of the cervix by sharp or blunt dissection (Fig. 1.5). The plane just above the cervix is relatively avascular, but it is safer to be too close to the cervix than to traumatize the base of the bladder where the trigone and ureters are located.

If there is distortion from disease, tumor, or previous surgery, it is important to be positive about the location of the cervix. Its position can be felt from behind the uterus so that the dissection does not wander off laterally to one side or the other; dissection of the base of the bladder is to be avoided. Lateral to the base of the bladder and cervix is Santorini's plexus which frequently has large dilated vessels that bleed profusely when traumatized. Control is difficult and hazardous because of the proximity of the ureters. When encountered, use of large transfixion sutures or blind clamping must be avoided. Pressure and suction should be used to control bleeding and to permit visualization so that only the involved vessels are ligated. Hypogastric ligation may be necessary and may be accomplished with virtually no risk. An additional method of salvage is the use of ring forceps as described in the chapter on ureteral damage (see Fig. 4.24).

Although the bladder must be taken down past the cervicovaginal junction, it should not

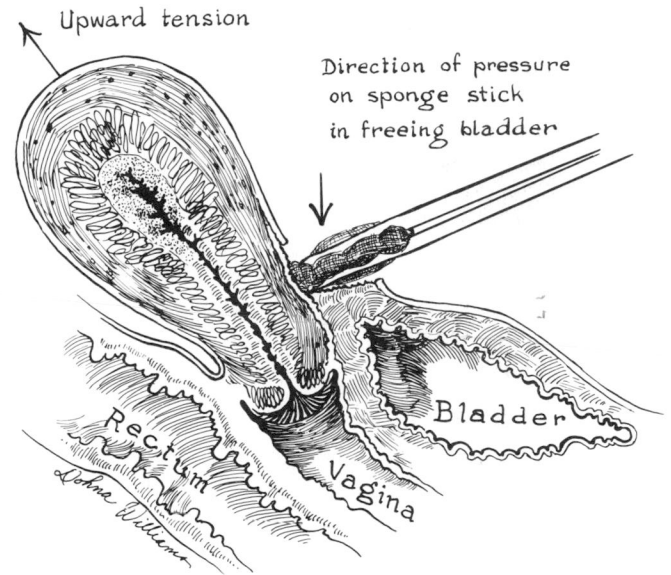

Upward tension

Direction of pressure
on sponge stick
in freeing bladder

Bladder

Rectum

Vagina

Fig. 1.5. Blunt dissection of bladder from lower uterine segment and cervical area.

be taken any further than is necessary to remove the cervix and to reconstruct and suspend the vagina. Wide and unnecessary dissection only increases the bleeding and the chances for bladder and ureteral damage with subsequent fistula formation. When extrafascial hysterectomy is required, however, further dissection is necessary because the pubovesicocervical fascia must be removed in continuity with the specimen as noted in preceding paragraphs.

After the bladder has been freed, the uterine vessels are ligated. Skeletonization of the vessels is indicated to avoid the error of too large a pedicle that cannot be tied properly. This may be done either by sharp or by blunt dissection, freeing the posterior peritoneal leaves of the broad ligament and the loose fatty areolar tissue over the vessels. This dissection should stop, however, when the veins and arteries are encountered in order to avoid trauma and bleeding. The vessels are then triply clamped, cut, and ligated with double sutures (Fig. 1.6).

The clamps are placed so that the tips are at the base of the fundus, near the level of the internal os and top of the cervix. The third clamp merely controls the back-bleeding from the fundus and is placed higher on the uterus so that the incision between the clamps is facilitated. Double suture ligation is used, tying each ligature separately behind each of the clamps in turn. Double ligation of these vessels provides a safety measure to avoid subsequent bleeding. If the pedicle is large, one must be sure that the ties are snug. Opening the clamps may be required to determine that there is no extra tension on the tissue preventing a snug knot. When exposure is poor, only two clamps may be possible; the two sutures are then placed distal to the single clamp as just described. Each suture should be placed just beneath the tip of the clamp rather than transfixed and tied on both sides. This takes less time and allows a snugger tie, which is fixed in place as a safeguard but prevents vessel perforation and minimizes hematoma formation.

If hematoma results from vessels slipping back into the broad ligament or from laceration of the vessels, control should be carried out promptly. If the vessel can be located easily, it then may be clamped individually and tied. If exposure is poor, however, it is far safer to drop back to the hypogastric artery and ligate the uterine vessel at its origin rather than damage the ureters with large sutures or blindly placed clamps. One should stay close to the fundus to have the most room possible between the surgical area and the course of the ureter. Prompt salvage avoids more extensive dissection.

Ligation of the uterine vessels is performed in a similar fashion on either side. The uterus is then attached by the cardinal ligaments laterally, the uterosacral ligaments posterolaterally, and the vagina inferiorly. When the procedure is being performed for benign disease or when the

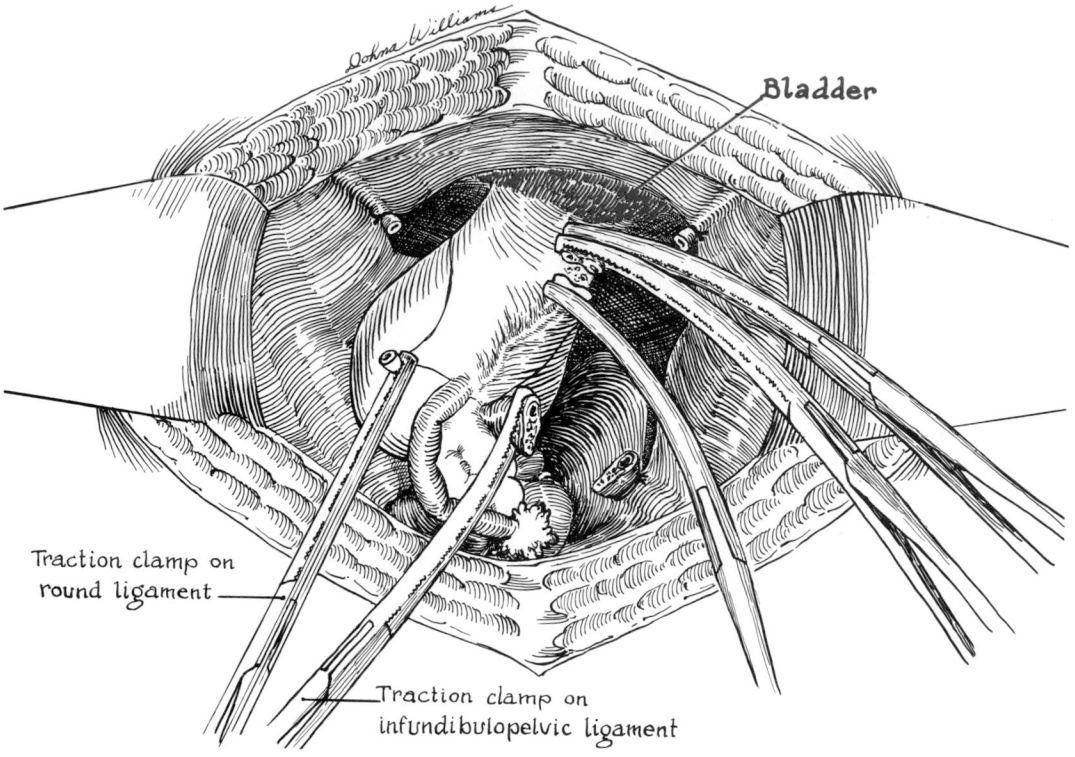

Bladder

Traction clamp on
round ligament

Traction clamp on
infundibulopelvic ligament

Fig. 1.6. Triple clamping and cutting of uterine blood vessels.

lymphatics of the pubovesicocervical fascia are of no significance in spread of the disease, then intrafascial hysterectomy is safest. The pubovesicocervical fascia spreads from the cardinal ligaments over the surface of the cervix. Between these fibers more laterally or through the base of the cardinal ligament runs the ureter from the pelvic wall toward the bladder. By staying within this fascial plane, damage or kinking of the ureters can be avoided. When operating for cervical or endometrial carcinoma, however, lymphatics run in this fascial layer and it must be sacrificed, accepting the additional risk to the ureters in a cancer operation.

The intrafascial component is initiated by making a superficial V-shaped or curved incision through the fibers of the pubovesicocervical fascia (Fig. 1.7). When the uterus is held cephalad on tension, the fibers will spread apart as they are incised. The plane beneath them can be freed by sharp or blunt dissection sweeping the tissue from the anterior surface of the cervix in a perpendicular fashion toward the pubis. The handle of the scalpel serves admir-

ably for this purpose (Fig. 1.8). Whatever instrument is used, care must be taken not to let it slip and drive into the back of the bladder. Dissection is carried down until the vagina is reached. The tissue of the vagina is whiter than the surrounding fascia, and the vagina tends to balloon when the fascia and bladder are freed from it. If the tissues are particularly bloody, dissection of the pubovesicocervical fascia should be done in steps, controlling bleeding and clamping the cardinal ligaments in turn.

When the fascia has been developed, the cardinal ligaments may be clamped, cut, and sutured. Large Ochsner's clamps are excellent for this and should be placed almost parallel to the axis of the cervix and allowed to squeeze off the cervix to give the most lateral room and protection to the ureters (Fig. 1.9). Since the blood supply has been controlled, a single clamp suffices and the incision is made, slightly at first, into the cervical stroma and then down to the tip of the clamp so that there is a fair amount of fibrous tissue left beyond the clamp (Fig. 1.10). The suture ligature is then placed within the fascia and beneath the tip of the

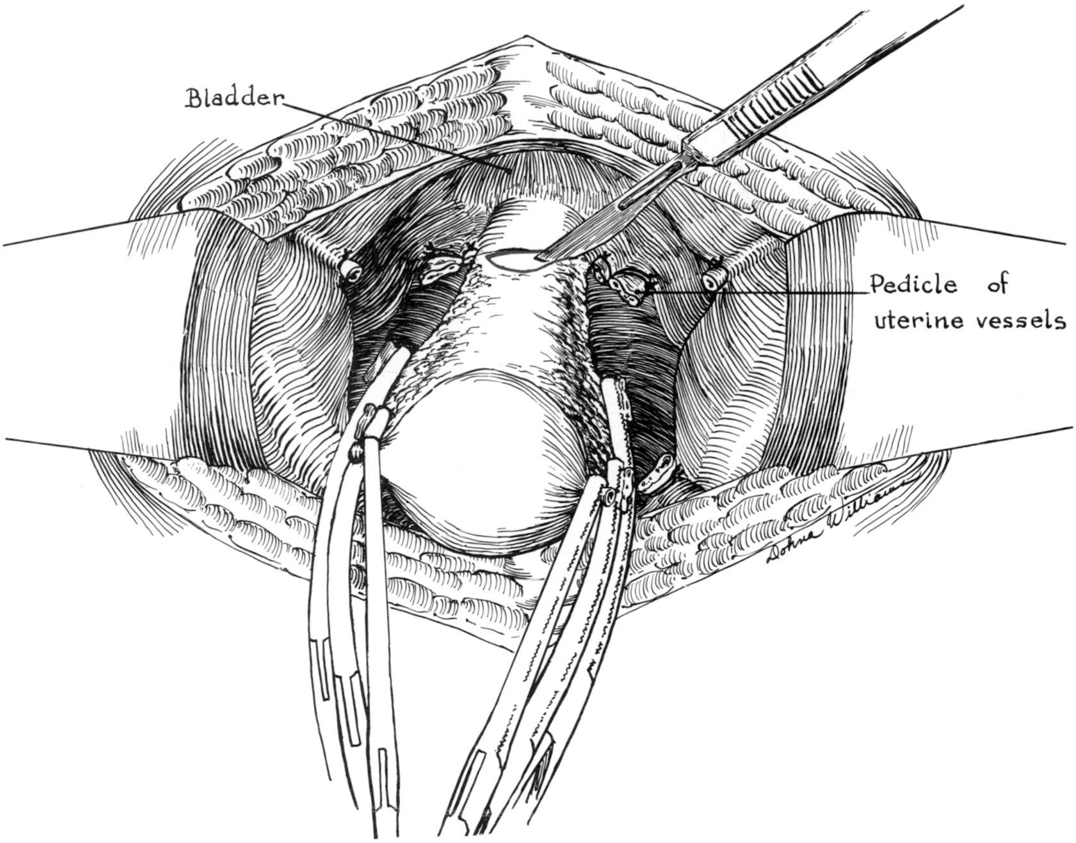

Bladder
Pedicle of
uterine vessels
Dohna Williams

Fig. 1.7. Incision of pubovesicocervical fascia.

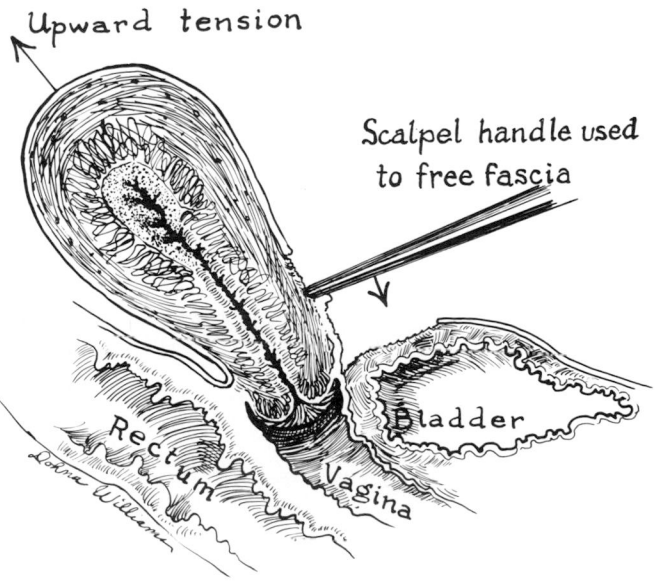

Upward tension
Scalpel handle used
to free fascia
Bladder
Rectum
Vagina
Dohna Williams

Fig. 1.8. Downward dissection of pubovesicocervical fascia.

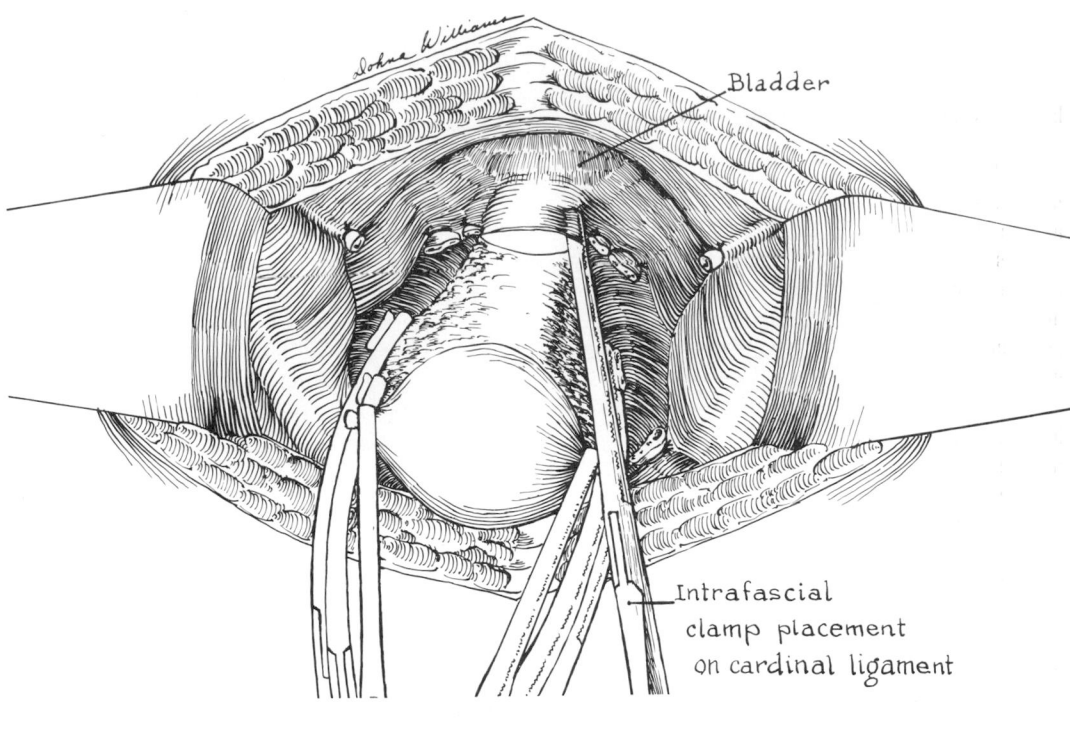

Fig. 1.9. Intrafascial clamping of cardinal ligament after development of the pubovesicocervical fascia.

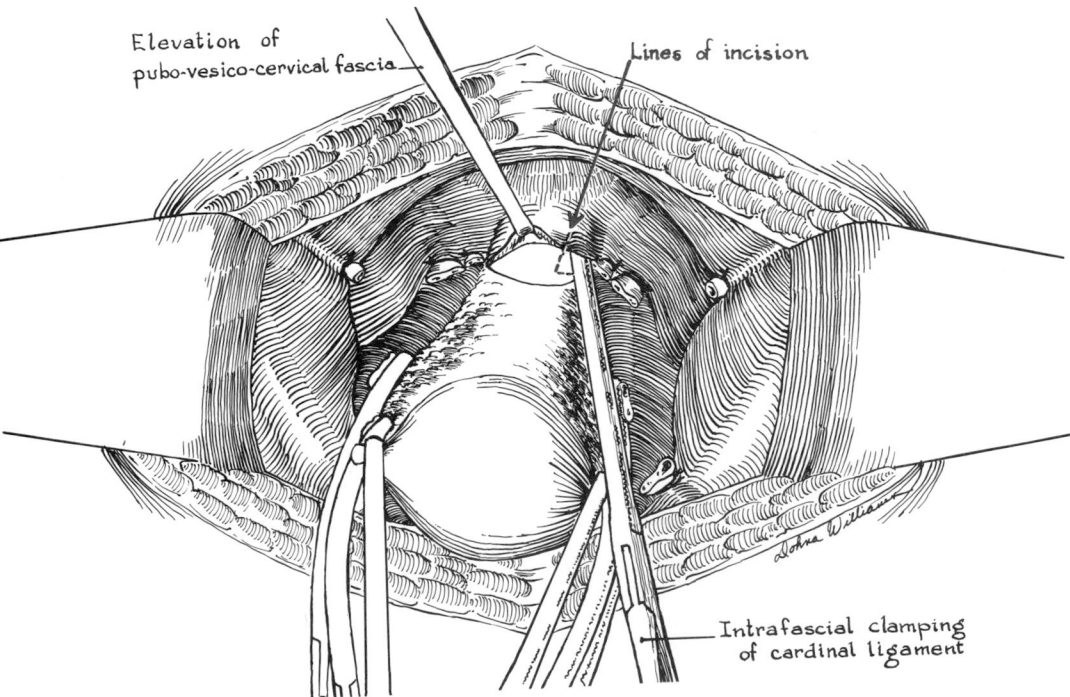

Fig. 1.10. Method of incision to leave pedicle on cardinal ligament.

clamp, tying directly behind the clamp, which is gently released as the suture is snugged tight. A single tie suffices and the nubbin of tissue leaves a satisfactory area distal to the tie which can be used in suspension of the vaginal vault.

It is important not to drop the tie back toward the pelvic wall, as this only diminishes the safety factor for the ureter. This step is repeated on each side until the lower end of the cervix is reached. The same precautions are carried out with each step and the number of ties required will be in proportion to the size of the uterus and the length of the cervix.

Attention then may be turned to the posterior portion of the uterus and the uterosacral ligaments. Endometriosis, infection, and adhesions may have obliterated the cul-de-sac. If this is the case, the bowel may be adherent to the back of the fundus and, on occasion, almost to the top. When freeing such bowel adhesions, it is better to have a patch of uterine serosa in the bowel than *vice versa*. Once the cul-de-sac is free, the uterosacral ligaments can be clamped, cut, and sutured (Fig. 1.11). Curved Ochsner's clamps serve well and should be placed as close to the uterus and cervix as possible, joining up with the posterior incision from the cardinal ligaments. One clamp and one bite are usually all that are required, but if adhesions have been a problem, several smaller ones are safer.

The ligament is cut with the scalpel; a portion proximal to the clamp is left so that it will not pull out to retract and become lost but will be available for use in reconstruction (Fig. 1.10). The suture is placed directly beneath the tip of the clamp and is tied directly behind the clamp. Because of the tension, the stump of the ligament is likely to pull out of the heel of the clamp; the tie should then be dropped down to include this area. Bleeding from this area is generally not a problem, but it occurs frequently enough to justify control and minimization of blood loss.

When both uterosacral ligaments have been suture-ligated (Fig. 1.11), the peritoneum between them is incised and dissected downward. This is best done with curved dissecting scissors as the uterus is held forward toward the pubis. Then the space between the vagina and the rectosigmoid can be further developed with the fingers. It will be found that the cervix is attached only by the vagina. Palpation should be performed to confirm this. If further

dissection is necessary, it should be carried out at this point so that only the vagina needs transection to remove the specimen. No further dissection than necessary should be done for this, because troublesome bleeding and tissue damage will result in unnecessary vaginal shortening, a useless error.

Pertinent points to be observed in management of the supporting cervical ligaments involve performing all dissection and reconstruction as close to the uterus as possible to increase the distance between adjacent organs and to lessen the chance of damage to them. Adhesions should be freed first, utilizing sharp and blunt dissection. Sutures and ligatures also should be placed as close to the clamps as possible, and if one slips or breaks it should be replaced under direct vision. Large mattress or figure-of-eight sutures should never be placed blindly into tissues; they should, in fact, be avoided. Bleeding is controlled best by pressure, hot packs, or more proximal ligation of the hypogastric vessels if necessary. If the intestinal or urinary tract is damaged, repair should be made promptly.

Removal of the uterus is most safely accomplished under direct vision while the adjacent bladder is held toward the pubis. The vaginal sponge should be removed and the vaginal wall grasped with a clamp for tension and traction. This makes it easier to incise and the problem of retraction beneath the bladder is avoided. Once incised, the remaining circumference of vagina is cut and the specimen is removed, as the lateral angles and the midpoint of the anterior and posterior walls of the vagina are grasped with clamps for exposure and identification.

Bleeding will occur from the vaginal mucosa but it is most profuse at the angles. With open removal of the cervix, the lateral angle clamps may be placed to control the bleeding. Care must be taken to include the full thickness of the vaginal wall but no other tissue. Figure-of-eight or mattress sutures are best at the vaginal angle to provide good hemostasis. These sutures may be held to provide traction and simplify the subsequent suspension.

Cross-clamping of the vagina or the "closed" technique carries an increased risk of damage to the bladder or the bowel and is best avoided. Even when the bladder and rectum have been dissected downward, portions may be included

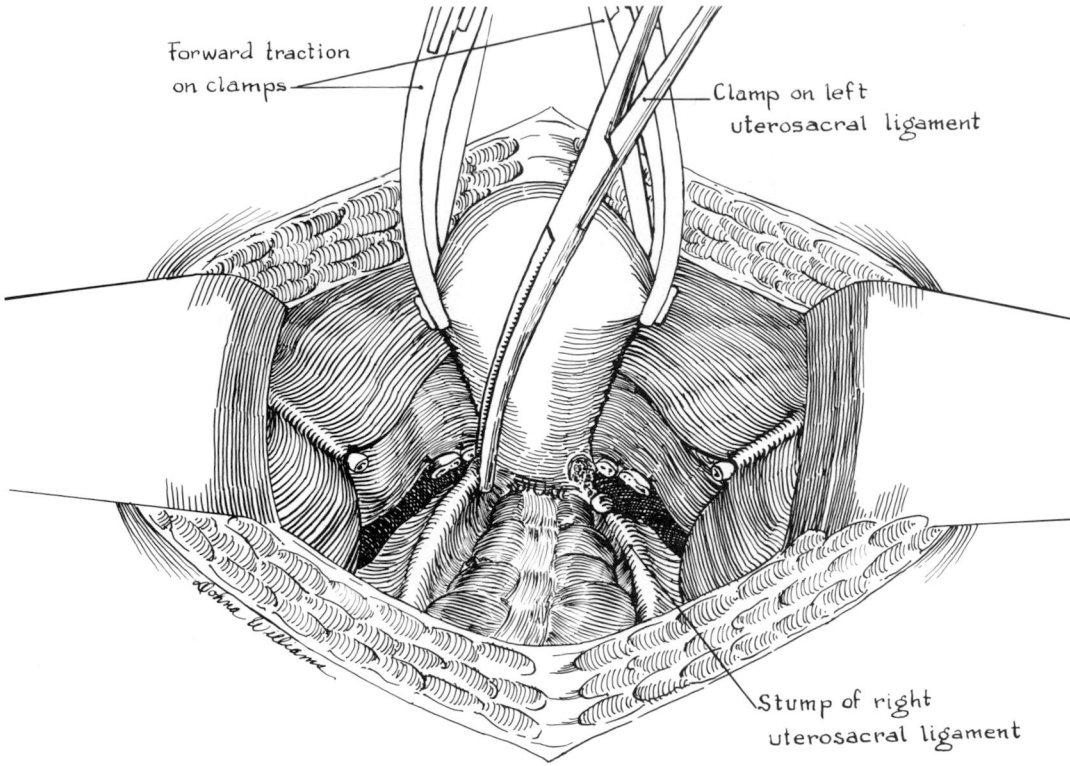

Forward traction on clamps

Clamp on left uterosacral ligament

Stump of right uterosacral ligament

Fig. 1.11. Clamping of uterosacral ligaments.

in the clamp and the damage goes unrecognized when the vagina is closed. If the bladder or rectum is incised under open vision, damaged areas can be recognized and repaired without untoward effect. A curved clamp may be placed just on the angle of the vagina without clamping the entire width (Fig. 1.12). Mattress sutures behind this will give good hemostasis, but placement of both clamp and suture is critical and requires more dissection and causes greater risks.

After removal of the specimen, it seems most logical to close the vagina. Any one of the several methods may be used with equal success. The vagina may be left open, utilizing a continuous suture in the edges to provide hemostasis. In the event that drainage is indicated because of hematoma, infection, or abscess, this method is useful. The edges of the vagina may be approximated in a submucosal fashion, which seems to leave more vault granulation and is more subject to vaginal cuff bleeding in the postoperative period. It seems simplest to use figure-of-eight sutures through the whole thickness of the vagina to provide

snug anatomic approximation and excellent hemostasis (Fig. 1.13).

If the angle sutures and the suture in the midline are held under tension, suspension of the vagina to the ligaments is facilitated. The most important supporting structures are the cardinal and uterosacral ligaments, which should be sutured to the angles of the vagina. It is wise to include the pubovesicocervical fascia as well in this suture to improve anterior support and to control bleeding from the fascia itself.

The suture is started from the front and goes through both anterior and posterior vaginal walls (Fig. 1.14). It then incorporates the pubovesicocervical fascia followed by the angles of the vault with care taken to place the needle distal to the previous suture to avoid pulling it out of the tissue. The same suture of 1-0 atraumatic chromic catgut is next carried to the cardinal ligaments and thereafter the ends of the uterine vessels are picked up and pulled into the extraperitoneal portion of the suspension. If the round ligaments and infundibulopelvic or utero-ovarian ligaments will reach the vault

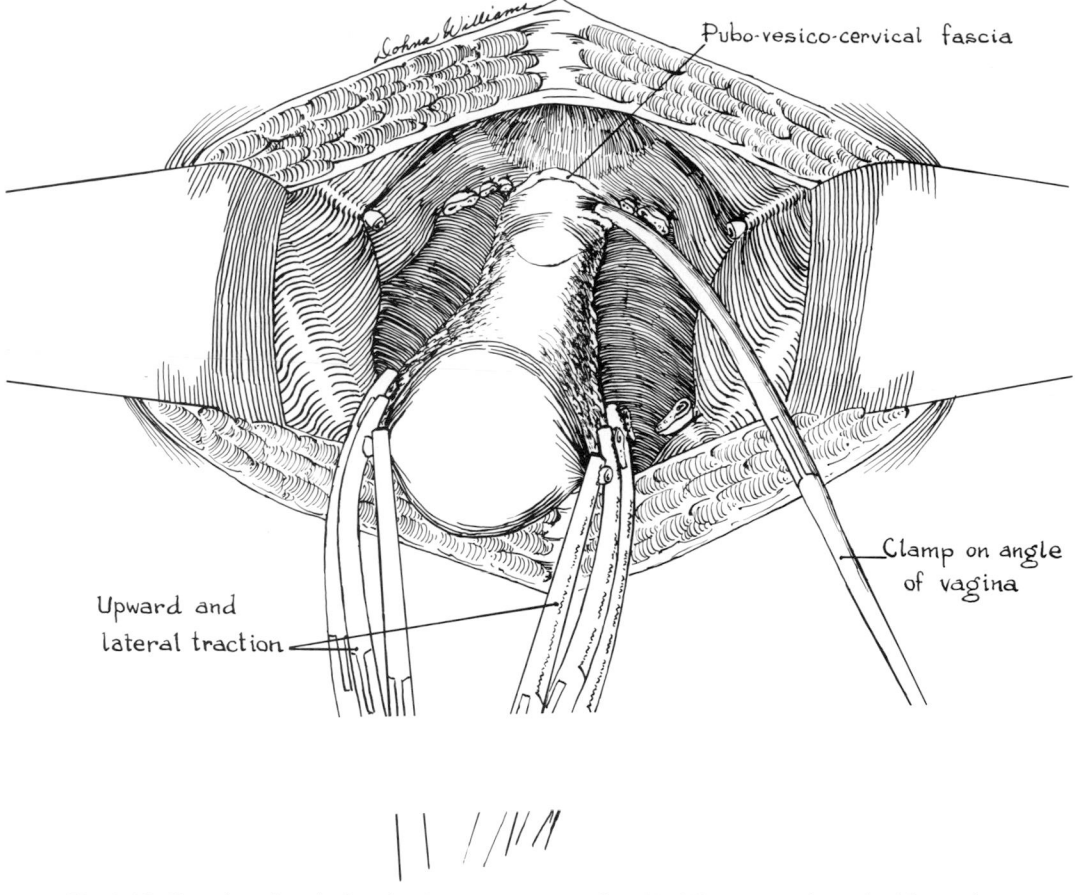

Fig. 1.12. Clamping of vaginal angle after management of cardinal ligaments prior to incising vagina.

without undue tension, they, too, may be included. In all instances it is important to place the suspension suture distal to the previously placed ligatures. In this manner, bleeding will be avoided, as well as possible damage to the ureters or bladder. The utero-sacral ligament is then included in a similar fashion.

When all the structures to be approximated have been included, the suture is passed through the vagina again, drawn tight, and secured. Care must be taken to avoid extreme tension, which will tear the suture from the tissues or cause subsequent pain. It may be necessary to release the tension on the retractors in order to tie the suture snugly. The end-effect is that of a vertical purse-string suture from the vaginal vault through the supporting structures of the uterus (Fig. 1.14).

The round and infundibulopelvic ligaments provide little in the way of support to the vault, but their inclusion facilitates subsequent peritonization and hemostasis and minimizes raw surfaces.

Peritonization is the important final step to provide complete hemostasis, to cover the incised areas, and to prevent subsequent adhesions. If the patient is in poor condition and speed is essential, hemostasis should be secured, the sigmoid placed over the vault, the omentum brought down, and the incision closed. These maneuvers usually will supply appropriate peritonization as a last resort.

However, anatomic closure is more surgically aesthetic and is preferred with 3-0 atraumatic catgut providing the peritoneal approximation and hemostasis. Closure is best started laterally. The raw stump of any cut ligaments such as the infundibulopelvic or utero-ovarian is inverted with a purse-string suture, which is continued to the vaginal vault approximating the peritoneal edges. Careful placement of the needle

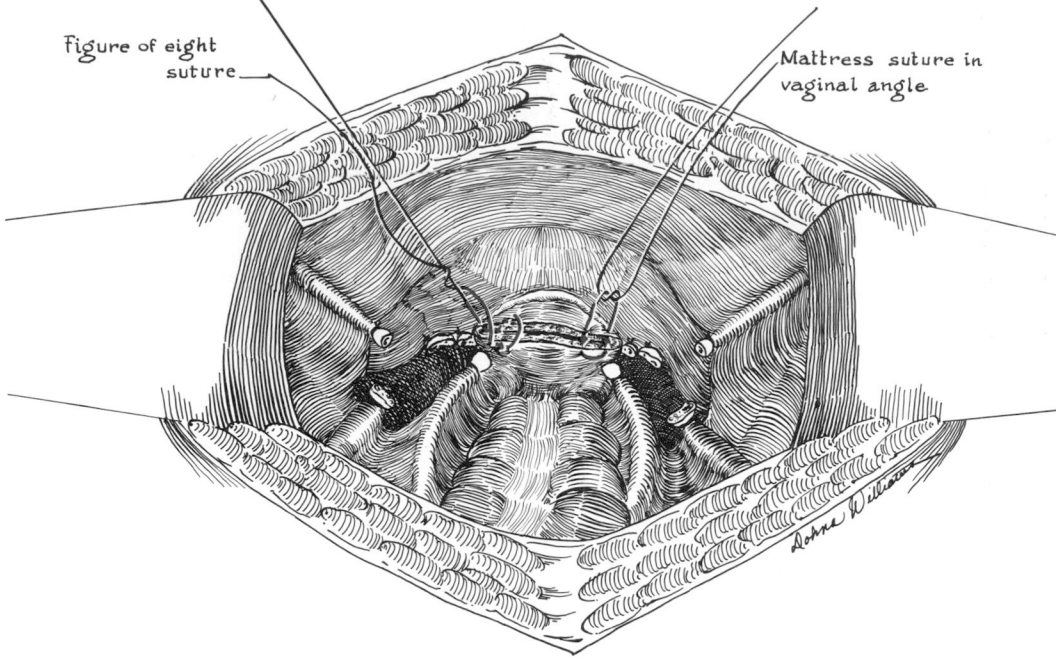

Fig. 1.13. Figure-of-eight and mattress sutures to close vagina.

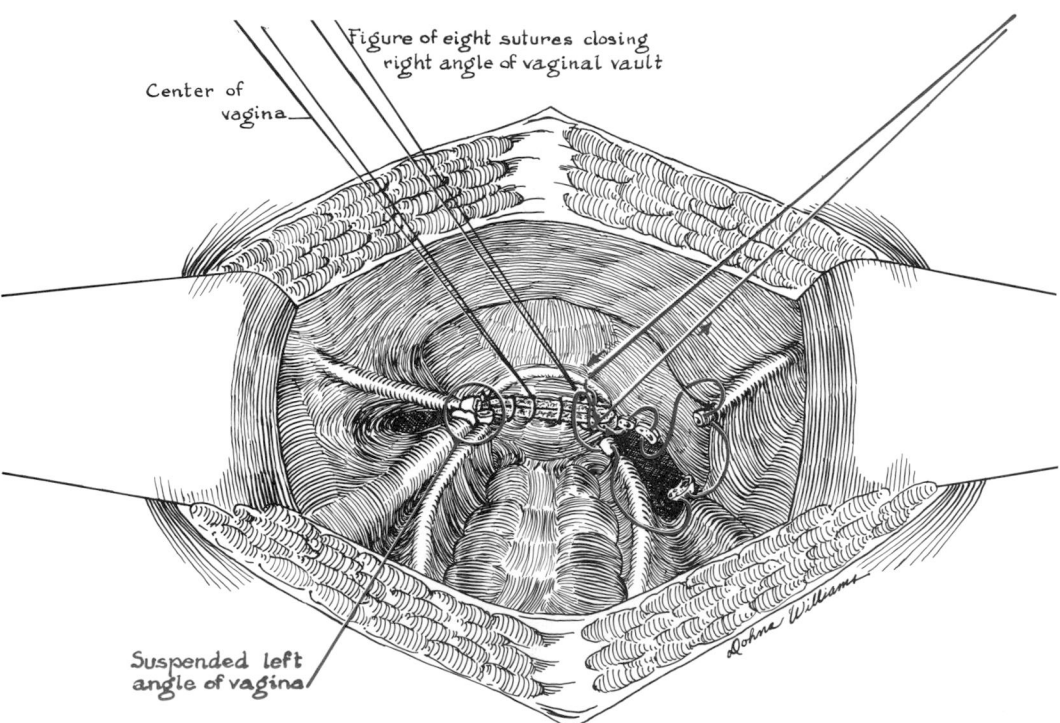

Fig. 1.14. Detail of suspension of vaginal vault.

posteriorly is required to avoid the ureter. Placement should include any bleeding points in order to control bleeding and to prevent hematoma formation. Each lateral pelvic wall may be managed in a similar fashion.

The vaginal vault must be covered as well. Continuing from the angle, the bladder peritoneum is picked up with a similar suture and incorporated with the pubovesicocervical fascia, the vagina, and the peritoneum posteriorly between the uterosacral ligaments. The stitches then are continued across the width of the vagina further securing the suspension, obliterating dead space, and providing excellent hemostasis.

Properly performed, there is smooth approximation of the peritoneum. All large vessels that may bleed are extraperitoneal so that if mishap occurs, the bleeding will be into closed extraperitoneal space, where it is more amenable to diagnosis and salvage than is intraperitoneal hemorrhage in a postanesthetic patient. No raw areas are left to which adhesions may form nor are there any defects for subsequent herniations. Tension on blood vessels or ureter, which might cause bleeding or kinking of the ureter and obstruction, is avoided.

The operative site should be carefully inspected for any bleeding, oozing, or hematoma formation. Bleeding must be controlled under direct vision and on occasion may require taking apart the peritonization and suspension. Hematomas likewise should be evacuated and the source controlled directly. Large sutures or clamps should never be placed blindly in attempts to control bleeding. Hypogastric artery ligation may be required to avoid such trauma and to control the bleeding satisfactorily.

Once the surgical team is satisfied, the sigmoid may be placed over the vault for further protection in preventing adhesions and subsequent obstruction to the small intestine. If adhesions, infection, endometriosis, and tumor or the like have required extensive dissection, there may be persistent oozing from the peritoneal surfaces of the cul-de-sac and parietal peritoneum. Packs and pressure help to control oozing during the operation. If the ooze is still significant on completion of the procedure, Oxycel or Gelfoam may be left against the area to minimize blood loss and serum collection. As a final step, the omentum should be brought down to the vault for further protection of the vaginal and abdominal incisions from adhesions to the intestines.

Accomplishment of abdominal hysterectomy, as outlined, minimizes complications and lends itself to efficient surgical teamwork. The dissection is always anatomic, bleeding is always under prompt control, and modifications because of pelvic disease are easily undertaken.

Incisional Closure. The closure of the abdominal incision includes certain aspects that are important regardless of the type of incision selected. Although en bloc closure may be utilized as an emergency procedure, layer-by-layer closure is stronger, more anatomic, and less prone to infection, dehiscence, and herniation.

The peritoneum is closed first and, in the instance of longitudinal incisions, will incorporate the posterior rectus sheath in the upper portion of the incision. Care must be taken to close the ends of the incision completely to prevent a defect for occurrence of subsequent herniation. The closure is always started at the top of the incision while there is good exposure. The posterior fascial layer is not dissected away but is included in the peritoneal closure. This attachment prevents adequate approximation except at the beginning of closure, since the error of a blindly placed suture can only cause problems. Free peritoneum over the bladder is abundant at the lower end of the incision so that closure at this end is rather simple with minimal risks, and herniation is less common in this area as well.

Continuous atraumatic suture is utilized and it is important that the peritoneal surfaces are in approximation. Fatty or other tissue should not intrude between the edges or hernia may result. Everting types of suture placement serve as a safeguard to prevent this problem. Additional rents or tears in the peritoneum should be repaired or supported with sutures. To obtain exposure, it is sometimes necessary to extend the peritoneal incision laterally along the dome of the bladder. In such instances, it may be necessary to start closure of the peritoneum at both ends and meet in the middle. This is far more preferable than would be a blind attempt to get the lower edge of the peritoneum and in so doing include the bladder in the suture or miss approximation of the peritoneal edges completely.

The prime area of strength is the fascial layer. Permanent interrupted sutures are recommended. Catgut sutures may be used but because of known disease or unexpected postoperative complications in which healing may be delayed, permanent sutures are best. Teflon-coated sutures seem to handle somewhat better than silk or other material and also cause less tissue reaction. Fine wire is good, but pain and reaction are greater and may require subsequent removal. Continuous sutures are to be avoided, since any weakness in the suture compromises the entire closure and is a ridiculous sacrifice to speed. Figure-of-eight sutures are useful in closure and provide better hemostasis than do single interrupted sutures.

The fascial edges should be approximated by the sutures without strangulation and necrosis. Undue tension will cause distortion and puckering and is to be avoided. Again, it is important to avoid including fat or peritoneum between the fascial edges. The sutures should leave no more foreign material in the body than is necessary for good approximation. If factors that might compromise healing are known, retention or stay sutures are advised, as, for example, in patients with anemia, cancer, and debilitative conditions requiring prolonged surgery. Other factors are cortisone, radiation, and elderly or obese patients, for which heavy sutures incorporating the skin, fat, muscle, and fascia should be used. Because of subsequent tissue edema, they should be tied somewhat loosely to prevent cutting into the skin and causing infection and discomfort. Prevention of dehiscence and evisceration, however, is a far more satisfactory safeguard than treatment and salvage subsequent to these conditions.

The fascia should be approximated in an anatomic manner and the ends should be closed first while there is good exposure. As mentioned earlier, the fascia should not be denuded, as this affects the blood supply and promotes dead space, hematoma, and collection of serum with infection and compromise of the entire incision. The subcutaneous fat is best approximated also in order to prevent dead space. Interrupted or continuous sutures are satisfactory since there is no tension or hemostatic component to the suture. In slender patients with normal subcutaneous fat, no suture will be required in this layer. In obese patients several layers may be required for proper approximation.

The skin edges should be approximated to avoid inversion of the edges and distortion of the scar. Vertical mattress sutures are best for this because the superficial bite ensures approximation of the cut edges. Subcuticular suture provides a finer scar and is best utilized with transverse incisions. Continuous sutures are somewhat faster to place and never difficult to remove; they provide excellent closure when a mattress component is used. Subcutaneous bleeders often may be controlled by the skin sutures, but, because of the edema, should never be tied in a necrotizing fashion; instead they should be gently approximated.

Any collections of blood should be evacuated and, if the incision is dry, a snug dressing should be applied promptly. Support during the first 24 hours is an aid to immediate postoperative respiratory care but adds little to the strength of a properly sutured incision. Removal of the dressing within 24 hours ensures appropriate care of the incision and avoids failure to recognize hematoma or abscess. Prompt recognition of such problems allows immediate and appropriate therapeutic measures minimizing morbidity and hospitalization.

Comment

The most common error to be anticipated with abdominal hysterectomy is that of failure to recognize the various tissues of the pelvis, bladder, bowel, uterus, ureter, and blood vessels. Each has different characteristics, but disease may have distorted the anatomic position of the various organs as well as their identifying features. The most serious error is failure to recognize and repair damage to these organs. The safeguard is knowledge of the surgical area and avoidance of blind manipulation in unrecognized areas.

Myomectomy

The indication for this surgical procedure would seem to be comparatively simple and logical: the presence of uterine fibroids causing subjective discomfort or infertility in patients who are desirous of maintaining childbearing potential.

The young, unmarried woman with enlarging

or symptomatic fibroids certainly deserves the opportunity to retain her pelvic organs and reproductive function if this is technically feasible. Similarly, the woman with infertility whose only related abnormality is significant fibroids is deserving of a chance to improve her reproductive potential.

Conversely, in women with extreme distortion and enlargement, rapid tumor growth, or other evidence of degeneration, careful thought and consideration are necessary before one accepts any increased risk of conservative surgery. Preservation of a nonfunctioning uterus is unjustified but so is the acceptance of increased risk to the life and well-being of a female patient for social reasons only. As women increase in age, the risk of a complicated pregnancy increases. Although it is difficult to set any specific age above which myomectomy is contraindicated, only in extraordinary situations should this operation be considered in women older than 35 years.

Since the diagnosis is based on pelvic examination, consideration of other possible diagnoses and necessary operations must be carefully and thoroughly discussed beforehand. As stressed before, it is unwise to plan on a major surgical procedure in which there are specific restrictions placed on the surgeon. Tumors, benign or malignant, may be found in the ovary as well as in the uterus and may necessitate definitive and complete pelvic surgery. Infection of the pelvic organs and inflammation of adjacent organs likewise may predicate against any attempt at conservative management of the female pelvic organs. Thorough and factual discussion as to the probable and possible diagnoses, along with the projected and planned but necessary procedures with aims and results, is necessary. Each patient should understand that the surgeon will do his best to abide by her wishes, but that in all events her life and medical welfare must come first.

Although myomectomy is often considered a relatively minor procedure, it is a major operation with all of the attendant risks. Indeed, the mortality rate is in excess of that for abdominal hysterectomy performed for benign disease. This surprising fact is related to the problem of postoperative hemorrhage. If the incised uterus bleeds after the operation, it bleeds into the peritoneal cavity, often with little or no warning, particularly in the post-

anesthetic patient. More rigid and more frequent evaluation of these patients is required during the immediate postoperative period. Any change in the vital signs suggestive of continuing loss of blood must be immediately and aggressively evaluated and treated.

Preoperative preparations are similar to those discussed earlier from the hospitalization until the completion of abdominal incision. Because of the necessity to know about the fertility status, a hysterosalpingogram will be necessary to confirm tubal patency. In addition, this test will provide information relative to size or distortion of the uterine cavity from tumors. If submucous fibroids are present, they are often associated with infection, and antibiotic coverage is indicated. Surgery should be done during the proliferative phase of the menstrual cycle so as to minimize blood loss. Likewise, the possibility of early unknown and unsuspected pregnancy is avoided.

Exploration and evaluation of the contents of the abdominal cavity are performed as in all procedures. After the patient is placed in mild Trendelenburg's position and the intestines packed away from the pelvic region, the pelvic organs are evaluated.

The diagnosis of myomata uteri must be confirmed, as well as the normalcy of tubes and ovaries. The size, position, and consistency of the fibroids are pertinent, and it must be technically feasible to remove the fibroids and reconstruct the uterus without compromising the tubes and ovaries or the uterine blood supply. Evidence of active infection contraindicates myomectomy, and violation of the intestinal continuity is to be avoided at all costs, including appendectomy.

Once myomectomy is considered feasible and there are no contraindications, certain basic surgical factors must be followed. Anatomic exposure is imperative and deviation of the tissues due to tumor distortion must be considered at all steps. Tension, traction, and adequate dissection with hemostasis and visualization of the entire operative field are necessary *at all times* to avoid damage to other adjacent organs.

As mentioned earlier, postoperative hemorrhage is a significant problem. Uterine incisions should be placed so that subsequent peritonization is feasible. Similarly, a minimal number of incisions should be made and as many of the fibroids as possible should be removed through each incision. Incision into the uterine cavity should be avoided, if possible, yet all tumors need to be removed. Even though the hysterosalpingogram does not show evidence of distortion or submucous fibroid, the slightest suspicion at the operating table requires that the surgeon be positive, and incision into the uterine cavity may be necessary for confirmation.

The uterus should be held under tension for better exposure and so that the bleeding may be minimized with pressure at the same time. Areas that must be avoided with the incision are the cornual region near the uterine portion of the tube and the utero-ovarian vessels. Likewise, dissection into the lateral surfaces of the uterus near the uterine vessels should be minimized.

Mobilization of the bladder peritoneal flap will provide better coverage of raw areas. The use of round and broad ligaments to suspend and cover such denuded regions also should be considered. The uterine incisions should be placed to avoid such dangerous areas as the tube or uterine vessels and to take advantage of the other tissues that are present.

Bleeding during the procedure is often heavy and annoying and is usually brought under complete control only at the end of the procedure. Certain suggestions have been made in attempts to minimize this problem. The use of vasoconstrictor drugs gives good control of the smaller vessels when the drug is injected directly into the adjacent myometrium. However, mechanical compression of the myometrium and major vessels is thought to be safer. The vasoconstrictors will function for varying times, and it seems preferable to control bleeding at the operating table when it can be identified rather than to accept the risk of subsequent vessel dilatation and bleeding after the incision has been closed.

Rubber shod clamps have been designed for use on the uterine vessels. Tourniquets around the lower uterine segment provide a similar effect. Some authors have used large ring forceps to control both the ovarian and the uterine blood supply simultaneously (Fig. 1.15). With good exposure, manual traction and vessel compression allow the procedure to progress smoothly and the bleeding can be controlled adequately and promptly as it is encountered.

An *elliptical incision through the superficial myometrium* on the surface and carried down to the tumor will allow for more aesthetic anatomic reconstruction of the uterus. There should be a reasonably good plane of cleavage between the fibroid and the adjacent myometrium so that blunt dissection is most satisfactory.

Allis clamps are useful for small tumors, while towel clamps and sutures will provide a good grasp on the larger ones. Compression will control the bleeding from the operative sites until all of the tumors from the particular incision are removed. Reconstruction of that portion of the uterus can then be carried out.

The sutures should be large enough to avoid cutting the myometrium when tied and strong enough to approximate the muscle and also give hemostasis. Atraumatic chromic catgut (0-0 or 1-0) is usually best. For a small incision a figure-of-eight suture is best, while for larger defects, continuous sutures will be required. It is important to obliterate dead space and avoid hematomas. In some instances, there may be enough myohypertrophy to require two layers of sutures for adequate closure. A lock suture is also useful to improve hemostasis on the surface.

If the uterine cavity is entered, it is best to avoid placing a suture through the endometrium. Care should be taken to obtain good approximation of the endometrial edges without having suture material through the mucosa. Particular care must also be taken to avoid placing a suture through the cornual region where it might occlude the tube or isthmic portion of the tube. After closure of all incisions, each should be reinspected to be sure that it is dry and without evidence of significant bleeding. The tubes and ovaries also should be reinspected for damage to the blood supply or from the operation.

The incisions should then be covered with peritoneum wherever possible to prevent subsequent adhesions to the raw surfaces. The use of the bladder flap and broad ligaments such as with a Coffey suspension is helpful. The omentum should be used in an attempt to cover the incisions and to separate the uterus from the small intestines. Minimizing the possibility of adhesions will avoid postoperative obstruction to the intestines as well as pain and discomfort secondary to such adhesions.

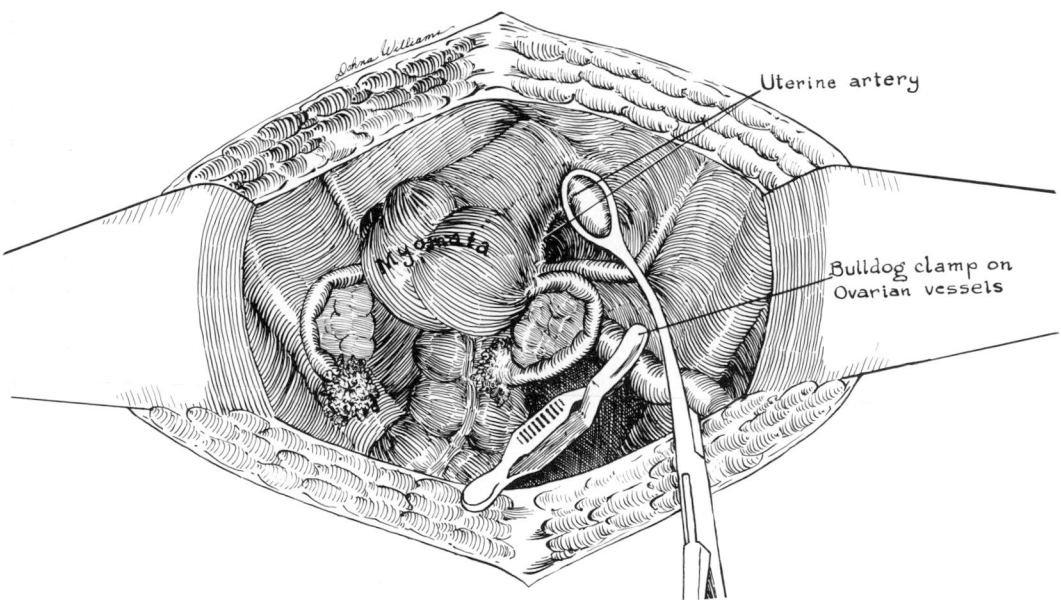

Uterine artery

Myomata

Bulldog clamp on Ovarian vessels

Fig. 1.15. Clamp placement for controlling uterine blood supply in myomectomy.

At this point, the procedure has been completed and the incision closed in the usual fashion. Particular and frequent attention must be paid to the vital signs during the immediate postoperative course so that any intraperitoneal bleeding can be diagnosed and controlled. This point cannot be stressed too frequently.

Presacral Neurectomy

This operation requires interruption of the nerves to the pelvic organs. The valid indication would seem to be dysmenorrhea of such severity as to be incapacitating and uncontrollable by medical means, including non-narcotic analgesia and hormone therapy. It is important that any psychiatric overtones be evaluated preoperatively. Endometriosis is the organic condition most frequently associated with this operation, although malignancy may be helped in some instances. A specific point should be made regarding the expected results, and the patient must understand that there can be no guarantees as to the effectiveness or completeness of relief from pain.

The selection and making of the incision for presacral neurectomy must be modified by the particular area to be reached during the procedure. A midline incision is best, inasmuch as it allows better exposure of the region over

the sacral promontory than does a transverse suprapubic incision. A transverse incision may be made beneath the umbilicus, but it cannot be extended easily if circumstances require. Exposure and packing away of the bowel are carried out after complete abdominal exploration, as previously described.

Individualization of the procedure is required, and indeed, presacral neurectomy and uterine suspension frequently are associated with operations for endometriosis. The use of neurectomy, however, should be predicated on the necessity for relief of uterine pain in the particular patient. Injection of the uterosacral ligaments with local anesthetic agents may give a clue as to the possible efficacy of the operative section of the presacral nerves; in fact, some have recommended injection of the fourth and fifth lumbar nerves before operation in order to gain some idea of the benefit of surgical excision.

Exploration of the pelvic organs should precede presacral dissection. Any surgery for ovarian cysts, fibroids, endometriosis, and similar conditions should be carried out first; then, on completion of suspension and the like, attention may be turned to the neurectomy. The sigmoid colon is drawn to the left and the pelvic organs toward the pubis, so that there is complete visualization of the sacral area.

A longitudinal incision is then made into the peritoneum from the level of the bifurcation of the aorta downward toward the hollow of the sacrum. The edges of the peritoneum may be held under tension with sutures to improve lateral exposure. Dissection is carried laterally toward each ureter, which must be carefully identified (Fig. 1.16).

Small nerve fibers cling to the underside of the peritoneum and these are stripped away and excised. The major portion of the plexus lies against the sacrum and all of the tissue between the two ureters should be freed. This is best done by blunt dissection isolating the bundles of nerve, plexus, and fibrous tissue. It generally can be easily removed from the dense ligament on the anterior surface of the sacrum.

Care must be taken to avoid damaging the ureters and the middle sacral vessels, which lie snugly against the sacrum almost in the midline. Pressure often will control bleeding from the vein, but it is troublesome and easier to avoid than to control. Suture ligation or a silver clip may be required, incorporating the superficial part of the anterior spinal ligament to gain hemostasis. The inferior mesenteric and superior hemorrhoidal vessels toward the left side also must be avoided so that there is no compromise to the sigmoidal and rectal blood supply.

After the nerve bundles are isolated they are clamped, cut, and tied near the level of the promontory. This may be done on either side of the pelvis to minimize chances of injury to the midline sacral vessels. The inferior end of the tissue bundles should be freed down past the inferior hypogastric plexus (about the middle of the sacral hollow), which also should be clamped, cut, and tied.

The tissue should be sent to the laboratory to be sure that nerve has been identified. The area is then carefully inspected for bleeding: if present, it must be controlled; if absent the peritoneum is approximated with fine continuous atraumatic suture.

Two additional areas might be considered in the management of dysmenorrhea. Nerves extend through the infundibulopelvic ligaments along with the ovarian vessels; section and ligation with reapproximation of these structures may afford some relief from pain. More important, however, would be similar management of the uterosacral ligaments.

The uterosacral ligaments may be clamped, cut, and tied; a specimen can be removed from them, after which they should be reapproxi-

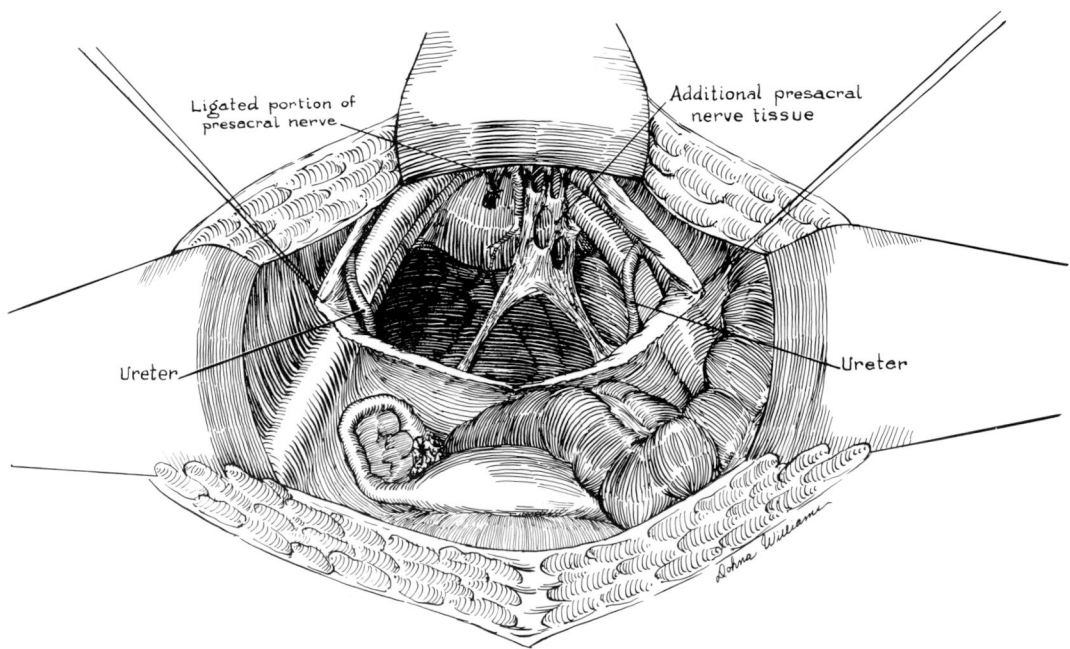

Fig. 1.16. Retroperitoneal space in presacral neurectomy.

mated and plicated to afford further improvement of the uterine position and suspension if previously performed.

After completion of these steps, the operative sites are reinspected, the sigmoid is replaced in the pelvis, the omentum is brought down, and the incision is closed as described earlier.

If the bowel is damaged, it must be repaired as described separately. If there has been compromise of the blood supply to the sigmoid, resection should be performed as soon as the extent is outlined. The ureters should also be inspected and, if damaged, managed as outlined.

If there is true neurogenic dysmenorrhea, relief should be dramatic. However, one may expect satisfactory results or improvement in about three-fourths of the patients, if properly selected. Side-effects as far as bowel and bladder function and control are not seen, nor is there effect on orgasm. The pain of uterine contraction and cervical dilatation is often completely absent after this procedure, and close attention to progress in subsequent labor is necessary.

Management of Associated Problems and Complications

Bladder Injury

The anatomic position of the bladder subjects it to increased risk during pelvic operations. Inasmuch as pelvic operations require low abdominal incision, the relationship of the bladder to the lower portion of the abdominal wall necessitates extreme awareness. This is true both in making and in repairing the incision. The intimate relationship between the cervix and the bladder also requires gentle dissection to avoid trauma during the required separation of these organs.

The end-result of damage to the bladder is urinary incontinence caused by formation of fistulae. Urinary ascites or urinoma may occur and significantly increase the morbidity of the postoperative patient. Even if the patient survives the immediate complications of infection and loss of blood associated with vesical injury, the continual wetting, tissue maceration, and urinous odor are a horrible and unnecessary fate. Proper knowledge of anatomy and opera-

tive technique will avoid this. *Recognition and repair* of any bladder injury are mandatory.

In every vesical injury that I have seen there has always been a warning beforehand and obvious evidence of the injury. It is only when the surgeon is oblivious to the tissues with which he is working and ignorant of the possibility of damage that disaster befalls.

The surgeon should always be alert to certain warning signs. Foremost of these is the history of previous pelvic surgery that might have affected the anatomic relationships of the bladder. The operation that was performed is immaterial. Any incisional closure may have elevated the fundus of the bladder even more than its usual position so that it is more likely to be affected by subsequent incision.

Any operation in which vesical peritoneum is likely to be utilized increases the risks of injury to the bladder. Cesarean section, wherein the peritoneal flap is used to cover the uterine incision, is the most frequent of these operations. Additional adherence between the uterus and the bladder itself is encountered in such instances. Uterine suspension presents similar problems; often the bladder has been advanced to the top of the uterine fundus obliterating the anterior cul-de-sac except for the bladder itself.

Disease processes that further distort the anatomy will, likewise, cause annoying positional changes. Endometriosis and infection may elevate the bladder on the uterus and may obliterate space between these two organs. Fibroid tumors present similar problems, particularly when they occupy the lower uterine segment and broad ligament areas. History and pelvic findings of such conditions always alert the surgeon to the need for particular attention to the bladder in order to minimize the chances for injury and to recognize any damage that may occur.

At times, anatomic distortion and adhesions make incision into the bladder mandatory in order to proceed with the dissection. It is only the failure to recognize the organs with which one is dealing that must be condemned. Once recognized, appropriate repair and subsequent management of the bladder will avoid unsatisfactory results. It is the failure to recognize, repair, and properly manage that leads to increased morbidity with subsequent postoperative fistulae and complications.

With all abdominal procedures, the first step

in bladder management is to ascertain that the bladder itself is collapsed and empty. The patient is relatively dehydrated because she has had nothing by mouth since the night before operation; she also was instructed to empty the bladder prior to going to the surgical suite. Despite this, one cannot assume that the bladder is empty. The presurgical examination under anesthesia will allow evaluation of the bladder contents. With the intravenous use of fluids, however, an empty bladder may fill to an annoying degree during the time required for cleansing, preparation, and draping. Even if the bladder is empty when the incision is made, gradual filling may hamper further dissection and the incisional closure. Therefore, a urethral catheter is inserted not only to empty the bladder but also to ensure a continued collapsed state until the operation is completed. The catheter may be connected to a closed drainage system, so that the flow of urine can be monitored. It is important that proper sterile precautions be utilized with the catheterization, a factor often neglected in the operating room. After catheterization, bimanual compression is required at the time of the examination under anesthesia and vaginal preparation. A free flow of urine should be established and maintained after the patient is placed in the operative position. Kinking or obstruction of the catheter will negate all of the advantages to be gained from catheterization. If postoperative bladder drainage is anticipated, a retention catheter should be used to avoid future unnecessary bladder intubation.

In considering the times at which the bladder may be injured, the first is at incision. The peritoneum should always be opened at the upper part of the incision as far away from the bladder as possible. Dissection should be performed with good surgical technique and bleeding should be controlled. Blind manipulation and blundering in a puddle of blood can only lead to complications.

After the fascia has been incised and the muscles separated, dissection in the lower portion of the incision should be avoided until the peritoneum is opened. The consistency of the bladder muscularis is distinctive, as is the appearance of the muscular fibers themselves. Bleeding is increased and should alert one to proximity of the bladder. If the bladder is entered, the thickness of the wall, the vascu-larity, the mucosal lining, the presence of urine, and the catheter are unmistakable. If the exact location of the bladder in relation to the region of dissection is questionable, it should always be assumed to be near until proved otherwise.

Proper use of the surgical instruments and proper surgical technique serve to alert one to changes in tissue consistency. Once the peritoneum is opened, the incision in it can be extended toward the pubis under direct vision taking care to cut only the peritoneum. If the preperitoneal fat is freed from the area to be incised, visualization of the bladder is simplified. Palpation of the dome of the bladder will identify its position exactly.

Dissection scissors, correctly used, will avoid damage to the bladder and even alert the surgeon to its presence. The proper method is to use the tips of the scissors as though they were opposed cutting blades and to push gently against the peritoneum as it is held under tension. If the bladder is adherent, the change in the feel of the tissue will alert the surgeon that more than the peritoneum is present. Conversely, use of the scissors in a guillotine fashion allows one to cut into the bladder before becoming aware of its nearness. If additional room is required at the lower end of the incision, the peritoneum may be incised diagonally along the dome with greater safety than directly downward beneath the bladder musculature. Such a maneuver minimizes the risk of subsequent peritoneal closure and is a possibility always to be considered.

If the bladder is entered while making the incision, the dissection should be completed and then the bladder closed. It is best not to repair the bladder until the possibility of further damage is gone. It is foolish to repair one bladder defect only to make another as the incision is extended to its necessary length for proper exposure.

In addition to incision, the bladder also may be sutured while attempting to control bleeding or it may be crushed in a clamp. If a suture is placed into the bladder, the surgeon must be sure that it does not enter the bladder mucosa itself, particularly when permanent sutures are used, because encrustation and infection may ensue. No suture should be placed so deeply as to transfix the entire bladder. If the mucosa has not been entered, the suture may be left in place without harm.

Crushing of the bladder in a clamp is a similar example of poor tissue technique. Such crushing should be supported by atraumatic catgut sutures in the adjacent muscularis. Interrupted or continuous suture of 2-0 or 3-0 chromic catgut is satisfactory and supplies necessary hemostasis as well. A purse-string suture will do well and a single layer will suffice in most such instances.

If the bladder wall is transected, dissection should be completed and extended for adequate exposure. The bladder muscularis is then approximated with a continuous suture of 3-0 atraumatic catgut, taking care to avoid the bladder mucosa and also to invert the mucosa into the bladder. This closure should then be supported by an additional layer of suture. A third row of sutures is seldom required. When the incision is closed, snug peritoneal approximation will prevent any leakage into the peritoneal cavity with resultant urinary ascites. Catheter drainage is required to rest the bladder and a small drain should be placed extra-peritoneally at the area of repair. Although this is often unnecessary with the proper repair and subsequent bladder rest, it will serve as a safety valve in the case of catheter obstruction and subsequent bladder distention. Although use of a drain may be rejected, it must always be considered; failure to use it carries a calculated risk.

The bladder is always placed at rest after injury to permit healing of the suture lines without the tensions of a distending bladder. An indwelling catheter is inserted into the bladder and connected to straight drainage. Great care must be taken to ensure that the catheter does not become obstructed or removed. By monitoring the output closely, one is able to minimize chances of obstruction and to avoid distention and dehiscence of the suture line.

The bladder may be damaged in the dissection from the cervix, and if the trauma region is unrecognized and unrepaired, fistulae probably will form. Careful attention is required in evaluating the anatomy and in correcting any adhesions or distortions prior to starting the operative procedure. If the bladder has been advanced, it is taken down so that the peritoneal incision is made in the proper plane.

Careful incision of the peritoneum, starting at the round ligaments, opens into the loose areolar tissue between the leaves of the broad ligament and above the bladder. The incision is connected between the two round ligaments and the bladder may be swept gently downward from the cervix. This is an avascular plane, and bleeding that occurs will be from either the bladder or the underlying fascia. The appearance of longitudinal muscle fibers in this area can only be from the bladder, and the dissection should be redirected deeper into the pubovesicocervical fascia to avoid further trauma to the bladder.

Previous surgery or adhesions may require sharp dissection to free the bladder from the cervix. Although the surface of the cervix will bleed, it is better to have extra fascia attached to the bladder than to remove part of the bladder with the specimen. By developing the layer of the pubovesicocervical fascia, one protects the bladder and makes it easier to avoid damage. If a defect is made into the muscularis, it should be supported by atraumatic suture, avoiding the mucosa. Subsequent bladder rest allows healing to proceed without complications.

Incision into the base of the bladder requires repair as soon as the area is freed enough for visualization. The mucosa should be inverted so that no suture is left in the interior of the bladder. Two layers are best for adequate closure. Here one must be sure not to include the ureters in the sutures; if there is any doubt as to the position of the ureter, a ureteral catheter (5-F to 7-F) should be inserted through the open bladder. Palpation of the catheter will simplify ureteral identification and so avoid further complications.

With bleeding but no clue of bladder damage because of poor exposure, absence of urine spill, or catheter visualization, further diagnostic steps must be considered. Indigo carmine given intravenously or methylene blue injected through the indwelling catheter will provide a diagnostic contrast medium. Any suspicion of bladder damage must be either confirmed or disproved, as the time to repair the damage is at the initial operation when it occurs.

After closure of the bladder, the operation should be completed, the vagina closed, and suspension carried out. Peritonization should be done carefully to separate the bladder incision from the vagina. A drain may be left down to the incision retroperitoneally and brought out through the incision. If the reconstruction has not been entirely satisfactory, a suprapubic cystostomy should be made to serve as an adequate safety valve to avoid distention. A period of 10 to 14 days of bladder rest is sufficient for healing.

Some authors have recommended leaving the cervix in place if the bladder is damaged during dissection for hysterectomy. It has been their feeling that vesicovaginal fistulae cannot develop subsequently unless there is a vaginal incision and that after healing the cervix may be examined periodically or removed if necessary. Such management does present a conservative safeguard against vesicovaginal fistula when the bladder is opened during the procedure. Recognition and proper repair with postoperative bladder rest, however, should give good results without the necessity of further cervical surgery.

Clamping or suturing of the bladder is managed similarly, regardless of where or when it is done. Cystotomy to delineate damage is preferable to uncertainty of damage and subsequent development of fistulae. Particular care is required at the base of the bladder to avoid ureteral damage or obstruction. When the vaginal or abdominal incision is closed, sutures may inadvertently be placed through the bladder. The surgeon should always be positive of the anatomic position, and if not sure, he should not proceed without positive identification. Before abdominal closure is completed, the bladder region should be reinspected to make certain that the bladder is intact and that the peritoneum only is approximated with no bladder included in the sutures.

If bladder damage is unrepaired, three complications may occur: (1) intraperitoneal leakage will cause urinary ascites and a profoundly ill patient; (2) vesicocutaneous or vesicovaginal fistulae will eventuate if the patient survives the immediate postoperative period; or (3) extraperitoneal leakage may dissect into the tissues forming a urinoma, which will eventually localize with fistula formation. This last condition is particularly likely to develop with an unrepaired defect in the dome of the bladder associated with opening or closing the incision. Vesicovaginal fistulae usually appear after damage to the base of the bladder with leakage through the relatively inflamed vaginal cuff.

In all three instances, morbidity may precede by some days the appearance of the fistula. Clues to unrepaired bladder damage are diminution in urinary output, bloody urine, mass in the abdominal wall or pelvis, and abdominal swelling with intra-abdominal urine. Despite these clues, diagnosis is likely to be delayed until the appearance of vaginal or cutaneous urine. Cystoscopy, cystogram, or dye such as indigo carmine or methylene blue may aid in making the diagnosis.

Unfortunately, diagnosis in the foregoing conditions is made at the time of maximal tissue reaction, and attempts at definitive correction are contraindicated. Prompt diagnosis is important so that treatment can be started. There are two specific aims: to promote healing and to minimize subsequent complication. An excretory urogram is important, since ureteral injury may be involved and the upper tracts must be protected from further damage. The bladder should be catheterized to put it at rest and to increase the chances of spontaneous healing. The frequent association of infection usually will require antibacterial coverage as well.

Use of the Bradford frame should be considered if the damage is at the base of the bladder. The prone position should help to keep urine away from the defect at the base of the bladder, which will increase the chance of spontaneous healing. From 10 to 14 days will be required for this. If leakage is persistent, catheter drainage for as long as 30 days should be carried out. Under these conditions, spontaneous closure is possible without further surgery and morbidity.

If the fistula is small, it may close spontaneously or cauterization may promote closure without surgical intervention. Catheter drainage will diminish the patient's discomfort. Cutaneous fistulae will always close and dressings will keep the leakage to a minimum. If a vesicovaginal fistula persists, a vaginal cup often is more satisfactory than diapers and rubber pants. The cup is connected to a catheter and supplies reasonable comfort. Low pressure suction seems to hasten closure of cutaneous fistulae.

Definitive surgery for persistent vesicovaginal fistulae should be deferred until maximal tissue reaction has resolved. This generally requires 3 to 6 months. Attempting to reoperate prior to this time will diminish the chances of success and make subsequent attempts more difficult. Since some fistulae will close spontaneously, such an interval supplies this chance as well. Cortisone does not provide any better healing and adds the risk of potent endocrine medication. It is not considered worthwhile.

To summarize, there is little excuse for damage to the bladder and none for failure to recognize and repair such damage. Knowledge of anatomy, proper surgical precautions and technique, and careful reconstruction will minimize this problem.

Intestinal Damage

Damage to the intestines may occur with any intra-abdominal procedure, and certain disease processes encountered in pelvic surgery may predispose to this complication. Whenever symptoms are referable to the intestinal tract, preoperative evaluation is wise. X-ray study and proctoscopy can be used to rule out such disease and to alert the surgeon to likely complications. If use of a difficult procedure that may involve bowel resection is anticipated, preliminary preparation is helpful.

Any barium used in testing must be evacuated before surgery. If it is allowed to remain in the intestine during the postoperative period, intestinal atony, extreme hardening of the barium, and obstruction may result. Routine cleansing enemas are given to all patients, not only to empty the lower part of the bowel but also to minimize the chances of contamination from defecation during anesthesia.

Chemotherapeutic medications are recommended if bowel resection is to be part of the surgical procedure. For difficult or complicated cases, wherein bowel involvement is likely, additional preparation of the bowel with neomycin or a sulfonamide such as phthalyl-sulfathiazole (Sulfathalidine) is useful. Excessive dosage should be avoided, however, as pseudomembranous colitis and secondary septicemia have significant morbidity and mortality. Many surgeons recommend only mechanical cleansing and careful peritoneal toilet to avoid this complication, reserving antibiotics for infection, if it appears despite mechanical precautions. This carries the least risk to the patient as well as giving satisfactory cleansing.

Injury to the bowel may occur while making the incision. It is important to tent the

peritoneum and be sure that there is no intestine included in the peritoneum. As the scalpel is used at this point, it becomes obvious when the bowel wall is reached and the dissection is discontinued and started at another area. In secondary incisions, special care is required and the incision should be extended upward toward a new area if there is significant adherence. Herniation must be checked for as well, so that a hernial sac with intestine is not encountered unexpectedly above the fascial layers.

The dissection should be gentle and the changes in resistance of the tissues will warn of the presence of other organs. Adhesions secondary to previous operations or disease will part in the plane of least resistance, which is usually the adherent area. Sharp and blunt dissection thus allows one to avoid undue trauma to the intestinal wall and prevents entering the lumen of the bowel itself.

Damage to the intestines may be partial or complete according to the involvement of the layers of the intestinal walls. If there is only serosal laceration, this may be supported with inverting sutures of fine atraumatic catgut. Continuous or interrupted sutures work equally well, depending on the size of the tear. It is usually best to repair such areas promptly so that they do not become lost or forgotten. However, if further extensive dissection is required, it should be completed before repair because damage and disease may be so extensive as to require resection to obtain the best results. With larger serosal tears it is important to use the safeguard of transverse closure to avoid constriction of the lumen and subsequent obstruction.

When the lumen of the intestine has been entered, the rest of the abdomen should be promptly packed away in an attempt to minimize contamination. Continuous fine atraumatic catgut is used to approximate the mucosal edges. The serosal coat is then approximated with interrupted stitches of fine permanent suture in order to invert the wall and give serosa-to-serosa closure. One such layer is usually adequate, although an additional layer of support is desirable if radiation, infection, and other conditions which jeopardize healing are anticipated.

With incision or excision of the intestine, it is important to avoid constriction of the lumen and to check for patency after closure of anastomosis is complete. Drainage is best, particularly with defects in the large bowel, to serve as a safety valve and minimize peritoneal contamination if there is separation of the intestinal sutures. All patients who have undergone extensive intestinal surgery should have the bowel placed at rest during the immediate postoperative period. A Miller-Abbott tube may be placed preoperatively, if resection is planned, or during the operation, if required. This will minimize the pressure of gas and bowel secretions on the suture line. After the bowel has recovered motility, feeding should be gradually increased; low residue diets will give an additional margin of safety.

Most bowel adhesions to pelvic organs may be seen and managed under direct vision. The posterior cul-de-sac, however, may be an exception, particularly if the uterus is large. In such cases, it is best to perform subtotal hysterectomy and then remove the cervix later in the procedure. In this manner, one will be able to visualize the cul-de-sac when the sigmoid is frequently elevated and adherent. If damage does occur, it should be repaired promptly as outlined. Portions of uterine serosa may be better left on the sigmoid than in the opposite situation. Sump or extraperitoneal drainage should be used if there has been a large defect in the rectosigmoid area.

The appendix is often removed during routine gynecologic procedures; this is a reasonable procedure, unless uterine, ovarian, or tubal surgery for infertility is performed. Although there is no evidence to suggest less morbidity with inversion of the stump, this is recommended. It gives an additional margin of safety relative to the ligature on the appendiceal stump and minimizes chances of adhesions and postoperative obstruction. Fat or mesoappendix may be included as a patch over the closure for further coverage. The viability of all areas of intestine damaged or operated on should be rechecked prior to closure of the incision.

During the closure, the omentum is brought down to help protect the bowel from being included in the sutures and to avoid adhesions between the abdominal wall and bowel. The peritoneum should always be closed under direct vision and no sutures placed deep to this closure subsequently.

If evidence of damage to the bowel appears after the operation, prompt diagnosis is required. Re-exploration with repair or short-circuiting procedures may be necessary unless drainage is spontaneous. If this occurs, surgery is deferred until the patient has recovered and can tolerate such a procedure. Suction and exteriorization of fistulous areas are helpful, and protein and fluid intake must be kept optimal. Hyperalimentation is often useful in such patients and several good commercial preparations are now available. This is best managed by conservative means, but obstruction requires prompt re-exploration and correction. Bowel rest will be required until the incisions have healed.

Vascular Damage

Damage to the large vessels of the pelvis is a complication that should not occur in gynecologic surgical procedures. Only in the most radical procedures does the field of dissection approach such vessels. An operation of such extreme difficulty should not be undertaken unless the surgeon is prepared to cope with the problem. Whenever such procedures are anticipated, a large and efficient hospital team must be available. Anesthesiologists and an effective blood bank are primary needs.

Bleeding from vessels which branch from the internal iliac artery or vein is controlled by clamping of the vessel and subsequent ligation. It is imperative to have adequate exposure and to clamp only the bleeding vessel. Blind clamping in a pool of blood can only lead to further damage. If the bleeding is arterial, pressure and suction by the assistants will enable the surgeon to locate the vessel and control it.

Further control may be obtained with pressure to stop the local bleeding and by dissecting the uterine or hypogastric artery and ligating it. Ligation of the smallest vessel necessary to provide adequate hemostasis seems logical. In some instances, however, ligation of the hypogastric artery may be required and even bilateral ligation may be necessary, particularly in association with pregnancy or postirradiation malignancy. No significant sequelae will develop from such ligation and revascularization will occur.

In venous bleeding, pressure alone often

provides satisfactory control while vessel contraction and clotting occur. The packs may be rather warm and should be placed snugly over the bleeding area compressing the vessels firmly against the bony pelvis. It is important to keep the pack under pressure for 5 to 10 minutes during which time attention can be turned to another part of the surgical procedure. When sponging it is important to "pat" rather than wipe the tissues. In this way, one will avoid removing the clots in vessels that have stopped the bleeding.

In rare instances bleeding may be so profuse and diffuse that hypogastric ligation is of no avail. A snug pack may be left in place retroperitoneally as a tamponade to be gradually removed in 48 hours. Even clamps may be left in place in such a fashion and gradually released and removed in 48 hours.

Pressure on the aorta or iliac vessels may cause enough decrease in the frank hemorrhages so that localization of the bleeding point is facilitated. Brief use of atraumatic bulldog clamps will occlude the greater vessels while adequate dissection and exposure are obtained.

Of special value, when working deep in the pelvis with small but profuse vessels, are silver clips such as those used by the neurosurgeons on the dura. When one can stop the bleeding with a clamp but cannot place a ligature behind it, nonreactive clips may be used with great success. Even with large vessels in inaccessible places, large clips similar to those used for cerebral aneurysm are effective.

Whenever great vessels are seriously damaged, prompt consultation with a vascular surgeon is required. Pressure usually will control a small area of trauma to the external iliac or common iliac vessels, particularly the veins. An incision or defect in the external or common iliac artery is more likely to require repair. Pressure on the aorta or proximal portion of the artery will allow placement of vascular occlusive clamps for repair of the defect. Atraumatic vascular sutures (5-0) may be used for the closure with heparin injected proximally and distally to the clamps to prevent clotting until completion of the repair. The peripheral pulses should be checked to be sure the vessel is patent. Arterial continuity must be maintained and confirmed prior to closure of the incisions. The common iliac and great vessels may be managed in a similar fashion.

A defect in the vessels may require a patch or prosthesis. Techniques should be utilized that will avoid the loss of a leg and these are best performed by a vascular surgeon. As mentioned at the beginning of this section, unless complete support facilities are available, some surgical procedures should not be attempted but should be referred to an appropriate medical center.

All bleeding must be under control before the operation is considered complete. The surgical field should be dry; if it is not, hemostasis should be obtained rather than ignored. Despite careful and meticulous attention to these details, bleeding will occur after operation. If the bleeding is intraperitoneal, it may not be recognized and the patient may die from exsanguination. For this reason, all large vessels should be doubly ligated. The tissue ligated should not be so large that it cannot be snugly tied, and the large vessels should be placed retroperitoneally. This will have the effect of bleeding into a closed space should hemorrhage occur. Although the peritoneum will be dissected, the pressure and tension will cause significant pain and alert the staff that something is unusual. On occasion, the tamponade effect of the pressure and clot will stop the bleeding. On all occasions there will be a palpable mass from the hematoma. Fall in blood pressure and rise in pulse may be associated and eventuate in shock if allowed to progress.

Proper management requires prompt exploration and control of the bleeding. Transfusion to replace the estimated blood loss is started immediately. On exploration, the first matter is control of bleeding. The peritoneum may be opened and the clot evacuated. If a specific artery is easily visible, it should be clamped carefully and the field should be inspected for other bleeding points. Unless the vessel is immediately visible, attention should be turned to proximal ligation of the uterine or hypogastric artery. The tissues are friable and anatomic landmarks are poorly defined. Under no circumstances should extensive exploration be performed in the region of the hematoma. The clot should be evacuated and the area drained.

Such hematomas are often midline so that it is difficult to determine the site of origin of the bleeding vessel. In such cases, bilateral uterine or hypogastric ligation may be required. It is important to remember that the blood will extravasate into the adjacent tissues as well as form a hematoma. Such dissection will particularly affect the bladder so that clots and hematuria may be present. Catheterization and bladder rest are important and, unless there has been previous vesical damage, fistulae are not likely to develop. Measurement of urinary output is important as a parameter of the patient's renal status, particularly if shock ensues. A large catheter is necessary to prevent plugging from clots, and irrigation is often necessary to keep the catheter open.

When hematomas are discovered late in the postoperative course, the bleeding has stopped and three courses are likely: (1) the mass may be entirely asymptomatic and may resolve spontaneously with no sequelae; (2) a low grade temperature is likely; and (3) an infection of the hematoma may follow. Heat and antibiotics will allow the hematoma to regress or to drain spontaneously. Continuation of the therapy is all that is required. A persistent symptomatic and infected hematoma that does not resolve or drain should be drained extraperitoneally when it becomes fluctuant. Use of heat and antibiotics should be continued for an adequate time. Infections of such degree often take considerable time to heal and under no circumstances should further surgery be undertaken until all tissue reaction is gone.

Nerve Damage

A note on nerve damage is appropriate even though it is rarely encountered. In the usual process of abdominal hysterectomy, presacral neurectomy, or myomectomy, no significant nerves are encountered in the operative field in which sacrifice is not planned. With radical procedures, the ilioinguinal nerves may be encountered, but seldom does resection laterally require their removal. However, any nerve that lies within the field of dissection in radical operations for malignant disease should be removed with the specimen.

Damage to the femoral nerve may occur if dissection is carried beneath the psoas muscle. Although this is not planned in the procedures under discussion, trauma to the nerve may occur in any lower abdominal operation. Self-retaining retractors are commonly used and the lateral blades must be carefully checked to see that they do not rest on or below the psoas

muscles. This is particularly true in thin asthenic patients with a thin abdominal wall. Retractors that have deep blades are particularly dangerous in this respect. When the retractor is placed, the surgeon must make sure that no bowel is caught between the abdominal wall and the retractor, and that the blades of the retractor do not rest on the posterior part of the pelvis. Likewise, he must be sure that the assistant does not use the retractor as a resting place and so force it down onto the nerves or deeper tissues. Paralysis will result but can be easily avoided by careful placement of the retractor. Once such trauma has occurred, physiotherapy is required to minimize muscle degeneration and contraction until the nerve recovers.

Transection of such a nerve requires neurosurgical consultation and approximation of the sheath so that regeneration has its optimal chance.

Thromboembolic Disease

"Thromboembolic disease" is an inclusive term for vascular clotting problems and their sequelae. In this particular discussion, the postoperative complications of thrombophlebitis and pulmonary embolization are of particular concern.

It is well recognized that stasis and hypotension will promote formation of clots. Increased clotting follows all major surgery and is particularly prevalent with pelvic operations. The proximity of the surgical procedure to the large pelvic vessels, packing that compresses the vena cava or iliac vessels, and inflammation serve to increase the possibility of distal clot formation. If the clots embolize, sudden death may ensue.

Certain conditions increase the risks of thrombophlebitis and pulmonary emboli. Recognition of these conditions and the patients in whom they may occur will allow special steps to minimize these risks. Any woman with a history of thrombophlebitis or pulmonary embolus has an increased risk of recurrence of the complication after major surgery. Because varicose veins so often follow repeated pregnancies, women are in particular jeopardy, especially with pelvic surgery. The incompetent and dilated vessels promote stasis with subsequent clot formation, inflammation, and embolization. Such patients should have support and compression to these dilated vessels during the operation and in the postoperative period.

If surgery is entirely elective, surgical treatment of varicose veins should be carried out prior to major pelvic surgery to minimize the complications of phlebitis and embolization. Often this is not feasible, and in these instances the use of Ace bandages or vascular support hose before, during, and after the surgery is indicated.

Other conditions that may promote increased clotting should be evaluated before the operation. Malignancy is the most commonly encountered condition in the female pelvis promoting clotting. Indeed, thrombophlebitis may be the only sign of an occult pelvic cancer.

Recognition of high risk patients and preventive measures are the most important aspects when dealing with this complication. Because of these risks, and the frequency with which parous women have varicose veins even though of minor degree, it has been sound policy to use wraps or supports on the legs of all patients undergoing pelvic surgery. Antiembolism support hose for the calf may be satisfactory for patients who do not have varicosities. However, wrapping of the entire leg is required if there are large and numerous varicose veins. Anemia should be corrected and infection treated. Obesity almost doubles the risks of such complications.

During positioning of the patient for surgery, care must be taken to avoid local pressure on any veins of the legs which might traumatize them and cause subsequent thrombophlebitis.

The same precautions are necessary during the operation itself. With adequate anesthesia and mild Trendelenburg's position, the intestines will fall cephalad and leave the pelvis free. Snug packing of the intestines not only promotes postoperative ileus but also puts increased pressure on the vena cava and large pelvic veins and, hence, should be avoided. The Trendelenburg position promotes better venous return from the legs. Large pelvic veins must not be traumatized by instruments or especially by retractors. The nurses' instrument tray must not rest on any part of the body of the anesthetized patient and the surgical assistants should not be allowed to lean against the patient.

Similar careful attention must be paid during the movement of the patient after surgery. As the patient recovers from the anesthesia she should be encouraged to move her legs, as well as to turn, to breathe deeply, and to cough. Use of the bandages or supports should be continued until the patient is returned to her full activities. During convalescence, pressure, crossing of the legs, prolonged dependent position, and acute flexion of hips or knees should be avoided to minimize obstruction or kinking of vessels that might diminish flow rates and promote clotting.

Early ambulation is considered particularly beneficial in prevention of thromboembolic complications. Many patients may be out of bed the day of operation, and all should be ambulatory by the next day. Movement of the legs stimulates venous return and decreases stasis. Ambulation and leg movement are to be stressed, particularly in patients with varicosities and those with a history of thromboembolic problems. Indeed, for these patients, it is wise to keep the foot of the bed slightly elevated as well, in order to improve the venous return when the patient is supine.

Because of the frequency with which thromboembolic phenomena are encountered in patients who have undergone pelvic surgery via the abdominal route, the use of anticoagulants after operation is worthwhile. Studies have shown considerable decrease in thrombophlebitis and pulmonary emboli under such a routine. Although risk is involved with the use of any medication, care and common sense will minimize complications.

The use of anticoagulants as therapy for specific medical and surgical complications is well established. The prophylactic use of anticoagulants has had more varied acceptance, particularly as a routine procedure after major pelvic operations. The risks of development of thromboembolic disease after major pelvic surgery were well documented by Barker and his associates in 1940 (35). The incidence of significant thromboembolic complications was three times that of surgical laparotomies. Significant reduction in these complications is noted with the use of prophylactic anticoagulants.

Unfortunately, few references report the pure effects of anticoagulants and of early ambulation in such a way that they can be compared, and there is even less in the way of a definitive prospective study. Available reports distinctly support early ambulation and the use of anticoagulants for prevention of thromboembolic complications.

It has been the policy to start routine use of anticoagulants on the third day after *all* major pelvic laparotomies except in those patients who have a specific contraindication, such as a history of ulcers, bleeding complications, infection, cortisone usage, renal insufficiency, hepatic disease, or neurosurgical procedures. In patients in whom thromboembolic risk is exceptionally high, there is history of pulmonary emboli, prosthetic cardiac valves are in use, or similar problems are present, anticoagulants may be started or resumed the night of operation.

Sodium warfarin (Coumadin) has been the medication of choice, unless immediate anticoagulation is required. In all instances the blood must be monitored daily by means of the prothrombin time so that the dosage may be adjusted as required. If heparin is used, the clotting time also should be followed until the effect of the Coumadin is apparent.

Caution must be exercised in selecting the proper dosage of Coumadin for the postoperative patient. Its effect, as measured by the prothrombin time, seems to be augmented during the postoperative period. It is possible that this is due to the effect of the anesthesia on the liver and the way it handles this portion of the clotting mechanism. A fourth of the recommended dosage is often enough to push the patient well into therapeutic range. Certain other medications, such as chloral hydrate, also seem to augment anticoagulant activity. Maintenance of a range of 30 to 35 per cent has seemed satisfactory. An initial dose of 10 mg of Coumadin often will accomplish this with maintenance dosages of 2.5 to 5 mg daily.

Hemorrhagic complications may occur with this regimen. They are rare, however, in the absence of other factors that may predispose to bleeding and are unlikely if the required observations of the prothrombin time are utilized. The morbidity from such bleeding complications is almost always related to some other factor rather than to hemorrhage alone. The risk exists but is not a valid contraindication unless the specific problems outlined earlier are present.

The medication is continued until the patient is on full activity and dismissed from the hospital to care for herself. When maintenance of anticoagulation is required for medical reasons, the necessary blood tests must be continued until stable levels are reached and easily controlled. Unless the prothrombin time has risen to abnormally high levels, the medication may be discontinued on hospital dismissal and the prothrombin time allowed to drift gradually into normal range as the patient increases her activities. Medication should be discontinued and the prothrombin time should be stabilized or decreasing before the patient is allowed to leave supervision. The use of vitamin K for rapid decrease of the prothrombin time should be reserved for those patients in whom bleeding has occurred or reoperation becomes necessary. Otherwise, it is better to allow the body to stabilize itself gradually without abrupt changes in hemostatic mechanisms.

When thrombophlebitis occurs, prompt treatment is indicated. Any elevation of temperature after operation should be evaluated. Appropriate work-up should include checking the legs for evidence of thrombophlebitis and the calves for tenderness and for Homans' sign. If equivocal information is obtained, the circumference of the leg should be measured. This may provide additional information and also serve as a baseline for future evaluation. Varicosities or redness or tenderness of specific vessels may be noted and when a clinical diagnosis is made, treatment should be started promptly.

If the patient has not been treated by anticoagulants, administration of heparin and Coumadin should be started simultaneously. The heparin should be continued until the Coumadin reaches therapeutic ranges. If anticoagulants have been given, the blood should be checked to be sure that therapeutic ranges have been reached and maintained.

The legs should be elevated and the patient should rest in bed. It is important that the patient not be allowed to have the head of the bed upright since hip flexion will negate the effect of elevating the legs. Heat by means of moist hot packs or a heat cradle should be utilized but with care to avoid burns. Infection should be treated promptly with appropriate antibiotics.

The heat, elevation, and rest in bed should continue until the pain or tenderness has resolved. Support of the legs should be continued during this period, particularly if there are any predisposing factors. After the patient becomes ambulatory the legs should be elevated whenever possible. Use of anticoagulants, however, should be continued until all signs and symptoms are gone and the patient has become fully active.

Two other associated complications are infection and embolus. It is difficult to cleanse the vagina even in the absence of pelvic infection or contamination. Septic pelvic thrombophlebitis may occur and be resistant to conservative management. A high, spiking fever in the absence of an obvious focus of infection that is unresponsive to antibiotic medication is common in such instances. Examination may suggest fullness and tenderness on the lateral pelvic walls in the region of the iliac vessels. Septic emboli may result and further complicate the postoperative course. If there is response to massive antibiotic therapy, then resolution is likely. However, if there is no response, ligation or clipping of the vena cava is required for control. Even ligation of the ovarian vessels is necessary when these are dilated and involved in the disease process. These patients are extremely ill; additional surgical procedures are risky, yet required; and the results are often dramatic.

More common than prominent septic thrombophlebitis and septic emboli are emboli with silent inflammation and clotting. In many instances, there is no warning or previous evidence to suggest thrombosis. Yet, a clot may have formed, broken off into the veins, and proceeded to the chest. If massive, there is sudden obstruction to the pulmonary artery and death almost immediately with a sudden cough, chest pain, and subsequent collapse. Chest pain, fever, and pulmonary changes may follow smaller clots as lesser branches are occluded and smaller portions of the lung are affected.

If the diagnosis is suspected, roentgenograms of the chest, an electrocardiogram, and preparation for embolectomy should be made immediately. Arteriograms may be of value but should not delay pulmonary embolectomy. Immediate thoracic consultation is required and effective teamwork must ensue if the patient is to survive the insult. Consideration also must be given to clipping or ligation of the vena cava to prevent subsequent embolization.

Careful attention to the vessels before, during, and after surgery should avoid trauma to them and should decrease the stasis that leads to clotting. Support and ambulation are important measures and postoperative anticoagulants further diminish the risk of thrombophlebitis and pulmonary emboli. Such measures are strongly recommended unless there are specific contraindications.

Summary

To summarize areas of common errors, one may list the following points relative to abdominal hysterectomy: (1) failure to make the incision in the midline so that anatomic landmarks are obscured; (2) damage to the bowel or bladder when making incision due to failure to recognize the differences in these tissues; (3) damage to the bladder when freeing the uterus from the bladder, particularly when there is scarring from serious injury or disease; (4) damage to the ureters while dissecting and clamping the infundibulopelvic ligament caused by distortion with tumor or previous surgery; (5) damage to the ureters when, in clamping cardinal or uterosacral ligaments, clamps are placed extrafascially or too far from the cervix; (6) damage to the rectosigmoid when clamping the ureterosacral ligaments; (7) damage to the ureters or bladder while peritonizing by including these organs in the sutures; (8) adhesions and obstructions from failure to peritonize and cover raw areas; (9) hernia or fistula from inclusion of bladder or bowel in the peritoneal closure; and (10) hematoma or abscess with failure to obliterate dead space and obtain good hemostasis with incisional closure.

Most significant of these errors is the failure to recognize and repair any damage which may have occurred.

Bibliography

Hysterectomy

1. American College of Surgeons: Manual of Preoperative and Postoperative Care, 2nd ed. W. B. Saunders Co., Philadelphia, 1971.
2. Burchell, R. C.: Arterial physiology of the human female pelvis (editorial). Obstet. Gynecol. *31:* 855, 1968.
3. Burchell, R. C.: Physiology of internal iliac artery ligation. J. Obstet. Gynaecol. Br. Commonw. *75:* 642, 1968.
4. Burchell, R. C., and Olson, G.: Internal iliac

artery ligation: Aortograms. Am. J. Obstet. Gynecol. *94:* 117, 1966.

5. Everett, H. S.: Urology in the female. In Urology, Vol. 3, 3rd ed., edited by M. F. Campbell and J. H. Harrison, p. 1957. W. B. Saunders Co., Philadelphia, 1970.
6. Pacheco, J. C., and Williams, T. J.: Unpublished data.
7. Pratt, J. H., Lee, M. J., Jr., Hasskarl, W. F., Jr., and Brandes, R. W.: Morbidity after total abdominal hysterectomy. Am. J. Obstet. Gynecol. *61:* 407, 1951.
8. Richardson, E. H.: A simplified technique for abdominal panhysterectomy. Surg. Gynecol. Obstet. *48:* 248, 1929.
9. Te Linde, R. W.: Operative Gynecology, 3rd ed. J. B. Lippincott Co., Philadelphia, 1962.
10. Ulfelder, H.: Gynecologic surgery. In American College of Surgeons: Manual of Preoperative and Postoperative Care, 1st ed., p. 412. W. B. Saunders Co., Philadelphia, 1967.

Myomectomy

11. Brown, A. B., Chamberlain, R., and Te Linde, R. W.: Myomectomy. Am. J. Obstet. Gynecol. *71:* 759, 1956.
12. Brown, J. M., Malkasian, G. D., Jr., and Symmonds, R. E.: Abdominal myomectomy. Am. J. Obstet. Gynecol. *99:* 126, 1967.
13. Davids, A. M.: Myomectomy: surgical technique and results in a series of 1,150 cases. Am. J. Obstet. Gynecol. *63:* 592, 1952.
14. Finn, W. F., and Muller, P. F.: Abdominal myomectomy: special reference to subsequent pregnancy and to the reappearance of fibromyomas of the uterus. Am. J. Obstet. Gynecol. *60:* 109, 1950.
15. Ingersoll, F. M., and Malone, L. J.: Myomectomy: an alternative to hysterectomy. Arch. Surg. *100:* 557, 1970.
16. Lock, F. R.: Multiple myomectomy. Am. J. Obstet. Gynecol. *104:* 642, 1969.
17. Malone, L. J.: Myomectomy: recurrence after removal of solitary and multiple myomas. Obstet. Gynecol. *34:* 200, 1969.
18. Munnell, E. W., and Martin, F. W., Jr.: Abdominal myomectomy, advantages and disadvantages. Am. J. Obstet. Gynecol. *62:* 109, 1951.

Presacral Neurectomy

19. Black, W. T., Jr.: Use of presacral sympathectomy in the treatment of dysmenorrhea: A second look after twenty-five years. Am. J. Obstet. Gynecol. *89:* 16, 1964.
20. Browne, O.: A survey of 113 cases of primary dysmenorrhea treated by neurectomy. Am. J. Obstet. Gynecol. *57:* 1053, 1949.
21. Colcock, B. P.: Presacral neurectomy for the relief of severe primary dysmenorrhea. Surg. Clin. North Am. *21:* 855, 1941.
22. Cotte, G.: La sympathectomie hypogastrique:

dans la thérapeutique gynécologique? Presse Med. *1:* 98, 1925.

23. Cotte, G.: Die Resektion des Nervus praesacralis: operative Technik. Zentralbl. Gynaekol. *57:* 77, 1933.
24. Counseller, V. S., and Craig, W. M.: The treatment of dysmenorrhea by resection of the presacral sympathetic nerves: evaluation of end-results. Am. J. Obstet. Gynecol. *28:* 161, 1934.
25. Curtis, A. H., Anson, B. J., Ashley, F. L., and Jones, T.: The anatomy of the pelvic autonomic nerves in relation to gynecology. Surg. Gynecol. Obstet. *75:* 743, 1942.
26. Erb, H., and Hauser, G. A.: Resultate der Cotte'schen Operation bei Dysmenorrhoe. Gynaecologia *148:* 357, 1959.
27. Henriksen, E.: The role of the superior hypogastric plexus in gynecology. West. J. Surg. Obstet. Gynecol. *49:* 1, 1941.
28. Ingersoll, F. M., and Meigs, J. V.: Presacral neurectomy for dysmenorrhea. N. Engl. J. Med. *238:* 357, 1948.
29. Keene, F. E.: The treatment of dysmenorrhea by presacral sympathectomy. Am. J. Obstet. Gynecol. *30:* 534, 1935.
30. Meigs, J. V.: Excision of the superior hypogastric plexus (presacral nerve) for primary dysmenorrhea. Surg. Gynecol. Obstet. *68:* 723, 1939.
31. Pemberton, F. A.: Resection of the presacral nerve in gynaecology. N. Engl. J. Med. *213:* 710, 1935.
32. Rutherford, R. N.: Presacral neurectomy: a gynecological and obstetrical follow-up. West. J. Surg. Obstet. Gynecol. *50:* 597, 1942.

Vascular

33. Allen, E. V.: The clinical use of anticoagulants: report of treatment with Dicumarol in 1,686 postoperative cases. JAMA *134:* 323, 1947.
34. Allen, E. V., Hines, E. A., Jr., Kvale, W. F., and Barker, N. W.: The use of Dicumarol as an anticoagulant: experience in 2,307 cases. Ann. Intern. Med. *27:* 371, 1947.
35. Barker, N. W., Nygaard, K. K., Walters, W., and Priestley, J. T.: A statistical study of postoperative venous thrombosis and pulmonary embolism. I. Incidence in various types of operations. Proc. Staff Meet. Mayo Clin. *15:* 769, 1940.
36. Barker, N. W., Nygaard, K. K., Walters, W., and Priestley, J. T.: A statistical study of postoperative venous thrombosis and pulmonary embolism. III. Time of occurrence during the postoperative period. Proc. Staff Meet. Mayo Clin. *16:* 17, 1941.
37. Belding, H. H.: Use of anticoagulants in the prevention of venous thromboembolic disease in postoperative patients. Arch. Surg. *90:* 566, 1965.
38. Beller, F. K.: Thromboembolic disease. In Davis' Gynecology and Obstetrics, Vol. 1, edited by J. J. Rovinsky, Chap. 57N, p. 11. Harper & Row, Hagerstown, Md., 1969.
39. Bruzelius, S.: Dicoumarin in clinical use: studies

on its prophylactic and therapeutic value in the treatment of thrombo-embolism. Acta Chir. Scand. *92 (Suppl. 100):* 1, 1945.

40. Burchell, R. C., and Olson, G.: Internal iliac artery ligation: aortograms. Am. J. Obstet. Gynecol. *94:* 117, 1966.
41. Burns, W. T.: Thromboembolic disease in obstetrics and gynecology: the value of early diagnosis and adequate treatment. Am. J. Obstet. Gynecol. *71:* 260, 1956.
42. Counseller, V. S., and McKinnon, D. A., Jr.: Factors influencing the incidence of postoperative thrombophlebitis in gynecologic surgery. Surg. Gynecol. Obstet. *75:* 114, 1942.
43. De Takats, G.: Anticoagulant therapy in surgery. JAMA *142:* 527, 1950.
44. Goldsmith, H. S.: The prophylaxis of thromboembolism. Surg. Gynecol. Obstet. *122:* 799, 1966.
45. Jennings, J. A.: Thromboembolic disease in obstetrics and gynecology. Henry Ford Hosp. Med. Bull. *11:* 289, 1963.
46. McCann, J. C.: Thromboembolism: a comparison of the effect of early postoperative ambulation and Dicumarol on its incidence. N. Engl. J. Med. *242:* 203, 1950.
47. Moss, N. H., Schafer, R. L., and Kirby, C. K.: Anticoagulant effect of Dicumarol at various prothrombin levels in dogs. Proc. Soc. Exp. Biol. Med. *69:* 143, 1948.
48. Schulman, H., and Zatuchni, G.: Pelvic thrombophlebitis in the puerperal and postoperative gynecologic patient: obscure fever as an indication for anticoagulant therapy. Am. J. Obstet. Gynecol. *90:* 1293, 1964.
49. Sharnoff, J. G.: Results in the prophylaxis of postoperative thromboembolism. Surg. Gynecol. Obstet. *123:* 303, 1966.
50. Spittell, J. A., Jr.: Thrombophlebitis and pulmonary embolism. Circulation *27:* 976, 1963.
51. Wright, I. S.: The discovery and early development of anticoagulants: a historical symposium. Circulation *19:* 73, 1959.

CHAPTER TWO

GEORGE W. MITCHELL, JR., M.D.

VAGINAL HYSTERECTOMY: ANTERIOR AND POSTERIOR COLPORRHAPHY; REPAIR OF ENTEROCELE; AND PROLAPSE OF VAGINAL VAULT

Vaginal hysterectomy has wide application in the field of gynecologic surgery, and the indications for its use seem to be constantly expanding. Part of this apparent increase in scope may be due to the boldness of a generation of gynecologic surgeons fortified by the excellence of modern pre- and postoperative care, which helps to make the patient safe for surgery. Although it is true that advances in the management of surgical problems apart from technique permit greater liberty in both planning and performance, the extension of indications beyond, or even to, the limits imposed by common sense constitutes the most common impediment to the successful completion of what should be a useful, safe, and easy procedure. To avoid falling into this obvious error, a review of the factors which might influence the selection of vaginal hysterectomy for a variety of different circumstances is necessary.

Indications

Of first importance are the experience and technical skill of the operator. Those who have been trained in institutions which have a volume sufficiently large to allow the performance of many operations of this type or who in their practices have acquired expertise through trial and error may stretch the indications a bit further than novices who are unfamiliar with the reversed anatomy and reduced exposure of the transvaginal route. A review of the anatomy of the pelvic floor or, if available, practice on cadavers is most helpful to the beginner in establishing the landmarks by which he is to be guided. Assisting experts, or vice versa, is also of great value in gaining confidence and avoiding error; and if this type of direct contact

is difficult to achieve, watching films is a satisfactory substitute.

The close approximation of the ureters to the field may be visualized by study of pyelograms and cystograms and can be further delineated by the insertion of ureteral catheters prior to surgery so that the relationship of the distal ureters to the placement of instruments may be repeatedly ascertained by palpation. By passing a Kelly clamp through the urethral meatus and directing its point downward toward the base of the bladder, the operator can readily see how close the bladder lumen is to the anterior wall of the cervix and the delicacy of the bladder muscle. By placing a finger protected by a second glove in the rectum during repair of the posterior vaginal wall, the operator can determine the relationship of the rectum to the course of his dissection and estimate to what extent his plicating sutures might encroach upon the lumen. With understanding and mastery, such simple maneuvers may be discarded until a tough case suggests their re-employment.

Uterine prolapse, which is often but not invariably associated with cystocele and rectocele, is probably the most frequent indication for vaginal hysterectomy. The classical symptoms are a bearing-down sensation in the pelvis, a feeling that the internal viscera are falling or protruding, and varying types and degrees of urinary dysfunction. Any one, all, or none of these may be present in any individual case and may not, in any way, correlate with the severity of the anatomic dislocation. Since many parous women who have been delivered vaginally have some degree of prolapse, the urge to correct such relatively minor anatomic defects must be repressed unless they can be correlated with specific symptoms. An exception to this would be a case in which the cervix or vagina protrudes beyond the introitus, incurring the risk of trophic changes and eventual severe urinary tract disability. In addition to obstetrical injury, conditions which predispose to prolapse include old age, congenital weakness of the pelvic floor usually in the form of prolongation of the posterior cul-de-sac, obesity, hard coughing, the wearing of tight supporting garments, and occupations which necessitate increase in intra-abdominal pressure. When one or more of these conditions are present, the probability of successful surgery is proportionately reduced, and other means of affording palliation should be considered.

Women in the fourth, fifth, and sixth decades of life who may have prolapse are also not infrequently prey to a variety of other ailments which they or their doctor may attribute to the position of their pelvic organs but which have no real cause-and-effect relationship. Of these, backache is perhaps the most common. The surgical salvage rate in women who suffer from neuroses is significantly reduced, and the surgeon should never assume that a successful anatomic repair will produce a good functional result. On the other hand, persistent symptoms can aggravate anxiety and depression, and the possible benefits to be gained by surgery must be weighed against its depressing effect and the chance of a poor result.

The presence of cystocele not associated with significant uterine prolapse may be an indication for vaginal hysterectomy in attempting repair in order to utilize the stumps of the uterine ligaments to buttress a repair which otherwise would depend upon plication of the adventitia of the bladder alone. The hysterectomy also provides sterilization and prevents the ruin of the repair by subsequent pregnancy and delivery. Large enteroceles are often associated with uterine prolapse in some degree and are usually best treated by vaginal hysterectomy combined with appropriate repair. Under certain conditions, however, especially in the elderly patient, the preservation of the uterus may be safer and even useful in effecting a different type of repair. Rectoceles without associated cystocele or prolapse are usually asymptomatic even if they protrude beyond the introitus. They are not a cause of constipation but when very large may interfere with the expulsion of feces and necessitate digital intravaginal pressure to defecate. Repair of rectocele and perineum alone can be accomplished quite effectively without vaginal hysterectomy unless concomitant sterilization is desired.

After defects of the pelvic floor, the most common indication for vaginal hysterectomy is abnormal uterine bleeding. This type of bleeding is of common occurrence in the fifth and sixth decades and does not always respond readily to treatment with appropriate hormones. Vaginal hysterectomy provides a definitive cure and obviates the necessity for frequent trips to the doctor's office and the inconvenience and anxiety associated with episodes of prolonged or irregular bleeding. The decision to perform an operation under these circumstances should not depend upon fear of a tissue committee's reaction to the removal of a "normal" uterus but upon consideration for the welfare of the patient. The reasons for the operation must be clearly documented in the record prior to surgery. Small submucous fibroids and endometrial polyps detected by hysterography may be similarly treated. In some areas, the use of vaginal hysterectomy has been extended to include large uterine tumors (1) and even adnexal masses. Although this is feasible by the morcellation technique, the correct diagnosis of large pelvic masses cannot always be made with certainty beforehand, and the vaginal approach may prove hazardous. Increased blood loss and postoperative morbidity are more likely.

Vaginal hysterectomy is an excellent operation for carcinoma *in situ* of the cervix when the involved areas in the cervix have been so diagnosed by cone biopsy and the adjacent tissues mapped by colposcopy. The time lapse between conization and vaginal hysterectomy should be less than 48 hours or more than 8 weeks to reduce the incidence of sepsis, and the remaining cervix should always be cultured preoperatively. The margin necessary to encompass the lesion can be delineated under direct vision and resected *en bloc* with the uterus. Radical vaginal hysterectomy for Stage I or II carcinoma of the cervix is a highly specialized procedure useful under very limited circumstances (2).

In the very obese patient, it is sometimes easier to remove a uterus containing carcinoma of the endometrium, either pre- or postirradiation, by the vaginal route; but obesity of the thighs and vulva may also preclude effective exposure, and the adnexa may be inaccessible.

Greater facility in vaginal surgery and the need for surgical sterilization as one means of population control have encouraged the performance of vaginal hysterectomy as a sterilizing procedure (3, 4). Further support for this concept comes from reports indicating a high incidence of secondary gynecologic symptoms and pathology following tubal ligation (5). In the presence of associated uterine dysfunction, vaginal hysterectomy seems the preferred method for sterilization provided that the other criteria are met.

Contraindications

Without expert assistance, the inexperienced surgeon should not attempt vaginal hysterectomy on patients who have had previous pelvic surgery or who are suspected of having other pelvic pathology, particularly chronic salpingitis. Careful assessment of the patient's pelvis under anesthesia should give the necessary information regarding size and mobility but cannot be depended on completely. The more experienced surgeon may tackle more difficult problems, such as patients who are nulliparous or who have had previous low cervical cesarean sections (6), but would be well advised to approach the fixed, or partially fixed, uterus with great caution. Once a vaginal hysterectomy is begun, however, the operator can, at any point and for a variety of reasons such as adherent bladder, unexpected adnexal pathology, or bleeding which is difficult to control from below, switch to an abdominal approach. There are some instances in which vaginal hysterectomy might seem the operation of choice for prolapse, but the possible presence of other pathology, either in the pelvis or elsewhere in the abdomen, requires laparotomy. Since repair of the pelvic floor cannot be successfully accomplished by an abdominal approach, circumstances such as these necessitate a combined operation.

Certain orthopedic and vascular disturbances, especially of the back and lower extremities, may be aggravated by prolonged suspension of the legs in stirrups or preclude the position required for proper exposure of the operative field. Such patients should be treated pallia-

tively for symptoms associated with prolapse or, in the event of uterine pathology, by the abdominal route.

As with any other type of surgical procedure, the general condition of the patient may be a contraindication to vaginal hysterectomy. Since many of the patients are in the older age group and subject to a variety of systemic diseases, careful personal evaluation of the patient by the surgeon and the members of his staff and the accurate recording of their observations in the chart are essential for the welfare of both the patient and the physician. When indicated, the opinion of consultants should be obtained with regard to specific organ systems, but the surgeon must take full responsibility in making the final decision as to whether the operation should be performed. The responsibility is the heavier because the operation is usually elective.

Preparation

Every surgeon has his own routine for preparing his patient for surgery. Some of these routines are rational and others simply ritualistic, having been passed down as folklore from the early days of surgery. All infections should be appropriately treated prior to surgery, and sufficient time allowed for the patient to recover completely. This is particularly true of infections involving the pelvis, urinary tract, vagina, or external genitalia. Infections in the genital and urinary tracts are best treated by antibacterial medication given either orally or parenterally. The local use of antibiotics is less effective and may cause tissue irritation. Estrogen by mouth is helpful in eradicating senile vaginitis and other vaginal infections prior to surgery, but its prescription for simple atrophy of the vagina to render it more amenable to dissection is seldom helpful and may increase the amount of bleeding at the time of surgery. Douches and suppositories may slightly reduce the bacterial count if used for at least 1 week preoperatively, but there is no evidence to indicate that this really reduces the postoperative morbidity from infection.

Once admitted to the hospital, the patient should have a complete general history and thorough physical examination, even though she is to be subjected to a specialized procedure. This is the patient's opportunity to have a careful survey of her condition, and neglect of this opportunity to her detriment will not easily be forgiven. Laboratory studies in addition to complete blood count, sedimentation rate, and routine urinalysis should include admission urine culture, random blood sugar, creatinine, urea nitrogen, proteins, and electrolytes. Chest X-ray and electrocardiogram are mandatory in most hospitals. On many services, intravenous urography and cystoscopy are performed on patients who are to undergo vaginal hysterectomy, especially those whose urinary tract disability is the chief indication for surgery. In the event of urinary tract dysfunction postoperatively, it is important to know the situation beforehand. When the problem is one of urinary incontinence, cystometrograms should be included (7). Since blood loss during vaginal hysterectomy when repair is done concomitantly can be heavy, the hematocrit should be at least 35 per cent preoperatively and, if not, should be brought to that level either by deferring operation and giving the patient appropriate medical therapy or by giving transfusions of packed red cells. At the time of surgery, the patient should be cross-matched with a minimum of 2 units of whole blood. All patients must have had a Papanicolaou smear and, when indicated, cervical biopsy.

Anesthesia

The choice of anesthesia should no longer be made by the surgeon, but he is perfectly justified in using his influence to achieve the desired results. Some anesthesiologists are under the mistaken impression that good relaxation is not an important factor in a vaginal procedure. General anesthesia must be accompanied by the use of drugs which relax the musculature of the abdomen and pelvic floor and allow the uterus to move downward with traction. Intrathecal spinal anesthesia is excellent for vaginal hysterectomy but has the drawback that it is inappropriate when residents and other beginners are performing the operation under supervision with ongoing instruction and advice. When epidural anesthesia is used, relaxants are necessary. A mirror set up at the end of the table at which the operator is working permits the anesthesiologist to observe the procedure, to understand the surgeon's

recommendations, and to estimate blood loss. Certain types of extraperitoneal vaginal surgery, such as perineorrhaphy, can be done under local anesthesia on a cooperative patient.

Positions of Patient, Surgeon, and Assistants

Proper positioning of the patient on the operating table not only provides better exposure but facilitates the entire procedure. Figure 2.1 shows the optimal position for the patient. She is first placed supine on the extended operating table; the stirrups are raised to the desired height and turned inward; and the legs are then slowly and simultaneously elevated until the feet can be fastened in the straps. The lower end of the table is then dropped, the buttocks are drawn just past the edge of the midsection of the table, and the sacrum is stabilized with a rubber pad (Fig. 2.1). The placement of the buttocks is most important in order than the weighted speculum which will eventually be inserted in the posterior vagina can hang freely beyond the edge of the table (Fig. 2.3). The position provides maximal access to the pelvic viscera; allows the assistants

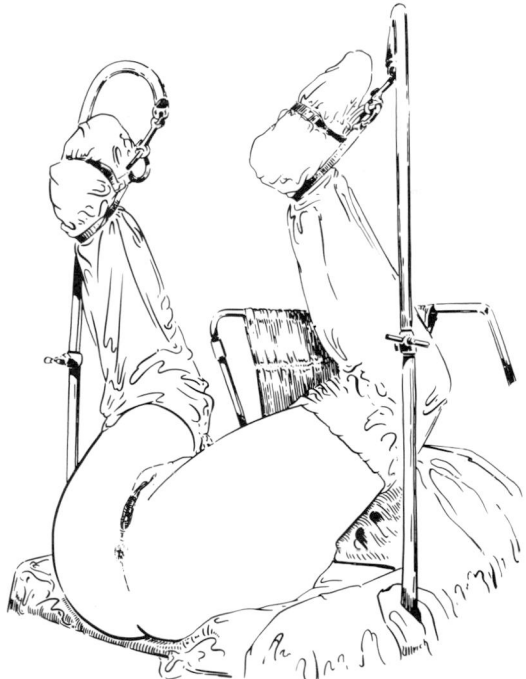

Fig. 2.1. Patient's position for vaginal hysterectomy: thighs flexed, legs extended, buttocks beyond table edge.

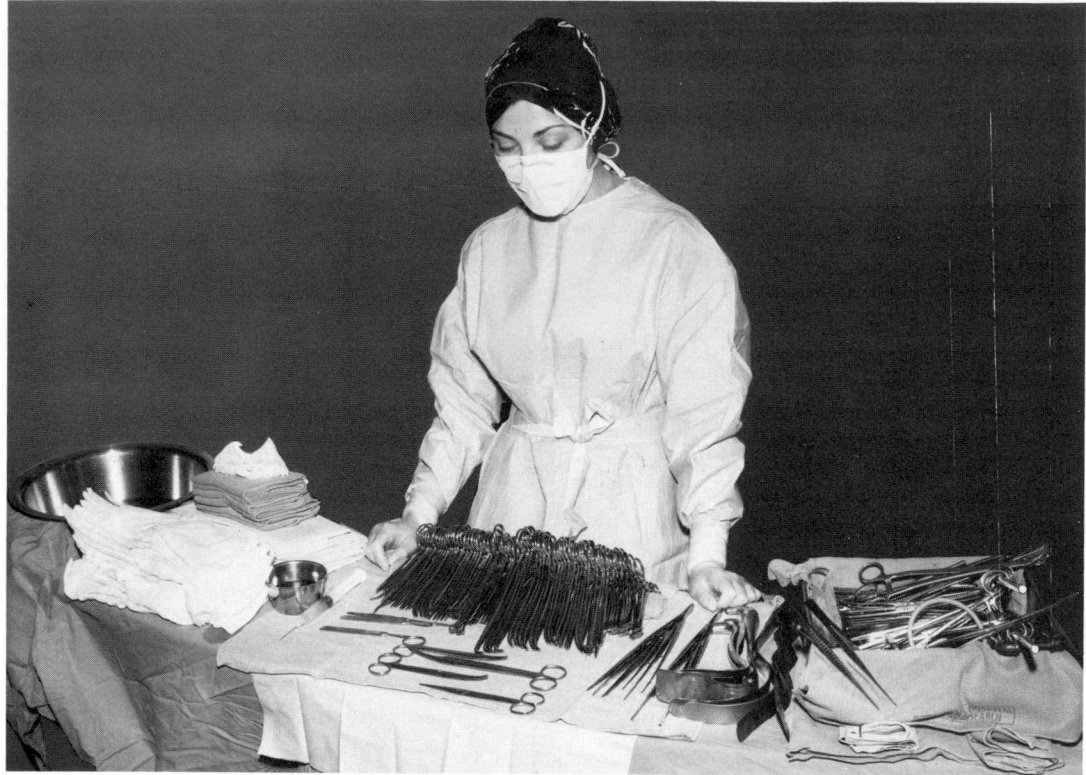

Fig. 2.2. Instrument table with instrument nurse beyond concave margin.

to work below and inside of the legs without having thigh, knee, and foot interfere with their activities; and permits the scrub and circulating nurses a clear view of the field. Tired or incapacitated assistants may sit on high stools on either side of the patient and function efficiently. The operator sits on a comfortable stool arranged at the height best suited to the length of his legs. The height of the table is then raised or lowered according to the surgeon's preference. Ordinarily the patient's urethral meatus should be approximately at the level of the surgeon's eyes. The surgeon should sit approximately two-thirds of an arm's length away from the end of the table and about midway between the two legs so that both hands can be used without interference. Unless he has a well trained team on which he can depend, the surgeon is well advised to enter the operating theater prior to the completion of the patient's preparation in order that he may assure himself that the details described above have been carried out to his satisfaction. Changing the patient's position after the drapes

have been applied or proceeding with the operation under unsatisfactory conditions is both time-consuming and dangerous.

Instruments

Two instrument tables are desirable. The first is preferably a low, narrow, curved table on which the routine instruments are arranged in the middle, and those less frequently used on the wings (Fig. 2.2). If a scrub nurse is available, she stands in the concave portion of the curve and passes the instruments across the table, which can also be pushed close to the surgeon's right side and made available to him and his first assistant when no scrub nurse is available. Larger, rectangular tables necessitate the nurse's working with her back to the operation or having to lean far forward to pass instruments. The second table is a low Mayo stand on which are placed a pair of curved Mayo scissors, a scalpel, a dressing forceps, a toothed forceps, and at least three marked sponges. This stand is more stable than a lap tray and offers immediate access to a few important instruments. The first assistant keeps a pair of straight suture scissors, and each assistant has available several marked sponges, which are kept on the patient's lower abdomen. Draping is best accomplished by using two separate booties for the legs and two half sheets, the upper one of which extends from the pubis over the anesthesiologist's frame, and the lower one from the patient's buttocks almost to the floor. If no instrument nurse is available and only one assistant, as occurs in many community hospitals, the assistant and the surgeon can turn from the instrument table back to the operating field without changing position, and the surgeon keeps a larger number of instruments on his stand. During the operation, the nurse should remove unnecessary instruments from the surgeon's stand and keep it free of blood. Proper arrangement of instru-

ments on the stand is most important in order that the surgeon need not search unnecessarily for what he wants. There are many different preferences regarding instruments, and many surgeons have given their names to instruments of their own design. For practical purposes, the essentials to be kept on the curved table are a dilation and curettage kit; two cervical tenacula, preferably of the crushing type, since single-toothed tenacula tend to pull through soft cervices when traction is applied; two needle holders and needles; at least a half dozen heavy clamps with box locks for securing the principal uterine ligaments; a half dozen hemostats, straight and curved; approximately eight Allis or T clamps; a weighted speculum; and two short right angle retractors. Also handy in case of emergency are small right angle clamps of at least 8 inches length for grasping high bleeders which may have escaped ligature, Sims

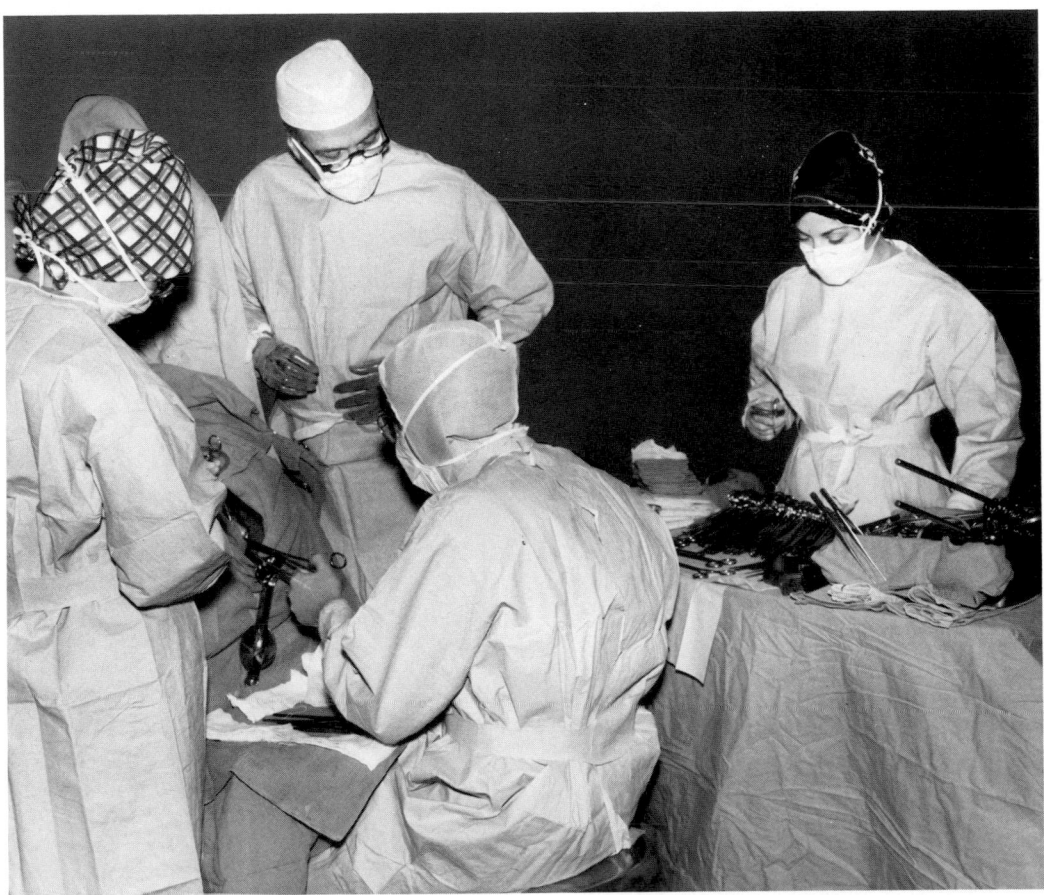

Fig. 2.3. Arrangement of tables, nurse, and assistants during operation.

and Deaver retractors, and long-toothed forceps. One or two spot lights usually provide better illumination than the overhead light.

Clean-up

The type of cleansing agent used in the preparation of the operative field is not important. A significant reduction in bacterial count cannot be attained at this time, and the chief object is to remove debris. Of great importance, however, is gentleness in prepping the vagina to avoid tearing delicate tissues. Vigorous scrubbing can even tear uterine arteries when the mucous membrane is atrophic.

Procedure

The injection of hemostatic solutions into the paracervical tissues and the anterior and posterior vaginal walls at the beginning of the operation has been alleged to reduce blood loss and assist in the dissection of tissue planes. This is a matter of preference but is unnecessary if the correct steps are followed and the proper planes entered. Dilatation and curettage is routine, if not previously done, to rule out pregnancy or endometrial carcinoma. If the tissue obtained is suspicious, it should be sent for rapid section diagnosis. The old dictum that endometrial tissue in the unfixed state is unsatisfactory for pathologic examination is not true, and it is most unfortunate for the patient's prognosis if the diagnosis of carcinoma is not made until after the procedure is over. When pregnancy is present, the surgeon may elect to discontinue the operation, complete the abortion by curettage, or proceed with hysterectomy. Vaginal hysterectomy as a means of abortion up to 16 weeks of pregnancy has recently been reported but can be recommended only to the boldest (8).

If a hysterectomy and repair are to be done together, it is best to do the hysterectomy first. The surgeon does not have to contend with the blood draining from the anterior repair during the hysterectomy and need not maintain undesirable traction on the repair. When suprapubic drainage of the bladder is to be instituted, the catheter should be inserted prior to beginning the hysterectomy. A #18 Foley catheter is placed in the urethra and the bladder filled to approximately 400 cc. The trochar is then pushed into the bladder percutaneously from a point 2 inches above the pubis, and the appropriate catheter passed through the trochar until good drainage ensues. The trochar is withdrawn, and the catheter fixed to the skin and connected to a drainage bottle. Doing this procedure first insures that it is performed under the direct supervision of the surgeon when the team is fresh. It also prevents placing undue strain on the suture line of the anterior repair by stretching the bladder. The Foley catheter may be left in the bladder as a guide for the plication of the vesical neck and should be occluded and fastened to the drapes suprapublically during the early part of the procedure.

The pros and cons of suprapubic, as opposed to transurethral, postoperative drainage remain a source of controversy. The chief problem in using suprapubic catheterization is that it necessitates a well educated team of nurses and residents on the floor to monitor the catheter and make sure that it is working properly. It has the distinct advantages that the patient can attempt to void at any time postoperatively and that it serves to measure residual urine after voiding, making repeated catheterizations unnecessary. Whether it is also helpful in reducing the incidence of postoperative urinary tract infections is debatable. Several of the newer types of suprapubic catheter kits obviate some of the inherent disadvantages of the method by reducing the complication rate. The Ingram catheter is a good model (9).

To provide good exposure, the labia minora are sutured to the adjacent skin of the thigh at a point which will provide good traction without tearing the delicate tissues. Fine cutting needles are used for this. Bleeding encountered as a result of these transfixion sutures nearly always stops spontaneously or with a little pressure and can usually be ignored. The cervix is placed on traction by two crushing clamps, one on the anterior and one on the posterior lip. If the cervix is quite small, as in the case of an elderly patient, the entire cervix may be grasped with a single tenaculum, but this should have at least two teeth in order to prevent tearing. Laceration of the cervix by single-toothed clamps early in the procedure causes the surgeon to lose his best hold and makes the entire subsequent operation more difficult. The cervix is then circumcised with a scalpel at a point approximately 3 or 4 mm below the lowest extension of the bladder. When it is not obvious, this point of extension is ascertained by passing a Kelly clamp through the urethral meatus down to the junction of bladder and cervix or by elevating and lowering the bladder with an Allis clamp so that the bulge above the cervix may be readily seen. Upward traction on the bladder during the circumcision of the cervix is highly desirable to avoid damage and to give a clear view of the submucosal tissue planes as they are being divided. As the incision progresses from anterior to lateral to posterior surface, the cervix is drawn first down, then sideways, then up in keeping with the principle of countertraction to allow separation of tissues in the planes of least resistance and to provide good visualization. If exposure is poor because of a high perineum, a perineotomy is done, and a sponge and the weighted speculum placed over the incision to lower the bridge. The blade of the weighted speculum should be approximately 3½ inches long, a length which permits the cervix to come down to or beyond the introitus with traction. A longer, weighted speculum is necessary when the vagina is unusually deep and is useful after the posterior peritoneum has been opened. The depth of the incision around the cervix necessary to reach the proper tissue plane varies with the individual and cannot be stated in terms of millimeters. This is a problem for the beginner, who finds difficulty in entering the anterior plane which permits dissection of the bladder from the uterus. Instead, he may inadvertently penetrate the bladder wall or plough into the uterine muscle. To prevent this, the end of the handle of the scalpel should be wedged into the incision at a point between eleven and one o'clock, and the divided tissues pushed upward in the midline keeping the handle pressed firmly against the cervical isthmus and with maximal traction on the anterior lip (Fig. 2.4). The bladder attachments and endopelvic fascia will divide smoothly, and the dissection can then be carried up with minimal pressure to the peritoneal reflection. This step is taken only in the midline, since similar stripping only a few millimeters lateral to the midline will avulse the vascular pillars of the bladder. When the attachments of bladder and cervix have been severed, a small right angle retractor is placed

beneath the bladder, keeping it on traction and out of harm's way during subsequent steps. The vaginal mucous membrane, which has been cut through around the cervix, is then pushed upward from the supporting ligaments of the uterus by one finger covered by a single layer of gauze (Fig. 2.5). This must be done quite superficially to avoid premature separation of the ligaments from the cervix and should be continued until the mucous membrane is well above the areas where clamps must later be placed.

Posteriorly, the mucous membrane is pushed upward between the uterosacral ligaments, exposing the peritoneum of the cul-de-sac for easy entrance (Fig. 2.6). During this step, the posterior lip of the cervix is maintained on firm traction toward the pubis. If the operation is being done for uterine disease rather than prolapse, even heavy traction sometimes does not bring the cervix low enough in the vagina for good visualization, and it is necessary to enter the posterior peritoneum blindly, with curved Mayo scissors pointed toward the uterus and in close proximity to the uterine wall. The posterior cul-de-sac does not reach its lowest point close to the uterus and, under ideal circumstances, can be opened 1 cm or so away from it. Failing direct visualization or blind entry, usually due to technical error, the rectum and unopened peritoneum can usually be wiped bluntly away from the uterus in the midline and pushed upward to clear the uterosacral ligaments for extraperitoneal clamping. Once the cul-de-sac has been entered, the posterior pelvis is explored manually for previously undetected disease and for adhesions which might interfere with hysterectomy.

If the findings are favorable, the first clamps are then applied at right angles to the cervix and from below upward (Fig. 2.7). A heavy clamp of the Heaney type is best for this because of the large wad of tissues to be crushed. The inner blade of the clamp should be within the peritoneum, unless penetration has not been possible, and the outer blade should extend around the uterosacral and cardinal ligaments, as well as the pillar of the bladder on that side. Some surgeons prefer to clamp these structures separately, but with good exposure, experience, and the right kind of clamp, the principal supporting structures can be clamped together, cut, and sutured

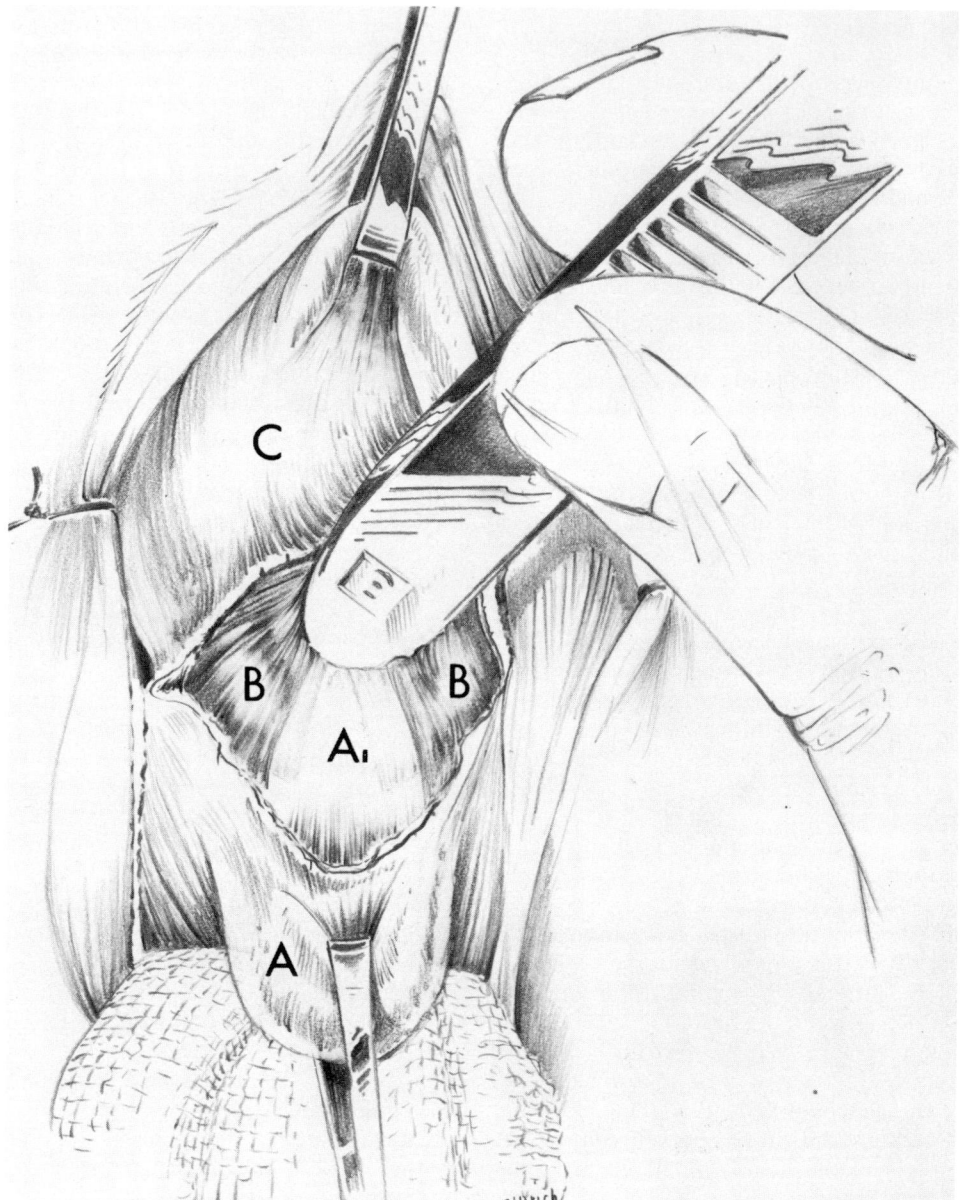

Fig. 2.4. Separation of bladder from cervix. Blunt dissection with pressure against the cervical isthmus as well as upward while heavy traction is maintained on cervix. A, Cervical portio; A₁, cervical isthmus; B, bladder pillars; C, vaginal mucosa.

without difficulty. In the interest of speed, a single clamp can be used on each side, but this is not recommended. Heavy chromic catgut, #1 or #0, is used for this and the other main ligaments. Since the ligament is to be held and subsequently used in the repair, it is important to set two clamps in order that one may be

replaced with a suture for hemostasis and the other with a suture for traction. If only one clamp is used, it is imperative that it be replaced with a mattress or hook suture of a type which is not likely to slip. The technique of passing a suture carrier around the ligaments without prior clamping is helpful when it is difficult to mobilize the uterus and obtain adequate room but has the disadvantage that the ligament is more likely to slip out of the suture after being cut. The supporting ligaments of a high, relatively fixed uterus must be divided separately or piecemeal on a catch-as-catch-can basis, with full realization that there is greater risk of both immediate and delayed hemorrhage. A similar procedure is performed on the left side. If the operator is ambidextrous, a highly desirable trait in vaginal surgery,

these clamps can more easily be placed with the left hand. Once the ligaments have been secured, the ends of the traction sutures are fastened to the drapes laterally.

At this point, the weighted speculum, preferably a longer one, or a right angle retractor of the Simms type is inserted directly into the cul-de-sac, where it remains until the peritoneum is to be closed. After the uterosacral and cardinal ligaments have been severed, the cervix usually can be drawn into the lower vagina or

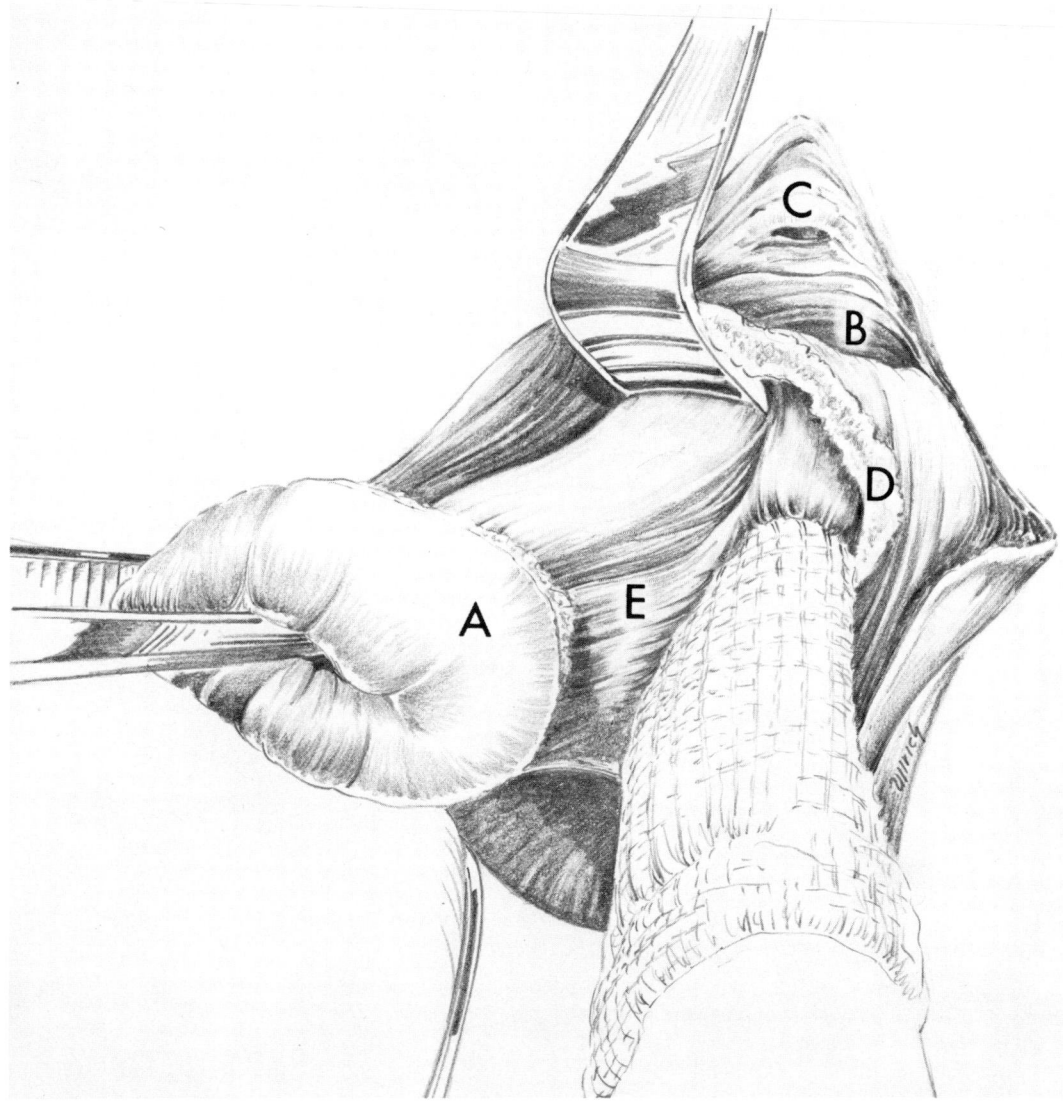

Fig. 2.5. Stripping back vaginal mucous membrane to expose supporting ligaments of uterus. A, Cervix; B, bladder; C, urethral meatus; D, vaginal mucosa; E, cardinal ligaments.

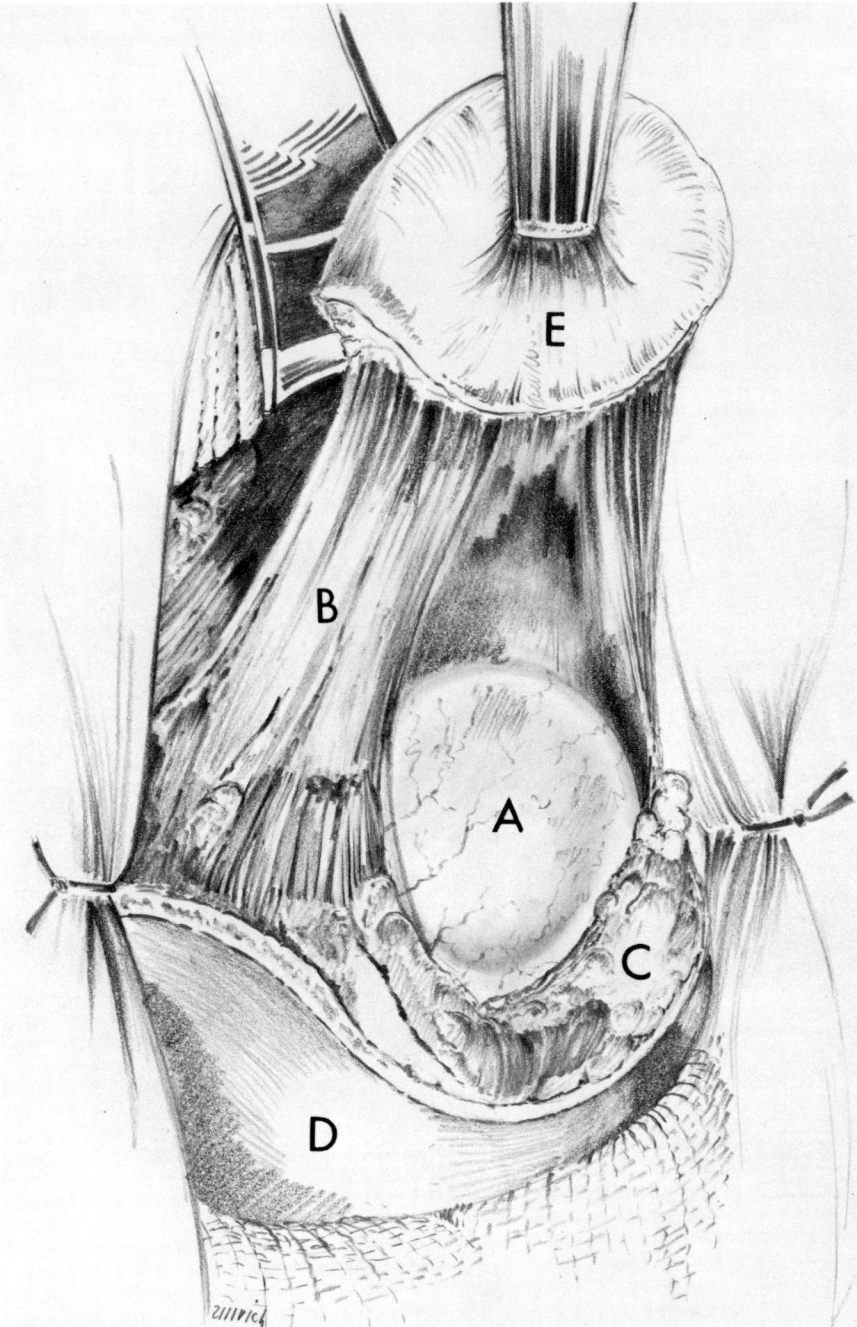

Fig. 2.6. Exposure of posterior peritoneum between uterosacral ligaments and rectum. A, Cul-de-sac peritoneum; B, cardinal and uterosacral ligaments; C, rectum; D, vagina; E, cervix.

beyond the perineum, exposing the uterine vessels. These are doubly clamped, cut, and doubly ligated, again placing the clamps at right angles to the uterus and from below upward (Fig. 2.8). The toes of the clamps should be close to the side of the uterus, and when cut free, the edge of the peritoneum of the bladder reflection is usually entered or clearly exposed. This saves a separate step of searching for and opening the peritoneum anterior to the uterus.

The bladder is up on the retractor and so cannot be damaged. The bladder retractor can then be shifted directly into the peritoneal cavity, and all subsequent clamping of uterine ligaments and vessels is done from one peritoneal surface to another. Once ligated, the uterine vessels are not held for fear they might shed their ligatures and also because they are not to be used in the subsequent repair. One of the common mistakes made during the early part of the operation is an attempt to deliver the uterus, either anteriorly or posteriorly, before adequate mobility has been achieved. Under these circumstances, the uterus acts as a plug preventing good exposure of the remaining supports and vessels to be dealt with. If the uterus is left in the horizontal plane, it is usually possible to continue to clamp successively up the side no matter how high or large

the organ is. The entire broad ligament must be clamped and tied. To attempt to cut through the clear space without clamping leads to bleeding from unseen or aberrant vessels, which are present just often enough to be dangerous.

When well mobilized, the uterus is usually most easily delivered posteriorly. If it is quite large, this can be done with the aid of traction by hooked clamps of the Leahy type attached to the posterior wall of the fundus. If the uterus is too large to be delivered, even with traction, it may be necessary to perform a morcellation operation, either by removal of individual fibroids, by splitting the uterus into two or more sections, or by taking a large V-shaped wedge out of the posterior wall (1). The remaining sections are grasped and pulled down with hooked clamps. Since the next step proceeds rapidly, bleeding can be temporarily

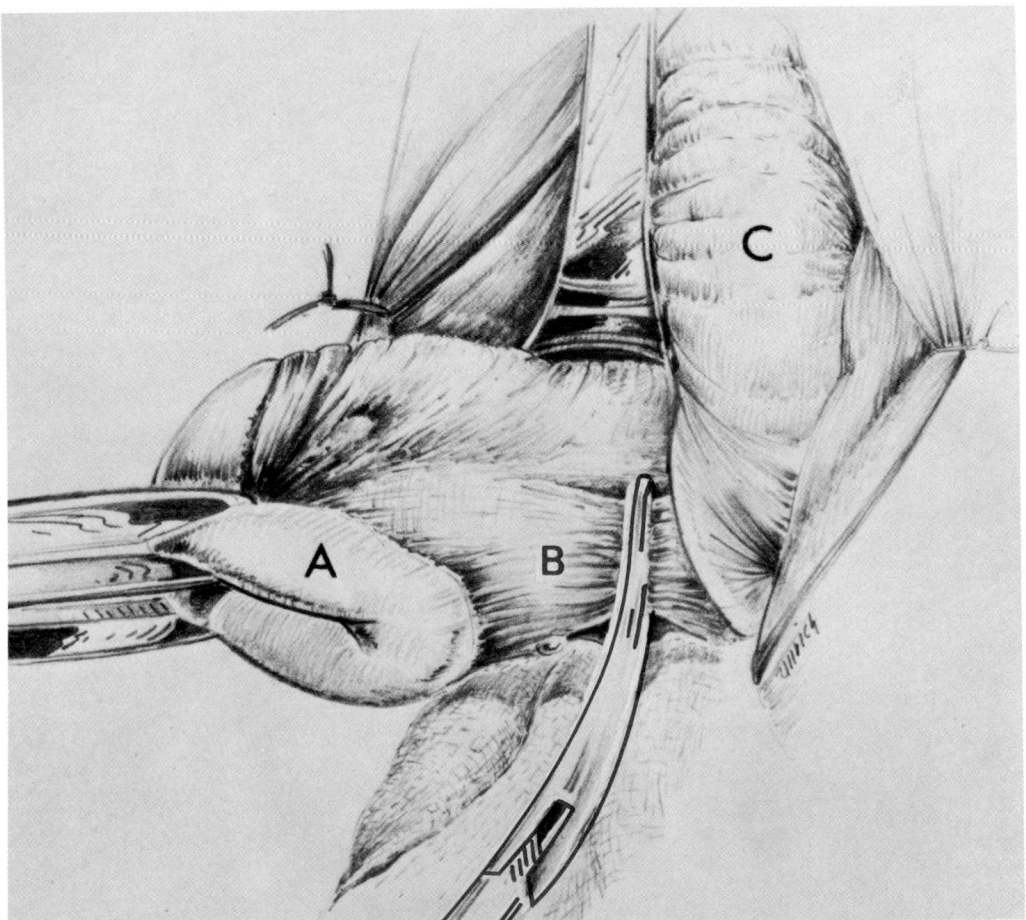

Fig. 2.7. Application of Heaney clamp to uterosacral and cardinal ligaments (B) so that they may be severed together. A, Cervix; C, bladder still covered with vaginal mucosa.

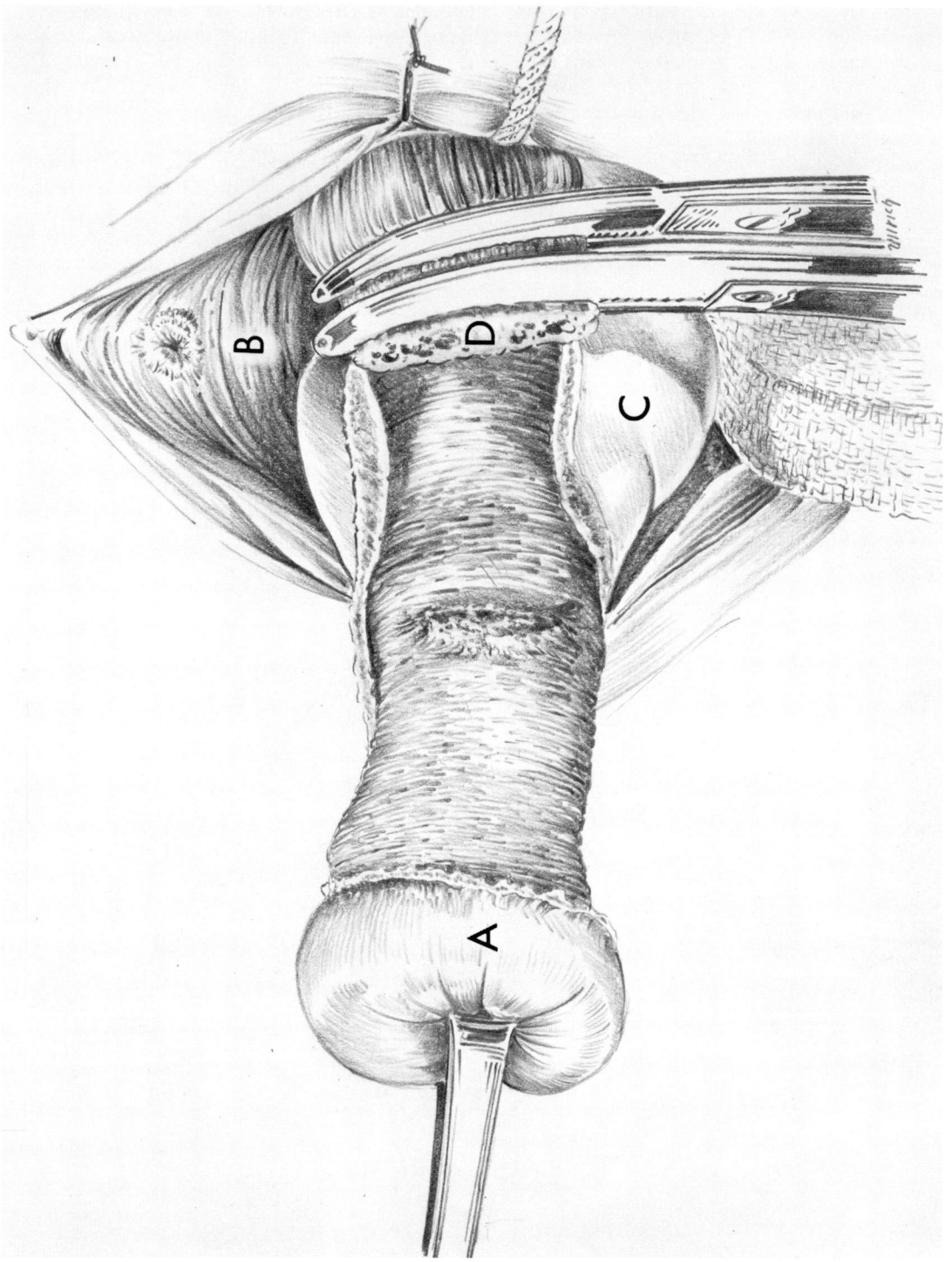

Fig. 2.8. Uterine vessels have been doubly clamped and cut and retract upward. A, Cervix; B, bladder; C, uterine fundus; D, stumps of uterine vessels.

ignored. Once the uterus has been drawn outside the introitus, the ovarian ligament, the Fallopian tube, and the round ligament are exposed. These structures are doubly clamped together, cut, and doubly ligated on either side (Fig. 2.9). If it is desirable to remove the adnexa, this can best be done separately with the uterus out of the way unless they descend readily into the field. If removal of the adnexa is not planned, they should be carefully inspected for pathology. To remove the adnexa, special instruments may be necessary, since the mobilization of these organs can be quite difficult. Deaver retractors and long, heavy, right angle clamps facilitate this procedure. Traction on the tube and ovary with long Allis or McBurney clamps is helpful, as is good relaxation to allow mobilization and packing of the bowel. Dense adhesions, poor exposure, or suspicious ovarian disease require an abdominal approach. The upper end of the broad ligament having been doubly ligatured, the second ligature is held laterally, providing, together with the uterosacral and cardinal, control of the entire broad ligament, which can be drawn down for inspection of possible bleeding sites.

The peritoneum is then closed in such a manner as to extraperitonealize the upper and lower ends of the broad ligaments. This closure need not take much time and can usually be done with one or two pursestring sutures incorporating the stumps of the broad ligaments at points approximately 1 cm from their cut ends. A meticulous running suture takes more time and is unnecessary. The exclusion of the stumps of the broad ligaments from the peritoneum channels any subsequent bloody drainage down through the vagina rather than into the peritoneum. When the peritoneum is about to be closed, after the pursestring sutures have been placed but not tied, a clean sponge is inserted within the peritoneal cavity to assess occult bleeding. If the sponge comes out reasonably dry, the sutures are tied. One other important step prior to closure of the peritoneum is to ascertain the length of the cul-de-sac. This can be done by inserting the forefinger from above downward into the posterior cul-de-sac and curving the finger into the operative field (Fig. 2.10). The peritoneal reflection will be seen attached to the superficial layers of the rectal wall. If the cul-de-sac

is more than 1 cm in depth, it should be resected to prevent the development of an enterocele at a later date. If an enterocele is already present, adherent bowel or omentum should be freed, the peritoneum mobilized from the rectal muscle by blunt dissection, and the sac resected as high as possible. The subsequent peritoneal closure will then be from the anterior peritoneum to the remains of the rectal reflection. Redundancy of the anterior peritoneum at the point of attachment of the bladder is very rare, but excess can be trimmed if necessary.

When repair operation is not to be associated with vaginal hysterectomy, the only remaining step is to elevate the stumps of the uterosacral and cardinal ligaments by traction from above the pubis while the uterosacral components are plicated back toward the sacrum. The last suture includes a portion of the anterior rectal wall (Fig. 2.11). Combined with the resection of excess peritoneum, this obliterates the cul-de-sac space and effectively walls off the posterior pelvis against enterocele. The vagina is then closed horizontally rather than vertically to prevent narrowing at the upper end, and the stumps of the broad ligaments can be sutured into the vaginal cuff at any point along the line of closure. It is simpler to use the same traction sutures for this, bringing the ends through opposite sides of the vaginal closure and tying them together where they seem to meet most conveniently. Closing the posterior pelvis by uniting the uterosacral ligaments shortens the vagina to some extent but not enough to impair future function.

If a concomitant repair is to be done, the anterior vaginal wall is grasped in the midline with two or three Allis clamps placed vertically from about 1 cm below the posterior margin of the urethral meatus to the apex and pulled up. The edge of the vaginal apex, where it has been severed from the cervix, is grasped in two places on either side of the midline and pulled down. The points of a pair of curved Mayo scissors are inserted between the vaginal mucosa and the bladder wall and gently forced upward while partially opening and closing the scissors in the traditional manner (Fig. 2.12). The importance of countertraction during this maneuver cannot be overstated, since with all of the tissues on the stretch there is much less likelihood of

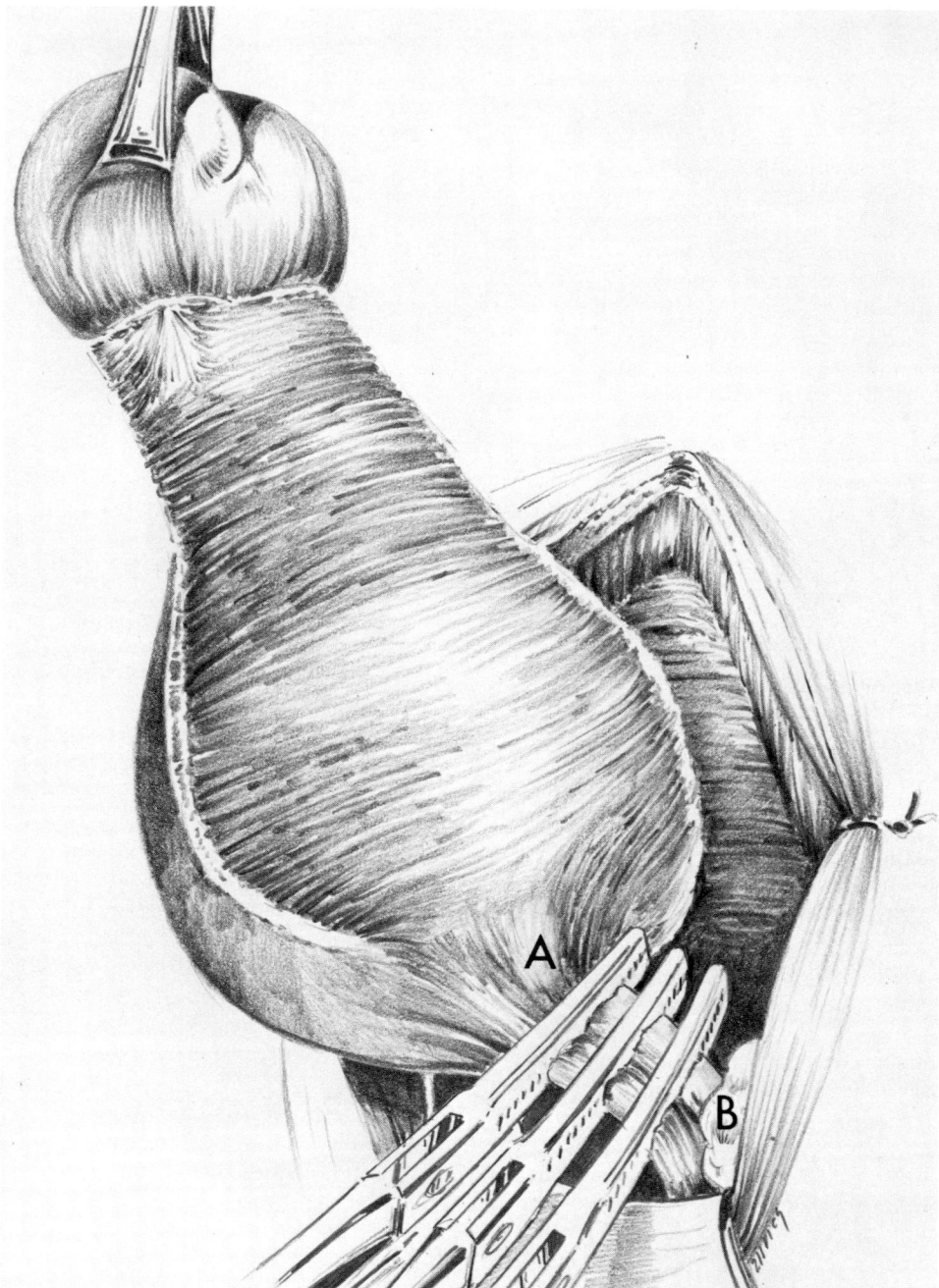

Fig. 2.9. Uterus delivered posteriorly. Clamps placed across pedicle including the Fallopian tube and the round and ovarian ligaments (B). A, Ovary.

perforation of adherent bladder wall. Unless the anterior wall is quite short, it is best to accomplish the dissection upward to the highest Allis clamp in two or three stages cutting the vaginal wall vertically in the midline when it is clear of the bladder. When the entire vaginal wall has been cut, the edges are grasped with T clamps and drawn laterally for further mobilization. Three or four of these T clamps on a side reduce tearing of the vaginal wall by misapplied traction. Subsequent dissection of the vaginal flaps and mobilization of the cystocele are best accomplished by turning the T clamps back across the forefinger of the left hand and incising the endopelvic fascia beneath the mucous membrane with the scalpel while constant traction is maintained superiorly and medially by the assistants (Fig. 2.13). The use of the finger beneath the vaginal flap adds the factor of proprioception in determining the depth of the cut and prevents buttonholing.

The same maneuver is performed on the left side, preferably placing the right finger beneath the flap, and making the incision and doing the dissection with the left hand. Stripping the bladder adventitia and the endopelvic fascia from the undersurface of the mucous membrane should be done chiefly by blunt dissection using a single layer of gauze on top of a forefinger but cutting those attachments that cannot be easily released. Such refractory attachments are often small blood vessels which

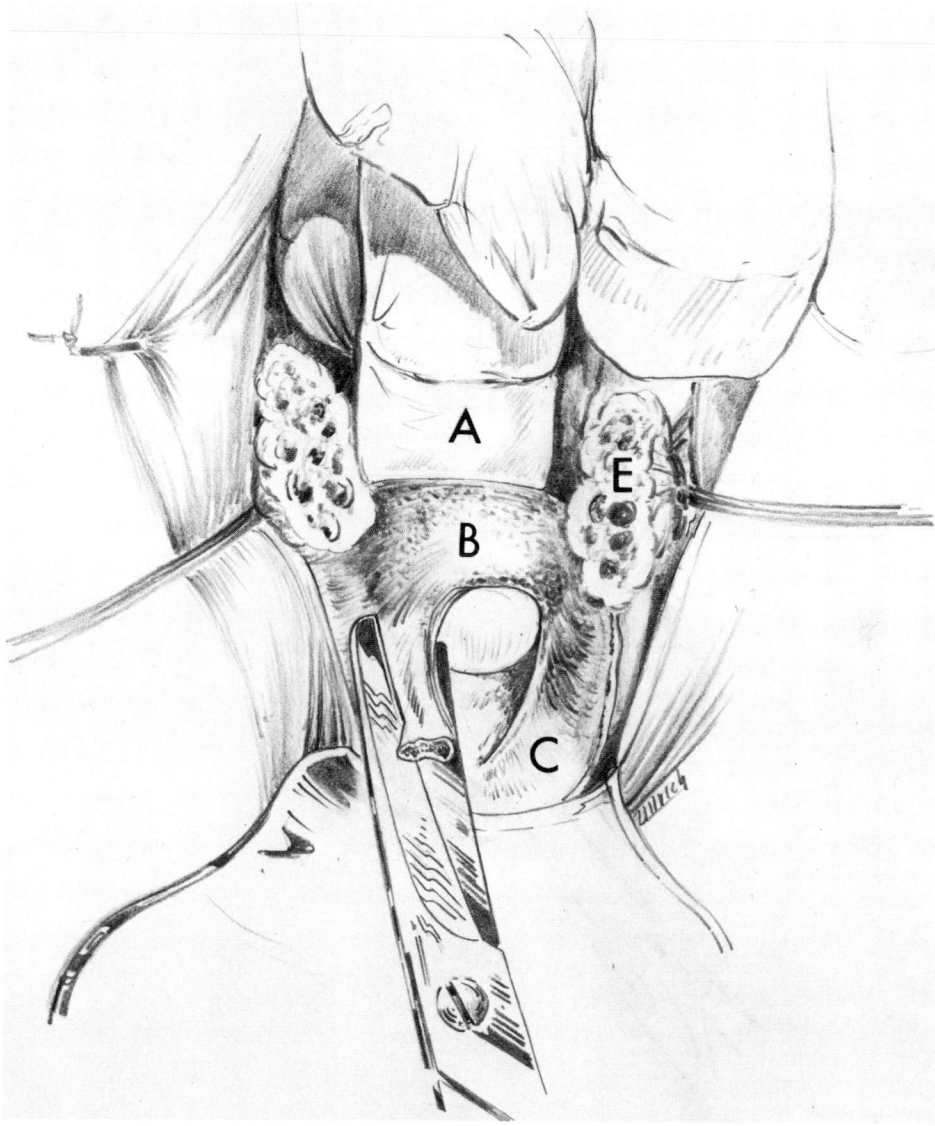

Fig. 2.10. Forefinger of right hand inserted in cul-de-sac (A) and keeping it on traction while excess peritoneum (B) is removed with scissors. C, Rectum; E, stumps of uterine ligaments.

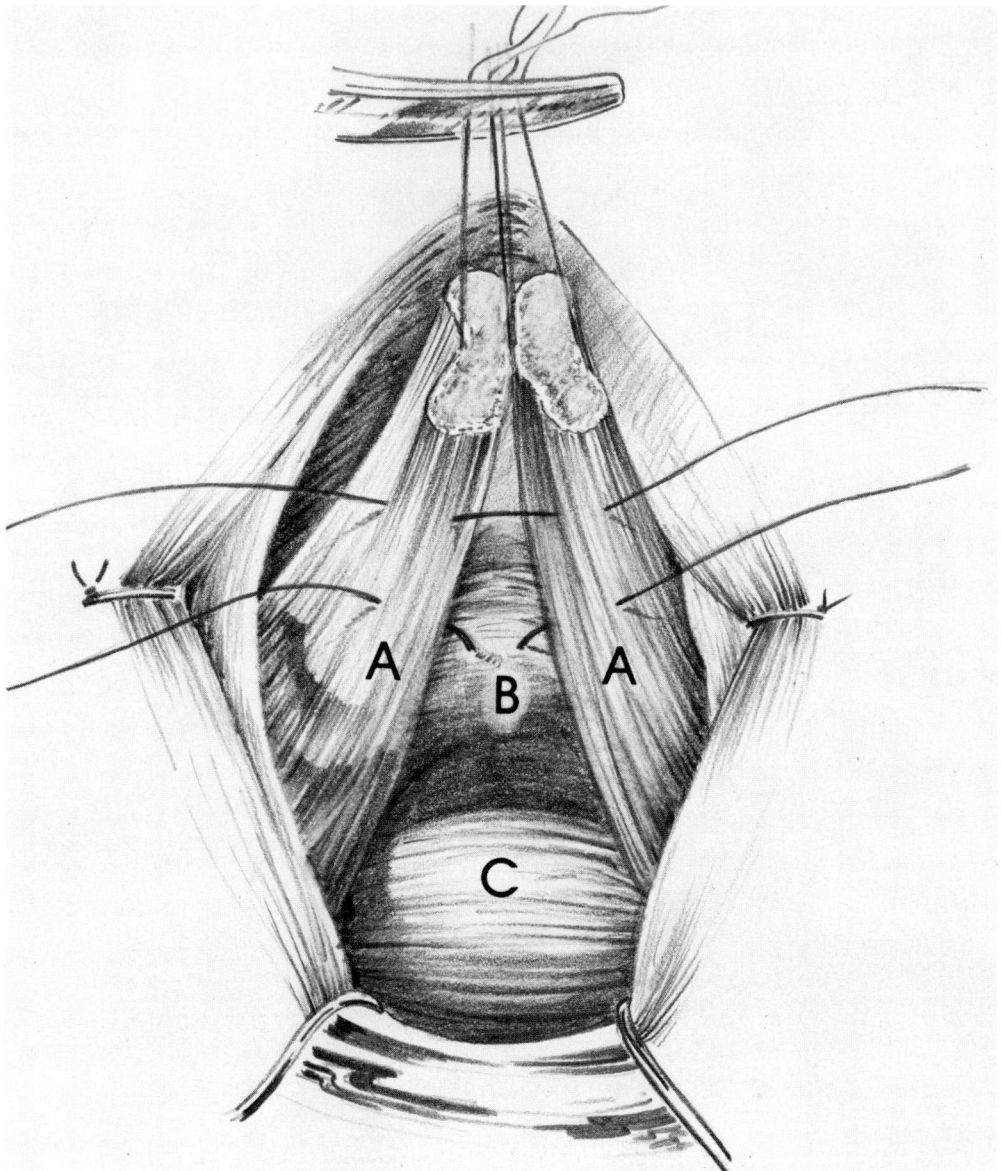

Fig. 2.11. Plication of uterosacral ligaments (A) below peritoneum (C) obliterating cul-de-sac. Highest suture includes rectal wall (B).

should be clamped prophylactically before being cut and ligated with fine catgut. If the bleeding is heavy and diffuse, the wrong cleavage plane has been entered, and an attempt should be made to move the dissection closer in to the underside of the vaginal flap. How far to carry the dissection around the bladder is a matter of judgment in each case, but a good rule of thumb is that it should extend to the level of the superior surface of the descending pubic ramus, which is a good landmark because it is so easily palpable. Freeing the bladder beyond this point may rupture the inferior fascia of the urogenital diaphragm above which is a complicated network of veins, the so-called "bloody angle." No advantage is to be gained by mobilizing the urethra and bladder to this extent. Electrocoagulation of bleeders in this inaccessible space, or elsewhere in the repair, is a helpful method of controlling hemorrhage. Near the apex of the vagina, lateral penetration should not be quite so deep, since thick anterior reflections of the endopelvic fascia from the cardinal ligaments are encountered, which are quite vascular and need to be preserved and utilized in the final suspension.

When the vaginal flaps have been developed and the cystocele delineated, the urethrovesical junction can be identified visually or by pulling the Foley catheter downward until the bulb obstructs in the vesical neck (Fig. 2.14). Repair should begin at this point unless a urethrocele is demonstrable. Plication of the urethra along its entire length may lead to stricture, loss of mobility, and subsequent urinary tract dysfunction and is contraindicated in the absence of urethrocele. Regardless of whether the patient suffers from urinary incontinence, plicating

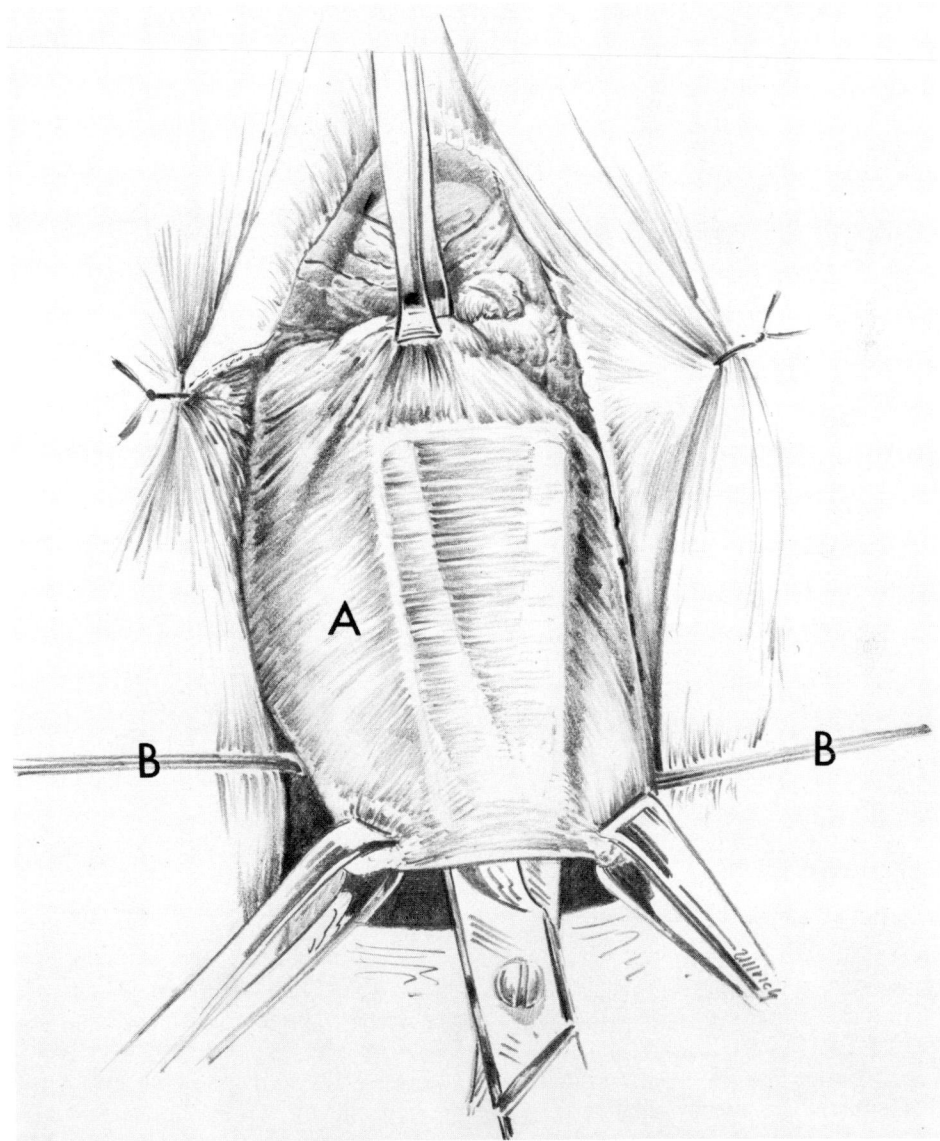

Fig. 2.12. Separation of vagina from bladder. Points of curved scissors are pressed toward the vaginal side as they are pushed upward. A, Vaginal mucosa; B, ties on stumps of uterine ligaments.

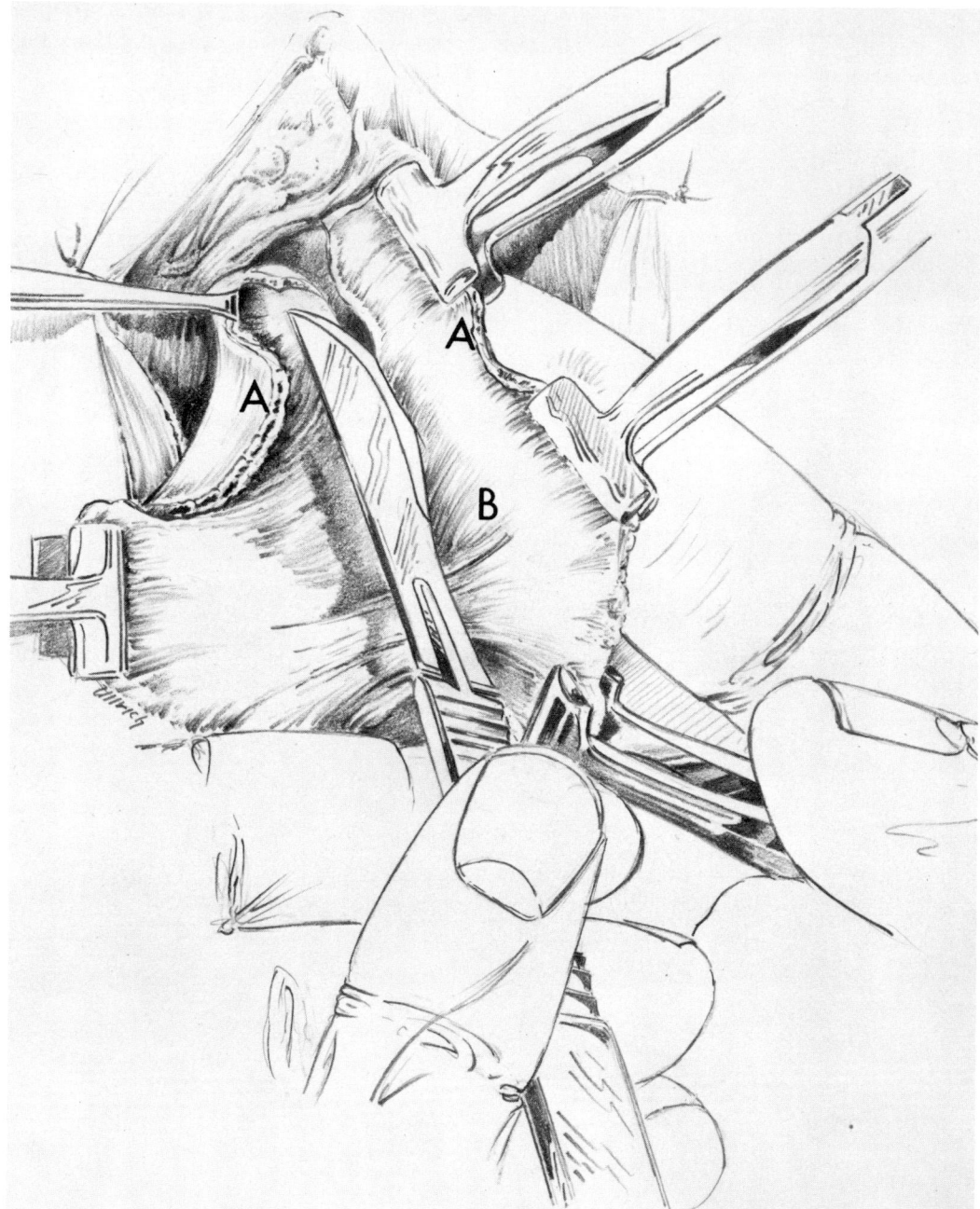

Fig. 2.13. Incising for dissection submucosal tissues (endopelvic fascia) over forefinger while traction on vaginal edges is maintained. A, Edge of vaginal mucosa; B, attachments of bladder to undersurface of vagina.

sutures at the urethrovesical junction should be somewhat tighter than elsewhere along the line of repair in order to preserve the posterior angle and insure that incontinence, if not present at the time of operation, does not develop subsequently. The vesical neck and cystocele are repaired by turning in the remains of the submucosal fascia and the bladder adventitia using vertically placed Lembert sutures (Fig. 2.15). A round Murphy needle is best for this because it is both thin and durable. It should not dip far below the surface but should encompass a section about 5 to 7 mm long. Smaller bites often pull out of the tissue when the sutures are tied, particularly when there is tension, and deeper bites might impinge upon the bladder or the ureters. The isthmic segments of the ureters lie lateral and superior to the point of plication but can be caught by an unusually deep suture. The bites on either side include a small portion of the tissue plicated in the previous suture and follow the course of the descending pubic ramus from above downward so that each successive stitch is further out from the midline as the largest protrusion of the cystocele is reached and turned in on itself (Fig. 2.16). If the cystocele is very large or if the vesical neck seems to require further

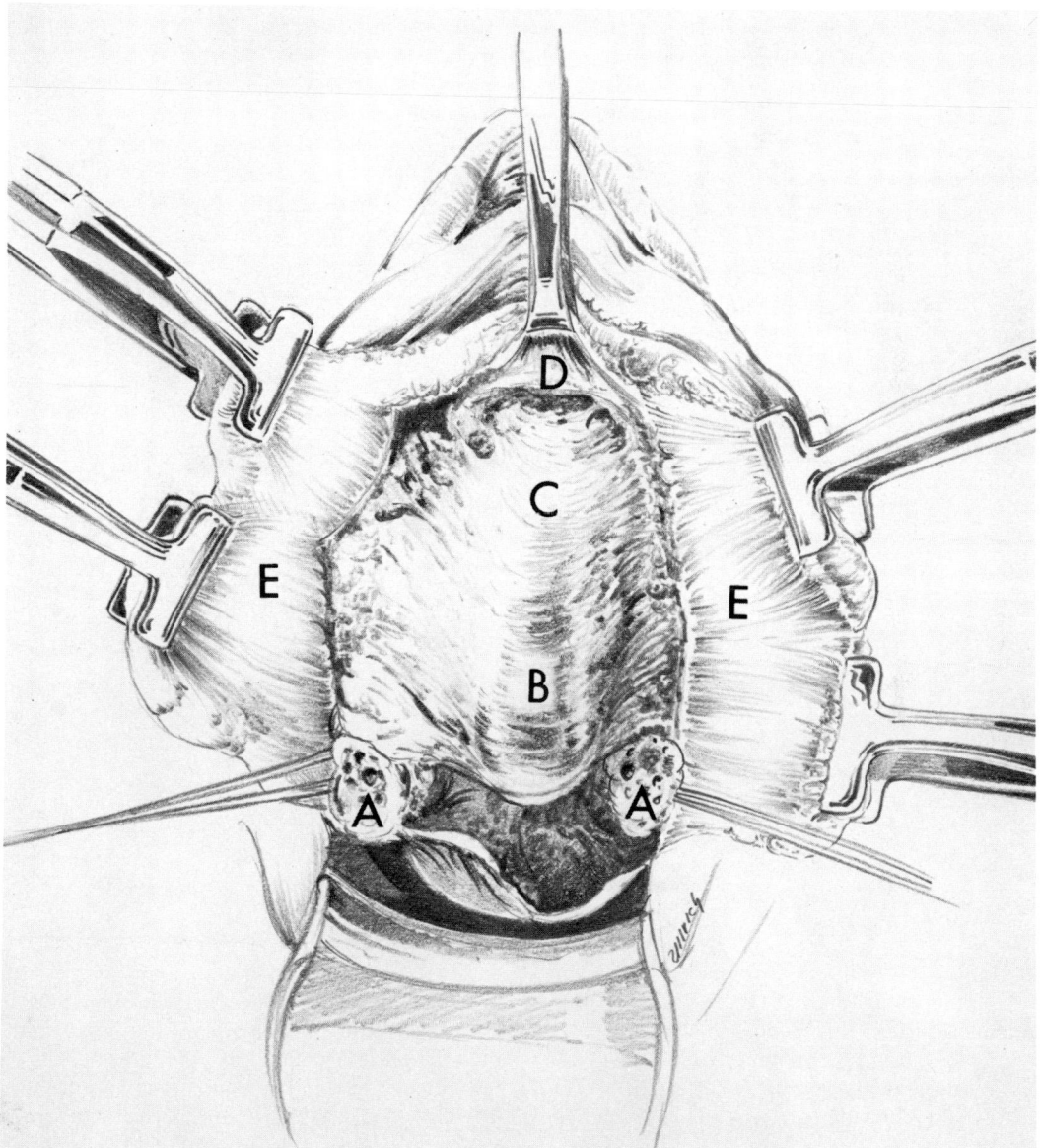

Fig. 2.14. Dissection of cystocele completed; bleeding controlled. The important layer of submucosal tissue (endopelvic fascia) has been reflected medially (E). A, Stumps of uterine ligaments; B, bladder; C, urethrovesical junction; D, proximal urethra.

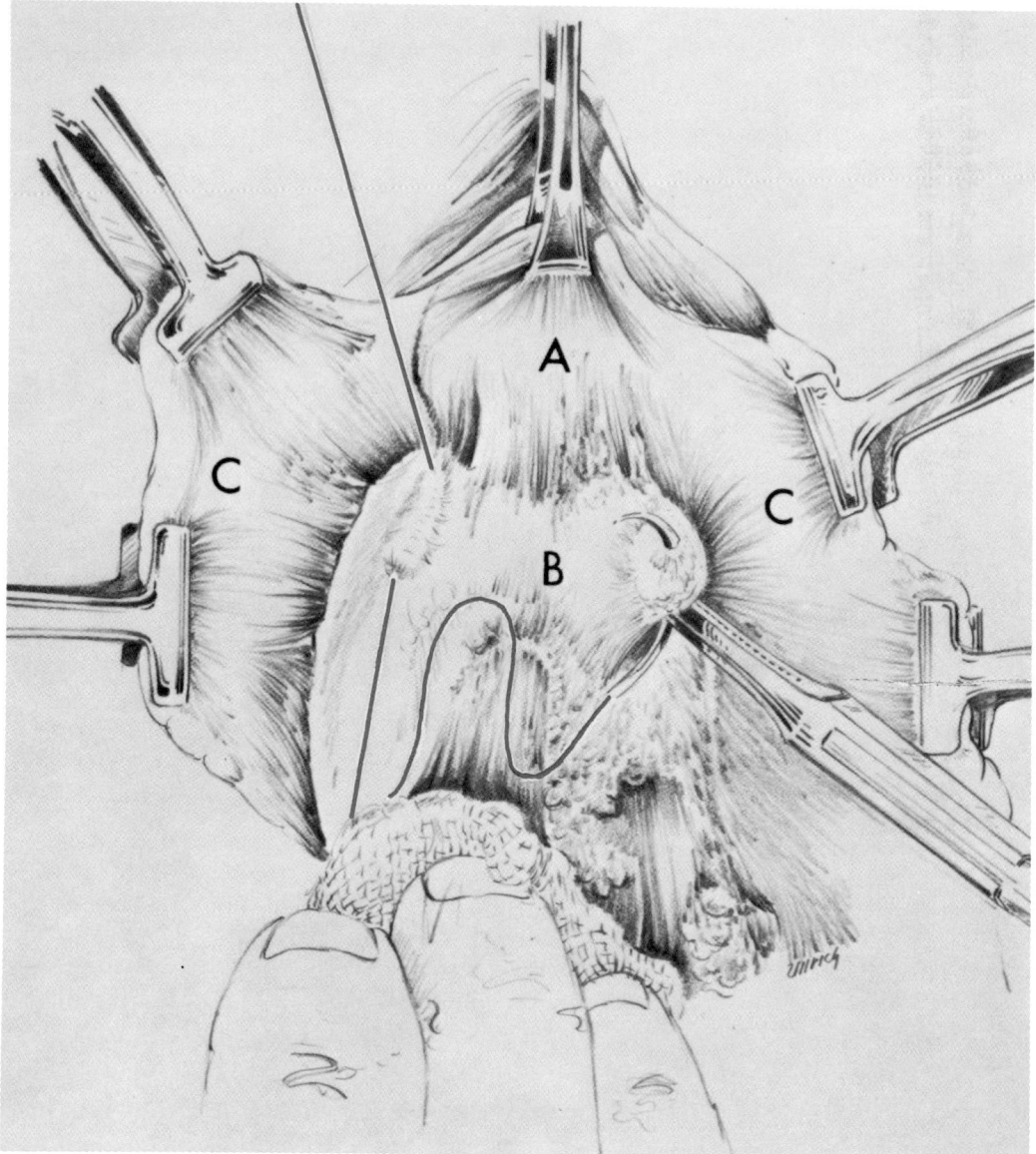

Fig. 2.15. First plicating suture being placed into paraurethral endopelvic fascia at urethrovesical junction. A, Proximal urethra; B, bladder; C, vaginal mucosa.

tightening, two layers of plicating sutures may be used provided that there is not undue tension on the suture line.

At this point, a number of variations in technique lend themselves to different types of problems. When the primary object is the cure of anterior wall relaxation, the stumps of the broad ligaments should be brought forward and fastened beneath the bladder in the midline either at the urethrovesical junction or further toward the apex, depending upon where additional support is needed. This maneuver is especially helpful when the tissues are atrophic or of poor quality. If the ligaments are redundant, they can be overlapped and fastened laterally to the fascia or the periosteum of the descending pubic ramus. Ordinarily, only the ends of the cardinal and uterosacral ligaments are devoted to this, but when all of the structures to be utilized in the repair are thin and attenuated, the upper ends of the broad ligament may be included in a similar manner provided that the ovaries are not brought too close to the vagina. When the pelvic floor is not notably weak, the stumps of the broad ligaments are sutured into the lateral margin of the vaginal cuff without relating them to the undersurface of the bladder. The tube and ovary should be allowed to remain high in the pelvis so that they do not become foci of postoperative inflammation or later cause dyspareunia. In all cases, the space between the uterosacral ligaments and the rectum should be closed to prevent enterocele.

Following the closure and buttressing of the fascia, an estimate is made of the amount of mucous membrane needed to cover the denuded area. This is best accomplished by

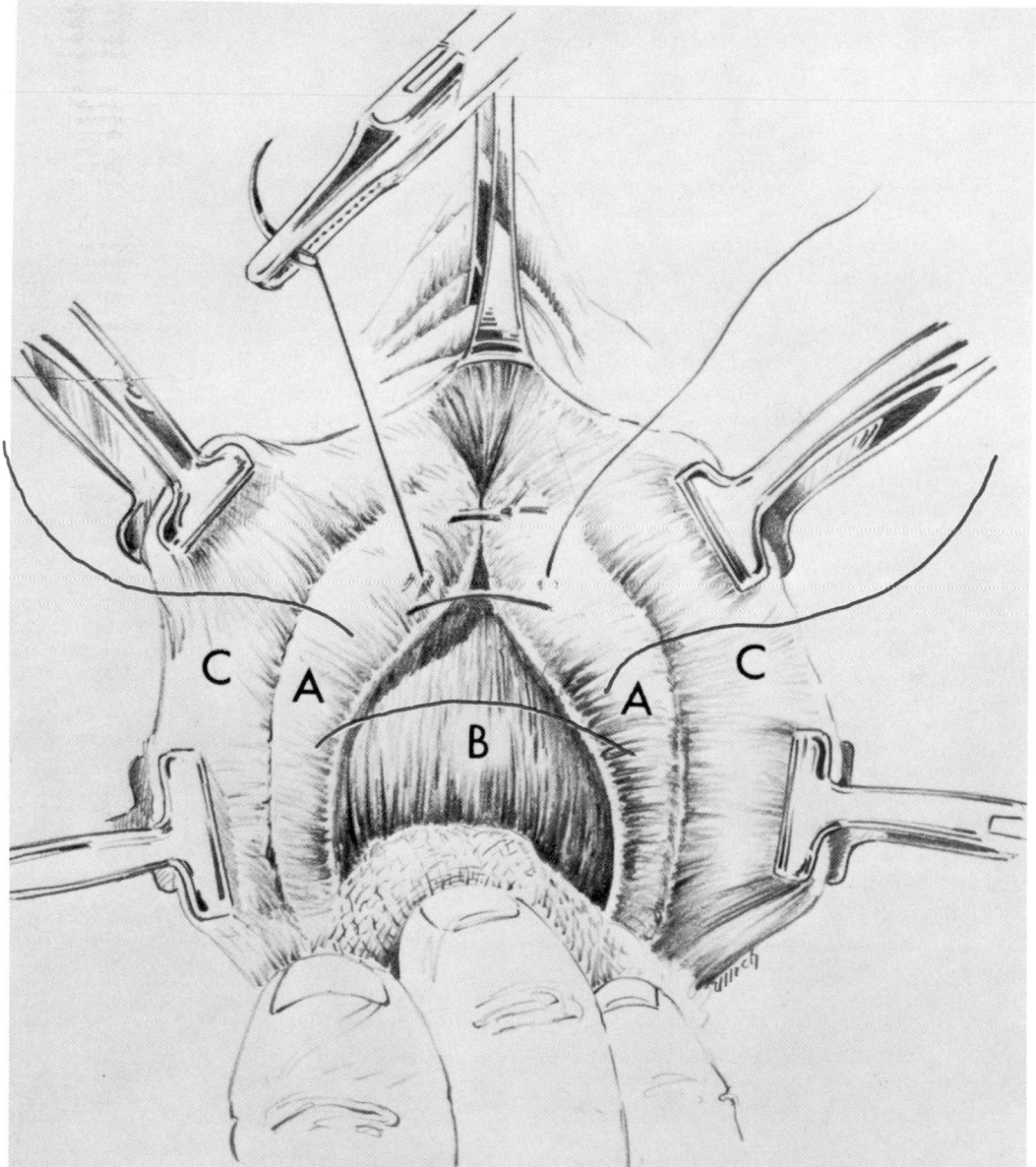

Fig. 2.16. Cystocele repair. Continuing plication of endopelvic fascia (A) from above downward placing each successive bite a little further from the midline. B, Bladder; C, vaginal mucosa.

pushing the vaginal flaps upward into the pelvis until the desired vaginal length is achieved. The area of mucous membrane to be resected in order to insure a snug closure can then be ascertained. A common error is to resect the vaginal flaps until they barely cover the corrected cystocele only to discover that the apex of the vagina is near the introitus at the conclusion of the repair. To facilitate resection, one flap is stretched out and drawn toward the opposite side. The blades of a pair of angled scissors with straight cutting edges are then introduced from below and used to cut upward obliquely toward the top of the original vertical incision (Fig. 2.17). Too little is removed rather than too much, as further trimming can always be done during the subsequent closure. After the mucosa has been trimmed, it is closed in the midline from the urethra downward using fine chromic catgut sutures placed at intervals of 3 to 4 mm. These sutures should always be interrupted because a continuous closure, though faster, will not permit the exudation or removal of blood postoperatively, and one or two sutures cannot be cut without the sacrifice of the entire closure. Inadvertent buttonholes in the flaps are usually of no concern but, if large, should be closed horizontally. At the vaginal apex, the edges of the flaps are pulled laterally, and the upper end is closed horizontally beginning in the fornices and approaching the midline. This avoids the formation of a narrow, pointed upper vagina. The closure then looks like a long inverted T, except that in the midportion of the cross-bar, the mucosa is not closed, leaving an opening about 2 cm in diameter. This opening permits drainage of blood postoperatively and provides manual access if identification of the vaginal apex is necessary during the posterior repair. Drains and wicks are more likely to act as plugs and provide an expressway for the invasion of bacteria if they remain more than 24 hours.

A small gauze pack or sponge may then be placed in the upper vagina loosely and brought out along the line of the closure. This provides pressure for hemostasis and protection from retractors during exposure for the posterior repair. If packs are applied properly, no sutures are needed to fasten the vagina to the underlying fascial repair to obliterate dead space, and the vagina will adhere to the deeper structures in a neat, symmetrical manner without distortion.

Posterior wall repair and perineorrhaphy need not invariably be a part of vaginal hysterectomy and anterior wall repair for prolapse. It should be done strictly on anatomic indications, or if considered essential to buttress the anterior wall repair. In many cases the posterior wall is relatively firm and the perineum high, and the operation may be concluded at the point described. The posterior repair, particularly the perineorrhaphy, is most painful during convalescence, and plication of the pubococcygeal and/or perineal musculature with resulting spasm interferes with the patient's ability voluntarily to lower the bladder neck and prolongs the time before satisfactory voiding. When significant rectocele is present, when the perineum is very low or the introitus is too large, a complete posterior repair is, of course, indicated. The operation is done in much the same manner described for anterior repair, placing Allis clamps on the vagina vertically from apex to perineum about 3 cm apart and using them for upward traction by an assistant while the surgeon maintains countertraction at the level of the introitus. A diamond-shaped section of the vaginal mucous membrane immediately adjacent to the introitus is first removed by sharp dissection. Some of the perineal skin may be included in the diamond to avoid tissue redundancy at the time of closure. The width of the skin and mucosal flap removed determines the height of the perineum and the caliber of the introitus. Prior to this denudation, it is advisable to mark the prospective margins of dissection with two Allis clamps and approximate them in the midline to measure the exact size of the future vaginal opening. Allowance must be made for rigidity due to scar formation and the atrophy of old age. The vagina may be shortened by one-third to one-half without interfering with normal coitus, but a relatively minor degree of narrowing, particularly at the perineal level, may obstruct intromission and cause distressing discomfort, anxiety, and involuntary muscle spasm.

A vertical incision is made in the midline of the posterior vaginal wall from the introitus to the crown of the rectocele by using scissors to separate the mucous membrane from the

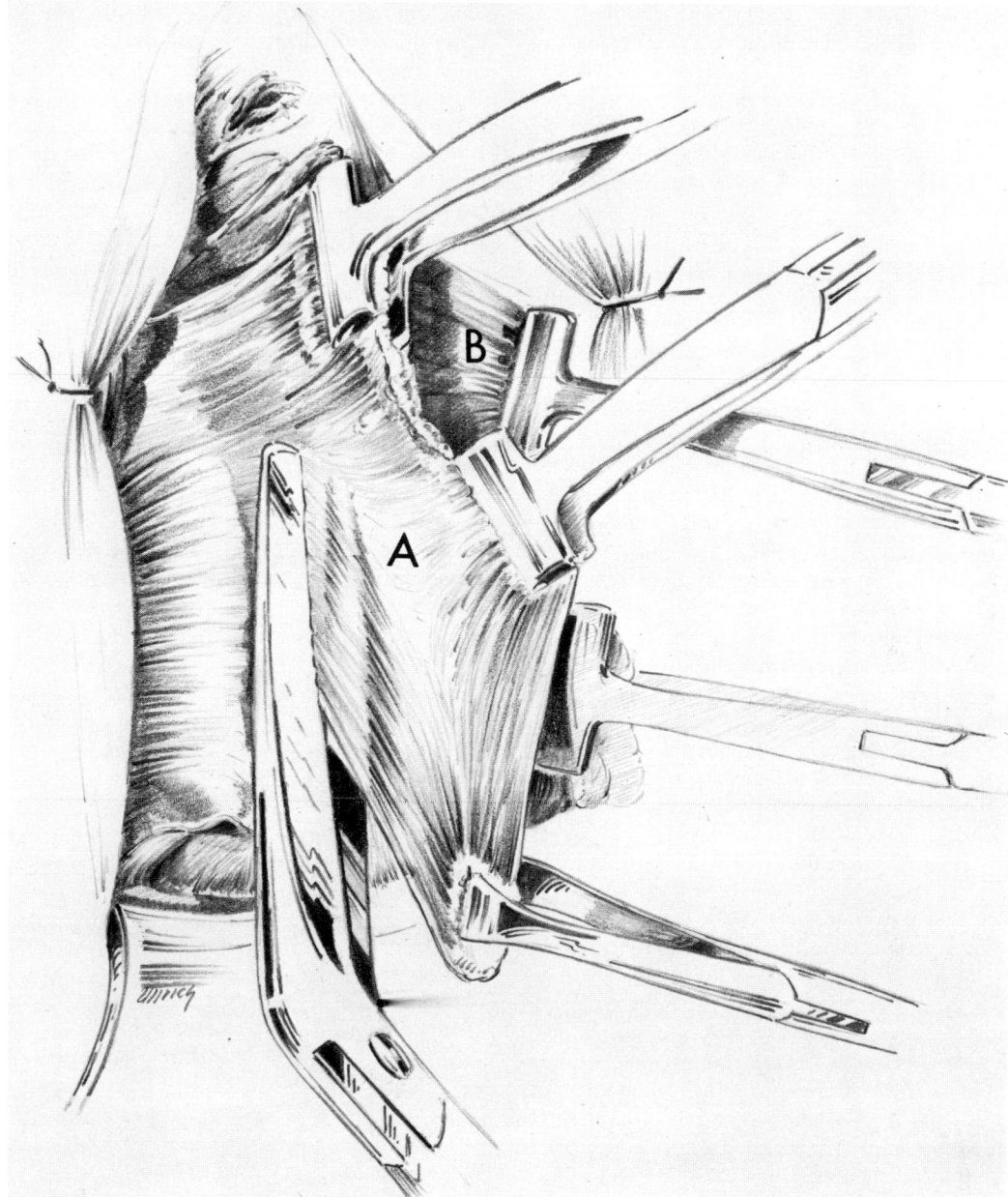

Fig. 2.17. Resection of excess vagina. Edge of flap is drawn toward the opposite side and stretched while oblique cut is made from below upward. Vaginal mucosa–(A) right flap, (B) left flap.

underlying fascia and muscle and cutting it in stages, as in the anterior repair. Extending this incision all the way to the top of the vagina is usually unnecessary for full exposure of recto-cele or enterocele and may cause adherence of the two suture lines after healing. The layer between vagina and rectum is mostly loose areolar tissue, which may be easily separated down to the perineal level, but the dissection must be accomplished by delicate blunt strip-ping under direct vision to avoid injury to the inferior hemorrhoidal veins, which frequently bulge into the operative field. Remaining close to the undersurface of the vagina and well away from the rectum protects these vessels against such a mistake. When the vessels are inadvertently damaged, they must be clamped and ligated immediately. Vascularity must not deter the surgeon from fully exposing the rectocele and the muscles of the levator sling and perineum.

The simplest way to correct the mobilized rectocele is to place a pursestring suture superficially in the rectal muscle around the crown of the hernia, bringing the ends out on either side of the upper end of the vaginal incision or submucosally through the undersurface of the previously plicated uterosacral ligaments. A pursestring at two or three levels is possible in the event the hernia is quite large. This maneuver effectively turns the rectocele in on itself and draws it upward away from the introitus. The soft perirectal tissues are poor stuff with which to attempt an alternative type of repair, and bringing together the pubococcygeus muscles over the rectum constricts the midportion of the vagina and produces an hourglass shape. On the other hand, the frequent failure of surgeons to carry the repair into the upper vagina leads to many persistent and troublesome high rectoceles. At a point about 4 cm within the introitus, however, the fascia overlying the pubococcygeus muscles may be plicated in the midline without forming too high a bridge (Fig. 2.18). When the sutures have been placed, the height of this bridge may be tested by crossing the ends of the sutures and pulling without tying. Sutures which are poorly placed or must be tied under tension are removed. After the rectocele has been turned in and the lower vagina effectively supported by plication of the pubococcygeus muscles, the mucous membrane is closed in the midline with interrupted sutures. Unless the rectocele is very large or the vagina very redundant, it is inadvisable to resect much of it, since this might cause areas of constriction. The vaginal edges may be freshened by snipping away ragged areas as the closure continues, insuring a neat, straight suture line without tissue deficiency. The perineotomy is closed with three or four sutures of heavy catgut taken deep through the perineal muscles, with care that the needle remains superficial to the rectum. These sutures can be placed earlier in the posterior

wall operation, but, if tied too soon, restrict exposure of the upper vagina. Beginning at the junction of the mucosal closure with the skin, a continuous subcuticular suture of fine chromic catgut covers the remaining distance to the bottom of the skin incision and is tied with a small knot or left long without typing in order to reduce postoperative discomfort. As a precaution, a finger is inserted into the rectum to detect the presence of sutures invading the lumen. When present, they may simply be cut transrectally or transvaginally, whichever is easier, and not removed.

Since hemorrhoids, both external and internal, are often associated with rectocele and the necessity to strain in order to defecate, the question of whether to do a concomitant hemorrhoidectomy must be resolved. Extensive resection of hemorrhoids or fissures should be done as a separate procedure in most instances because of the resulting increase in pain and the complication rate. The removal of external skin tabs which annoy the patient or two to three protruding symptomatic hemorrhoids at the time of posterior repair is acceptable practice if the patient wishes it and has given written permission. Both the skin and mucosal components of each hemorrhoid are elevated, clamped radial to the anal margin, and resected, ligating the base with catgut or oversewing the margins of the mucosal incision. After hemorrhoidectomy, the caliber of the anus is measured with a finger and, if not constricted, a small petroleum jelly pack is left in the rectum for 24 hours to provide pressure on the suture line and prevent bleeding.

When vaginal hysterectomy and anterior and posterior repair have been completed, another careful inspection for bleeding should be made. The end of a pointed hemostat is inserted between the sutures in the vagina in several places, and pressure in placed against the vaginal walls to force out retained clots and note any fresh bleeding. Uncontrolled arterial bleeding is more readily recognized, since it usually exudes persistently from the flaps or through the vaginal apex. When the bleeding remains excessive for several minutes after pressure has been applied, the repair should be partially, or completely, taken down immediately, and the bleeding points sought and ligated. To rely on packing to control heavy bleeding which continues after the operation is

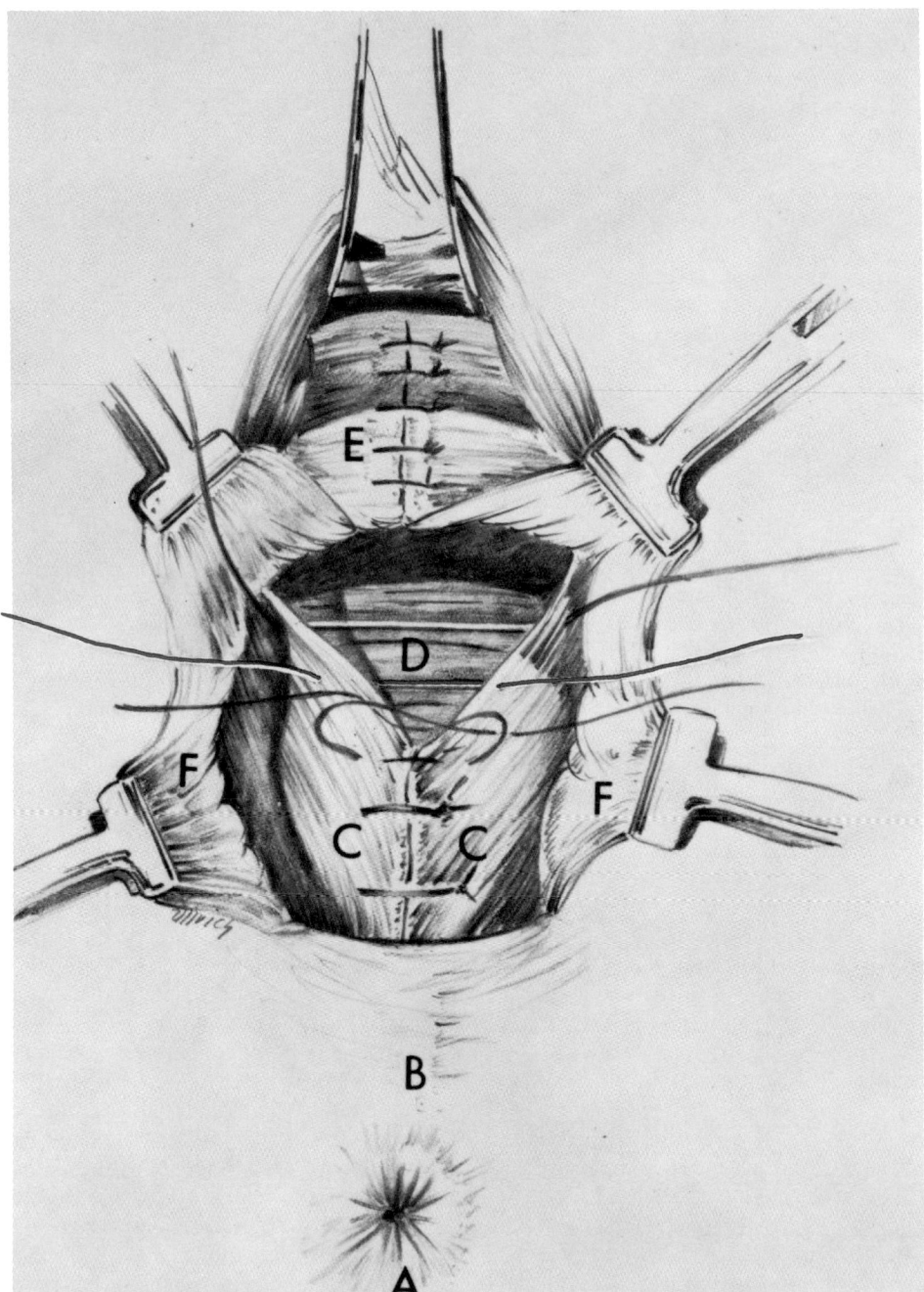

Fig. 2.18. Suturing levator muscles (C) together over rectum (D) near introitus. A, Anus; B, perineum; E, anterior closure; F, vaginal closure.

finished is one of the most frequent and gravest errors made in this procedure. It is safer to take the additional time necessary to control the bleeding while the patient remains under her first anesthesia.

If bleeding is absent or minimal, a gauze roll impregnated with Iodoform or Furacin is loosely packed into the vagina. Tight packing is undesirable, since it causes marked discomfort and may cause necrosis of the vaginal flaps. The purpose of the packing is to exert mild pressure against the suture line and permit good conformation of the vaginal flaps to the underlying tissues. Medicated packs have no advantage over nonmedicated in the prevention of infection but, to a certain extent, reduce unpleasant odors which can be objectionable both to patient and staff. Under no circumstances should these packs be left in longer than 24 hours, since they will lead to increasing discomfort and postoperative infection.

After the sponge count has been checked by the operating room nurse and the catheter has been connected to straight drainage, the end of the table is brought up and the patient's legs gently lowered, preferably by having one attendant on each side bring the legs down simultaneously to the supine position. Low backache is one of the most common nagging disabilities from which a postoperative patient suffers, and this can be due to improper positioning on the operating table or rough handling in moving the patient about. Particular care must be exercised for those who are known to have orthopedic disabilities. In the absence of an experienced assistant, the surgeon should attend to this personally. Constant suction by vacuum tube in the submucosal dead space has been used to prevent accumulation of blood and serum and thus reduce the incidence of postoperative infection. If bleeding has been adequately controlled and the apical cuff left open for the exudation of these accumulations postoperatively, special drainage should not be necessary, and ascending infection along the tubes can be avoided.

Complications

As in the case of any surgical procedure, large or small, the ultimate complication of vaginal hysterectomy is death. The exact mortality figures across the United States are impossible to ascertain, since late casualties may escape the notice of the surgeon and reported figures are usually derived from large services where the quality of care is excellent. On a first-class service an estimate of 0.1 per cent would probably not be far off the mark (10). Death may occur on the operating table as a result of factors beyond the control of the surgeon, but every surgeon must be prepared to play his role in the prompt resuscitation of

patients suffering from cardiac arrest, coronary occlusion, respiratory paralysis, etc. Postgraduate education in all hospitals must include the regular and constant repetition of the measures necessary to save the patient in an emergency and the individual responsibilities of the surgeon and the other members of the operating team. The availability of consultants affords no excuse for ignorance in this area. Deaths in the hospital during the postoperative course are usually the result of hemorrhage, infection, embolism, or intercurrent disease; later deaths can sometimes be correlated with urinary tract damage and/or pyelonephritis which had its inception at the time of surgery.

Vaginal hysterectomy is notoriously more likely to give rise to postoperative infection than abdominal hysterectomy (11), and the risk of postoperative hemorrhage at an early stage is also more common. For this reason, much attention has been devoted to means for preventing these problems or at least reducing them to an absolute minimum.

Every surgeon knows that different patients bleed in variable amounts regardless of the refinements of technique which he employs. Routine hematologic investigation beforehand cannot completely evaluate any individual patient's bleeding tendency; but a few simple questions concerning family history, bruising, reactions to previous operations such as dental extractions, and the use of a few additional laboratory tests such as Lee-White coagulation time, prothrombin time, and platelet count, will prevent subjection of individuals especially liable to heavy bleeding to elective surgery. During surgery, sponges should be weighed and blood loss estimated. The nurse or anesthesiologist is undoubtedly a better judge of this than the surgeon or his assistants. If a surgeon repeatedly incurs a blood loss of greater than 300 to 400 cc, he should ascribe it to faulty technique or poor selection of cases and take the steps necessary to re-educate himself. Blood loss greater than 500 cc should be replaced even if the patient starts with a high hematocrit, or the bleeding tendency may increase. An attitude of allowing continuous oozing of blood from denuded surfaces on the basis that it is uncontrollable is to be condemned. Heavy packing at the conclusion of the operation is no substitute for good technique and may dam blood back into the retroperitoneal space or the peritoneal cavity instead of allowing it to emerge from the vagina where it can be seen and treated. At least two postoperative evaluations of the hematocrit, one within 24 hours postoperatively and the other 2 days later, give the best assessment of blood loss and should be routine. Variations of 5 per cent or less may represent hydration factors but signal the need for further determinations.

Although secondary hemorrhage can be minimized, it cannot be entirely prevented. It is more likely when hemostatic solutions such as adrenalin have been injected into the retrovaginal space at the beginning of the operation. When it does occur, the amount and rapidity of blood loss must be critically evaluated without delay. If blood seems to be coming from the cut edges of the vagina or to be accumulating beneath the vaginal flaps, a slightly firmer packing may be instituted with the patient awake and remaining in her own bed. If the blood loss is brisk, the hematocrit is progressively falling, or clots are accumulating in the vagina, the patient should be immediately removed to the operating room and examined under anesthesia. When the bleeding seems to be chiefly local and not too rapid, some portion of the repair may be taken down, and an attempt made to find the bleeding point. This is usually extremely difficult, since the uterine ligaments have been fixed and are now obscured by blood, inflammatory reaction in the tissues, and their distorted positions. Bleeding from the edge of the vagina or the surfaces of bladder or rectum can be managed by oversewing the area with mattress sutures. When the hematocrit is falling, the patient shows signs of incipient shock, and vaginal bleeding is of relatively small amount, laparotomy is indicated. The bleeding most often comes from the infundibulopelvic or uterine vessels, but these may be difficult to expose without damaging the repair. Isolation of the bleeding point by painstaking dissection is essential to avoid injury to the ureters. The use of local agents such as oxycel- or thrombin-soaked gauze to promote clotting is of little advantage.

The most feared complication of vaginal hysterectomy is sepsis, and this occurs most commonly when blood loss has been heavy during the operation or when blood has accumulated behind the closure. The age and condition of the patient, the duration of the procedure, and the quality of the technique in avoiding massive necrosis of tissue are all of the utmost importance as predisposing factors. Since the operation is performed through a heavily contaminated area, a certain proportion of so-called cuff abscesses are unavoidable. Pre-existing inflammation in the Fallopian tubes may lead to acute salpingitis when the tubes are severed from the uterus and left *in situ.* Much controversy has arisen in recent years as to the value of prophylactic antibiotics in reducing the incidence of pelvic abscess and salpingitis postoperatively (12, 13). Unfortunately, the available studies have defects in experimental design or the patients have been inadequately followed. Good criteria as to what constitutes a diagnosis of infection have not been agreed upon. As a result, they do not provide definitive answers as to the desirability of using antibacterial medication on a routine basis beginning just prior to or during surgery, nor have they established rational guidelines as to the necessary dosage and duration of administration of the drugs to be used. In addition, the advantages claimed for prophylaxis must be weighed against drug reactions, the danger of superinfection by secondary invaders, and the development of resistant strains among the hospital and community populations. From a practical viewpoint, it seems logical to begin treatment, using therapeutic dosage levels at the time of surgery, and to continue it for not more than 72 hours. This will provide effective suppression of the organisms which enter at the time of surgery and will not last long enough to foster resistance or obscure the diagnosis of smouldering occult infections. In most cases, when the risk of infection is not great, patients should be individualized and infections treated therapeutically after documentation by culture and physical examination.

When pelvic abscess occurs, it should be promptly opened and drained transvaginally. This can usually best be done either by poking a long Kelly clamp through the central opening in the vaginal cuff or by cutting one or two lateral sutures with a long pair of scissors which are then passed further upward in the direction of the abscess and spread. When the mass is palpable per rectum, a finger in the rectum is helpful to guide the blind insertion of the instrument per vaginam. Even if pus is not encountered immediately, the opening usually insures eventual drainage. Acute salpingitis with associated pyosalpinx must be managed by transperitoneal resection of both tubes and ovaries, if the process does not respond to medical treatment. Very large abscesses may require trans- or retroperitoneal drainage.

Collections usually are not clinically apparent before the fourth or fifth postoperative day, and earlier signs of infection should be ascribed to pulmonary, vascular, or other causes. To keep pelvic sepsis localized, the liberal use of antibacterial medication appropriate to the organism is indicated and should be continued for a minimum of 10 days to 2 weeks regardless of the clinical improvement in the condition. If the patient is otherwise well enough to leave the hospital, she can continue her medication at home either orally or under the supervision of a visiting nurse.

Transient bacteriuria is the rule in individuals who have undergone any type of instrumentation or manipulation involving the urinary bladder, and occurs in at least 80 per cent of the cases (14). In the majority, the bacteria are eliminated by the patient's immunologic mechanisms, one of which is the regular rinsing of the bladder by the flow of urine. The use of an indwelling catheter, whether suprapubic or transurethral, is routine following vaginal hysterectomy and repair and, if retained longer than 72 hours, causes bacteriuria in nearly 100 per cent of the cases. For this reason, although the long term risk is small, when vaginal hysterectomy is done for uterine pathology and not in association with repair, the indwelling catheter is undesirable unless the patient cannot void during the first 24 hours. Attempts to keep the urine sterile by using antibiotics while the catheter remains *in situ* are often unsuccessful, and treatment should be reserved for those who have a positive urine culture with specific pathogens following removal of the catheter. During the period of catheterization, the catheter should be irrigated at least twice daily to prevent occlusion by clots and other debris and consequent retrograde flow and possible extension of infection into the upper urinary tracts. The irrigation can be best accomplished by a closed system technique employing an overhead drainage bottle connected to a three-lumen catheter which permits 30 cc of fluid to be run in and out of the bladder without contamination or interference with drainage of urine. The constant infusion of antibacterial drugs into the bladder through the indwelling catheter (15) has received a prolonged trial but has not been shown to have significantly reduced the incidence of late infection. Emphasis should be placed on postcatheter follow-up and treatment.

Lower urinary tract infections are asymptomatic in most patients on constant bladder drainage and do not cause significant elevation of temperature. There is a tendency to ascribe a fever of 100°F or more occurring in the first 2 or 3 days postoperatively to urinary tract infection, especially when a positive urine culture has been obtained. This is seldom the case, and the cause for the elevation should be sought elsewhere. When the urine culture is positive, with a significant colony count for a known pathogen following removal of the catheter, treatment for 10 days to 2 weeks is advisable, regardless of the absence of symptoms. An appropriate broad spectrum drug which has a high concentration in the urine is prescribed but can be changed, if necessary, according to sensitivity studies. An oral form of the drug should be continued after her discharge from the hospital. When the patient returns for her check-up in 2 to 4 weeks, the urine culture should be repeated. With or without treatment, most patients will be well at that time, and the urine will be sterile. Treatment, therefore, has been directed at the relative few who cannot accomplish their own recovery. Only a small fraction continue to have positive urine cultures at the 6-month check-up, but the test should be performed by the clean-catch technique to guard against the development of late pyelonephritis. When there is symptomatic or objective evidence of direct damage to either ureters or bladder as a possible consequence of surgery, cystoscopy and intravenous urography should not be delayed, since prompt relief from obstruction is vital in preventing long term damage.

Other types of infection complicating vaginal hysterectomy run the usual gamut following major surgery. A rough rule of thumb is to think of the chest the first 3 days, the wound the next 3 days, the belly the next, then the veins, and the urinary tract throughout.

Perhaps the most annoying postoperative symptom to patient and surgeon is inability to void, or incomplete voiding with retention of large amounts of residual urine. This can occasionally be related to the difficulty of the operation and the amount of trauma inflicted, at other times to the firmness of the posterior repair causing pain and inability to relax the levator muscles, and, not infrequently, to simple anxiety or neurosis. The opinion that satisfactory postoperative voiding is not possible because of partial occlusion of the bladder neck or urethra by edema is not valid, since calibration invariably shows that the lumen is adequate, and dilatation helps only indirectly. It is necessary to be certain that no surgical mistake is responsible for the inability to void; thereafter, time may safely be relied upon to encourage healing of the local condition or of the psyche, and the patient should be frequently reassured that function always returns. If a neurogenic bladder was not ruled out prior to surgery and is now suspected, cystometry must be performed. Repeated instrumentation or the passage of irritating solutions into the bladder have no place in the treatment of urinary retention. When it is necessary to reinsert an indwelling catheter because post-voiding residuals remain above 100 cc, it is advisable to leave the catheter for at least 48 hours prior to another attempt at voiding. One of the advantages of suprapubic catheterization is that it obviates the necessity of repeated catheterizations and enables the patient to void and test the residual urine without additional instrumentation. Occasionally, the patient will do better when removed from the hospital setting and sent home with a catheter attached to a leg reservoir for a week or more.

Very rarely, a needle is broken during surgery, and a part of it cannot be recovered among the paraphernalia of the operating room. This accident should not happen if heavy Mayo needles are used to transfix the tougher structures. X-ray localization usually discloses whether the needle is in the patient but by no means assures finding it. If the needle cannot be removed at the time, the patient must be informed of the fact before she leaves the hospital.

When the patient leaves the hospital, she should be supplied with a typed list of do's and don'ts and a description of the symptoms she is likely to experience, such as transient discharge, fatigue, and occasional lower abdominal pains. This saves many unnecessary telephone calls and is infinitely superior to the unremembered words spoken at the bedside prior to departure. Emphasis is given to the need for consultation if persistent pain, bleeding, or voiding disability occurs. Efficient bed utilization and economic factors have combined to reduce the length of hospitalization, but if the patient's safety remains the primary consideration, the stay should be for not less than 1 week. Rest and the avoidance of activities which increase intra-abdominal pressure until the first check-up allow healing of the hernia repair. Coitus is deferred until after the examination.

When the patient returns for her first postoperative check-up, there may be small pseudopolyps of granulation tissue in any of the vaginal suture lines. This exaggeration of the healing process is unavoidable in some cases, nor does it have any serious implications except for the anxiety associated with minor vaginal staining. The polyps should be removed by avulsion, and the bases cauterized with silver nitrate to stop bleeding. Complete separation of the vaginal flaps is most unusual, but when it does occur, can be remedied by light packing rather than resuturing. The flaps are actually pedicle grafts and adhere to the undersurface of the repair within 24 hours unless they become gangrenous. In the very unusual event that this complication occurs, the necrotic tissue is debrided, and time allowed for complete healing before making final assessment of the result and the necessary further steps. Occasionally, the fimbriated end of the Fallopian tube prolapses into the vagina (16) through a defect in the peritoneum and can be mistaken for granulation tissue. The diagnosis can be made if the red polypoid tissue persists in spite of excision and cauterization and if there is a constant discharge of serous fluid into an otherwise healthy vagina. The end of the tube may close spontaneously and eliminate the problem but it may be necessary to excise the distal end by opening the vaginal cuff under general anesthesia, mobilizing an inch or so of the tube, ligating it, and closing the incision beneath it.

Although proper precautions should greatly reduce the incidence of late complications of vaginal hysterectomy and repair, some will continue to occur, even in the best hands. The persistence of infections in the urinary tract has been mentioned, but emphasis should again be given to the need for repeating the urine culture at every routine check-up because of the occult nature of the process until the late stages. A significant incidence of prolapse of the vaginal vault follows operations for relaxation of the pelvic floor. This is usually due to uncorrected enterocele or failure to occlude completely the triangle formed by the uterosacral ligaments and the anterior wall of the rectum. Varying degrees of recurrent cystocele are quite common, often without functional impairment. The patient may notice a slight protrusion, but unless this is a source of major annoyance, no further surgery need be done. Urinary incontinence may occur following repair when it was not present before and is related to potentiating detrusor action by relocating the bladder within the pelvis while failing to tighten the urethrovesical junction relatively more than the rest of the repair. Since this symptom may be transient and is difficult to distinguish from the urgency of inflammation, a long period of observation is indicated, with the use of perineal exercises to strengthen the voluntary muscles of micturition. Adhesions occurring in the vagina a month or more postoperatively may obliterate one or both fornices or cause a midline septum by joining anterior and posterior suture lines. They should be lysed, and the patient seen at more frequent intervals to repeat the process. Early coitus, local lubricants, and, in the postmenopausal patient, estrogen either by mouth or locally are helpful both in preventing and treating this complication.

If the perineum has been raised too high or the caliber of the vagina much reduced by too generous a resection of the mucous membrane, apareunia or dyspareunia may develop. The use of estrogen and local dilatation combined with counseling of both patient and partner are the first recourse in this dilemma. If the problem persists and is primarily on a mechanical rather than a psychologic basis, an attempt at surgical correction may be necessary.

Prolapse

Vaginal hysterectomy, combined with repair of the pelvic floor, is the operation of choice for uterine prolapse, enterocele, and cystocele. Attempts to achieve the desired result by abdominal hysterectomy or suspension of the uterus without repair from below are contrain-

dicated, since they fail to correct the basic defects. When the uterus is much enlarged or there is associated adnexal disase which must be dealt with transabdominally, a combined vaginal and peritoneal approach may be necessary. This is preferable to an attempt to wrestle a large adherent tumor from below. Transabdominal cystocele repair by excising a wedge of the anterior vagina at the time the cervix is removed has been described. This places the operator at a disadvantage from the point of view of gaining adequate exposure during the separation of the bladder from the vagina and does not permit plication of the endopelvic fascia beneath the vaginal mucous membrane. When prolapse of the vaginal vault recurs two or more times following primary surgery, the vagina may be too narrow, and the supports too much obliterated for another attempt from below. A multitude of different types of transperitoneal suspension of the prolapsed vaginal vault have been devised, and one of these must be employed under such circumstances. The best method is to form a retroperitoneal sling, which descends from the fascia of the anterior abdominal wall through the internal inguinal rings to be attached to the vaginal cuff on both sides (17). When the patient's own fascia is in good condition, this is the preferable material for the sling. Under other circumstances, a variety of synthetic materials have been proposed, all of which have the disadvantage that they may act as a foreign body in the tissues. As an adjunct to this operation, it is often necessary to obliterate the posterior cul-de-sac completely by suturing the anterior wall of the rectum to the posterior wall of the vagina and, if possible, incorporating some of the lateral pelvic wall peritoneum. Great care must be taken not to injure the ureters in so doing, and they must be directly identified as each suture is placed. Rectal prolapse may be a corollary problem, and resection and/or suspension of the redundant rectum may have to be done at the same time.

Other types of vaginal operations which have been applied to the treatment of prolapse include chiefly the Watkins interposition, the Manchester-Fothergill plication of the cardinal ligaments, the Richardson composite interposition of the cervical stump, and colpocleisis, usually by the LeFort technique. All of these operations have the disadvantage that all, or a portion, of the uterus is left behind as a site for the future development of pathology and have, therefore, a very limited application. The Watkins operation, which requires transposition of the uterine fundus beneath the bladder, has, for all practical purposes, passed from the repertoire and has, as its only claim for recognition, that it works.

The Manchester-Fothergill repair, which is usually combined with amputation of the cervix and plication of the uterosacral and cardinal ligaments anterior to the cervical stump, may be used when the problem is predominantly one of cystocele repair and when the patient's general condition makes an intraperitoneal operation undesirable. This operation is absolutely contraindicated in the age group when pregnancy might occur subsequently.

The Richardson composite operation (18), which requires amputation of the cervix and fundus and the preservation of the cervical isthmus to be interposed beneath the bladder, produces results similar to those of vaginal hysterectomy but has the disadvantage that it is a more difficult procedure and likely to be attended by greater blood loss.

Most types of colpocleisis preclude the possibility of future coitus. For this reason, they should be reserved for the elderly and debilitated patient and performed only after the question of future sexual function has been thoroughly discussed with the patient and her husband. Because it is technically simple, does not require penetration of the peritoneum, and can be performed quickly with minimal blood loss, this operation is applicable to women in the seventh, eighth, and ninth decades. Some have advocated the use of local anesthesia, but light general anesthesia is preferable to allay anxiety and allow for proper positioning on the operating table without orthopedic disability. The operation is much more easily performed when complete, or nearly complete, prolapse has occurred. The tissues should be properly prepared beforehand by adequate cleansing, by treatment of local infection, and by temporary reduction of the prolapse through means of a pessary or binder to allow edema to subside. If trophic cervical ulceration is present, it may be best to amputate the cervix as a preliminary step. Presumably, cervical smears and/or biopsy have been done and found negative, but

curettage is essential to rule out endometrial malignancy. Very thin rectangles of vaginal mucous membrane measuring approximately 2 inches in width by 3 to 4 inches in length depending upon the size of the vagina are marked out with the point of a scalpel on the anterior and posterior walls of the vagina at a point beginning about 1 inch proximal to the cervix or cervical stump and are then resected. These flaps should be as thin as possible, leaving a maximal amount of the underlying fascial structures on the bladder and rectum.

On the anterior wall, a small vertical incision is continued upward from the midportion of the resection almost to the urethral meatus, and the urethra and vesical neck are separated from the undersurface of the vagina. This is a most important step, since it allows plication of the urethrovesical junction and reduces the likelihood that the patient will develop urinary incontinence when the prolapsed bladder is repositioned and its expulsive power increased (19).

Posteriorly, the pouch of cul-de-sac peritoneum is usually seen as the mucosa is resected downward toward the perineum, but this should not be entered if avoidable. About 1 inch of intact vagina is left proximal to the perineal skin. After bleeding is controlled and the vesical neck plicated, the two denuded areas are approximated by suturing together the cut vaginal edges and gradually pushing the uterus inward. It is not necessary to join the bladder and rectal musculature with sutures.

When the entire vagina has been inverted, two troughs of vaginal mucosa will remain on either side to allow for uterine drainage, and the repair will have progressed to the point where the superior and inferior margins of the denudation can be sutured horizontally. A routine perineorrhaphy is then done to increase posterior support and narrow the introitus. Some type of urinary drainage is usually necessary for a short time after this operation but should be discontinued at the earliest possible moment. A lateral view of the repair when completed is seen in Figure 2.19. Complications from this operation should be few, and prognosis excellent.

Summary

Every surgeon has his favorite operation, technique, maxims, and superstitions, and it is

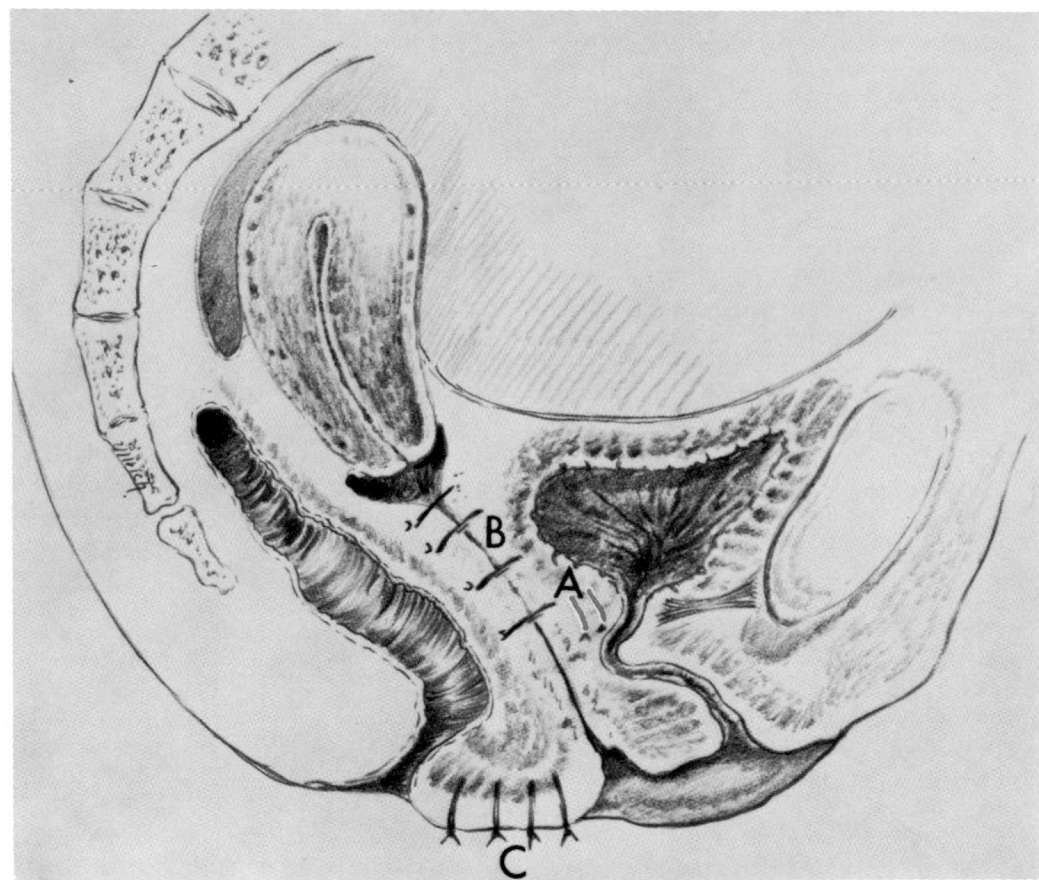

Fig. 2.19. Lateral view of completed colpocleisis (LeFort closure). Anterior and posterior vaginal walls sutured together closing midportion of vagina. Urethrovesical junction plicated. Perineum elevated. A, Suburethral "Kelly" plication; B, vaginal closure; C, perineorrhaphy.

best for his patients that this is so, since he continues to do what he does well. The risk is that he may lose flexibility, assume a posture of omnipotence, and become careless about the application of his expertise. Vaginal hysterectomy is not a big, nor ordinarily a dangerous operation, as long as it is employed according to well defined indications and not as a circus stunt to demonstrate technical virtuosity. Records of accidents, complications, and late results must be regularly reviewed by the surgeon and his peers to determine whether recognized standards of competence are being maintained. It is crucial never to lose sight of the fact that it is nearly always an elective operation.

References

1. Pratt, J. H., and Gunnlaugsson, G. H.: (title) Vaginal hysterectomy by morcellation. Mayo Clin. Proc. 45: 374, 1970.

2. Crisp, W. E.: The Schauta operation. Obstet. Gynecol. 33: 453, 1969.
3. Van Nagell, J. R., Jr., and Roddick, J. W., Jr.: Vaginal hysterectomy as a sterilization procedure. Am. J. Obstet. Gynecol. 111: 703, 1971.
4. Atkinson, S. M., Jr., and Chappell, S. M.: Vaginal hysterectomy for sterilization. Obstet. Gynecol. 39: 759, 1972.
5. Haynes, D. M., and Wolfe, W. M.: Tubal sterilization in an indigent population. Report of fourteen years' experience. Am. J. Obstet. Gynecol. 106: 1044, 1970.
6. Conlam, C. B., and Pratt, J. H.: Vaginal hysterectomy: Is previous pelvic operation a contraindication? Am. J. Obstet. Gynecol. 116: 252, 1973.
7. Mitchell, G. W., Jr.: Cystometry in the evaluation of urinary incontinence. Clin. Obstet. Gynecol. 1: 678, 1958.
8. Laufe, L. E., and Kreutner, A. K.: Vaginal hysterectomy: A modality for therapeutic abortion and sterilization. Am. J. Obstet. Gynecol. 110: 1096, 1971.
9. Ingram, J. M.: Suprapubic cystotomy by trocar catheter: a preliminary report. Am. J. Obstet. Gynecol. 113: 1108, 1972.

10. Gray, L. A.: Indications, technics and complications in vaginal hysterectomy. Obstet. Gynecol. 28: 718, 1966.

11. Ledger, W. J.: Postoperative pelvic infections. Clin. Obstet. Gynecol. 12: 265, 1969.

12. Allen, J. L., Rampone, J. F., and Wheeless, C. R.: Use of prophylactic antibiotic in elective major gynecologic operations. Obstet. Gynecol. 39: 218, 1972.

13. Ledger, W. J., Sweet, R. L., and Headington, J. T.: Prophylactic cephaloridine in the prevention of postoperative pelvic infections in premenopausal women undergoing vaginal hysterectomy. Am. J. Obstet. Gynecol. 115: 766, 1973.

14. Marchant, D. J., and Mitchell, G. W., Jr.: Urinary-tract infections in gynecologic disease. Obstet. Gynecol. 26: 752, 1965.

15. Thornton, G. F., Lytton, B., and Andriole, V. T.: Bacteriuria during indwelling catheter drainage. Effect of constant bladder rinse. JAMA 195: 117, 1966.

16. Ellsworth, H. S., Harris, J. W., McQuarrie, H. G., Stone, R. A., and Anderson, A. E.: Prolapse of the fallopian tube following vaginal hysterectomy. JAMA 224: 891, 1973.

17. Te Linde, R. W., and Mattingly, R. F.: Operative Gynecology, p. 524. J. B. Lippincott, Philadelphia, 1970.

18. Richardson, E. H.: An efficient composite operation for uterine prolapse and associated pathology. Am. J. Obstet. Gynecol. 34: 814, 1937.

19. Ridley, J. H.: Evaluation of the colpocleisis operation: a report of fifty-eight cases. Am. J. Obstet. Gynecol. 113: 1114, 1972.

CHAPTER THREE

LAWRENCE R. WHARTON, JR., M.D.

SURGERY OF BENIGN ADNEXAL DISEASE: ENDOMETRIOSIS, RESIDUALS OF INFLAMMATORY AND GRANULOMATOUS DISEASES, AND URETERAL INJURY

Although it is often thought that a considerable portion of gynecologic surgery deals with the uterus, the proper treatment of adnexal pathology frequently may be the most important aspect of a particular problem. The diagnosis and treatment of diseases affecting the Fallopian tubes, ovaries, their respective ligaments and blood supply, as well as adjacent organs and structures can lead even the most wary and careful pelvic surgeon into difficult predicaments from which he must extricate not only himself but especially his patient.

It obviously follows that utmost care must be exercised in establishing as accurately as possible the correct diagnosis prior to treatment. In addition the extent of the pathologic process—that is, what organs or structures are certainly affected and what others are likely to be involved, to what degree, and what are the implications of this—should be considered before treatment, surgical or nonsurgical, is undertaken.

In general, adnexal surgery is undertaken because of one or more of the following reasons: inability to exclude malignancy; symptoms which are best handled surgically such as pain, infertility, fever, *etc.*; the desire to operate to preserve rather than extirpate organs; and the interference by the disease process of the function of other organs, particularly the uterus, urinary tract, and gastrointestinal tract. In some situations the need for operative intervention is obvious; in others, the surgeon's knife should be stayed. On many occasions, however, operative or nonoperative treatment can be employed; it is here in particular where the gynecologist must exercise all his judgment and skill to obtain the optimal and desired result, with the ultimate goal being, "What is best for this particular patient?"

In approaching the problem of a patient who is found on examination to have a mass or masses in the region of the uterine adnexa, questions which first arise are, "What is the origin of this mass? Does it arise from the tubes, ovaries, the uterus, or even the intestinal or urinary tract? Could it originate from the retroperitoneal space or even the space of Retzius or abdominal wall?"

Obviously a careful history is most important in clarifying the problem. Often after an examination when the exact diagnosis is not certain, it is helpful to ask the patient further questions as to symptoms, their duration and severity in view of the findings or physical examination. Requestioning may shed more light on the problem and help the gynecologist decide on the proper course to follow.

In regard to the examination itself, it is of prime importance that the patient's bladder be emptied immediately before the examination. She should be instructed to void at that time even though she may insist that her bladder is empty. A distended or even partially distended bladder not only interferes with an accurate examination, but also increases the patient's discomfort during the examination making the examination more difficult. Finally, a full bladder many times has been mistaken for a pelvic tumor. This tumor is best treated with a catheter, and if there is any doubt that the bladder is empty, the patient should be catheterized and the bladder emptied completely.

It is also desirable to have the colon and rectum empty during a pelvic examination. This is not often achieved during a routine gynecologic examination. If one is not certain of the pelvic findings and the bowel is filled with feces, the patient should be given an enema and re-examined or advised to return at another time when there has been a thorough evacuation. The pelvic examination then is more accurate and masses may be felt more easily or may have disappeared.

The need for additional studies or examinations prior to laparotomy for adnexal disease requires considerable judgment on the part of the gynecologist. If the patient is within the age that menstruation normally occurs (neither prepubertal or postmenopausal) and the mass palpated is relatively small (less than 6 to 8 cm) and feels as though it were thin-walled and cystic, the possibility of a physiologic ovarian cyst (*e.g.*, follicle or lutein) should be considered and the patient should be re-examined in 4 to 6 weeks to re-evaluate the mass. Most such physiologic cysts will regress within this time and laparotomy will be unnecessary. If the cyst seems to be smaller at that time but still present, another similar period of observation is justified but if it is unchanged in size or becoming larger, one must assume it to be neoplastic rather than physiologic and proceed with the laparotomy.

In some instances, it is impossible to distinguish an adnexal mass which is firm and smooth from a pedunculated myoma. This may even be the case when the patient is examined under anesthesia. Assuming that there is no other indication for laparotomy other than an asymptomatic adnexal mass in a pelvis free from induration or obvious adhesions, culdoscopy or laparoscopy can be very useful in establishing whether the mass is indeed an asymptomatic pedunculated myoma which probably does not require laparotomy or is an ovarian neoplasm requiring its removal. In most instances culdoscopy or laparoscopy is not needed, but in carefully selected cases it can be a very useful procedure.

In most instances of unilateral or bilateral adnexal tumors or masses, elaborate preoperative studies will not be necessary. As much judgment is required to know when additional studies are not essential as to determine when they are. If the mass is of moderate size or is adherent or fixed in the pelvis, pressure on a ureter and possibly hydronephrosis should be considered. In such instances, a preoperative intravenous pyelogram is essential to determine whether there is pressure on a ureter and kidney damage but also the status of the opposite kidney. Is it normal? Does it function properly? Is it present at all? Is there an anomaly such as a pelvic kidney instead of an adnexal mass? The correct answers to these questions are essential when one anticipates possibly difficult adnexal surgery. If abnormalities are found in the intravenous pyelograms, cystoscopy, ureteral catheterization, and retrograde pyelograms may be indicated. If only one kidney is seen on intravenous pyelograms, it is important to know whether the other is congenitally (or surgically) absent or nonfunctioning because of ureteral obstruction and also if it is not functioning at that time, whether function can possibly be restored.

At other times evaluation of the intestinal tract, particularly the descending colon, sigmoid, and rectum are vital. In the case of a left pelvic mass particularly, one must be aware that it could arise from the bowel and might be a bowel carcinoma or diverticulitis rather than an ovarian tumor. It is also quite possible that the large bowel may be involved in the pelvic pathology whether it be inflammatory endometriosis or neoplastic, and a barium enema and sigmoidoscopy are particularly valuable in evaluating these problems (see Fig. 3.2). At times even a tumor of the small bowel or ascending or transverse colon will drop into the pelvis and be confused with adnexal disease, making small bowel X-rays quite useful.

Preoperative Preparation

In most instances other than insuring that the patient is in as good physical condition as possible, nothing other than the ordinary preparation procedure prior to sending the patient to the operating room is needed. If, however, preoperative studies have shown ureteral compression or displacement or if by examination, despite normal intravenous pyelograms, the surgeon might expect difficulty in identifying one or both ureters or fears that there might be an increased risk of damage to a ureter during surgery, one or both ureters— depending on the situation—should be catheterized preoperatively with #6 or #7F ureteral catheters. The ureteral catheters may be held in place by taping them to a Foley catheter inserted into the bladder as a retaining device.

The use of ureteral catheters in pelvic surgery is somewhat controversial for some feel that they increase the risk of not only urinary tract infection but also ureter injury by decreasing its mobility and making trauma more likely. Certainly routine ureteral catheterization is unnecessary, but it is very reassuring to the surgeon to be able to palpate a ureter and to identify it with certainty when dissecting from it a densely adherent endometrial cyst or inflammatory mass. In addition, the ease with which the ureter may be identified can save considerable operating time and unnecessary dissection. Unless there is trauma or fear of trauma to the ureter during surgery, the catheters, having served their purpose, are removed at the completion of the operation.

The other consideration before operation is the preparation of the intestinal tract. In most instances nothing other than the usual "nothing by mouth" and cleansing enemas are necessary. There are situations, however, when it is likely or probable that the bowel may be involved in the pelvic disease or possibly be the primary site of pathology. Despite careful preoperative evaluation, one cannot always exclude these possibilities, and when such an event seems possible, preoperative bowel preparation for 24 hours with neomycin and Sulfathalidine, Kanamycin or other measures of bowel "sterilization" are wise precautions. Then, should a bowel resection be needed or the bowel opened unintentionally or intentionally, the risk will be substantially reduced.

Should major bowel surgery be contemplated such as formation of a urinary ileal conduit or similar surgery, the passage of a long intestinal tube such as a Miller-Abbott or Cantor tube prior to surgery may be a wise precaution. In emergency cases in which intestinal obstruction is suspected preoperatively or paralytic ileus is likely postoperatively as in a ruptured tubo-ovarian abscess, passage of the intestinal tube and beginning decompression of the intestinal tract is desirable.

Preparation in the Operating Room

When the patient is brought to the operating room for surgery for adnexal disease, a few remaining precautions are still in order before actually picking up the knife. First the bladder should be catheterized and emptied. Whether a Foley catheter is left in the bladder during or after the procedure in most instances will depend on the desires of the operator, the estimated duration of the procedure, and the operation to be undertaken. It is imperative that the bladder be completely empty. First *it is essential to examine the patient under anesthesia* to re-evaluate or confirm the previous finding encountered without the benefits of the relaxation afforded by a good general anesthesia. One may find that the situation is quite different from what was expected. A cyst or mass may have disappeared entirely making laparotomy unnecessary, or additional masses or induration may change the surgical approach comtemplated. Secondly, a full bladder is easily incised when making the laparotomy, particularly a Pfannenstiel incision; and finally, a full bladder during surgery continually gets in the operator's way and interferes with proper exposure. It is also much more likely to be injured during the procedure.

Generally after catheterizing the bladder and examining the patient under anesthesia, a surgical cleansing of the vagina is advisable. Often it is unwisely omitted when the surgeon expects to remove only an ovarian cyst and not the uterus. In most instances the operator will do what is intended, but at times he may encounter more pathology than anticipated requiring a hysterectomy rather than removal of an ovary. The few minutes required to prepare the vagina for this possibility is time well spent.

Incisions

Most adnexal surgery is done by means of a laparotomy. There are times when the vaginal approach may be used. Vaginal tubal ligation is a very satisfactory operation under proper circumstances and should be considered when interval rather than puerperal sterilization of a multipara is indicated. Exploratory colpotomy at times may be preferable to exploratory laparotomy, and it is feasible to remove early tubal pregnancies by this route. The vaginal approach should not be used when ovarian neoplasms, pelvic inflammatory disease, or a significant degree of endometriosis is expected. The latter two conditions may obliterate the cul-de-sac making colpotomy difficult and bowel injury likely. In the case of a suspected ovarian neoplasm, benign or possibly malignant, the surgeon should endeavor to remove the tumor without rupturing it. This is best done abdominally.

There are a variety of lower abdominal incisions which one may use. The two most commonly made are the low midline and Pfannenstiel. The latter's main virtue is cosmetic. It cannot give the exposure of the low midline or transverse muscle cutting incisions, and therefore should not be used for anything other than rather simple adnexal problems such as small tumors, ovarian wedge resections, tuboplasties, and the like. Because of the lack of exposure, it should not be used when a presacral neurectomy is planned nor for large or adherent adnexal masses. Because of the separation of the rectus fascia from the muscle and the larger area for contamination, it is not a good incision for treatment of active pelvic inflammatory disease. Nevertheless, the Pfannenstiel incision has its place and the patients like it.

For most pelvic surgery the low midline incision is preferred by most gynecologists. In emergencies it can be done more rapidly than most other incisions. It gives good exposure to the entire pelvis and can be extended upward around the umbilicus as far as necessary to deliver large unruptured ovarian tumors and to remove the omentum should one encounter ovarian cancer. Its main defect is that in healing it perhaps is somewhat weaker and more subject to hernia or disruption than a muscle-splitting incision, but nevertheless it is still the most satisfactory incision for pelvic surgery. A paramedian or rectus incision is naturally stronger when healed, but good exposure of the adnexa and pelvic wall of the opposite side is sacrificed.

In making a low midline or Pfannenstiel incision in all low abdominal incisions, great care should be taken in opening the peritoneum. Again the importance of an empty bladder is emphasized for if it is not empty, the bladder rather than the peritoneal cavity may be entered. To avoid bladder injury, the peritoneum should be incised near the upper portion of the incision. If there has been prior low abdominal surgery, the bladder may be fixed higher on the anterior abdominal wall than usual. Furthermore, the peritoneum should not be entered until the patient is properly anesthetized. If she is straining, coughing, or not properly relaxed, bowel injury is

very likely, or the bowel will billow out of the incision making further progress impossible. It is far better to give the anesthesiologist time to do his job properly.

The surgeon cannot always have the patient in optimal condition for laparotomy. The abdomen may be distended by tumor, blood, ascites, or distended bowel which cannot be remedied except at operation. Distention obviously increases the possibility of injury to bowel on opening the peritoneum but also later will impair exposure and make closure of the incision more difficult if not relieved. Care should also be taken to avoid bowel adherent to the peritoneum from prior surgery, inflammation, or tumor. This is not always easily accomplished. The peritoneum should be picked up carefully by the operator and his assistant. The preperitoneal fat and scar tissue should be cleaned away from the proposed point of peritoneal entry so that only the peritoneum remains; if lightly elevated between two pairs or forceps and folded over the knife handle, the handle can be seen through the intact peritoneum. It then is safe to incise the peritoneum and insert a finger through the small opening. The posterior surface of the peritoneum can be felt, and if adherent bowel or omentum is found, it can be avoided.

The inferior portion of a low midline peritoneal incision is limited by the presence of the bladder. As emphasized previously, it is most important that the bladder be completely empty. Nevertheless, since the bladder may be pushed upward by a pelvic mass or in an abnormal location because of prior surgery, the initial peritoneal incision should be in the upper portion rather than in the lower near the bladder. By elevating the peritoneum between two clamps or between two fingers of the operator, the thin peritoneum can be opened under direct vision. Transillumination of the peritoneum is a great aid. With the peritoneum elevated and the overhead operating light shining through it, by looking from the posterior side the edge of the bladder can then be found and avoided. If the bladder limits the incision in the midline, at times the incision can be extended along one of the lateral edges of the bladder to obtain more room and better exposure.

A key step in any laparotomy is the evaluation of the peritoneal surfaces and fluid.

This should be done immediately on entering the peritoneal cavity. If there is fluid present, what is its character? Often a small amount of thin, straw-colored serous fluid is present, but a large amount obviously is abnormal. Is the fluid clear or turbid, purulent, blood-tinged, or grossly bloody? Samples should be taken immediately for culture and cytologic examination. If either is found to be superfluous later, it can be discarded at the end of the case but if not obtained at the time of peritoneal entry, may not be obtainable later. The peritoneal surfaces should be inspected next. Are they smooth and glistening, thickened and inflamed, or thickened and studded with tumor implants or tubercles?

Next the bowel surfaces are checked and adhesions or other abnormalities are noted and attended to if needed. The upper abdominal viscera then are palpated checking particularly the liver, gallbladder, kidneys, and periaortic areas where enlarged lymph nodes may be encountered if a malignancy is present. Generally the exploration of the upper abdomen should precede pelvic exploration. If tumor or infection is present in the pelvis, one prefers not to disseminate either any more than necessary.

Adnexal Tumors

With the patient in Trendelenburg position, the bowel can be packed away from the pelvis gently, and the pelvic organs inspected and palpated to determine the nature and extent of the pathology to confirm or deny the preoperative diagnosis. It is at this point that the operator must decide what sort of operation is to be done and how he can best accomplish his purpose. When dealing with adnexal tumors, the operator must determine whether the tumor is benign or malignant. Most gynecologists with a good foundation in pathology are able to acertain this point, but when in doubt a representative area of a solid tumor or cystic tumor, or a tumor implant can be sent for frozen section. Since the objective is to remove cystic tumors intact without rupturing and spilling their contents, such tumors cannot be opened until they have been removed from the patient's abdomen, but they should be opened in the operating room so that their contents and inner surfaces can be inspected.

When dealing with ovarian carcinomas, solid or cystic, the preferred operative procedure is removal of the uterus, tubes, ovaries, and omentum when possible even if only one ovary is apparently involved. Microscopic tumor frequently is found later in the grossly normal ovary. This then is the minimal extent of the procedure in attempting to cure ovarian cancer. When the tumor is more extensive with implants on the pelvic peritoneum, at times removal of these—if they are not too numerous or extensive—may be done, but obviously the prognosis will be poor and the primary objective of the operation will be the removal of the bulk of the tumor with the hope that later chemotherapy and/or irradiation can control the remaining tumor implants.

Too often, however, the surgeon will encounter widely disseminated tumor with invasive tumor implants or masses involving all the pelvic structures including the pelvic peritoneum, bladder, colon, and small bowel. When the case is clearly inoperable, several biopsies from different sites should be taken to confirm the diagnosis of carcinomatosis. There have been far too many instances in which an operable case or a benign tumor with necrosis or inflammation has been thought to be inoperable and the abdomen closed without the correct diagnosis or operative procedure accomplished!

On the other hand, it is equally imprudent in the face of extensive plaques of tumor-agglutinating loops of bowel and tumor to attempt an extensive dissection ending either with hemorrhage, which is difficult to control from many areas of torn tumor, or multiple bowel lacerations. Again, it is better to recognize that the task is impossible, obtain confirming biopsies, and close the abdomen doing as little harm as possible. It might be possible with postoperative irradiation and chemotherapy that an inoperable tumor may shrink and become sufficiently mobile to be operable at a second laparotomy. Unfortunately, this is an infrequent occurrence.

One of the most difficult decisions to make in the surgery of adnexal tumors is the determination of what to remove and what should be left in each case. Generally with bilateral benign solid or cystic ovarian tumors, removal of the uterus and both adnexa are in order. In younger women, particularly those very anxious to retain or enhance their child-bearing potential, attempts may be made to resect the cysts or solid tumors, such as fibromas or dermoid cysts, provided a healthy functioning portion of at least one ovary can be preserved with unimpaired blood supply. Control of bleeding from the retained ovary is important. Generally the defect in the ovary is closed with a running lock suture of 000 chromic catgut after bleeding points have been ligated. At times when the resection has extended near the ovarian hilum leaving two rather broad flaps of ovary to be sutured together, additional sutures through the ovarian stroma will prevent or control hematoma formation within the ovary.

In the case of an obvious but operable ovarian carcinoma regardless of age, the chance for cure should not be compromised by less than a total hysterectomy and bilateral salpingo-oophorectomy and preferably omentectomy. But what of a girl in her teens or early 20's with a unilateral nonadherent granulosa cell tumor or dysgerminoma? About one-third of these tumors are malignant, and most gynecologists would tend to take a small risk and remove only the involved ovary and tube. Such patients should be kept under careful observation thereafter with frequent examinations.

On the other hand, one occasionally is confronted with findings of carcinoma microscopically in an ovarian tumor thought at laparotomy to be benign and for which only that tube and ovary were removed. The question then arises, what should be done next? Certainly, the removal of one tube and ovary is not considered adequate surgery for ovarian cancer, and the usual and proper treatment is reoperation removing the uterus and remaining tube and ovary. All of us probably have made exceptions to this usual form of treatment. The patient, if sufficiently mature to understand the problem, should be told of it. She should not be forced to make the decision of reoperation. That is the gynecologist's responsibility not to reoperate but to observe the patient carefully. If the small amount of peritoneal fluid which had been sent at the time of laparotomy for cytologic examination is negative for tumor cells, then the decision not to perform additional surgery is on firmer around. The chances are, however, that if the tumor was thought to be benign at the initial operation, the fluid was not obtained for cytology.

Many ovarian tumors, parovarian cysts, and tubo-ovarian inflammatory masses may reach rather large size and often are either adherent to the lateral wall and posterior broad ligament or may even be found enveloped by the anterior and posterior layers of the broad ligament. All such adnexal masses can present considerable technical problems in their removal. The infundibulopelvic ligament often is considerably shortened, and the cyst or tumor wall may lie against both the ureter and the iliac vessels. If this is suspected prior to laparotomy, preoperative intravenous pyelograms and passage of a #6 or #7 ureteral catheter up the ureter on that one or both sides immediately prior to surgery are very wise and often very helpful precautions. With these the ureter can be identified much more rapidly and with greater certainty during the adnexal dissection; the catheters can serve as a splint should the ureter be injured, and if all goes well be removed at the end of the procedure (Fig. 3.1).

When removing the intraligamentary masses, the round ligament should be divided near its insertion in the uterus. The uterovesical fold is then divided, and the bladder is dissected downward from the anterior surface of the uterus as far as needed for the procedure planned. Care should be taken in this dissection not to injure or tear the uterine vessels or any other collateral vessels which may have developed to supply the tumor. A plane of cleavage then can be developed between the anterior leaf of the broad ligament and the tumor (Fig. 3.3). The broad ligament is divided upward until the ovarian vessels are reached. These often are quite large in very vascular or large tumors. They can be isolated and individually clamped, divided, and ligated under direct vision. If this step is taken, the danger of ureteral damage at this point is obviated. Frequently this plane once developed can be continued around the mass superiorly and then down the posterior surface dividing only the attenuated peritoneal covering. With careful blunt dissection the mass can be peeled off the lateral pelvic wall and from the iliac vessels and ureter. When this has been accomplished and the mass has been delivered from between the leaves of the broad ligament, the ureter and vessels can

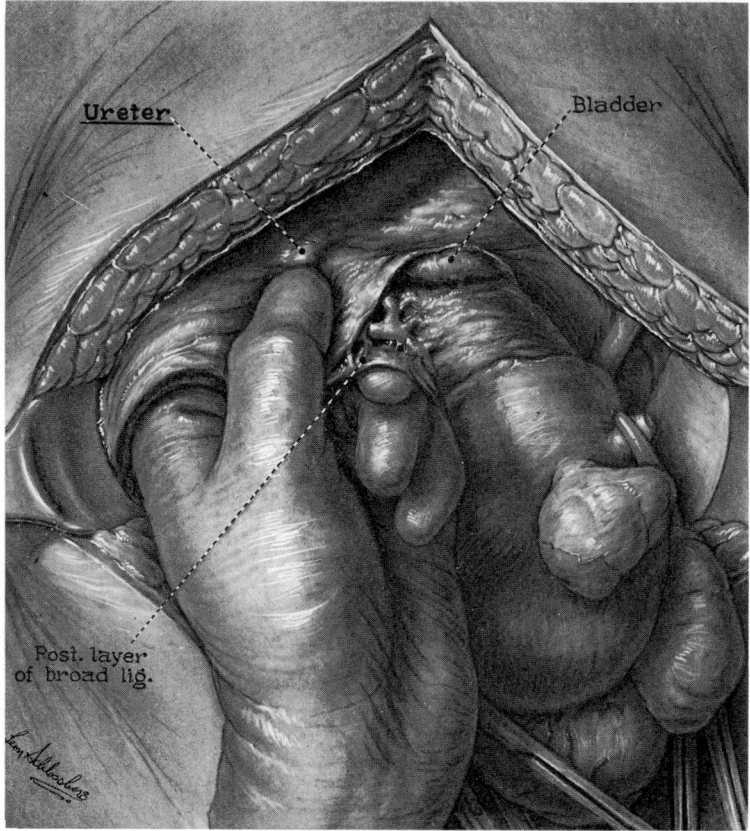

Fig. 3.1. Determining the position of the ureter in the lower pelvis by rolling it between thumb and index finger. (From Wharton, L. R.: Gynecology Including Female Urology, 2nd ed., p. 566, Fig. 302. W. B. Saunders Co., Philadelphia, 1947.)

be checked for damage, and the remainder of the planned operative procedure (*i.e.,* hysterectomy) can be completed.

In dissecting masses from their intraligamentary position or in dissecting adnexal masses adherent to the broad ligaments, the surgeon must be cognizant of the possible displacement of the ureter from its normal course as shown in Figure 3.1. Usually the ureter is attached loosely to the posterior sheath of the broad ligament and is displaced laterally and posteriorly by such masses (see Fig. 3.3). This is the area where the ureter should be sought. If it is not found there, a more medial position should be sought and confirmed before more extensive dissection is continued. It is in such cases that preoperative intravenous pyelograms and/or ureteral catheterization may be quite advantageous.

If the cyst is quite large and interferes with good exposure of the remaining pelvic organs, it is very helpful to remove it separately from the uterus and then proceed with the remainder of the operation unimpeded by the large mass. Such a maneuver had two additional advantages. It eliminates the inadvertent rupture of the cyst thereafter, and it takes a large mass off the abdominal wall making the task of the anesthesiologist easier.

Surgery for endometriosis, ovarian carcinoma, and chronic pelvic inflammatory disease presents many similar problems. Frequently both adnexa are involved and both are adherent to the cul-de-sac, peritoneum, uterus, colon, and even small bowel. Carcinoma and endometriosis implant and invade adjacent structures obliterating the usual planes of cleavage. Subacute or chronic tubo-ovarian abscess can create the same effect with the inflammatory reaction and scarring. The sigmoid colon is

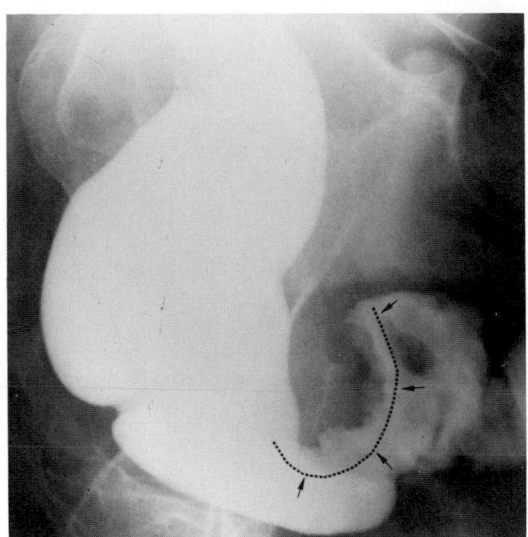

Fig. 3.2. Barium enema showing lesion in recto-sigmoid suggesting either adenocarcinoma or endo-metriosis, diagnosed only by microscopic section as endometriosis.

involved by the pressure of the masses, particularly those arising from the left adnexa or the bowel wall, and may be inflamed or infiltrated narrowing the lumen. Small bowel also can become adherent, invaded, angulated, or obstructed by these processes. The basic approach to bowel involvement by these processes differs somewhat. Adhesive bands and angulations, particularly of small bowel, should be released whenever found to prevent or relieve obstruction. Whenever the bowel wall is involved in an abscess cavity or an endometrial cyst, it is better generally to leave a bit of the cyst or abscess wall on the bowel, rather than damage the bowel wall. When dealing with a localized invasion of small or large bowel by ovarian carcinoma, if no other apparent tumor remains elsewhere, resection of the tumor with a portion of bowel wall is necessary to improve the frankly poor chances for cure. In some cases, the sigmoid colon may be so hopelessly invaded by tumor that obstruction is probable in the near future. In such situations a colostomy is usually made. When small bowel is invaded by ovarian carcinoma causing obstruction or making obstruction imminent, resection of the bowel should be done if there is a chance for cure, but if the case is incurable otherwise, the obstructed area may be by-passed.

Surgery for Endometriosis

The surgical treatment of endometriosis encompasses almost all of the problems encountered in adnexal surgery. Since this is nearly always benign and usually becomes inactive after the menopause, the decision to treat endometriosis must be based on the presence of significant symptoms which need alleviation or the presence of an adnexal mass, exact nature of which can only be determined by laparotomy. The fear that the mass may be malignant is a valid indication for exploration.

In surgery for relief of symptomatic endometriosis, the operator must decide which aspect of the treatment of the disease is most important to the patient. Is relief of infertility the prime objective or is pain relief most important? One usually tries to relieve all symptoms permanently if possible. In the case of infertility, there is always the possibility that endometriosis will become symptomatic later requiring another operation. This risk, however, is small (Gray, 4 per cent; Scott and Burt, 2.7 per cent; to McCoy and Bradford (19a), 21 per cent). Castration is definitive treatment for endometriosis but does little to help infertility.

In young women in whom the preservation or enhancement of reproductive potential is the prime consideration, every reasonable effort should be made to excise or destroy by fulgeration or resection all areas of endometriosis and release adhesions about the adnexa and uterus. When both ovaries are involved in the process, perhaps one-half or two-thirds of each ovary may need to be resected. Endometrial cyst frequently can be removed from an ovary with surprising ease considering the usual infiltrative characteristic of endometriosis. At times the cyst can be shelled out of the ovary leaving behind good ovarian tissue. Care must be taken to preserve the blood supply to the residual ovary and reconstructing the ovary as best possible. If necessary it should be suspended near the infundibulopelvic ligament so that it will not prolapse into the cul-de-sac again. The uterus also should be suspended usually by a Gilliam suspension to correct an adherent retroposition if present.

When a conservative procedure for endometriosis is done retaining childbearing capabilities, frequently a presacral neurectomy should be done particularly if dysmenorrhea is present. Good exposure is necessary for this procedure which is not generally available with a Pfannenstiel incision. Do not compromise the procedure for cosmetic reasons. A fairly long, low midline incision gives much better exposure to the retroperitoneal area over the sacral promentory. Here a 6- to 7-cm longitudinal incision is made in the posterior peritoneum starting just below the aortic bifurcation and extending downward over the sacral promentory to the hollow of the sacrum. In this area blunt dissection is best, and it is important to remove not only all the nerve fibers immediately beneath the peritoneum but also the deep layer overlying the periosteum which contains the main nerves for a distance of 4 to 5 cm. Care must be taken laterally since the lateral limits of the dissection are the ureters and iliac vessels which should be avoided. The inferior mesenteric artery and hemorrhoidal branches also should be avoided. The middle sacral artery usually is attached to the periosteum of the sacrum and can cause troublesome bleeding if injured. This is to be avoided if possible by careful blunt dissection; however, at times this vessel must be ligated for hemostasis. If, despite careful dissection laterally in the retroperitoneal space, the operator suddenly encounters severe bleeding, he first should try to control it with pressure from either a sponge on a stick or by a finger or fingers until the origin of the hemorrhage is found. Usually it is venous since veins tear much more easily than arteries because of their thinner walls. If the tear is in the side of a major vessel such as the common iliac which cannot be ligated, the rent can be repaired with fine arterial silk sutures while the vessel is compressed to control the bleeding. Other smaller vessels, both arteries and veins, in this area usually have anastamosing branches so that the bleeding point can be tied off without jeopardizing the blood supply to the sigmoid or rectum.

In this area when doing a presacral neurectomy, the error which leads to bleeding is in carrying the dissection too far laterally or anteriorly on the left side reaching the base of the mesentery of the sigmoid and injuring the vessels here. Control of bleeding first by pressure and then by careful clamping and ligation is important. Since this is in the retroperitoneal space, control of the bleeding by packing is at best a temporary expedient. If the bleeding point is not more specifically controlled, it can dissect further in the retroperitoneal space forming a hematoma which should be prevented.

At times, there is an ooze from the periosteum of the sacrum which is difficult to control with ties. Pressure will usually control this, and it may be helpful to leave a piece of Gelfoam, Oxycel, or similar material over this area. Then when the bleeding has been controlled, the posterior peritoneum is closed and rechecked before finally closing the abdomen.

Usually it is better to do the presacral neurectomy after the areas of endometriosis in the pelvis have been taken care of and peritonized but before doing the uterine suspension which requires shifting or removing the retractors and usually is the last part of the procedure to be done before closing the abdominal incision.

Endometriosis may involve many other sites usually in the pelvis, most of which can be treated by excision or fulguration if ovarian function is retained, or ignored if the ovaries are removed. This is particularly true of superficial serosal or peritoneal implants, but the bowel and urinary tract may present special problems. Frequently the anterior wall of the sigmoid is involved making it densely adherent to the uterosacral ligaments and posterior surface of the uterus. In dissecting the uterus or adnexa from the bowel, sharp dissection often is required and considerable care must be taken to avoid bowel injury. It is also most important to inspect the bowel at the end of the operation to be certain that no lacerations or injuries have gone unrecognized and untreated.

If a bowel injury occurs it should be repaired immediately to minimize the degree of fecal contamination. Small serosal tears are not important and frequently need no repair or can be closed with a few 000 chromic catgut sutures. If the laceration enters the bowel lumen, the extent of the damage must be determined. It may be so extensive that rather than trying to repair long, irregular laceration(s), resection of the area may be preferable. This is not often necessary. A two-layer closure is the usual procedure. The closure should be done transversely rather than longitudinally if possible so that the caliber of the lumen is not significantly reduced. The first layer should be a continuous suture of 00 chromic catgut closing the mucosa and muscularis. This should be followed by a second line of interrupted sutures of either 0 chromic catgut or 4-0 silk depending on the surgeon's preference. Often in the cul-de-sac no peritoneum remains. It is possible, however, to place the posterior vaginal wall against the anterior rectal wall to reinforce the damaged area. The open or sutured vaginal vault if a hysterectomy has been done should not, if possible, be placed over the repaired area of the bowel to avoid fistula formation.

Ordinarily these repaired lacerations do not require drainage. If there is extensive involvement of the sigmoid by endometriosis, frequently it is safer and better to remove the ovaries and uterus than to try to resect the scarred anterior wall of the sigmoid, particularly if the bowel has not been properly prepared before laparotomy. An exception to this is the presence of an area of constriction by endometriosis which may significantly narrow the bowel lumen and lead to bleeding from the endometriosis and obstruction. Resection of obstructing areas is necessary to correct such mechanical problems. Furthermore, menopause, surgical or natural, may lead to further scarring and constriction as the ectopic endometriosis becomes atrophic.

Small bowel endometriosis should almost always be resected. If this is done then it might be possible to retain ovarian function particularly in a young woman. In any event, if there is any possibility that such an endometrioma could cause obstruction, then it should be resected even if the ovaries are removed.

When there are deeply infiltrating endometrial implants in the bladder wall, these frequently cause bladder irritability and symptoms similar to cystitis. Such areas generally are best treated by local excision.

When there is extensive endometriosis about the uterosacral ligaments or bases of the broad ligaments, the ureter may be drawn medially toward the uterus making it more liable to injury during the operative procedure particularly if a hysterectomy or uterosacral ligament resection is done. The surgeon in his preoperative evaluation of the patient must consider this possibility; frequently intravenous pyelograms are an essential part of this evaluation. His pelvic examination is often a better guide as to the expected degree of difficulty of the contemplated operation, and preoperative catheterization of the ureters may save considerable operating time, extensive dissection, or ureteral injury.

Endometriosis, like carcinoma, may invade, constrict, or obstruct a ureter. If the compression is due to an endometrial cyst or mass which is removed, the problem is solved, but if the ureter passes through an area of extensive endometriosis near the bladder and the ureter shows evidence of partial or complete obstruction, then reimplantation of the ureter into the bladder should be done provided the kidney has not been so extensively damaged and hydronephrotic that it is not worthy of salvage. A nephrectomy then would be the procedure of choice to remove a nonfunctioning kidney.

Surgery for Residual Pelvic Inflammatory Disease

In general, acute episodes of pelvic inflammatory disease are best treated medically with antibiotics, avoiding surgery. However, many women will have recurrent flare-ups of these infections with fever, pain, and pelvic masses. Such attacks may severely incapacitate the patient making it difficult for her to keep a job or function as a mother if she is fortunate enough to have had her children prior to her infection. In such instances, despite the frequent youthfulness of the patient, a "pelvic cripple," surgical intervention is indicated with the expectation of performing a total hysterectomy and bilateral salpingo-oophorectomy.

Having decided that removal of the uterus and adnexa is indicated, the physician's next important step is proper timing of the laparotomy. The optimal time for such a procedure is between flare-ups when the disease is quiescent rather then when it is acute and the patient is ill. The procedure is much easier technically at that time, and the patient is in better general condition. This means that when the decision to operate is made usually after a series of attacks, the most recent attack is again treated with antibiotics and rest, if possible; the patient then is admitted about 6 weeks later for surgery. In theory this works well. In practice it is often difficult to achieve. The nature of the inflammatory process and the character of the patient frequently make optimal treatment impossible. The patient when feeling well erases from her mind the bouts with fever and pain and does not return when directed, or just when everything is arranged to proceed with the operation, the pelvic inflammatory process becomes hot again. When events conspire against optimal treatment, the operator must make the best of the situation. When another acute exacerbation of symptoms occurs, the patient should be hospitalized and treated intensively with antibiotics until afebrile for at least a few days and then proceed with surgery. In addition, there will be other instances when despite intensive antibiotic therapy the patient does not respond remaining febrile and in considerable discomfort. Such patients under treatment should be watched carefully and examined regularly, preferably by only one individual who can evaluate the changes, if any, from day to day. Too many or too frequent examinations only tend to stir up the pelvic inflammation and serve no useful purpose.

At times a pelvic abscess will localize in the cul-de-sac, and when it begins to dissect the rectovaginal septum and become fluctuant, a posterior colpotomy and drainage of the abscess are indicated. This procedure is best done under a general anesthesia so that a thorough examination can be done to evaluate the pelvic findings as best as possible. The operator may be able then to feel other higher and more lateral pelvic masses not palpable before because of the pain. The operator can also be certain that the abscess is suitable for drainage. Prior to this the bowel should have been emptied by an enema and antibiotic coverage continued. Many pelvic abscesses are composed of many locules, and when the first has been entered, cultured, and drained, other locules should be perforated by a long Kelly clamp to allow them to drain through the vaginal incision. Several large cigarette drains should be left in the colpotomy incision since more pus may drain through this area later.

If drainage of a pelvic abscess by way of posterior colpotomy is successful, the problem may well be solved and extensive abdominal surgery made unnecessary. Usually with evacuation of the abscess, the patient will become afebrile and asymptomatic. The situation should then be evaluated 6 weeks later to determine the extent of the residual pelvic inflammatory disease and the need for additional surgery. Should tender pelvic masses remain at that point, removal of the uterus and adnexa may be done.

In operating upon patients with residual pelvic inflammatory masses, preoperative evaluation of the patient is most important. One expects the masses to be adherent and fixed, but if there is considerable induration present in the pelvis suggesting that the process is still subacute, it might be better to delay the operation for a few more weeks in the hope that further resolution will follow. If this does not occur, several days of antibiotic therapy should precede surgery, and it is often advisable to pass ureteral catheters prior to operation.

When the abdomen has been opened with care since bowel or omentum probably are adherent to the abdominal wall, the omental and bowel adhesions are dissected free from the pelvic structures. When the tubo-ovarian inflammatory masses or abscesses can be identified, a good point of attack must be found. Sometimes a good plane of cleavage can be obtained between the uterus and the abscess and the abscess and cul-de-sac. If such is the case, it may be possible to deliver the mass out of its usual cul-de-sac position and gain access to the ovarian vessels so that they may be safely clamped, divided, and ligated. On other occasions when such a posterior approach does not seem to be going easily, the round ligament and anterior sheath of the broad ligament can be opened and the ovarian vessels approached from this direction. In either case the major vessels against the pelvic wall, the ureter, and bowel must be checked with each step to avoid injury. It is here that a ureteral catheter may be of great help. The tissues are so thickened and indurated that it often cannot be found by palpation without a catheter in place. The only other alternative is to identify the ureter at the pelvic brim above the inflammatory process and trace it downward, dissecting it away from the abscess.

The operator should not be too worried about opening a pelvic abscess during the laparotomy. When pus is encountered, it should be cultured, but many times no organisms will be identified. It is a good precaution when operating on pelvic inflammatory disease to pack off the upper abdomen so that as little contamination as possible will result from surgery.

The question of drainage upon completion of

the operation is still debatable. In many cases it will not be necessary. If, however, parts of abscess wall remain on the sigmoid or pelvic walls and there is considerable raw area, several cigarette drains through the vaginal vault are very helpful and effective. These can be tagged in the vagina with a suture or clamp so that they are not lost in the abdomen and can then be removed 2 or 3 days after surgery.

Postabortal pelvic abscesses in general are similar to postgonococcal pelvic inflammatory disease in many ways. The gonococcus involves the endosalpinx initially; however, the post-abortal infection often due to streptococci causes broad ligament cellulitis. These abscesses initially are broad ligament abscesses rather than tubo-ovarian. They may localize in the cul-de-sac and be drained by this route, but at times they may rise up out of the pelvis and point in the region of the inguinal canals. When this is the case and drainage is indicated, this can be accomplished by an extraperitoneal approach through a McBurney type incision over the abscess. A Kelly clamp can then be passed into the abscess without entering the peritoneum, and the abscess can be drained by leaving in several large drains through the incision.

Tuberculosis salpingitis no longer seems to be a major problem. Most cases initially should be treated by chemotherapy such as streptomycin, isonicotinic acid hydrazide (INH) and para-aminosalicylic acid (PAS). Surgery should be considered only when adnexal masses fail to resolve after at least six months of such therapy. It is no longer necessary to operate on the wet or ascitic forms of tuberculosis perito-nitis nor the fibrocaseous type where the loops of bowel and omentum are matted together and the risk of fistulae is considerable. Chemo-therapy has effected a profound change and it is no longer necessary to operate on such cases and to expose them to such high risk. Proper chemotherapy may obviate all this and make surgery if necessary later much safer and easier.

Gynecologic Emergencies Due to Adnexal Disease

There are three basic problems producing acute catastrophic conditions arising from the adnexa. They are 1) hemorrhage from ectopic pregnancy or corpus luteum hematoma, 2) torsion of entire adnexa or ovarian tumor, or 3) ruptured tubo-ovarian abscess. Each represents a somewhat different clinical picture and requires definitive surgical intervention.

Hemorrhage from the Adnexa. A ruptured tubal pregnancy immediately comes to mind when this is considered, and certainly is the most common cause of intraperitoneal bleeding of any significance from either the tube or ovary. However, ovarian pregnancy, early ab-dominal pregnancy, or hemorrhage from a corpus luteum may produce the same clinical picture of intra-abdominal hemorrhage and shock. Unfortunately, there rarely seems to be an entirely typical case of ectopic pregnancy or anything else for that matter. The symptoms will be for the most part dependent on the duration of the extrauterine gestation, the location of the gestation, and whether it has ruptured and if so the rapidity of intraperi-toneal bleeding. The most important thing is to be "ectopic conscious," that is, to be thinking of the possibility of ectopic pregnancy in any case with abdominal pain, menstrual irregu-larities, and adnexal tenderness. An adnexal mass is present in less than half of the cases of tubal pregnancy, and then in many instances it is the cystic corpus luteum of pregnancy which is felt rather than the ectopic pregnancy. It is therefore most important not to rule out this diagnosis by the absence of an adnexal mass.

The patient who is brought to the emergency room with the classical picture of a sudden onset of acute lower abdominal pain, a delayed or missed menstrual period, prostration, and shock does not require elaborate diagnostic procedures, but resuscitation. Intravenous flu-ids should be started immediately with Ringer's lactate followed by blood volume expanders such as low molecular weight dextran, plas-manate, and whole blood as soon as available. Replacement therapy should be monitored by measurement of the central venous pressure to prevent overtreatment. Laparotomy should fol-low as soon as possible after this, not necessar-ily awaiting the return of a normal blood pressure, for this may not occur until the hemorrhage has been controlled. This is one of the few situations in gynecologic surgery where speed can be of critical importance. One should enter the abdomen by the fastest route avail-able, a low midline incision, and not waste time with a Pfannenstiel or other cosmetically orientated incision. Nor should the operator spend time at first evacuating the blood and clots from the abdomen, but rather he should search immediately for the source of bleeding. If it originates from the tube, a Kelly clamp across the mesosalpinx and at the isthmus will immediately control the bleeding. If the ovary is hopelessly involved in the tubal pregnancy, then clamps are placed across the infundibulopelvic ligament as close as possible to the ovary to avoid injuring the ureter. If the pregnancy is a cornual or interstitial one, pressure on the bleeding sites will control the bleeding temporarily so that the surgeon can decide how best to handle the situation.

In reaching this decision the patient's age, parity, and desire for additional pregnancies are important, but the prime factors are the patient's general condition, the area involved, and the extent of the damage to the tube, ovary, or uterus in addition to any incidental pathology such as myomata, prior salpingectomy for ectopic pregnancy or sterilization, or ovarian disease.

It is always amazing to see how quickly a patient will respond with blood replacement (provided irreversible shock has not developed), once the bleeding points have been controlled. Then the operator must decide whether only the pregnancy can be removed and the tube repaired (about 5 per cent of the cases) or whether the tube should be removed. The removal of the ipsilateral ovary is a debatable point. Certainly if it has been significantly involved, it is safer and better to remove it. In the case of a cornual or interstitial pregnancy, usually a hysterectomy is the best procedure, but at times it may be possible and desirable to salvage the uterus by excising the cornu and repairing the defect.

There is no unanimity about the matter of the hemoperitoneum. Some take great pains to wash out the peritoneal cavity removing all blood and clots while others leave the blood. Our choice has been generally to remove the blood and clots which can be done easily but not to worry about a complete peritoneal toilet or irrigation.

Postoperatively blood, intravenous fluid, and electrolyte replacement should be continued and monitored by central venous pressure until the vital signs are once more stable. The urinary output should be watched and measured carefully. Also abdominal distention frequently occurs after laparotomies for hemoperitoneum making intestinal decompression by a nasogastric tube desirable until bowel sounds begin to return.

Adnexal bleeding usually is not so dramatic; however, it takes but a few drops of blood to irritate the peritoneal cavity and produce rather severe attacks of pain. In these milder more atypical cases, more diagnostic ability is required. Culdocentesis, examination under anesthesia, culdoscopy, laparoscopy, and exploratory colpotomy are various procedures short of laparotomy which may be used to establish the presence or absence of intraperitoneal blood and identify its origin.

Torsion of Adnexa. While a normal tube and ovary or even a hydatid of Morgagni may twist about itself or an adhesion and become infarcted, this is a rather rare occurrence. More commonly a freely movable ovarian cyst or tumor will stretch the infundibulopelvic ligament to form a long pedicle upon which it then twists obstructing the venous return and leading to hemorrhagic infarction. This produces a sudden sharp pain in the abdomen which becomes increasingly more severe and continuous. Following this are signs of peritonitis, fever, and leukocytosis. At other times, there may be intermittent partial torsion. With either, there is a tender abdominal mass and the need for immediate laparotomy. The involved adnexa should be removed, and additional surgery done if the original pathologic condition warrants it.

One frequently hears that the twisted adnexa should be removed without untwisting the pedicle. At times, the degree of torsion and edema will shorten the pedicle so that the ureter can also be damaged when the pedicle is clamped unless it is untwisted.

Ruptured Tubo-ovarian Abscess. This constitutes one of the most serious of all gynecologic emergencies and should be distinguished from peritonitis due to acute salpingitis or a leaking pyosalpinx. Usually it follows a long history of pelvic inflammatory disease ending in acute spontaneous intra-abdominal rupture of an abscess. The pain that ensues is usually acute in onset and progressive, followed by a generalized peritonitis which is in turn followed rather rapidly by septic shock.

As soon as the diagnosis is reasonably tenable, the patient should be prepared for operation with all possible speed. Central venous pressure monitoring is essential, and emergency blood chemistries must be obtained. Immediate intravenous fluids should be started containing large doses of penicillin, tetracycline, or sodium cephalothin (Keflin). Plasmanate also should be used until blood is available to combat shock. A Cantor tube should be passed as far as possible to decrease abdominal distention and the adynamic ileus which follows, and a Foley catheter placed in the bladder to record the hourly urinary output.

As soon as a reasonable degree of stability is achieved, the patient should be taken to the operating room. The longer the delay between rupture of the abscess and surgery, the higher the mortality which reaches almost 100 per cent in cases treated without surgery or by drainage alone (25) but can be reduced to about 5 to 10 per cent with intensive therapy and surgery. Nebel and Lucas (20) have found more postoperative problems and longer hospitalization after a delay of 12 hours following admission to the hospital. The critical number of hours, literally signifying life or death, between rupture of the abscess and surgery probably is between 18 and 24 hours. This is the time required to develop endotoxin shock which may be irreversible by any treatment.

The purpose of surgery is to remove the intra-abdominal pus and the abscesses. Usually this is best accomplished by removal of both tubes and ovaries since both usually are involved and a subtotal hysterectomy. Under the circumstances, this is a more rapid, less shocking procedure even in the most skilled hands than a total hysterectomy. Usually there remains at the end of the operation a considerable amount of ragged necrotic abscess wall adherent to bowel and therefore drainage either through the posterior cul-de-sac or abdominal stab wound is desirable. Cultures should be taken during the procedure, but usually the organisms are of the enteric group, usually *Escherichia coli.*

The postoperative period requires continued vigilance. Shock should be vigorously combatted with blood, plasmanate, and intravenous fluids to correct acidosis and electrolyte inbalance. Norepinephrine may be needed intravenously, and large doses of intravenous antibiotics should be continued. Central venous pressure monitoring, urinary output, and drainage from the Cantor tube should be watched closely. Intestinal decompression should be continued until bowel sounds have returned, and the patient begins to pass gas per rectum. Even then the Cantor tube should be clamped and suction discontinued for at least 24 hours before removing the tube to be certain that normal intestinal peristalsis will continue.

The chief error in the handling of a ruptured tubo-ovarian abscess usually is the failure to recognize the seriousness of the situation early. With aggressive treatment to correct shock and infection and above all prompt laparotomy, the dismal prognosis can be turned into a very favorable one. Speed in getting the patient to surgery and rapid but careful surgery are the keys. These patients are desperately ill and their surgery should not be delegated to a partially trained house officer. Experience is required to remove the abscesses and the uterus swiftly without injuring the bowel which usually is partially matted together and adherent to the pelvic organs. Leave parts of abscess wall adherent to bowel so long as they do not produce kinks or angulation leading to obstruction. Good hemostasis is obviously important. Ooze from raw areas usually can be controlled by packs. Do not waste time picking bits of abscess wall off the pelvis so long as most of the abscess has been removed and completely evacuated.

Postoperatively, care must be taken not to overload the patient with blood and intravenous fluids causing pulmonary edema. The central venous pressure measurement serves as a guide for this; however, the patient may have lost a large amount of water and electrolytes in the intestinal tract and by vomiting so that a rather large fluid deficit may need to be corrected.

The Ureter in Adnexal Surgery

Injury to the urinary tract is one of the major complications in gynecologic surgery and often is preventable. The only gynecologist who has not injured a ureter or bladder is one who has done little surgery. If you do enough cases, you will at some point run into this problem, but it should not happen very often.

The true incidence of urinary tract damage in

gynecologic surgery is difficult to ascertain. Bladder injuries and fistulae are obvious, but more subtle changes such as denervation or fixation of the bladder after radical hysterectomy are less obvious. Ureteral injuries resulting in fistula also are obvious, but it is certain that many ureters are unintentionally ligated and never produce symptoms nor are they recognized. Everett and Mattingly (11) reported 31 ureteral injuries, with 19 recognized at surgery in 16,100 abdominal and major vaginal gynecologic operations at Johns Hopkins Hospital as an incidence of 0.19 per cent. Bunkin (3a) estimates the incidence of ureteral injury in all gynecologic procedures for benign disease to be between 0.5 to 3 per cent although the higher figure seems rather unreasonable in the hands of competent gynecologists.

Prevention of injury to the bladder and ureter should be the aim of every pelvic surgeon. This requires first a thorough knowledge of the normal anatomy of the urinary tract and its possible anatomic variations, such as ureteral reduplication, pelvic kidney, or absence of a kidney congenitally or surgically (Fig. 3.4). In other words, as much information as practical should be obtained before pelvic laparotomies. This does not mean that every patient must have cystoscopy, intravenous pyelograms, ureteral catheters, and a bladder full of methylene blue before surgery. It does require, however, that sound judgment be used to determine which patient is likely to be technically difficult or have the urinary tract involved in the pathology to be treated and hence a likely candidate for trouble with the urinary tract at surgery (Fig. 3.5). Certainly with large, probably adherent and fixed adnexal

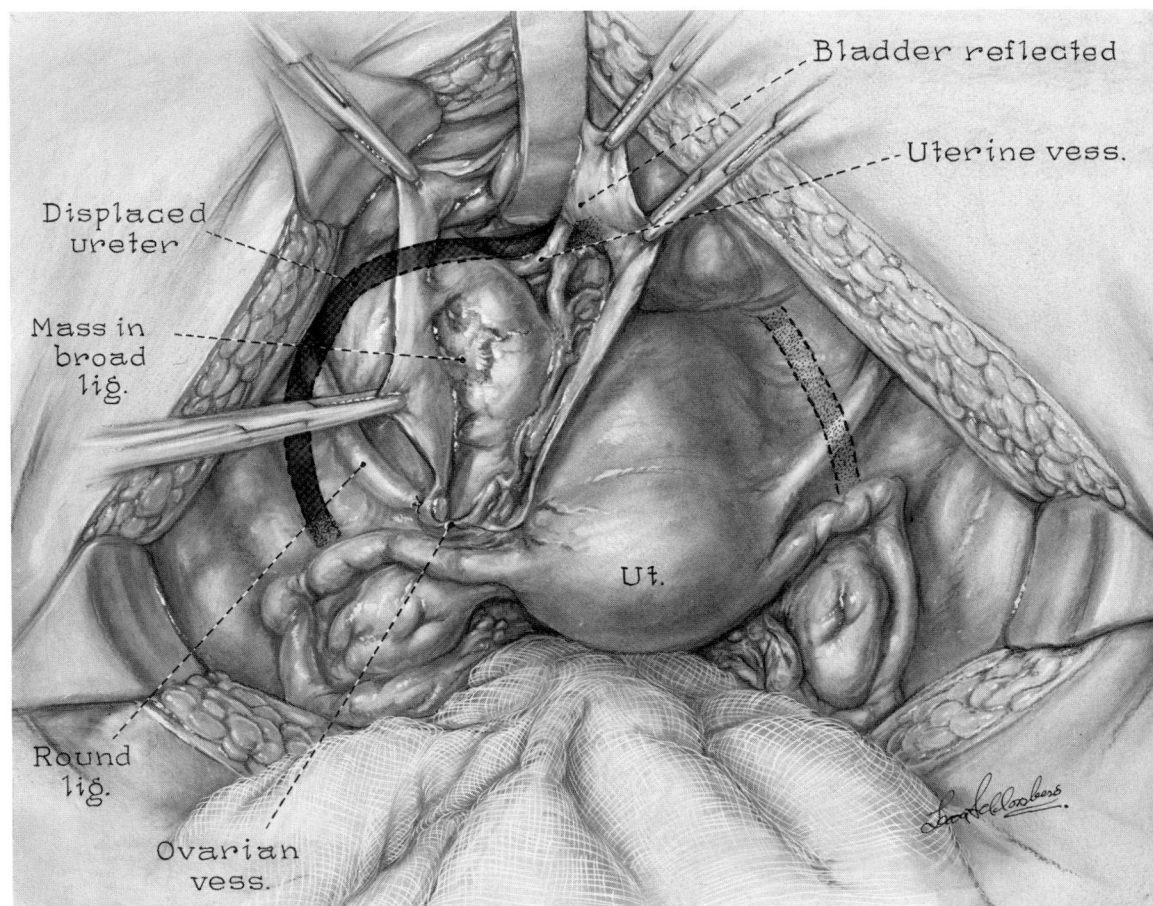

Fig. 3.3. Exposing a left intraligamentary adnexal mass. The round ligament has been divided and the anterior leaf of the broad ligament opened. Note the lateral displacement of the ureter.

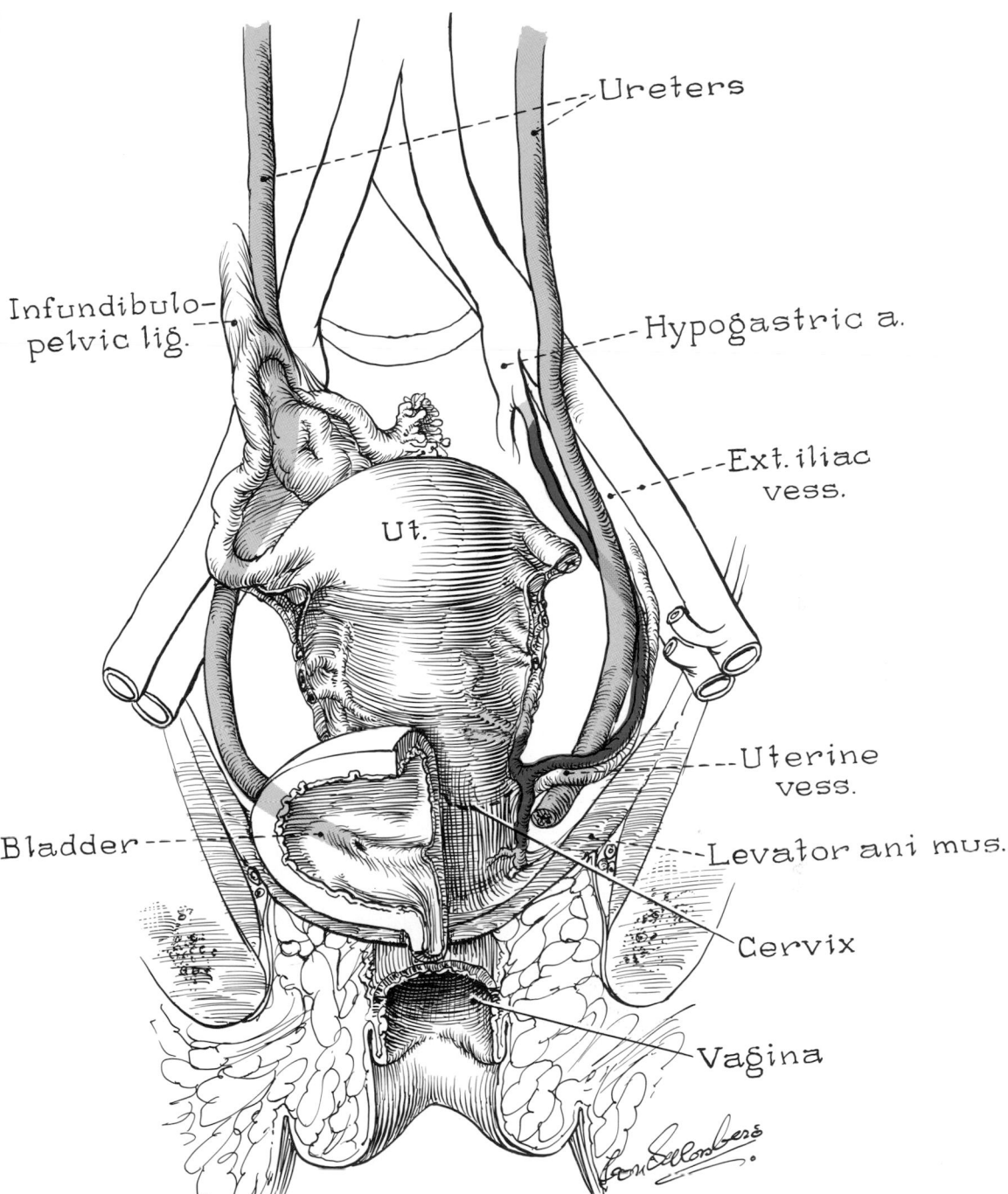

Fig. 3.4. Normal anatomy of the ureters and their relations to other pelvic organs encountered in gynecologic surgery.

masses, or probable intraligamentary cysts or tumors, preoperative intravenous pyelograms are most useful in determining not only the normalcy of the urinary tract but also if the ureters are in an abnormal position or the existence of any degree of ureteral obstruction (Figs. 3.6 through 3.12).

If the operator expects the case to be

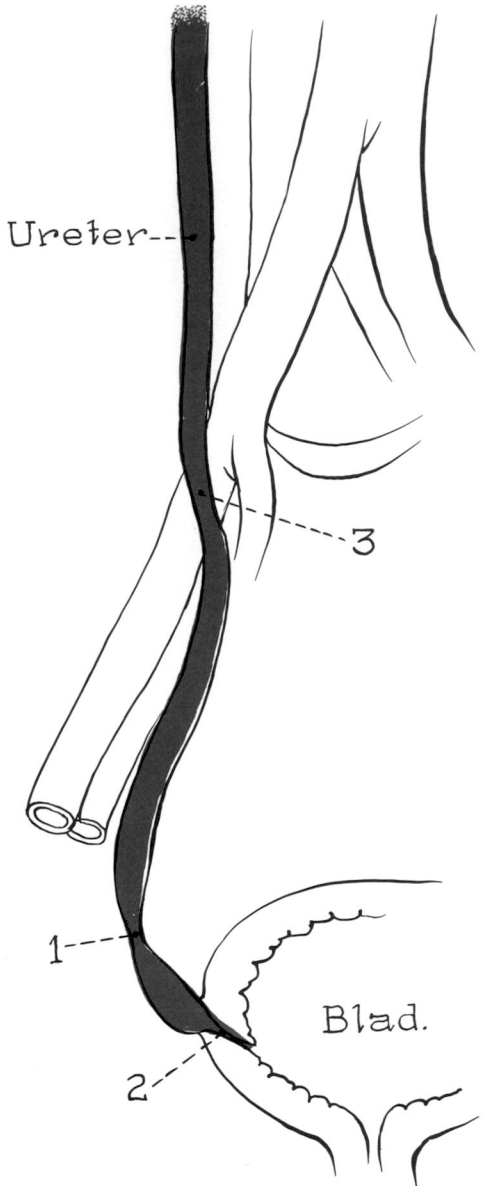

Ureter--

3

1---

Blad.

2-

Fig. 3.5. Most common sites of ureteral injury in gynecologic surgery: (1) pelvic wall lateral to uterine vessels, (2) area of uretero-vesical junction, (3) base of infundibulopelvic ligament.

ters are difficult to feel and do not drain as well. These are kept in place by taping them to a Foley catheter placed in the bladder; each ureteral catheter should be identified (right and/or left) so that the side can be identified later should the need arise. These are connected separately to straight drainage until they are later removed at the end of the operation having served their purpose.

The bladder should be empty at the beginning of the operation. The patient may be catheterized to accomplish this, and if it is likely to be a lengthy procedure, an indwelling Foley catheter is usually left in place.

Although the operator should have established by careful history and examination his preoperative diagnosis before scheduling the patient for surgery, an *examination under anesthesia immediately before laparotomy is essential.* The findings of this examination are correlated with the preoperative investigations and preparations of the patient for surgery, and then if the surgeon's total evaluation of the patient indicates it, the laparotomy should begin. The operator's first step usually is to evaluate the pathologic process present in the pelvis and to determine what procedures or steps are to be taken to correct it. Which organs are to be removed, retained, or repaired; and what organs are involved? Before proceeding further than releasing adhesions and exposing the pelvic structures, the position and course of each ureter should be known. Generally it is easiest to identify the ureter first at the pelvic brim where it crosses the iliac artery (see Fig. 3.4). It can then be traced down into the pelvis beneath the adnexa and ovarian vessels, then along the pelvic wall as it turns medially crossing under the uterine vessels to enter the bladder. It may be difficult to see through the peritoneum at this point, but it can be palpated usually by rolling the base of the broad ligament between the thumb and fingers as illustrated in Figure 3.1. If the position of the ureter is uncertain because of the pathology, the posterior peritoneum just lateral to the ureter at the pelvic brim should be opened; the ureter identified; and the dissection continued downward until the true position of the ureter is known.

As each step is made in the procedure, the position of adjacent structures should be checked. Bowel usually can be packed away

technically difficult with probable involvement of the ureters by inflammatory reaction, endometriosis, or tumor or if preoperative pyelography indicates this to be the case, then cystoscopy with passage of a #6 or #7F Teflon catheter up the ureter immediately prior to laparotomy is a wise precaution. Small cathe-

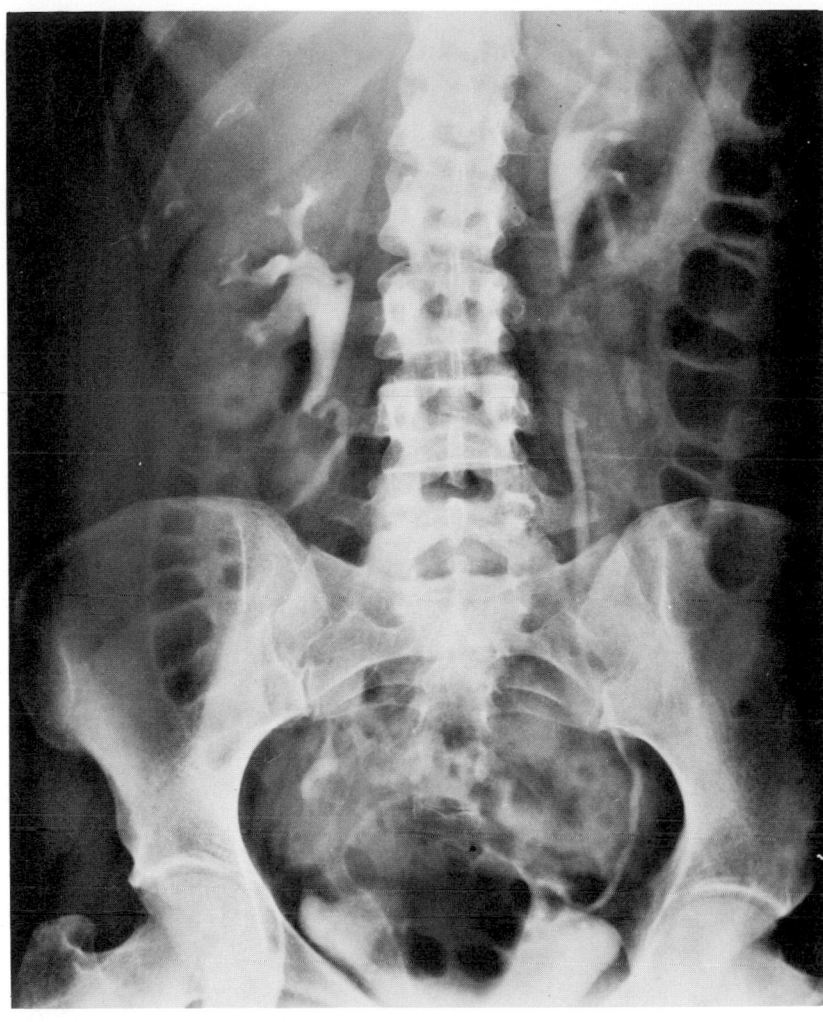

Fig. 3.6. Filling defect of lower right ureter without obstruction due to extensive endometriosis.

after any adhesions have been released and the ureter identified by palpation or dissection. If the clamps and sutures are not placed carefully on the infundibulopelvic ligaments, the ovarian vessels, and the cardinal ligaments or if the iliac vessels are torn or cut during the dissection, hemorrhage inevitably follows and must be controlled. It is this type of situation which may lead to injury to the ureter or bowel. If the operator can visualize clearly the bleeding point and control it with a clamp, the situation is under control, but if the clamps are placed blindly about bleeding areas, then the ureter can be also clamped or ligated. Most bleeding can be controlled by digital pressure until the operator can check his landmarks and then clamp the bleeding point. It may be necessary then, if the ureter is very near or possibly involved, to check its position by palpation or dissect it free before final ties or sutures are placed.

Injury Recognized at Surgery

Despite reasonable care, every competent gynecologic surgeon is going to injure a ureter sometime. If it is his misfortune to do so, it is better to recognize it immediately during the operation rather than later. The simplest injury consists of a clamp suture placed on, about, or through a ureter. If the ureter has been clamped and the clamp immediately removed, it is possible that very little damage has resulted. If the ureteral wall does not seem to have been damaged at all, nothing need be done; if there is any question of crushing the ureter or a portion

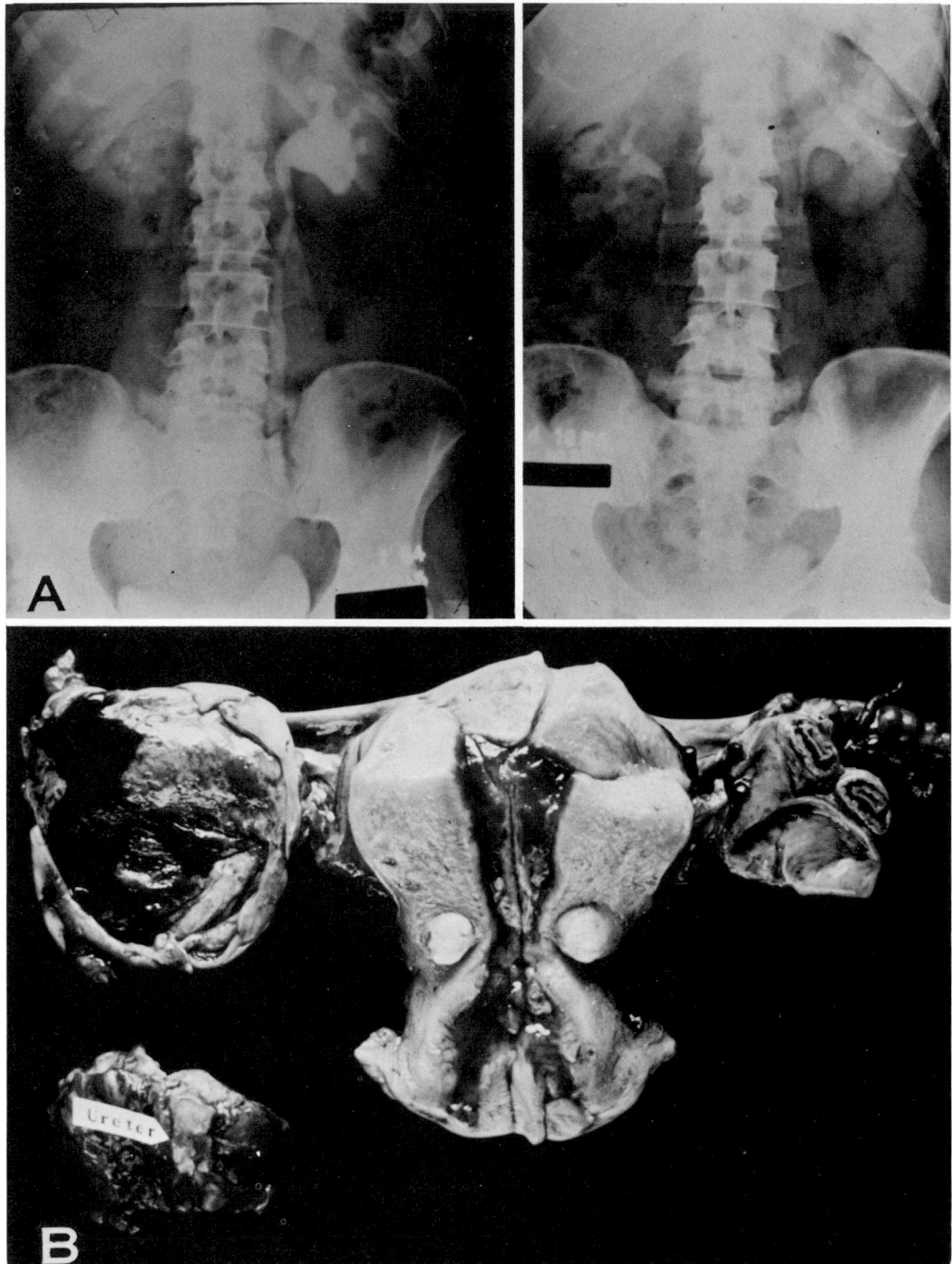

Fig. 3.7. Top, Serial pyelograms showing blockage of ureter by endometriosis and recovery toward normal function after resection of the affected ureteral segment in the true pelvis.

Bottom, Gross specimens removed at same operation showing extensive endometriosis in the resected, partially blocked ureter, and in the adnexa. (Courtesy of Dr. Joseph H. Pratt, Mayo Clinic, Rochester, Minn.)

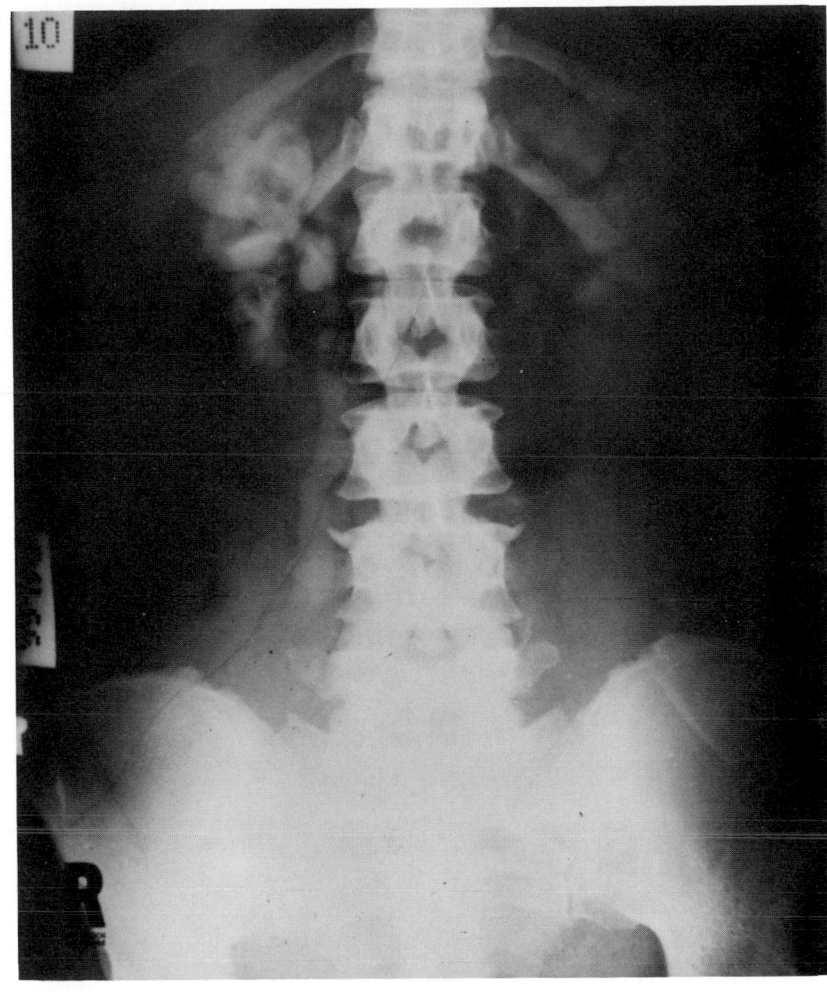

Fig. 3.8. Bilateral hydronephrosis due to large myomata uteri and left tubo-ovarian abscess. (Courtesy Dr. H. S. Everett.)

of it, extraperitoneal drainage should be done to prevent intraperitoneal or vaginal drainage of urine and to allow any urinary leakage to escape.

A suture about the ureter or through it should be removed and in this situation as with a crushing or perforating injury, a catheter should be passed up the ureter to the kidney either by cystoscopy immediately after surgery or the bladder can be opened and the ureter catheterized under direct vision at the time of surgery. The ureter may be opened by a small longitudinal incision 3 to 4 cm above the injury (Fig. 3.13), and a catheter may be passed downward and upward from here. The catheter is then brought out through the urethra, anchored by a Foley catheter, and left in place as a splint for about 10 days to allow the ureter to heal. In addition, a drain should be placed near the ureter draining the retroperitoneal area.

At times the ureter may be partially transected or crushed. If at least one-third of the ureteral circumference is intact, any traumatized portion can be resected and the divided portion loosely sutured with 4-0 chromic catgut interrupted sutures leaving a ureteral catheter in place and draining the area as well (Fig. 3.13). This usually will heal without fistula or stricture formation.

When the ureter has been transected or a segment removed or so devitalized as to likely slough, a greater problem arises and a more difficult decision must be made as to how the injured ureter should be treated. First the operator must decide how much ureter has been lost or damaged and must be resected since devitalized tissue will not heal. The next

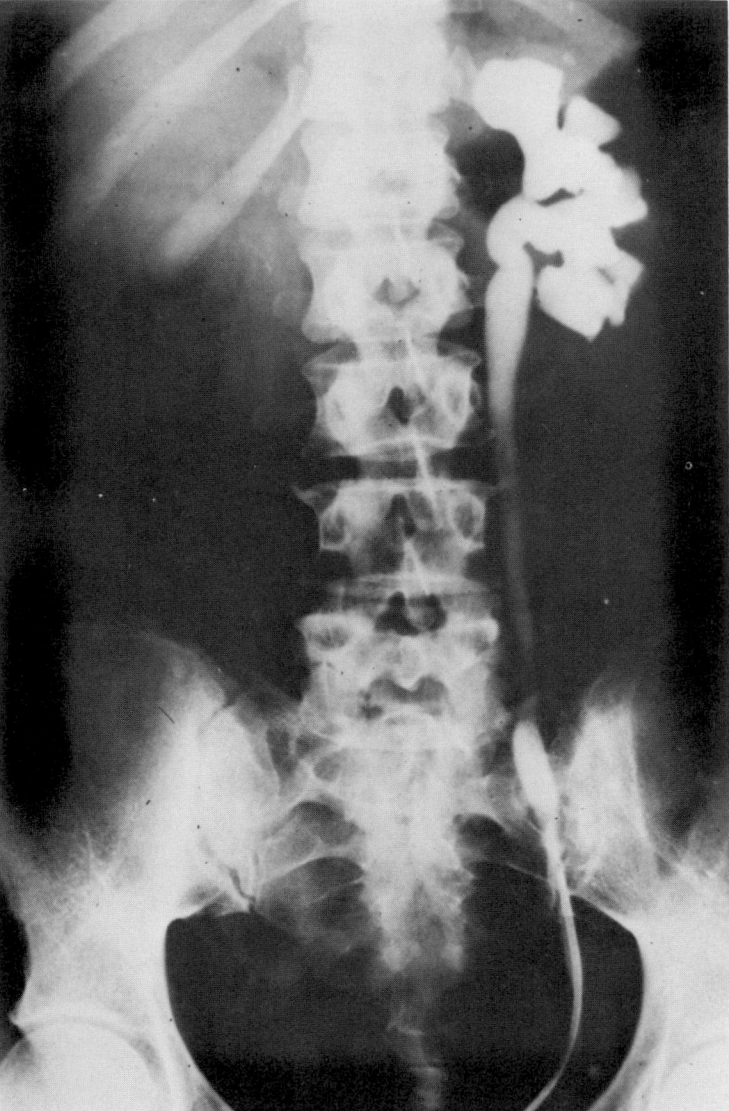

Fig. 3.9. Persistent left hydronephrosis 9 months following operation. (Courtesy Dr. H. S. Everett.)

important point is the level at which the ureter has been injured and the length of the ureteral defect. Finally the general condition of the patient at that point in the operation and her ultimate prognosis as indicated by the pathology present will determine the advisability of undertaking what may be an additional 30 to 60 minutes of operative time. If the patient has extensive carcinoma or other malignancy making a long term survival improbable and the other kidney seems to be normal, the wisest course is to ligate the ureter unless the defect can be repaired easily. If the kidney is not infected, the ligated kidney rapidly ceases to function and rarely causes trouble.

Ureterovesical Anastomoses

In correcting defects in the lower ureter, it is generally believed better to anastomose the ureter to the bladder rather than do a ureteroureteral anastomosis. The bladder wall has a better blood supply, will hold sutures better, and the anastomoses is more likely to heal without stricture formation. There are a variety of methods of effecting a ureterovesical anas-

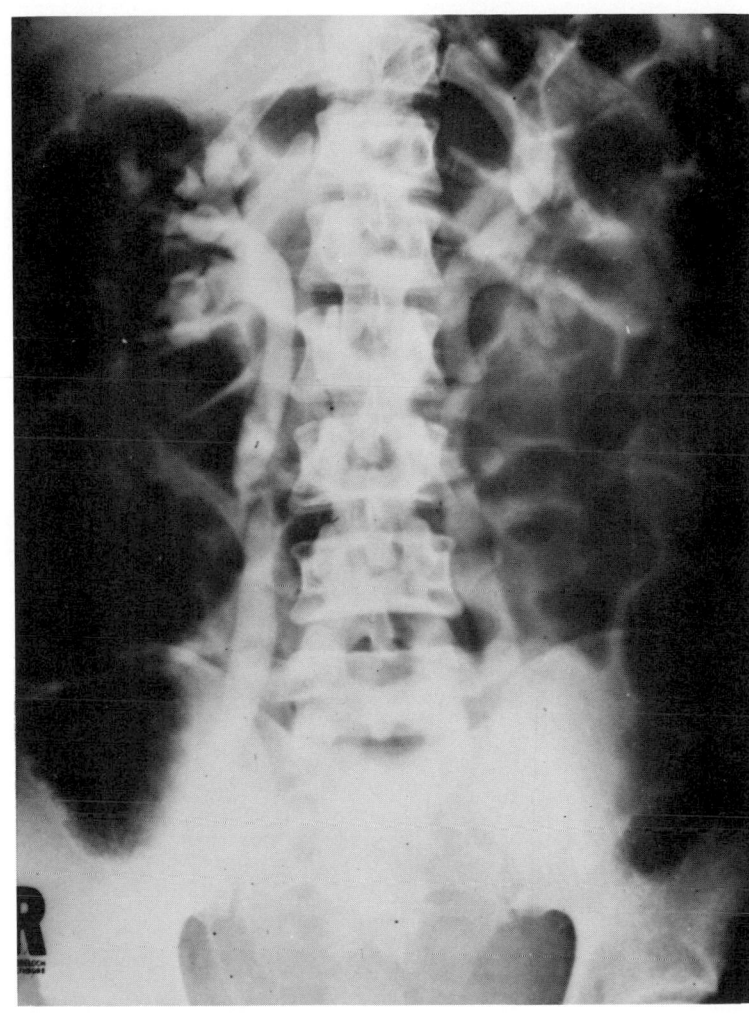

Fig. 3.10. Large pelvic abscess, before operation. Bilateral hydroureter and hydronephrosis. (Courtesy Dr. H. S. Everett.)

tomoses. The simplest is to bring the proximal end of the ureter to the nearest point in the bladder wall that can be reached without tension. At times the bladder must be mobilized to some degree to do this, but it is surprising how much the bladder can be shifted laterally and upward to avoid tension on the suture line. When this is done the bladder should be fixed by sutures to the pelvic wall and the psoas muscle to maintain its new position. An incision sufficiently large to accommodate the ureter easily is then made directly through all layers of the bladder wall at the selected spot. A # 7F Teflon catheter, polyethylene or silastic tube if available of comparable size is passed up the ureter to the kidney pelvis, and the distal end of the catheter is passed into the bladder where it can be coiled

and retrieved later by cystoscopy. Preferably the end of the Foley catheter can be pulled upward through the bladder incision and the end of the ureteral catheter tied to its tip so that the ureteral catheter may be withdrawn through the urethra at the end of the operation or even during the procedure under direct control so that the catheter is not withdrawn from the kidney pelvis.

Two longitudinal slits each about 1 cm long are made in the end of the ureter "fish-mouthing" it (Fig. 3.14). A suture of 000 chromic catgut is placed through the middle of each of these ureteral flaps leading the end of the ureter into the bladder and then bringing the ends of the sutures out through the bladder wall on either side of the incision. Any defect in the bladder wall is closed with 00 chromic catgut

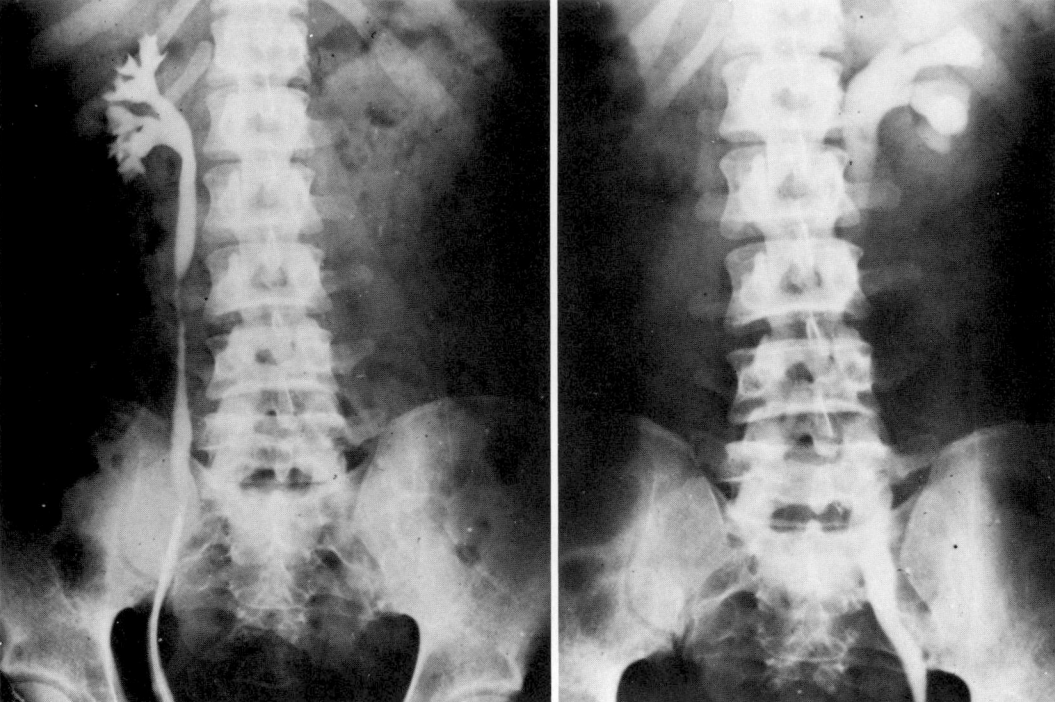

Figs. 3.11 (left) and 3.12 (right). Same as Figure 3.10. Postoperative, showing marked improvement on right but less improvement in left kidney with moderate residual hydronephrosis. (Courtesy Dr. H. S. Everett.)

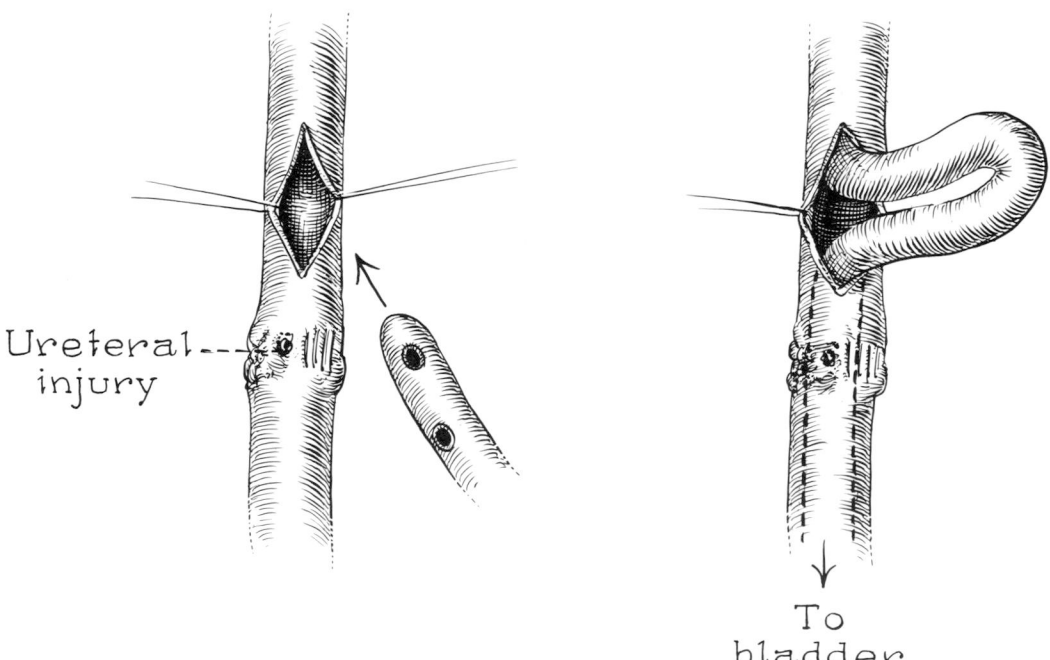

Fig. 3.13. Splinting an injured ureter. A longitudinal incision is made in the ureter 3 to 4 cm above injury and catheter passed up to kidney pelvis, and down through the injured area into the bladder.

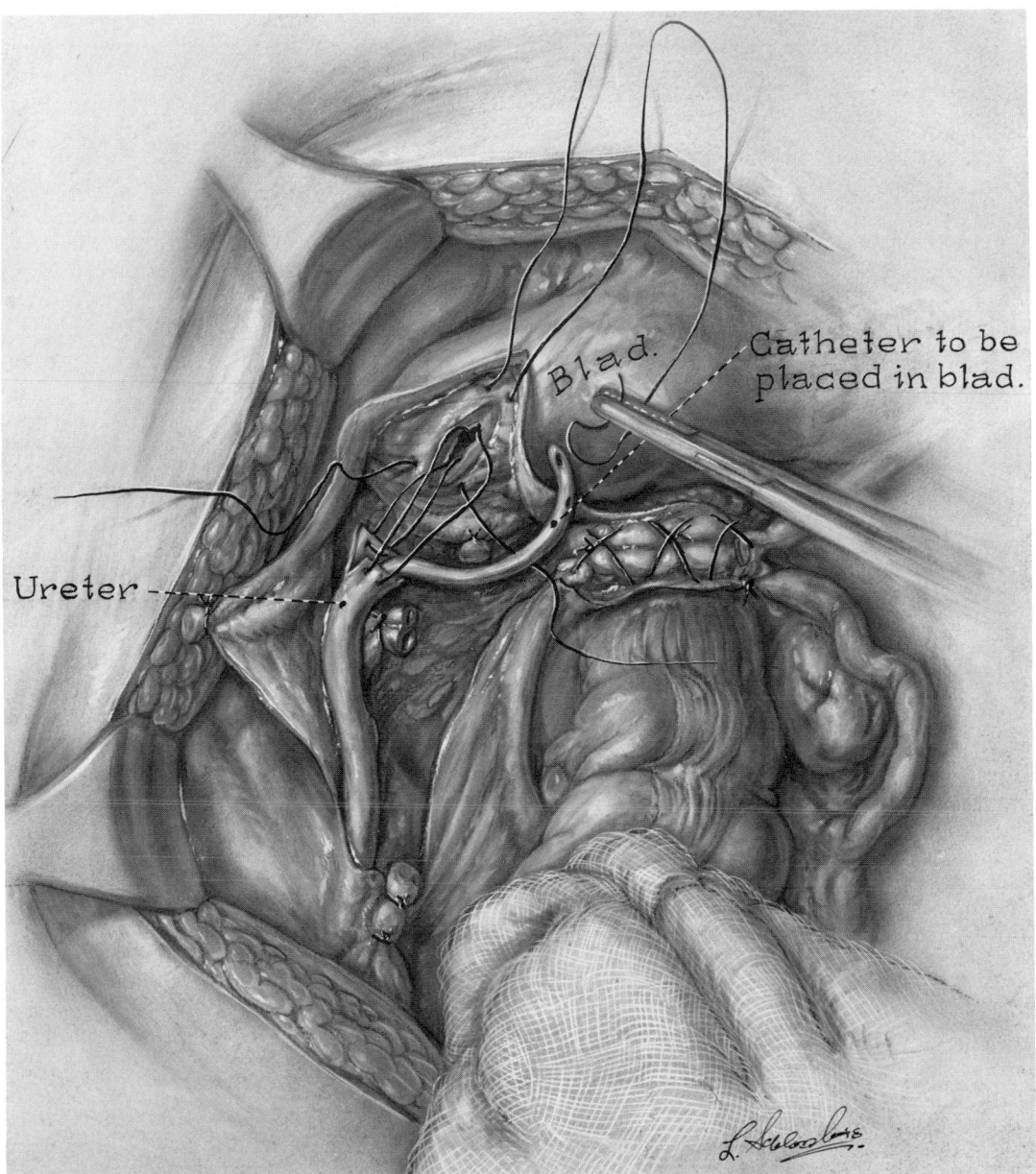

Fig. 3.14. Beginning ureterovesical anastomosis.

interrupted sutures (Fig. 3.15). The ureteral wall is then anchored to the bladder wall to prevent tension with interrupted 000 chromic catgut sutures through the ureteral and bladder serosa. The area should be drained and the ureteral and Foley catheter left in place about 10 days.

One objection to this simplest ureterovesical anastomoses is that it may permit vesicoureteral reflux and renal damage. This seems to be an infrequent problem, and often the simplest and shortest method of correction is the wisest course. An oblique tunnel may be made in the bladder wall through which the end of the ureter may be passed. Another incision is required in the bladder wall to allow a mucosa-to-mucosa anastomosis between ureter and bladder (Fig. 3.16). Additional serosa-to-serosa reinforcing sutures should be placed, and as before the anastomosis should be done with a ureteral catheter left in place. This is a somewhat more lengthy operative procedure and requires a little more ureter to effect the repair but does create a valve-like action which helps prevent vesicoureteral reflux.

If the ureter is too short to reach the bladder without tension even by mobilizing the bladder, then the possibility of creating a bladder flap as described by Ockerblad (21) to bridge the gap should be considered. At times 3 to 5 cm of flap can be obtained by this manner and is probably preferable to a ureteroureteral anastomosis (Figs. 3.17 through 3.19).

Ureteroureteral Anastomoses

When the area of ureteral damage is above the point where it is not possible or practical to join the ureter to the bladder, the preferred method, then ureteroureteral anastomosis is the next best choice provided the gap between the divided ends is not too great. The damaged

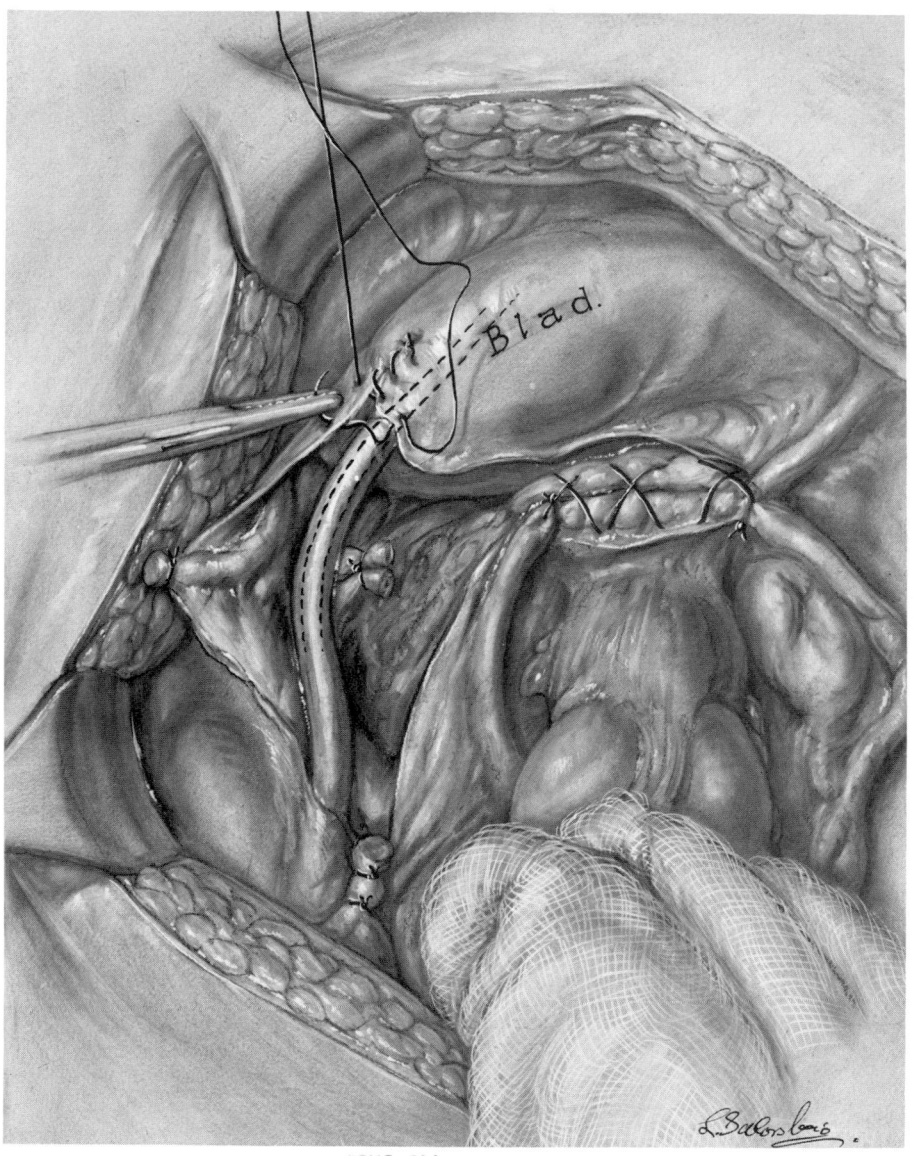

Fig. 3.15. Completion of ureterovesical anastomosis.

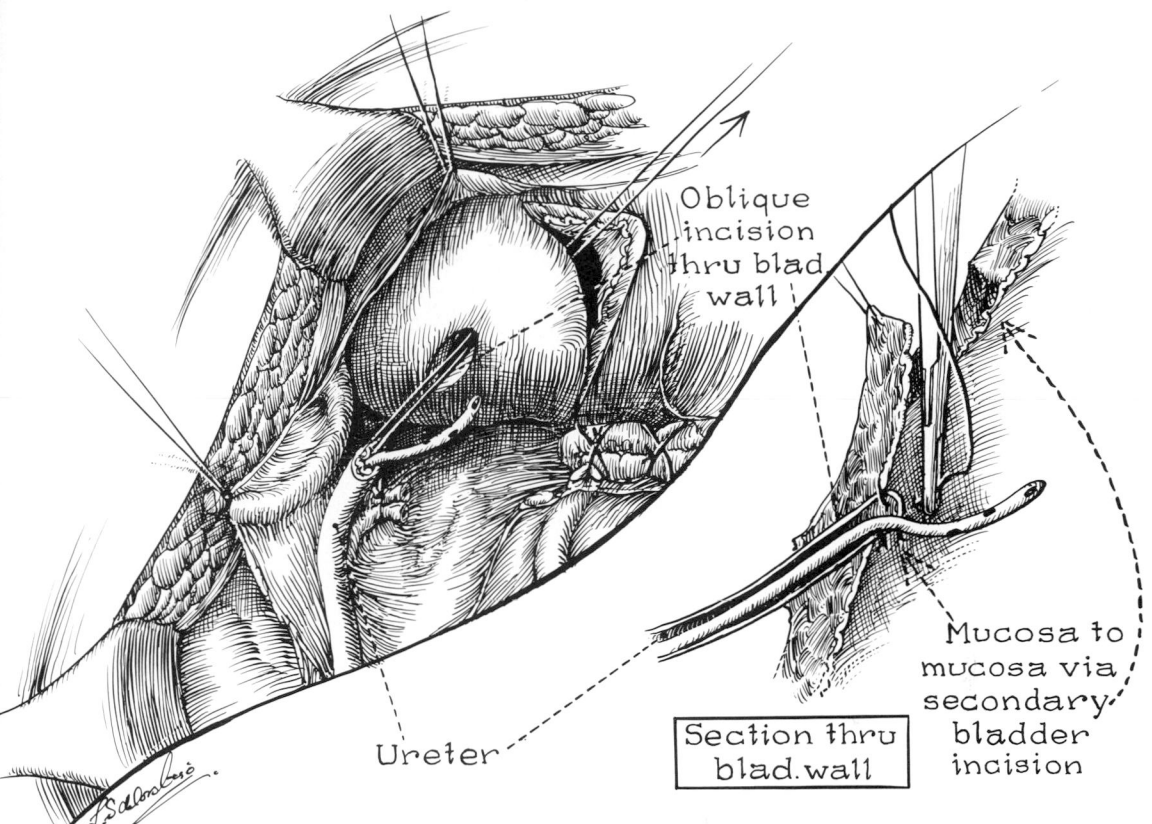

Fig. 3.16. Alternative oblique ureterovesical anastomosis.

portions of the ureter should be excised and the ureter mobilized only if additional length is needed. Excessive dissection may jeopardize the blood supply. Many techniques of uretero-ureteral anastomosis have been described, but generally the preferred method is an end-to-end anastomoses making the suture line oblique rather than directly across the ureter. It should be done with 000 or 0000 interrupted chromic catgut sutures, and there is general agreement that extraperitoneal drainage of the site is essential although the drain should not touch the ureter.

Most operators prefer to use a ureteral catheter as a splint for about 10 to 14 days afterwards, but other possibilities are a ureterostomy above the suture line, splinting the anastomosis with a T tube. Weinberg and Siebens (27) have shown, however, that ureteral peristalsis is better when no splinting catheter passes through the anastomosis, and the former prefers a ureterostomy about 5 cm above the injury with drainage by a T tube which does not pass through the anastomosis.

If ureteroureteral or ureterovesical anastomosis is unwise because of the patient's physical condition or impractical because of the length or level of ureteral division and the surgeon intends to repair the injury at a later date rather than ligate the ureter, a tubed ureterostomy can be done leaving the ureter in place and conveying the urine to the abdominal wall through the retroperitoneal space by way of a catheter. This is preferable to a cutaneous ureterostomy, another alternative, since the latter requires some dissection of the ureter and later will require some loss of ureteral length when repair is attempted. The tubed ureterostomy does not sacrifice any of the ureter which may be needed later.

Ureteral Injury Recognized after Operation

It is certain that many ureters have been ligated during pelvic surgery and never have produced symptoms or been recognized. A

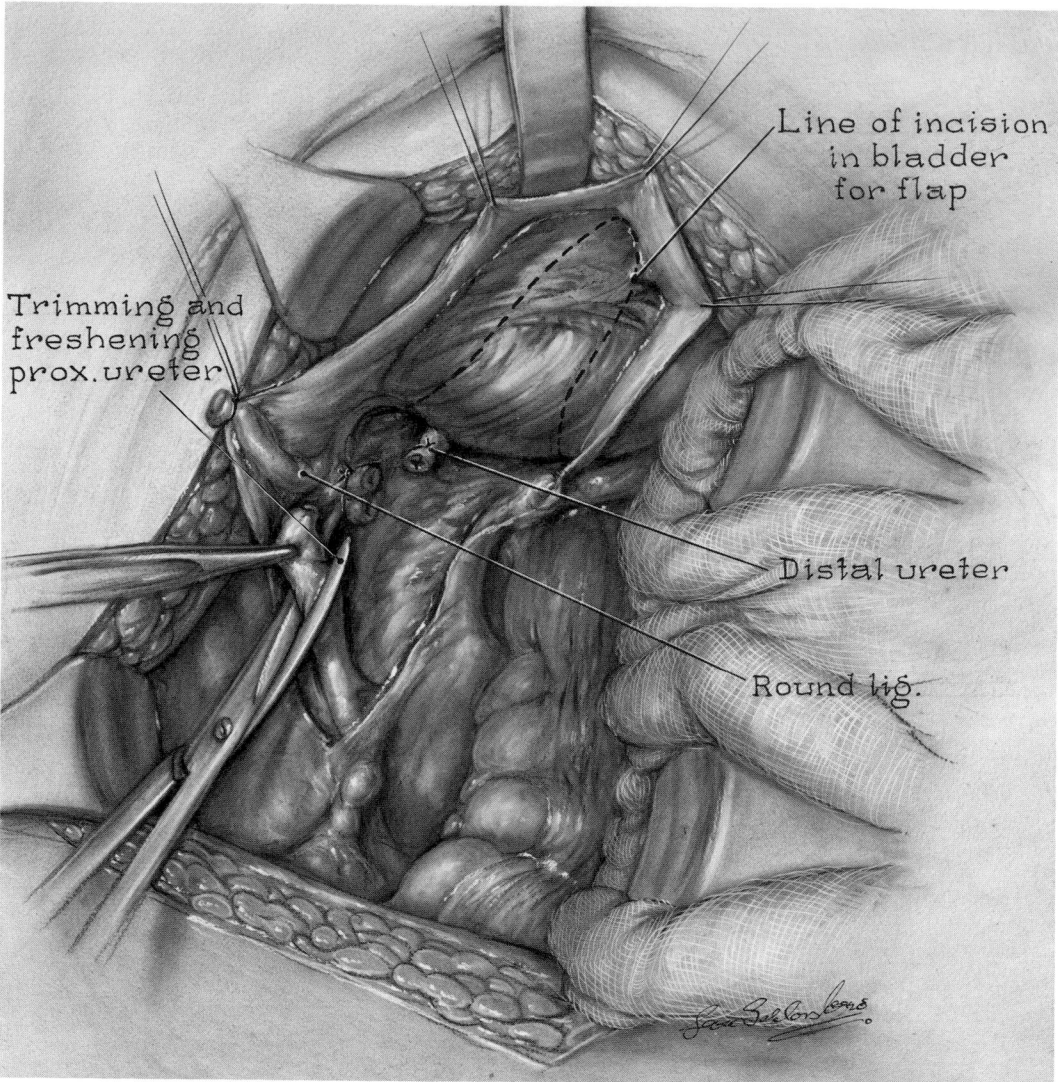

Fig. 3.17. Incision outlined to begin a bladder flap to bridge defect between end of injured ureter and bladder.

partially obstructed ureter is more likely to produce symptoms than a completely occluded ureter unless the kidney becomes infected. Postoperative fever, chills, possibly pyuria, and flank pain suggest urinary tract infection, and if prompt response to appropriate antibiotics does not occur, the urinary tract should be investigated by intravenous pyelograms. Bilateral ureteral ligation naturally produces anuria.

Ureteral fistulae make their appearance usually anywhere from 4 to 21 days after operation. The possibilities are ureteroperitoneal, ureteroretroperitoneal, ureteroabdominal, and ureterovaginal fistulae. Progressive distention and ascites may indicate a ureteroperitoneal fistula with urinary ascites. Fever, gaseous distention, and an abdominal or lateral pelvic mass could indicate a retroperitoneal mass which might be a hematoma, abscess, or urine extravasation. The retroperitoneal collection of urine ultimately may drain through the abdominal incision's drainage site, if one has been made, or vaginally. Drainage of urine through the incision or vagina often originates from ureteral injuries, but the possibility of a bladder fistula must be considered also.

When such possibilities exist, the origin of the fistula should be identified. The first and easiest step is to instill a methylene blue solution into the bladder watching for its emergence through the fistulous tract. If this does not occur, the bladder probably is intact. Indigo carmine should then be injected intravenously, and its appearance through the fistulous tract confirms the presence of a urinary fistula probably of ureteral origin. Intravenous pyelograms then should be obtained. From these it can be determined which ureter is involved and equally important whether there is any significant obstruction to the ureter and beginning hydronephrosis. It is important to remember that in some cases both the ureter and bladder may be injured or that the ureter may be damaged at the ureterovesical junction creating both ureterovaginal and vesicovaginal fistulae.

If injury of either the bladder or ureter is suspected, cystoscopy should be the next step in the diagnostic process. The bladder should be checked carefully, but if the problem arises a short time after a difficult surgical procedure, the bladder wall may be edematous, inflamed, or distorted by perivesical inflammation or masses and a fistula may be difficult to see. The ureter on the affected side should be catheterized if possible. The catheter should be passed as far as possible to determine the point of ureteral damage or ligation. Occasionally one will be fortunate and able to pass a catheter beyond the point of injury or obstruction to the kidney. If one has such good fortune, leave the catheter in place splinting it with a retaining Foley catheter for at least 2 weeks or longer. Drainage of urine through the fistula should then cease and the fistula will probably close. The possibility of subsequent stricture formation at the site of injury must be considered and follow-up intravenous pyelograms should be obtained over the subsequent months.

At times when ureteral catheterization is unsuccessful, which is usually the case, the vaginal drainage of urine may cease in a few weeks. It is possible that spontaneous closure of the fistula has occurred but intravenous pyelograms should be obtained promptly to be certain that with the closure of the fistula, the ureter has not also been obstructed and that renal function has been preserved.

If the ureterovaginal fistula persists with little or no damage to the kidney, attempts at surgical correction should be postponed for at least 6 weeks to allow the other pelvic tissues to heal and the patient to recover from her operation. She should be watched carefully but as long as there is satisfactory drainage of urine, irreparable damage to the kidney is unlikely. Then when the pelvic tissues and the patient are in better condition, repair of the ureterovaginal fistula usually by ureteroneocystotomy can be undertaken with a good chance of success.

The treatment of ureterovaginal fistula, although at times complicated, is less difficult than the treatment of a ligated or obstructed ureter which is not draining because there is no fistula. It is certain that there will be progressive damage to the affected kidney and that if the obstruction is not relieved within a matter of a few weeks, the kidney will no longer function. It is not certain how long this will take, but if infection is present in the kidney at the same time, the matter becomes quite urgent.

It should be kept in mind, however, that in many instances there may be some postoperative ureteral dilatation without ureteral injury. This frequently occurs after extensive ureteral dissection as in a radical hysterectomy and may occur with a pelvic cellulitis, abscess of hematoma, or the ureteral dilatation may have existed prior to surgery. There may be some edema and angulation of the ureter, and it is quite probable that the ureter eventually will be more or less normal without further surgery.

It is imperative that the degree of patency or obstruction of the ureter be determined by cystoscopy and ureteral catheterization. If the catheter passes the point of obstruction, it should be left in place to allow the periureteral inflammation to subside or the suture part way through the ureter to disintegrate, assuming it is catgut.

If a catheter cannot be passed through the obstructed area, it becomes essential that the obstruction be relieved promptly. It is even more urgent if both ureters are obstructed. The means of effecting this remains controversial. There are two basic choices to be made: (1) immediate laparotomy with removal of the suture and repair of the ureter if necessary or (2) diversion by means of a nephrostomy or pyelostomy with repair of the ureter at a later date.

The thought of immediate deligation is appealing in that it solves the problem and another operative procedure is not required. Furthermore, it has been successfully accomplished in a few isolated cases. Unfortunately, most patients with ureteral ligation or injury have had difficult surgical procedures from which they still have not stabilized, much less recovered. Also the local reaction about the ureter must be considered. The tissues certainly will be edematous and possibly necrotic with hematomas or exudate.

The suture encircling the ureter may also contain blood vessels and its release may lead to hemorrhage again. Also while attempting to remove the suture, the ureter may be torn or cut. The operation then would be a failure since the condition of the tissues would doom to failure a ureteral anastomosis or even a ureteroneocystotomy. Also, if there is loss of a portion of the ureter above or below the ligature, successful reconstruction is most unlikely.

For these reasons it is generally advisable to divert the urine by means of a nephrostomy or pyelostomy. After this, the suture may be absorbed, the edema may subside, and the ureter heal in a month or two. This should be confirmed by antegrade pyelography before **removing the nephrostomy** tube. Furthermore, if the ureter remains obstructed, the area can be explored electively when the patient is in optimal condition and the urinary diversion will protect the site of repair.

The type of repair will then be done under more favorable conditions, and the level at which the ureter is obstructed can be determined before surgery by cystoscopy and ureteral catheterization. An estimate can be made of the ureteral defect to be bridged or replaced. The reimplantation of the ureter into the bladder still remains the procedure of choice even if a flap or bladder is needed to reach the ureter. An end-to-end ureteral anastomosis should be done if the level of transection is too high to reach the bladder by any reasonable means. Anastomosis, usually end-to-the-side of the injured ureter to the intact opposite ureter, is a possibility, but should this not heal properly, then both ureters are damaged. The other possibility is the use of a segment of ileum to bridge the gap between the end of the

injured ureter and bladder. This procedure has considerable merit when a relatively long ureteral gap must be bridged and the only alternative is a nephrectomy. The latter should be done only when the other kidney is normal and the involved kidney seriously damaged or nonfunctioning. In short, every reasonable attempt should be made to salvage a good kidney in a patient with a normal life expectancy. Extensive reconstructive surgery is hardly worthwhile in a patient dying of ovarian cancer or some equally malignant disease.

In all forms of ureteral repair, ureteroureteral anastomosis, ureterovesical anastomosis, ureteroileovesical anastomosis, the results should be excellent but the adequacy of the reconstruction should be followed by intravenous pyelograms prior to discharge from the hospital, at 3, 6, and 12 months later provided the repair is functioning well. Stricture and obstruction at the point of repair or anastomosis may develop many months later and if found early, can be remedied by ureteral dilatations. The importance of postoperative follow-up cannot be emphasized too strongly. Nephrectomy should be reserved for cases in which bridging of the ureteral defect cannot be done, a previous attempted repair has failed, or a prior diversion procedure was done because of inadequate knowledge of the function of the contralateral kidney. It also should be done in cancer patients in whom cure is impossible and in repaired cases with continued serious pyelonephritis, ureteral obstruction, cortical abscesses, or stones.

Postoperative Anuria

Failure of the patient to pass urine after an operation may be due to:

1. Urinary retention
   a. Nonfunctioning bladder
   b. Catheter obstruction
2. Shock
3. Dehydration, electrolyte inbalance
4. Bilateral ureteral obstruction

The monitoring of the urinary output of a patient after any operation is one of the keystones of good postoperative care. It represents the summation of the fluid, blood, and electrolyte balance; the stability of the cardiovascular system; and the integrity of the urinary tract.

Probably the most frequent reason for postoperative failure to pass urine is bladder atony and urinary retention. This may be encountered after any surgical procedure even in those completely unrelated to gynecology or urology with adequate fluid replacement. If there is no spontaneous voiding in 8 hours after surgery or if the patient complains of bladder pressure or discomfort at any time, she should be catheterized and the bladder emptied whenever necessary. In most instances bladder function returns promptly provided overdistention is not permitted and the nursing staff recognizes the importance of postoperative bladder care.

In all critically ill patients, those with extensive operative procedures and those with operations affecting the bladder (cystocele repair, vesical sphincter plication, Marshall-Marchetti operation, Goebell-Stoeckel operation, vesicovaginal fistula repair, and repair of bladder laceration), an indwelling Foley catheter and/or suprapubic cystotomy, and drainage of the bladder are advisable. Thus the hourly urinary output may be followed and bladder distention prevented.

If even with an indwelling catheter or suprapubic cystotomy tube or catheter, there is little or no urinary output after 4 to 6 hours, the possibility of a misplaced catheter or catheter obstruction should be considered. The catheter or cystotomy tube should be irrigated with sterile normal saline or water ascertaining that the tubing is patent and not obstructed by blood clots or kinks and angulation. The operator must be certain that the catheter, particularly a cystotomy tube, is in the bladder. It may have been improperly inserted. The end of the cystotomy tube may be in the abdominal wall, perivesical space, or peritoneal cavity. Particularly in obese patients the end of the tube may have just penetrated the bladder wall and later have retracted out of the bladder. A Foley catheter is less likely to be improperly inserted, but it is conceivable that a false urethral passage may have been created at the operation or during insertion of the catheter and the end perforates the urethra and lies in the perivesical space. In such instances when the catheter is irrigated, there is no return of the irrigating fluid. The position can be checked by instilling a small amount of urographic dye solution and an X-ray taken. If the catheter is not in the bladder, then a new one should be used and free drainage of urine ascertained.

If the bladder indeed contains little or no urine, then the cause of the anuria or oliguria must be determined promptly. Any urine present should be checked for pH, specific gravity, protein, color, and microscopic urinalysis. Serum electrolytes, urea nitrogen, and bilirubin determinations should be obtained immediately. If the patient has been transfused, the possibility of a transfusion reaction or prior hypertension with renal damage must be considered. Providing fluid and electrolyte replacement has been adequate at that point, subsequent fluid replacement should be limited to insensible fluid loss and measured fluid loss such as urine, vomitus, and gastric suction. No potassium should be given to avoid hyperkalemia, and fluid should be replaced by 10 percent dextrose in water alone until kidney function returns.

The possibility of inadequate blood and fluid replacement must be considered also. The patient may have been hypovolemic before surgery due to blood loss, vomiting, diarrhea, or fluid trapped in the bowel due to obstruction or ileus and peritoneal fluid with peritonitis. Blood volume measurement may be helpful and packed red cells used to correct the deficit. To prevent overloading, the central venous pressure should be followed carefully with volume and rate of blood and fluid replacement guided by this, the electrolyte studies, fluid loss, and urinary output when it returns.

In many instances there may be multiple possible reasons for oliguria or anuria. These usually are seriously ill, complicated cases probably having fluid balance problems, shock, hemorrhage, transfusions, infection, and extensive and often difficult surgery. The possibility of bilateral ureteral obstruction must also be excluded by passing a catheter up one ureter to establish its patency. If one ureter is patent, the anuria then is due to a cause other than ureteral obstruction and the other ureter should not be catheterized. If the catheter will not pass up one ureter, the catheterization of the other should be attempted. Occasionally a catheter will pass through the area of obstruction whether it be due to edema, angulation, or an encircling suture. In such a fortuitous event, the ureteral catheter should be left in place.

When it is clear that both ureters are obstructed, an immediate nephrostomy or pyelostomy should be done. Since such patients are usually in rather precarious condition from their surgery, it is generally more prudent to do a unilateral nephrostomy on the better kidney if the preoperative status of either kidney is known. Urinary output then is established at least from one kidney and in a few days when the patient's condition is improved, the other kidney can be operated upon to relieve its obstruction by nephrostomy.

Then with both kidneys functioning well, the patient can recover from her operation, the damage to the urinary tract can be evaluated, and final repair or reconstruction can be attempted 6 to 8 weeks later when the chances of success are greater.

Intestinal and Adnexal Surgery

The bowel, both large and small, frequently are involved in and complicate adnexal surgery. This is equally true prior to, during, and after surgery and also in the terminal stages of malignancy, particularly ovarian carcinoma or following irradiation therapy.

Preoperative

The preoperative bowel problems a gynecologist is most likely to encounter are usually the result of peritonitis particularly from a ruptured tubo-ovarian abscess or the exacerbation of old pelvic inflammatory disease. A ruptured extrauterine pregnancy producing varying degrees of ileus is a relatively minor factor when compared to the intraperitoneal hemorrhage and shock. Also a patient with extensive ovarian carcinoma may present herself with marked abdominal distention due to ascites, but in addition there may be some degree of intestinal obstruction. These bowel problems, although secondary to the primary pelvic pathology, require remedy and complicate the management of the patient.

Accompanying the peritonitis of pelvic inflammatory disease will be varying degrees of ileus depending on the duration of the acute process, and in addition there frequently is an obstructive factor as loops of small bowel adherent to the pelvic abscess develop angula-

tions, adhesive bands, and partial or complete obstruction follows. With this, hypovolemia follows and, in addition, hypochloremic alkalosis with protracted vomiting. In any case laparotomy cannot be delayed very long since the mortality rises rapidly with the passage of time. A Cantor or Miller-Abbott tube should be passed immediately to start intestinal decompression; intravenous fluids, usually 5 percent glucose in normal saline or 0.45 percent normal saline, with large doses of penicillin or cephalothin (Keflin) added should be used until more specific electrolyte replacement can be determined by the serum electrolyte values. Blood may be needed to combat shock or anemia, and surgery should follow as soon as possible.

Operative Problems

Both the large and small bowel present problems which every gynecologist should be prepared to handle in pelvic surgery. The most common one involves adherent loops of small or large bowel adhesions. These are almost always present in pelvic inflammatory disease and frequently follow prior operations, endometriosis, and ovarian cancer.

In many instances the adhesive bands can be divided easily with Metzenbaum scissors. At other times the operator may encounter a tangled mass of bowel totally obscuring the pelvic organs. Such situations require patience to release the entangled loops with sharp dissection to the point where the pelvic organs can be identified and the proposed pelvic surgery eventually started. Particularly in the case of acute or subacute pelvic inflammatory disease and even more so in tuberculous salpingitis, extreme caution is needed. The bowel wall often is inflamed, edematous, possibly distended, and even partially or completely obstructed. Rough or careless handling will then lead to rents in wall, possibly considerable damage to the bowel, further peritoneal contamination, and possible fistula formation.

Small serosal lacerations usually require no repair but whenever the muscularis and/or the mucosa is torn, repair should be done immediately to prevent peritoneal contamination. The repair if possible should be made transversely rather than longitudinally to avoid as much as possible any narrowing of the lumen. A two-layer closure is made if possible using 000 chromic catgut on the mucosa and muscularis and 000 or 0000 interrupted silk sutures on the serosa. At times the bowel wall may have been so badly damaged or the blood supply compromised that it must be resected.

Often the sigmoid colon and rectum are adherent to adnexal masses and the posterior surface of the uterus or they make up part of the wall of pelvic abscesses. One should not try to remove all the abscess wall from the bowel. It is much better to leave abscess wall on the bowel than remove bowel wall with the abscess. Ragged areas can be trimmed but do not expect to leave a neat, tidy pelvis. Peritonize as well as possible. Often this can be best accomplished by obliterating the cul-de-sac and using the sigmoid to cover this area to keep small bowel out of the pelvis.

In inflammatory processes in the pelvis, usually only the serosa is involved, but when endometriosis or carcinoma is present, the bowel wall may be invaded deeply or extensively. In the case of endometriosis, if both ovaries are removed and the bowel lumen is not narrowed, the area can be left alone. On the other hand, if the patient is young and ovarian function is retained, it is better to resect the area of endometrial involvement. If this is not done, the endometrioma may increase in size and lead to intestinal obstruction. At times when there is extensive bowel infiltration by endometriosis causing narrowing of the lumen, this area should be resected even if the ovaries are removed. It is quite likely that further fibrosis and scarring with castration will cause more narrowing of the lumen and obstruction (Figs. 3.18 and 3.19).

An incorrect interpretation of preoperative abnormalities can lead many pelvic surgeons astray. Just as the differential diagnosis of right lower quadrant pain in a woman can be a considerable challenge, so may the presence of some pelvic masses, particularly those in the left adnexal region. Of particular importance is the differentiation of adnexal disease from diseases of the intestinal tract, particularly of the sigmoid colon. Diverticulitis with or without perforation and abscess formation and carcinoma of the colon frequently may feel like ovarian tumors or inflammatory masses and in many instances the patient will not have any symptoms pointing to a bowel problem.

Of course, preoperative sigmoidoscopy and a barium enema are very important studies and should help distinguish bowel lesions from adnexal disease. Such studies should be done whenever it is suspected that such a problem may exist. Nevertheless, there still will be occasions when the gynecologist will find that his ovarian tumor in fact is sigmoid diverticulitis or cancer and that his preoperative diagnosis is wrong. How should he proceed at this point?

The course he chooses will be affected by many factors. One is the operator's own experience and ability to handle the problem himself; two is the immediate availability of advice from a surgeon competent himself in this area and above all how are the best interests of the patient served? Although the patient should have had her lower bowel well cleaned out by her preoperative enema, the bowel has not been prepared with preoperative antibiotics such as neomycin, Sulfathalidine, of kanamycin as one normally would do in anticipation of a possible bowel resection.

If the gynecologist must fall back on his own resources in the absence of a surgical consultant (they are not always available, particularly when you need them most), he must elect one of several options open to him. First he must establish the diagnosis. Is the lesion inflammatory or neoplastic and is it resectable? If cancer, are there metastases? Whatever course he elects, this information is essential.

His choices are basically to determine first if the lesion is operable or not. If it can be removed, the gynecologist then can:

1. Close the abdomen with the plan to have definite surgery done later after the bowel has been prepared.

2. Do a colostomy but no resection. This relieves any obstruction and allows the bowel to be prepared for later resection. The colostomy should not be done in such a way as to make a later resection and anastamosis more difficult. A transverse colostomy may be the best choice.

3. Resect the lesion and (a) do a primary anastomosis or (b) do a colostomy with the intention of closing the colostomy and reconnecting the bowel ends later when the conditions are better.

Which of these options he elects will depend on the patient's general condition, the type and

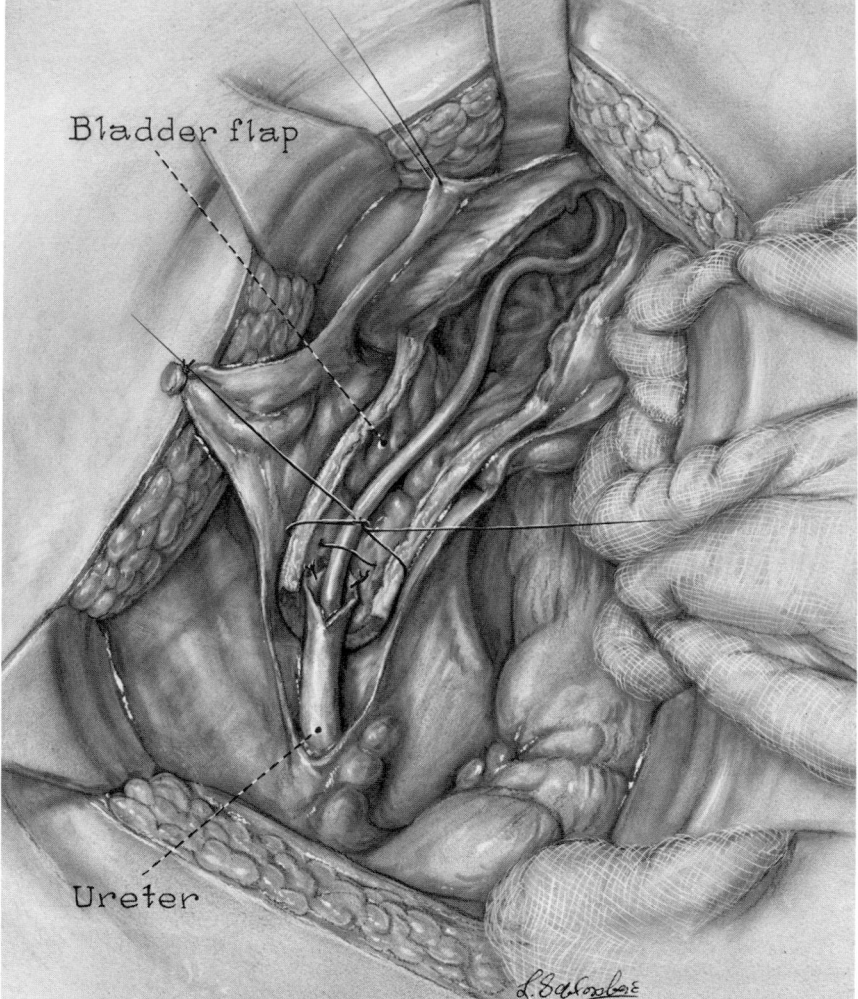

Fig. 3.18. End of ureter with splinting's catheter in place is sutured to superior portion of bladder flap.

extent of the pathology, and the operator's training and ability to handle the situation.

Postoperative Bowel Problems

Prevention of all postoperative nausea, vomiting, and distention would be utopia, but in most instances, serious problems can be avoided. The postoperative care of the intestinal tract must be individualized according to the type of surgery done, the condition of the peritoneal cavity (clean case *vs.* peritonitis or hemoperitoneum), the degree of bowel involvement at operation, and finally on the return of bowel sounds and the passage of gas per rectum.

In the simple uncomplicated pelvic laparot-omy, the patient's diet may progress in a matter of 2 or 3 days from water to clear liquids to a soft diet and ultimately to a regular diet. In cases in which distention is likely (peritonitis or hemoperitoneum), a nasogastric tube should be passed during or at the end of the operation and the patient maintained only on intravenous fluids until bowel sounds return. The same would be true for cases where the bowel has been injured, repaired, or resected except that it might be better to pass a Cantor or Miller-Abbott tube and leave it in longer to allow the bowel to heal.

When distention, nausea, or vomiting develop postoperatively, the possibility of intestinal obstruction instead of adynamic ileus must be considered. Usually obstruction develops later

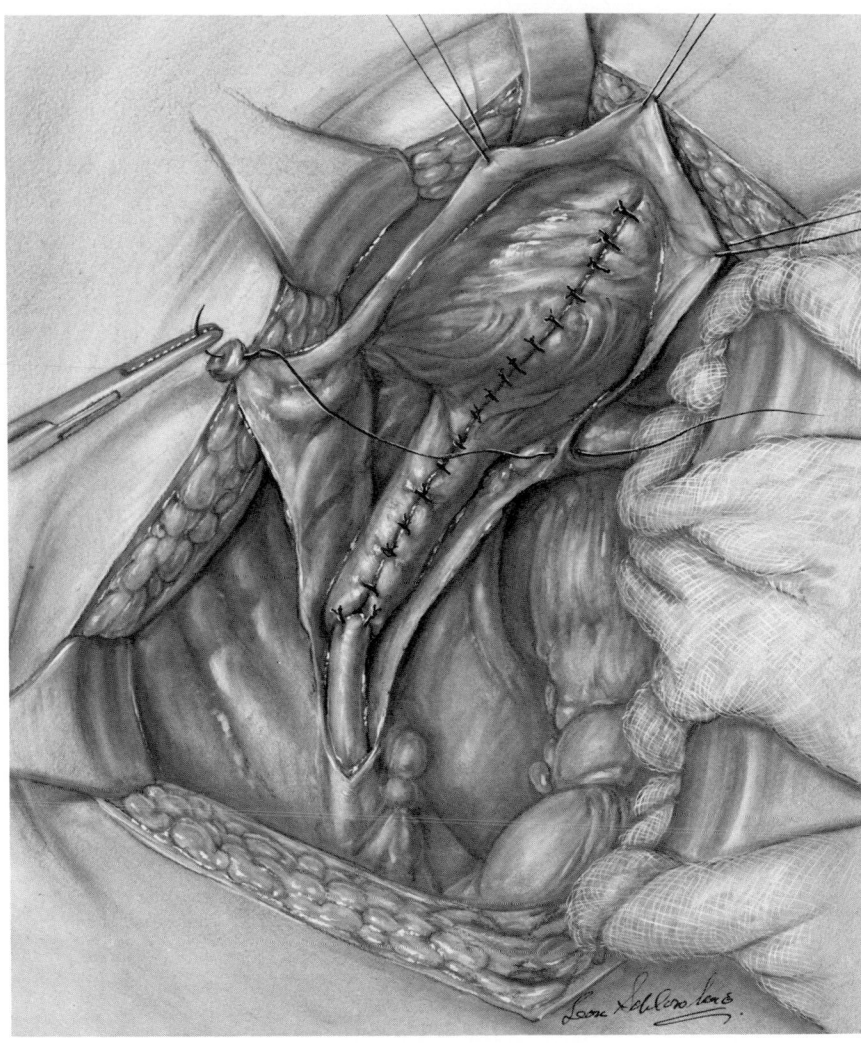

Fig. 3.19. Completion of Ockerblad flap procedure by peritonizing the area if possible.

after operation than ileus and differs in that there are cramping abdominal pains and abnormal bowel sounds with peristaltic rushes or high pitched tinkles. Also, flat and upright X-rays of the abdomen may show distended loops of bowel with fluid levels and little gas beyond the area of obstruction.

Nasogastric suction with careful control of fluid and electrolyte balance are important in the treatment of either. Rectal tubes, enemas, and often Prostigmin given at the proper time may speed the recovery from ileus but certainly the latter is not appropriate in intestinal obstruction. Often in gynecologic surgery, particularly in cases of pelvic inflammatory disease, loops of small bowel become adherent, inflamed, and edematous causing a partial

rather than complete obstruction. This frequently can be resolved by conservative treatment decompressing the distended bowel and allowing the edema and inflammatory reaction to subside. The possibility of complete obstruction must always be considered. If the patient's response to a conservative treatment is not satisfactory in a very few hours or she develops fever suggesting the possibility of gangrenous bowel, immediate laparotomy becomes essential.

Recapitulation of Common Errors

Adnexa

a. Failure to examine patient under anesthesia

immediately before laparotomy

b. Inadequate preoperative investigation and preparation

c. Insufficient incision for operative procedure to be undertaken

d. Failure to recognize exact pathologic process leading to excessive or inadequate surgery

e. Direct damage to bowel, ureter, or bladder during dissection of adherent adnexal masses

f. Delay in operating on ruptured tubo-ovarian abscesses and ectopic pregnancies

g. Failure to select optimal time to operate on chronic pelvic inflammatory disease

h. Inadequate or excessive fluid and blood administration before, during, and after surgery

i. Inappropriate antibiotic therapy

Ureter

a. Failure to know exact position of ureter at all times during pelvic surgery or placing clamps and sutures without knowing position of ureter

b. Failure to recognize ureteral injury immediately, incorrectly evaluating and repairing injury

c. Failure to recognize urinary tract injury after operation

d. Failure to insure adequate drainage for injury to urinary tract

e. Ureteroureteral or ureterovesical anastomosis done with tension on suture lines

f. Failure to protect kidneys from damage when ureter is injured

g. Selection of wrong time to correct urinary tract injury

h. Selection of wrong procedure or technique to correct urinary tract injury

Bowel

a. Prevention of bowel injury by careful dissection

b. Failure to recognize immediately and repair injured bowel

c. Pre- and postoperative bowel decompression when needed

d. Failure to prepare bowel before surgery which may involve bowel

e. Failure to distinguish between mechanical obstruction and ileus—at times very difficult

Anuria

a. Failure to recognize anuria or oliguria after operation

b. Failure to determine cause of anuria and to correct it

Bibliography

1. Abdel-Shahid, R. B., Beresford, J. M., and Curry, R. H.: Endometriosis of the ureter with vascular involvement. Obstet. Gynec. 43: 113, 1974.

1a. Beahrs, O. W., Hunter, S. J., Jr., and Schloss, P. T.: Intramural obstructing endometriosis of the ureter. Proc. Staff Meet. Mayo Clin. 32: 73, 1957.

2. Benson, R. C., and Hinman, F., Jr.: Urinary tract injuries in obstetrics and gynecology. Am. J. Obstet. Gynecol. 78: 467, 1955.

3a. Bunkin, I. A.: *In* Bergman, H.: *The Ureter*, Chapt. 23, p. 531. Hoeber Med. Div., Harper and Row, New York, 1967.

3. Burnes, E., and Peisa, I.: Treatment of urologic complications in gynecology. J. Urol. 75: 338, 1956.

4. Caughlan, G. J.: Ureterovaginal fistula. Repair of ureteral defect by use of a bladder flap. J. Urol. 58: 428, 1947.

5. Cavanagh, D., Clark, P. J., and McLeod, A. G. W.: Septic shock of endotoxin type. Am. J. Obstet. Gynecol. 102: 13, 1968.

6. Chin, J., Horton, R. K., and Rusche, C.: Unilateral ureteral obstruction as sole manifestation of endometriosis. Trans. West. Sect. Am. Urol. Assn. 23: 181, 1956.

7. Conger, K., and Beecham, C. T.: Ureteral injury in pelvic surgery. Obstet. Gynecol. 3: 181, 1956.

8. Coplan, M. M., Woods, F. M., and Melvin, P. D.: Surgical repair of the lower ureters and bladder which have been injured during pelvic surgery. J. Urol. 73: 390, 1955.

9. Counsellor, V. S., and Crenshaw, J. L.: A clinical and surgical review of endometriosis. Am. J. Obstet. Gynecol. 62: 930, 1951.

10. Everett, H. S.: Ureteroperitoneal fistula with urinary ascites. J. Urol. 78: 585, 1957.

11. Everett, H. S., and Mattingly, R. F.: Urinary tract injuries resulting from pelvic surgery. Am. J. Obstet. Gynecol. 71: 502, 1956.

12. Falk, H. C.: Urologic Injuries. F. A. Davis, Philadelphia, 1964.

13. Falk, H. C., and Bunkin, I. A.: Ureteral injuries. Prevention and management during gynecologic surgery for benign disease. Obstet. Gynecol. 4: 4, 1954.

14. Grayburn, R. W.: Ureteric obstruction due to endometriosis. J. Obstet. Gynaecol. Br. Commonw. 67: 74, 1960.

15. Hamm, F., Weinberg, S. R., and Waterhouse, K.: Repair of the injured ureter. A new technique for end-to-end anastomosis. Surgery 45: 575, 1959.

16. Lelly, H. A.: Resection and anastamosis of the divided ureter. JAMA 35: 860, 1900.

17. Kelly, H. A., and Bloodgood, S. C.: Uretero-ureteral anastamosis. Bull. Johns Hopkins Hosp. 4: 89, 1893.

18. Lee, R. A., and Symmonds, R. E.: Ureterovaginal fistula. Am. J. Obstet. Gynecol. 109: 1032, 1971.

19. Long, J. P., and Montgomery, J. B.: The incidence of ureteral obstruction in benign and malignant gynecological lesions. Am. J. Obstet. Gynecol. 32: 382, 1968.

19a. McCoy, J. B., and Bradford, W. Z.: Surgical treatment of endometriosis with conservation of reproductive potential. Am. J. Obstet. Gynecol., 87: 394, 1963.

20. Nebel, W. A., and Lucas, W. E.: Management of tubo-ovarian abscess. Obstet. Gynecol. 32: 382, 1968.

21. Ockerblad, N. F.: Reimplantation of the ureter into the bladder by a flap method. J. Urol. 57: 845, 1947.

22. Orkin, L. A.: Trauma to the Ureter. Pathogenesis and Management. F. A. Davis Co., Philadelphia, 1964.

23. Ratliff, R. K., and Crenshaw, W. B.: Ureteral obstruction from endometriosis. Surg. Gynecol. Obstet. 100: 414, 1955.

24. Rosenfeld, S. S., and Bergman, H.: Prevention of urological complications from injuries in gynecologic surgery. Obstet. Gynecol. 4: 562, 1954.

25. Vermeeren, J., and Te Linde, R. W.: Intra-abdominal rupture of pelvic abscess. Am. J. Obstet. Gynecol. 68: 402, 1954.

26. Weinberg, S. R., Peng, B., Kamhi, B., Ullman, A., and Hamm, F. C.: Improved regeneration of the ureter after division of the urine by proximal ureterotomy. J. Urol. 85: 749, 1961.

27. Weinberg, S. R., and Siebens, A. A.: Activity of the ureter after surgery. J. Urol. 80: 336, 1958.

CHAPTER FOUR

JOHN H. RIDLEY, M.D.

SURGERY FOR STRESS URINARY INCONTINENCE

Approximately 95 per cent of all clinically significant cases of stress urinary incontinence are seen in multiparous women. This suggests that the chief etiologic factor is tissue alteration by obstetrical trauma centered on the muscular and fascial structures about the bladder floor, bladder neck, and urethra. This original injury is further affected by the inexorable forces of gravity and aging. It is also aggravated by obesity, chronic pulmonary disease with cough, and extraordinary physical activity with abdominal straining. The remaining minority of cases of stress urinary incontinence, relatively few in number, is also due to tissue failure. However, these failures are caused by inherent weakness of the tissues and supporting structure—in effect, the gradual failure of tissue integrity.

Considering, therefore, that tissue alteration is the chief factor, reconstruction of anatomic changes and strengthening of weakened and torn tissues are the problems confronting the gynecologist. An assessment of the individual patient's particular problem will permit the surgeon to treat her by one of the several methods at hand.

This section will consider the three basic surgical approaches to the problem of stress urinary incontinence. Emphasis is placed on recognizing the potential points of error, how to safeguard against these errors, and how to salvage a failure or less-than-satisfactory final result.

Although there have been numerous modifications of the three basic procedures, the objectives and difficulties, which can affect practically all modifications, will be evaluated.

Historically, correction of stress urinary incontinence has been an interesting and well documented facet of gynecologic surgery for a hundred years. Also noteworthy is that the correction of stress urinary incontinence has never been completely satisfactory by any one means; and in a very small minority of cases, correction has defied all attempts even by the most competent surgeons. It has thus remained the challenge that we have today. Detailed historic reviews are to be found in many other textbooks, but in the interest of brevity a repetition of these reviews will not be undertaken except in instances in which a historic development is of technical interest.

In an appraisal of the success and failure of various efforts to correct stress urinary incontinence, certain basic principles of evaluation of the surgical problem at hand may have been abrogated and various technical errors may have been made.

An Adequate History

When the problem of stress urinary incontinence is presented, a careful and thorough questioning of the patient must be done. Under what circumstances is the leakage troublesome? Is it present only occasionally with violent abdominal muscular effort such as an explosive sneeze or cough, or does it occur more frequently with the ordinary straining during a usual routine day? Or is the stress incontinence nearly constant, necessitating the wearing of some protective clothing or pad? In some instances the patient leaks urine, not only with physical effort but at other times and even while sleeping, thus suggesting the possibility of a fistula somewhere in the urinary tract. Any one of these variations must be recognized and thoroughly understood by the operator.

Questioning must be done relative to the time of life of onset of the incontinence. Most likely it has followed, by some months or years, one or more vaginal deliveries. However, a patient with no obstetrical history may have the onset of stress urinary incontinence for no apparent reason or after some surgical procedure such as inappropriate transurethral resection of the bladder neck (1). Whatever the cause, it must be understood before a logical effort of correction can be done.

Differentiation of the type of incontinence is most important. Urinary leakage with muscular effort or stress is most frequently seen, and one may be erroneous in assuming that all cases of incontinence are due to simple tissue failure and anatomic alteration. However, urge incontinence, albeit relatively infrequent, is confusing and stubborn. Usually differential diagnosis can be detected by history alone, and one of the chief differential points of urge incontinence is that of having a nearly constant desire to void. On the other hand, stress urinary incontinence most frequently is not associated with a prodromal urge to void, but the patient leaks on muscular exertion. Failure to recognize urge incontinence is serious because no ordinary anatomic correction will cure it, a subject for full discussion below.

Neurogenic problems of micturition and continence are not to be overlooked. If these problems are not recognized and understood, the serious error or inappropriate surgical effort can aggravate the incontinence by further "obstruction" of the bladder neck with resulting increased bladder retention, atony, and overflow incontinence. An example is the complication of spina bifida occulta where improper motor and sensory innervation of the bladder is present. Usually not detected in earlier life and aggravated by the passage of time, spina bifida occulta is always suspect, even though a rare possibility. Its presence can be suggested by history and proven by simple urinary tract evaluation, to be discussed.

Urge incontinence, mentioned briefly above, deserves a more detailed discussion because of the ever present possibility of failure to recognize the condition. One must realize that urge incontinence, true stress incontinence, and fistulae may actually coexist in a single patient, although relatively rare.

The patient's history may reveal the presence of troublesome leakage, particularly during the day and under certain circumstances of environment or association. The mere thought of these emotionally distressing circumstances may cause the patient to have marked urinary frequency, urgency, and even incontinence. The consciousness of bladder distention is therefore heightened by emotional stress, triggering contractions of the detrusor muscle to the point of involuntary voiding. Therefore the gynecologist by careful history may find that he is dealing with a psychogenic situation not to be confused with true stress urinary incontinence.

In some instances, particularly in older women in whom stress urinary incontinence is seen more frequently, the condition of the spastic bladder, the generally contracted bladder, or the bladder of otherwise reduced capacity may be the confusing problem. This may result from the presence of the Hunner's ulcer of interstitial cystitis, or other inflammatory conditions causing reduced bladder capacity and increased bladder irritability. Not to be overlooked is the possible presence of urinary calculus, particularly of the bladder but also of the upper urinary tract; vesical neoplasms; and obstructive lesions. Urinary tract tuberculosis, albeit rarer now, can cause the bladder, by active process with resultant extensive scarring, to have marked urge incontinence. Whenever such pathology or derangements are even suspected, a comprehensive excretory and retrograde study must be done. Erroneous diagnosis of stress urinary incontinence therefore can result from inadequate and incomprehensive history evaluation.

Primary Physical Examination

This primary examination must be complete. Many findings other than those specifically of the urinary tract may be definitely contributory to the chief complaint of urinary tract dysfunction. The patient may exhibit pathology of the cardiovascular system with arteriosclerosis and hypertension. Definite emotional factors may be detected that would not only contribute to cardiovascular problems but also definitely to bladder dysfunction. Pulmonary tuberculosis may secondarily involve the urinary tract. Changes in the neurologic system may be detected by the ordinary gross neurologic tests that every practitioner should routinely do. An unusual finding will then alert him to seek further help from the neurologist.

Examination of the genitourinary system of the woman complaining of urinary incontinence must demand detailed evaluation of not only the history of other body systems but specifically of the abdominal and pelvic organs. The abdominal wall may reveal the scars of previous surgical procedures, some specifically directed to the urinary system, such as previous attempts to correct the very condition which is presented. There may have been a previous attempt at the retropubic urethropexy or a sling procedure, giving unsatisfactory results and causing subsequent difficulties by troublesome scar tissue formation. Incisions which might have been made for upper urinary tract pathology should alert the examiner to possible problems with bladder continence. Lower abdominal incisions, whatever the reason for their being, could give a clue to the problem of urinary incontinence whether it be of fistulous origin or of stress or urge origin. Varying amounts of postsurgical scarring will alter the bladder capacity and position, particularly of the trigone and bladder neck, and initiate bladder dysfunction. This is particularly true if the previous surgery was extensive, or possibly radical in nature.

Pelvic examination is, of course, the most important part of the evaluation. Vaginal relaxation is the most frequent finding in the patient who has complained of stress urinary incontinence, usually resulting from obstetrical trauma. The anterior vaginal wall support may show failure to a varying extent not necessarily proportionate to the amount of stress urinary incontinence. Indeed there may be scarcely a cystocele present, particularly in the nulligravida, but the amount of incontinence may be most troublesome (Fig. 4.1). Conversely, a pronounced anterior vaginal relaxation may have no stress leakage of urine at all (Fig. 4.2). Nevertheless, the presence of a cystocele, or the rarer cystourethrocele, is more frequently accompanied by the complaint of stress incontinence of varying degree. The presence of other changes in vaginal and uterine support, with different degrees of uterine prolapse, rectocele, or enterocele, may have a positive but secondary effect on bladder function. An error can be made technically in the failure to recognize and repair these concomitant failures of pelvic support. The presence of an enterocele can very easily go undetected.

Bimanual examination of the pelvis by abdominovaginal means, and, just as importantly, by abdominorectovaginal technique, will reveal pelvic masses of gynecologic or urologic origin which can cause altered bladder function. An overlying mass of a uterine myomata,

particularly with nodules growing beneath the bladder base (Fig. 4.3), or the pregnant uterus, either one can be a cause of a complaint. Ovarian masses causing ureteral and bladder displacement by the weight itself or by scar tissue formation can be contributory. Endometriosis is an offender which must not be overlooked in that it may directly affect the urinary tract itself. Manipulation of these pelvic findings, by application of pressure, displacement, or ballottement may duplicate the chief complaint, causing the involuntary loss of urine or creating the urge to void. This may be a factor not only in finding contributing pathology, but also distinguishing between urge incontinence and true stress incontinence. Another important point in making this distinction is the fact that true stress incontinence has no prefatory feeling of the bladder fullness and desire to empty the bladder whereas urge incontinence is preceded by this desire to void.

Evaluation of the Urinary Tract

This important part of the responsibility of the gynecologist does not transgress the domain of the urologic surgeon. To deal with all gynecourologic complaints, the competent gynecologist must be able to evaluate and treat the variety of urologic complaints that either arise from dysfunction or changes in the genital system, or are so interrelated anatomically, functionally, and physiologically that clear separation is impossible.

A midstream, clean-caught, voided bladder specimen is obtained from the patient at the time of the pelvic examination. She is then catheterized carefully, using adequate precautions. An aqueous solution of benzalkonium chloride (Zephiran) 1:750 is used about the external urethral meatus and vaginal introitus. The use of a small #16F metal or glass catheter minimizes trauma and the chance for introduction of pathogens into the bladder. Despite the condemnation in recent years of the use of the catheter (2-4), it is nevertheless a most important part of urinary tract evaluation, and when done properly, is quite harmless. The specimen is sent to the laboratory for the routine chemical and microscopic tests, and for bacterial culture and drug sensitivity tests for any organisms present. Catheterization also enables the examiner to determine what amount of

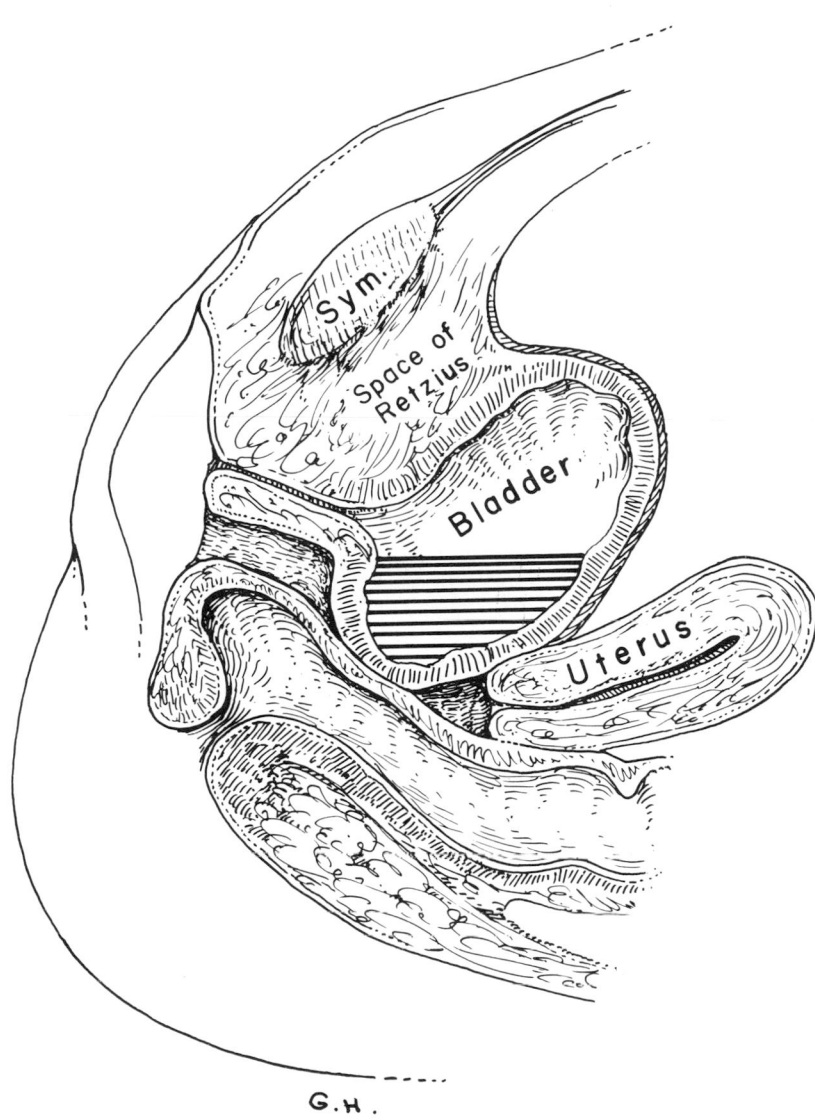

Fig. 4.1. Incompetent vaginal support with moderate cystocele, rectocele, and stress urinary incontinence. The urethra has lost the effective acuity of the posterior urethrovesical angle, and rotated downward relative to the axis of the symphysis pubis. It is necessary to correct the cystocele with the residual urine as well as re-establish the normal relationships and supports of the urethra.

residual urine is present in the bladder. The pelvic examination is then completed.

Cystometrogram studies are indicated in most cases in which stress urinary incontinence is the problem (Fig. 4.4). However, the test is usually unnecessary when confronting the most commonly seen type of uncomplicated stress urinary incontinence presenting itself with typical history and having had no previous surgical attempts at repair. Nor have we used chain cystourethrograms in all cases of ordinary uncomplicated stress urinary incontinence. However, although all of these more complicated tests must be available for use, they need

not always be used in the simple situation when vaginal relaxation is to be repaired with or without vaginal hysterectomy. Careful observation by the examiner as to the degree of anterior vaginal wall relaxation will reveal quite accurately the loss of support of the urethrovesical angle, and evidence of posterior rotation of the axis of the urethra as related to the vertical axis of the symphysis. This angle can be roughly estimated by observing the angle the straight catheter assumes to the horizontal with the patient in the lithotomy position. Figure 4.5 shows that if the external catheter tip points downward from the horizontal, then the

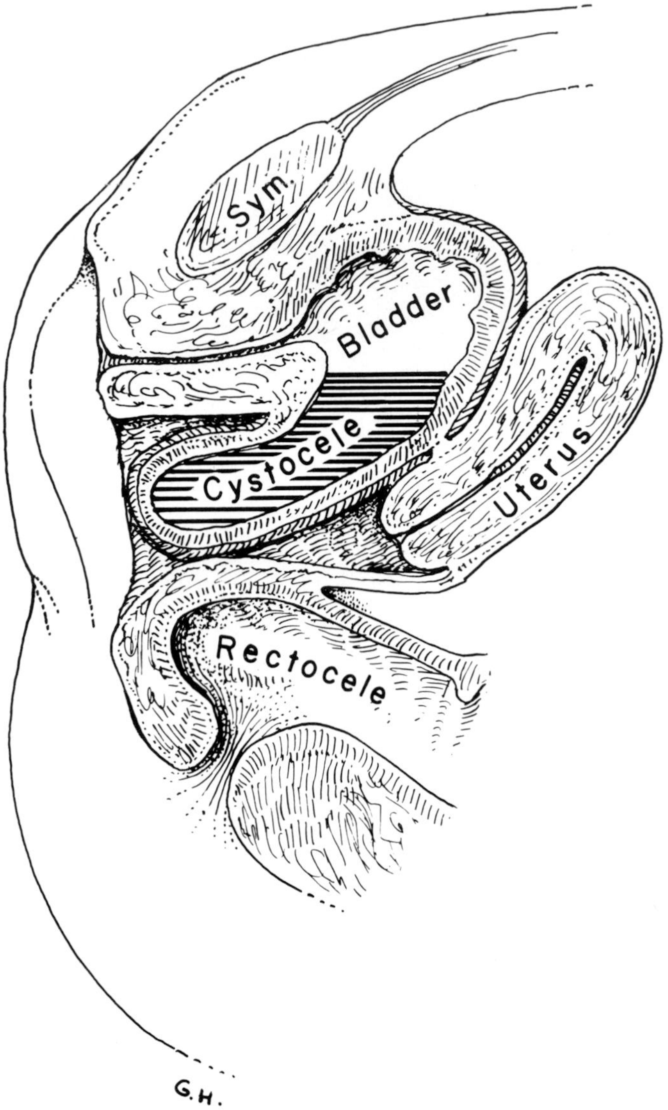

Fig. 4.2. Incompetent vaginal support showing prominent cystocele, beginning uterine prolapse, and rectocele. This is an example of a cystocele with residual urine and without stress urinary incontinence. The support of the urethra may yet exist with preservation of an effective posterior urethrovesical angle.

axis of the urethra is essentially normal. However, if the external catheter tip points upward from the horizontal, the urethral axis has rotated posteriorly away from the normal position. This suggests the Type II urethral position as described by Green (5). However, the presence of this type of urethral position with stress urinary incontinence does not rule out a simple anterior vaginal repair with proper plication for the chance for success is good, if properly done. This repair will be more fully described in discussion of technical efforts and errors.

The technique of chain cystourethrography has been fully described in other textbooks (13, 44) and has proven to be a valuable, easily performed, and a dependable adjunct to urinary tract evaluation. It will not be described in detail in this volume.

The cystometrogram, which evaluates bladder capacity, tone, and dynamics, is likewise of great value. However, the cystometrograph is not always available to the office of the gynecologist, or even in some hospitals. If the instrument is not available, we have used a simple technique which has proven very valu-

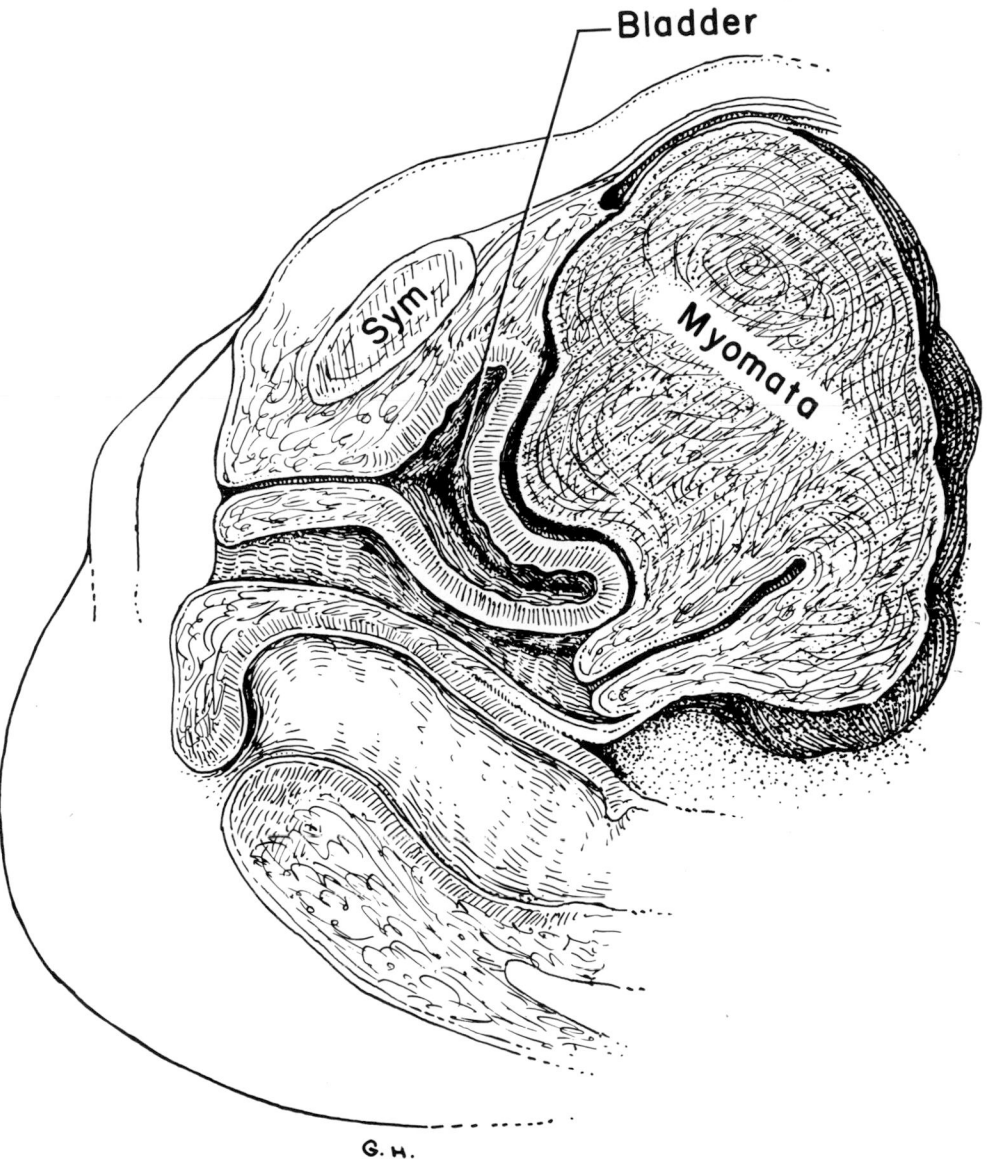

Fig. 4.3. Distortion of bladder by uterine myomatous mass, causing altered bladder capacity and function as frequency, urgency, and stress incontinence. Other pelvic masses may have similar effect.

able and gives essentially the same information sought by using the actual instrument.

The technique is a simple office procedure. The patient is allowed to void a specimen for chemical and microscopic examination. She is then placed in lithotomy position for catheterization. Adequate preparation and cleansing is done using sterile pledgets of cotton soaked with benzalkonium chloride (Zephiran) 1:750

in aqueous solution. A #16F or #18F Foley catheter with a 5-cc bag is passed into the bladder usually without any discomfort. Any residual urine is measured and sent to the laboratory for bacteriologic study and drug sensitivity tests. The catheter is now connected to a hanging flask containing 1000 cc sterile normal saline or distilled water warmed to about 90°F and hung about 36 inches above

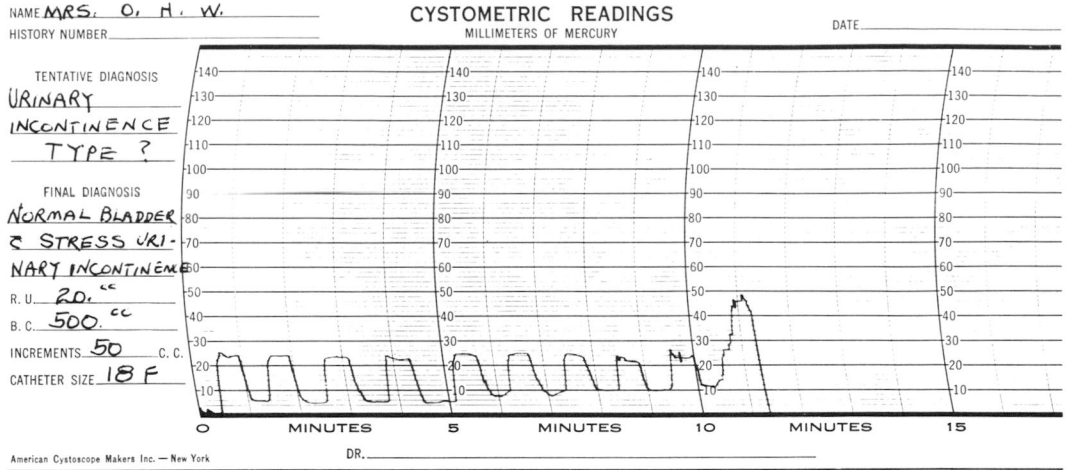

Fig. 4.4a. Normal cystometrogram tracing. There is a gradual increase of bladder tone as noted on the baseline until capacity of about 500 cc is reached. Micturition is then triggered, shown as both the voluntary and involuntary efforts are made.

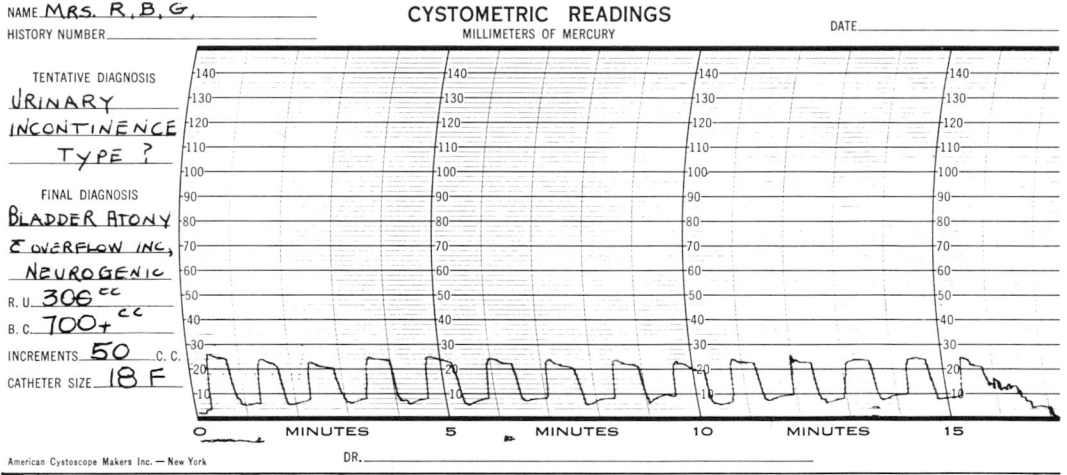

Fig. 4.4b. Cystometrogram of an atonic bladder. The bladder is filled with 700 cc+ showing no increase in tone or resistance, and the patient shows no voluntary or involuntary effort to void. This tracing suggests a neurogenic problem that must be further evaluated; until that is done, further bladder surgery is contraindicated.

the level of the patient's bladder. With the patient still in lithotomy position, relaxed, and reassured, the solution is allowed to gravitate into the bladder in increments of 50 cc. This is done intermittently about every 20 seconds until the patient voices the urge to void. The amount is recorded and the bladder is allowed to drain.

The capacity of the normal female bladder may vary from approximately 350 to 600 cc under ordinary circumstances. However, less than 250-cc capacity with sometimes a sudden

or "triggered" desire to void suggests a bladder of reduced capacity either due to spasm caused by intrinsic bladder pathology or unusual innervation, or some psychogenic stress. On the other hand, if the capacity exceeds 600 cc without complaint from the patient, one may strongly suspect some bladder hypotonicity or atony due to a neurogenic weakness. If the capacity exceeds 1000 cc and seems to be a simple "sac of water," a serious spinal cord lesion may be present.

If the bladder capacity and dynamics have

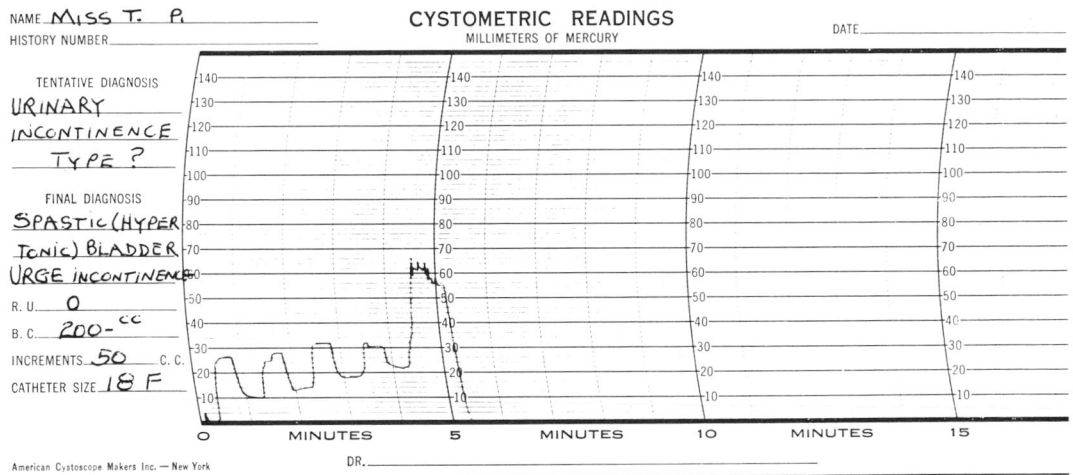

Fig. 4.4c. Cystometric tracing of a spastic or hypertonic bladder with which the patient's chief complaint was marked urge incontinence. The ordinary operations employed for stress urinary incontinence are here contraindicated. Further evaluation of the entire urinary tract must be done.

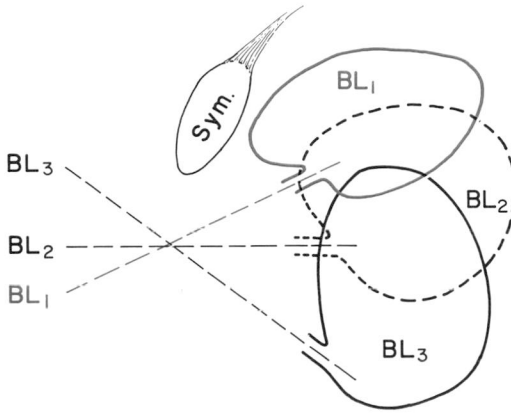

Fig. 4.5 Schematic drawing showing composite of various positions and relationships of the bladder, urethra, and symphysis pubis. BL_1, the normal position of the bladder and urethra with acute posterior urethrovesical angle and relatively close normal relationships of the axes of the urethra and symphysis pubis. This patient usually has no stress urinary incontinence. BL_2, borderline loss of urethral support with posterior rotation of the axis of the urethra and straightening of the posterior urethrovesical angle. This patient usually has moderate stress urinary incontinence. BL_3, pronounced posterior rotation of the axis of the urethra with loss of the posterior urethrovesical ange. This patient usually has a marked amount of stress urinary incontinence.

In the lithotomy examining position the gynecologist will note the position that the rigid straight catheter placed in the bladder, giving a good indication of the inclination of the angle that the urethra has with the perpendicular axis of the symphysis pubis.

been found to be normal, approximately 250 cc of the solution is left in the bladder for stress tests. The patient is asked to cough sharply, and the amount of urethral incontinence is noted. The bladder neck is then displaced upward and backward by the two gloved fingers straddling the urethra in a way as not to compress the structure, and the patient is asked to cough again. It is again noted whether this maneuver did or did not stop the stress incontinence. This displacement of the urethrovesical angle can also be done by grasping the locally anesthetized vaginal mucosa with a curved Allis clamp and displacing it gently backward and upward as described in the Marchetti stress test. If this maneuver stops the spurt of urine at the time of the physical stress, then the examiner could assume that creating a better support of the bladder neck and improving the posterior ureterovesical angle would cure or improve this type of incontinence.

If at any time there is an indication that intrinsic pathology exists within the urinary tract, a complete work-up should be performed including cystoscopy, retrograde pyelography, and excretory urography. In this type of study the gynecologist and urologist work as a team. This cystometric study may also reveal that there is neurogenic dysfunction of the bladder, and this must be evaluated by the neurologist. In any event, such pathology and dysfunction of the urinary tract is most likely to be discovered by this comprehensive preoperative evaluation, and thus obviate the serious error of performing an inappropriate operation for what might otherwise have been assumed to be stress urinary incontinence.

Therefore the pitfalls that must be avoided in assuming the care of the case of stress urinary incontinence are as follows:

1. Neoplasms, benign or malignant, of the genital tract
2. Neoplasms, benign or malignant, of the urinary tract
3. Fistulae
4. Chronic infection of the urinary tract including lithiasis
5. Chronic infections of the genital system
6. Granulomatous lesions
7. Endometriosis
8. Urge incontinence due to
   a. Reduced bladder capacity
   b. Psychogenic disorders
   c. Interstitial cystitis (Hunner's ulcer)
9. Neurogenic disorders
   a. Spina bifida occulta
   b. Degenerative neuropathy
10. Congenital anomalies
    a. Ectopic ureteral orifice
    b. Hypospodias
11. Cicatrix
    a. Postoperative
    b. Postirradiation

The presence of these conditions does not necessarily mean that corrective surgery cannot be ultimately undertaken; however, it is obvious that these conditions must be recognized and treated primarily, if possible, before definitive surgery for the stress urinary incontinence can be logically started.

Operative Technique

With few exceptions the correction of stress urinary incontinence is surgical. Since this disorder is primarily due to tissue damage, maldevelopment, or tissue failure, reconstructive surgery must be relied upon. Included in a small minority of nonsurgical cases are those in which the conscientious patient performs exercises of the pubococcygeal muscle hammock of the pelvis as advocated by Kegel (6). In addition, various pessaries and supporting devices may be applied in such a way as to support the anterior vaginal wall and improve the posterior urethrovesical angle. The measure of success of these makeshift means depends on the degree of cooperation by the patient, and enthusiasm of the gynecologist. In any event, the use of nonsurgical means to correct stress urinary incontinence, despite the limited success, is nevertheless necessary in those cases when surgery is contraindicated or must be postponed.

There are three basic surgical approaches to the correction of stress urinary incontinence. Although many modifications have been made in these techniques, nevertheless the fundamental principles remain (7): a) plication of the paraurethral and bladder neck tissues; b) sling procedures with application of various materials beneath the posterior urethra and bladder neck; and c) repositioning the urethra and bladder neck retropubically. Depending upon the problem at hand, a combination of two or even all three of these basic approaches may be employed. Hence, the competent gynecologist must be familiar with the use of any one or all of these and the various modifications. He must be able to fit his skills to the patient's problem rather than trying to correct all cases by any one favored technique.

The Plication Operation

The plication procedure is the basic operation for correction of stress urinary incontinence. In the great majority of instances it is the first operation that should be used in the attempt to correct the condition. It has been used longer than any other type of procedure, dating back to Schulte in 1870. It was described in classic detail by Kelly (8) in 1913. Since that time various modifications have been made but yet the basic principle has remained unchanged. The stretched and torn tissues about the urethra, bladder neck, and trigone are strengthened by the simple plicating mattress suture. Modifications have been suggested by Kennedy (9), in which procedure it is suggested that further peri- and paraurethral dissection be done in order to liberate any cicatrix that might have resulted from the previous trauma, whether it be from obstetric causes or from previous attempts at corrective surgery. With more recent understanding of the importance of augmenting the structural support of the bladder neck, and restoring more acuity to the posterior urethrovesical angle, subtle but important placement of the plicating sutures about these structures have given even better results with the plication operation.

Indications for the Plication Operation

In our experience the plication procedure is indicated, with a few exceptions, as the primary surgical effort to correct stress urinary incontinence in the female. The exceptions are:

1. The aged nulligravida who develops distressing stress urinary incontinence with or without coexisting uterine and vaginal prolapse. Primarily due to inherently weak tissues, this situation will not give the promise of success that one expects when dealing with tissues basically strong but torn by previous trauma. In these cases one usually elects to proceed directly to the sling procedure or the retropubic urethropexy.

2. Tissue changes of the anterior vaginal wall and bladder base which make local manipulation of the structure themselves unpredictable or impossible. This is seen in postirradiation changes following treatment for some neoplasm of the adjacent structures such as the cervix, uterus, or bladder.

3. Anatomic changes in which there may be partial or total absence of the urethra, bladder neck, and portions of the trigone. These may be seen in cases of obstetrical trauma causing actual destruction by forceps or by necrosis of these structures by ischemia due to prolonged second stage of labor for various reasons.

4. Conditions in which reconstructive surgery has been successful but urinary incontinence is yet a factor. This is seen in those cases of construction of the urethra, either absent congenitally or excised by surgical error (10). We must also include cases in which successful repair of a vesicovaginal or urethrovaginal fistula has been accomplished, but stress urinary incontinence still exists.

5. Coexistence of intra-abdominal pathology that must be investigated or corrected by abdominal visualization otherwise not feasible by vaginal approach. In this category we would recommend proceeding directly to the retropubic urethropexy as a part of the abdominal approach.

Technique of the Plication Operation

Although the description of the original procedure by Howard A. Kelly (8) of the Johns Hopkins Hospital is a classic example of conciseness and accuracy, there have been changes subsequently from his basic technique of this simple and dependable procedure. In the majority of instances the plication procedure is done as a part of vaginal repair, needed to correct the very frequently accompanying cystocele, rectocele, enterocele, and perineal relaxation. In addition plication is easily done when vaginal hysterectomy is being performed.

The description of the procedure will be limited here to the plication operation because detailed descriptions of the other steps and possible errors of the complete vaginal repair procedure are discussed elsewhere in this volume.

The patient is routinely prepared and draped in the lithotomy position. A weighted speculum with a medium vaginal blade is placed in the vagina and the cervix is grasped. The entire length of the anterior vaginal wall is grasped with Allis clamps at about 2-cm intervals from the anterior vaginal fornix to within 5 mm of the external urethral meatus. Care must be used here to avoid the error of tearing into the external urethral meatus, thus creating a problem of distortion by future scarring. The vaginal mucosa can be infiltrated along the midline by a vasoconstricting solution to minimize bleeding and facilitate dissection of the underlying fascial planes. Despite the controversy of defining this underlying tissue as true fascia or not, it is thus described as "vaginal fascia" to avoid confusion. We have used Neo-Synephrine, which gives satisfactory blanching of the tissues, in a weak solution of 1 cc diluted in 50 cc of sterile distilled water and injected sparingly but as needed along the mucosa where the incisions are to be made.

As inverted T-shaped incision is made. The horizontal position of the incision is made in the anterior vaginal fornix just above the cervix and extending from nine to three o'clock. The full depth of the mucosa is incised and dissected a short way anteriorly to expose the pillars of the bladder. Allis clamps are placed just to either side of the midline of the incised mucosa and curved Mayo scissors are inserted just beneath the mucosa, and by spread dissection carried anteriorly toward the external urethral meatus. As the scissors dissection proceeds, the vaginal mucosa overlying the outwardly turned tip of the curved scissors will blanch further, thus indicating to the operator that he is in the proper plane and least likely to injure the subjacent urethra.

It is advisable to have a #18 Foley 5-cc bag catheter indwelling in the urethra and bladder. This acts as a guide and safeguard without causing undue trauma by the periurethral dissection. If the urethra is injured by puncture or by resection, this error is more quickly discernible with the catheter in place. Always suspect the possibility of this error or accident. In the event that the urethra is thus injured, the defect is carefully delineated and closed with as little tension as possible, but in three layers: 1) the mucosa by an inverting suture, avoiding putting the sutures into the lumen of the urethra; 2) the muscularis; and 3) the overlying vaginal mucosa as the repair is completed. This is the principle of closure of any defect or injury of the urinary system. A 3-0 chromic catgut on a small atraumatic needle is most suitable for this repair. The integrity of the repair can be tested, for it is performed by transillumination layer by layer of the closure. Contrast liquid such as a weak solution of indigo carmine or sterile milk can also be used, just as we may employ these agents in the repais of vesicovaginal fistulae.

After the anterior vaginal mucosa has been divided longitudinally in its entire length, the subjacent fascia is dissected off, being careful to proceed in the correct plane (Fig. 4.6). A frequent error of the less experienced surgeon is splitting the mucosa, thus causing either unnecessary bleeding or perforation and inaccurate removal of the membrane. The proper incision is made 2 or 3 mm from the edge of the membrane and the entire length of the vaginal wall where the fascia must be developed. After getting into the proper plane, the fascia is gently dissected and condensed medialward with the gauzed finger tip. One must remember that the further lateralward the dissection is taken, the more likely the venous sinuses of the paraureteral spaces will be encountered. An advantage in the plication operation is to dissect to approximately two-thirds of the circumference of the urethra, freeing up previously formed scar tissue or taking full advantage, as may be possible, of the smooth muscle envelope of the structure. The procedure will interfere with the blood supply in such a way as to cause possible necrosis. An error can be made skeletonizing the urethra too extensively, leaving the possibility of a slough postoperatively (Fig. 4.7). Kennedy (9) has pointed out that this wider dissection, done carefully, enhances the chance for success of this plication procedure.

The plicating sutures must be properly placed. With 3-0 silk, mattress sutures are taken in sufficient numbers to plicate the entire urethra. The bites by the medium Mayo taper point needle are taken deeply in the paraurethral tissues, avoiding direct trauma to the urethra itself, which is identified by the indwelling retention catheter. The most posteriorly located suture is the most important one: this is taken as a semi-pursestring suture into the paraurethral tissues just lateral to and on either side of the location of the internal urethral meatus and over the trigone approximately 1 cm posterior to the bulb of the indwelling catheter (Fig. 4.8). By this suture, the smooth muscle, most well developed here, is plicated securely and is infolded to help restore the posterior urethrovesical angle. Further inspection postoperatively of this vital point will reveal by direct air cystoscopy that the closure of the posterior meatus is now more circular than eccentrical, as is so often seen in the case of stress urinary incontinence (Fig. 4.9). The proper placement of this semi-pursestring suture over the posterior urethrovesical angle or sphincter cannot be overemphasized. Although the entire length of the urethra is enveloped by a distinct layer of smooth muscle, there is a well developed muscle bundle about the circumference of the posterior third that can be easily demonstrated and rightfully called a sphincter (11).

The indwelling catheter is temporarily removed as the assistant enfolds the plicated area inward with a curved Kelly clamp; the mattress sutures of silk are tied successively, posteriorly to anteriorly.

The second layer of this plication is done in a

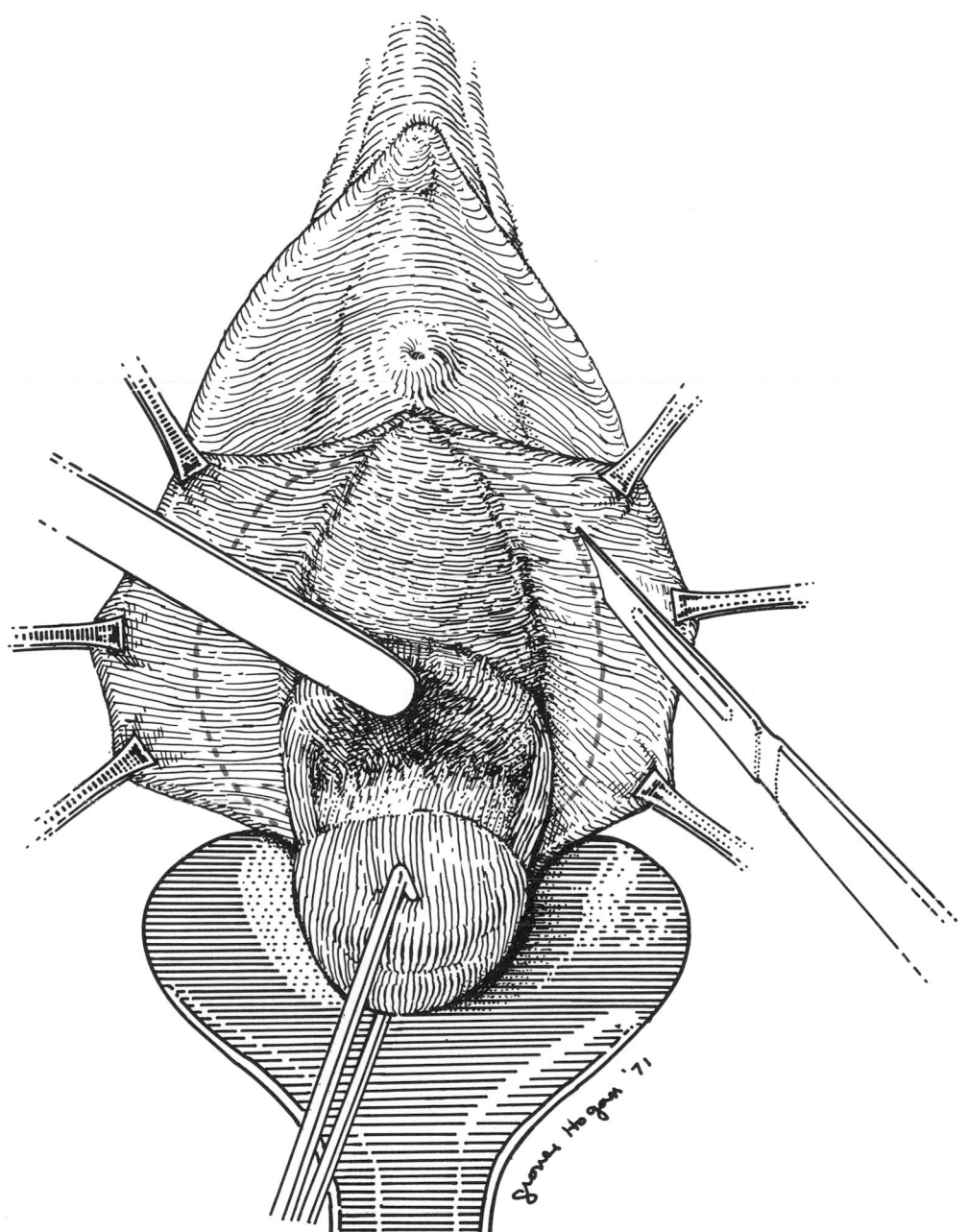

Fig. 4.6. Anterior colporrhaphy with plication of vesical sphincter. The anterior vaginal mucosa has been reflected lateralward and development of the subjacent pubovesicocervical fascia has begun. Incision (red) is made near edge of reflected mucosa and deep enough to enable operator to sweep the fascia medialward. A frequent error here is in making this incision too deep and thus splitting and buttonholing this vaginal mucosa. The dissecting end of scalpel is advancing the bladder on the anterior aspect of cervix and exposing the bladder pillars on either side.

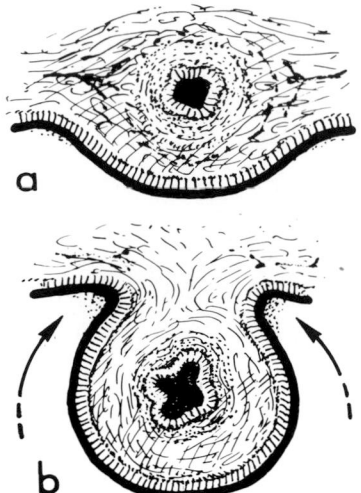

Fig. 4.7. Cross-section of mid-urethra showing preparatory dissection of paraurethral tissues for placement of the 3-0 silk plicating mattress sutures. An indwelling catheter is always used but not shown in this illustration. (a) Proper amount of dissection exposing the urethra without interference of the blood supply; and (b) error of dissection of the urethra too extensively skeletonizing urethra, interfering with blood supply and leading to possible necrosis and tissue failure.

somewhat similar manner using #0 chromic catgut (Fig. 4.10). Again mattress sutures are taken over the entire length of the urethra and again employing a semi-pursestring suture over the location of the posterior urethrovesical angle. Finally the pillars of the bladder are identified and sutured together in the midline without the interruption of these structures. This not only enhances the support of the bladder neck and advances the bladder, but also further augments the acuity of the posterior urethrovesical angle.

The redundant vaginal mucosa is trimmed away. The amount that is trimmed varies, of course, depending upon the size of the cystocele or cystourethrocele. An error can be made here of trimming away either too little or too much of the mucosa. If too little is trimmed away, one finds that full advantage of the repair attempt has not been obtained. If too much mucosa is trimmed away, one may unnecessarily narrow the vagina, particularly if the repair of the posterior vagina is also to be

done. Realizing that removal of any vaginal mucosa lessens the circumference of the vagina, one must be careful to accurately gauge the amount to be removed and yet give adequate vaginal support without constriction. The new edges of the resected vaginal mucosa are now reapproximated with interrupted sutures of #0 chromic catgut (Fig. 4.11). We prefer the interrupted suture because it is less likely to cause unnecessary shortening of the anterior vaginal wall and urethra. When suturing, care should be taken to obliterate any dead space beneath the mucosa and detect any bleeding. A vaginal pack of iodoform gauze is routinely put in the vagina snugly for 24 hours to act as a tamponade and remove any blood clot from the vagina when this pack is withdrawn.

The postoperative care of the plication procedure consists of adequate, constant drainage, and whenever practicable, early ambulation. Despite the simplicity of this plication procedure and the correct postoperative care, a patient might be unable to initiate micturition, more likely as a result of postoperative edema and involuntary muscle spasm rather than because of overcorrection of the posterior urethrovesical angle or actual obstruction of the urethra. If the patient is not voiding spontaneously and adequately at the end of the fifth postoperative day, the urethra is gently sounded and successively dilated with Hegar dilators from #6 (18F) to #9 (27F). This will not cause disruption of the plicating sutures because of the elasticity of the urethral wall, but will relax the spasm, help the edema to subside, and reassure the patient. Sitz baths given once or twice daily after the seventh postoperative day are a valuable adjunctive treatment.

The Sling Procedure

The sling procedure and the various modifications thereof constitute one of the three basic operations used for the correction of stress urinary incontinence. The other two, the plication procedure and the retropubic urethropexy, are discussed in detail elsewhere in this chapter. Although the plication procedure is our primary approach to the problem of stress urinary incontinence, we have found that there are nevertheless some indications to proceed

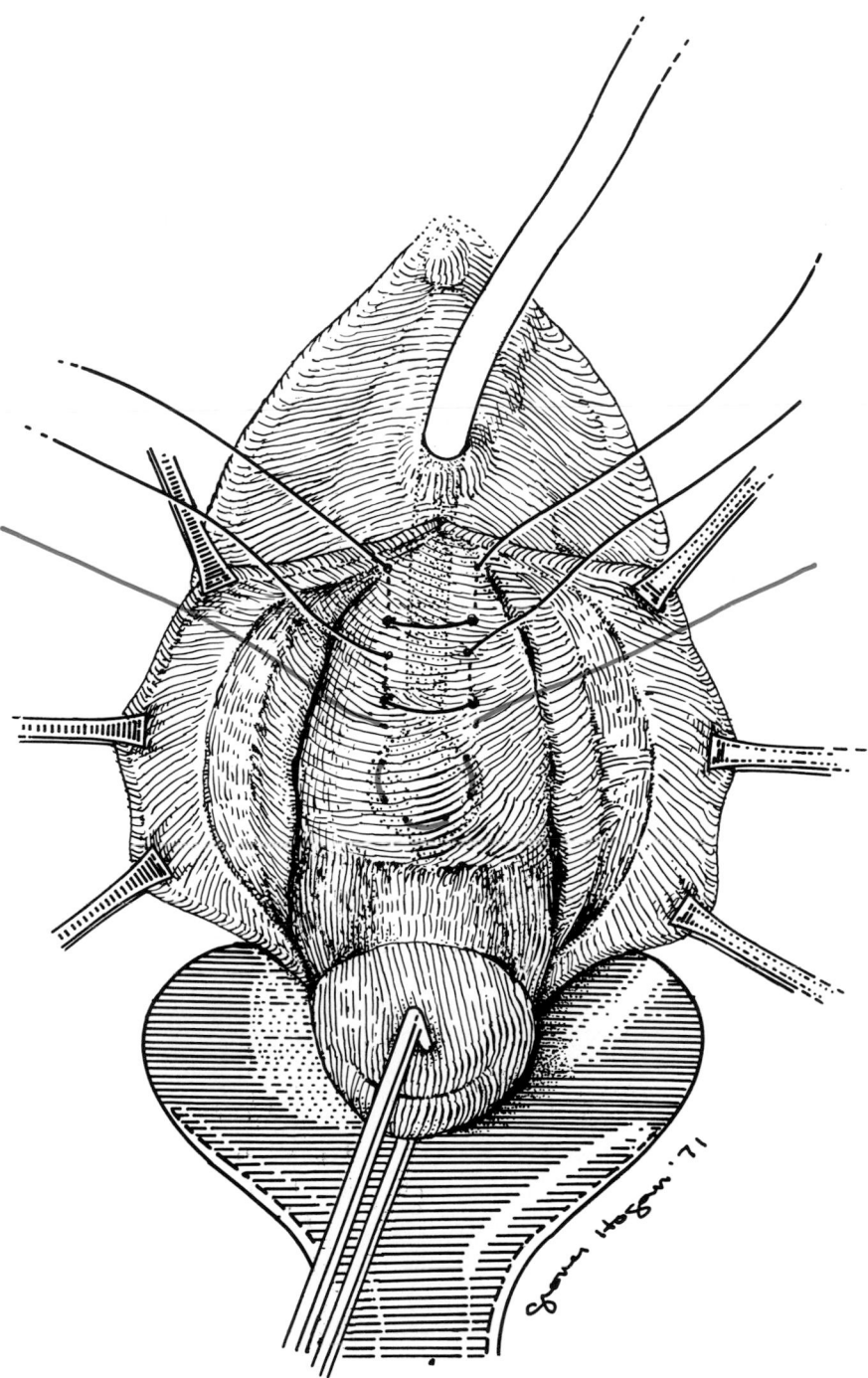

Fig. 4.8. The plicating sutures of 3-0 silk have been placed boldly into the paraurethral tissues of either side of the indwelling ballon catheter. The most important is a semi-pursestring suture (red) placed at the bladder neck marked by gentle traction on the ballon catheter. This suture plicates the tissue at the internal urethral meatus and tends to restore the posterior urethrovesical angle. All of these plicating sutures are tied over the tip of a Kelly clamp pressed into the midline. The fascia may be seen dissected from the overlying vaginal mucosa.

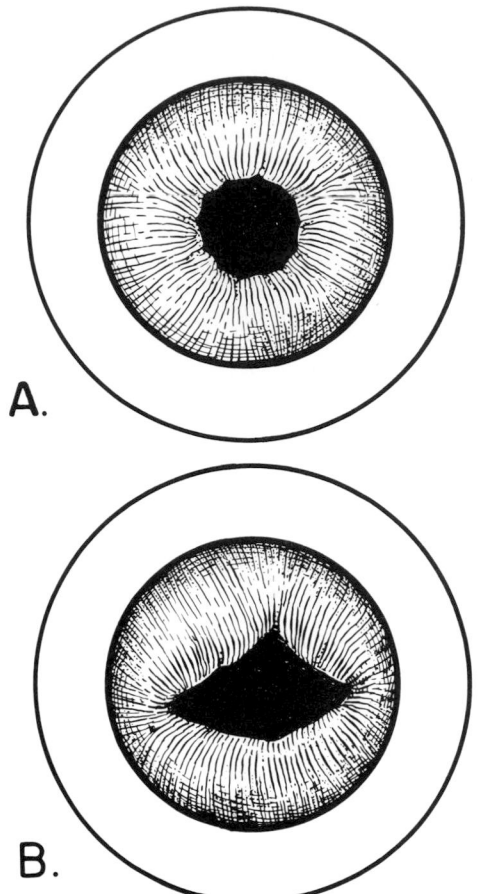

Fig. 4.9. Direct endoscopic view of internal urethral meatus using the simple Kelly air cystourethroscope. (A) Normal concentric sphincteric action closing over end of the instrument as it is slowly withdrawn from urethra; and (B) the incompetent internal urethral sphincter with eccentric action, sometimes failing to close at all as the instrument is withdrawn. This latter anatomic alteration may be seen with or without the altered position and urethrovesical angle in stress urinary incontinence.

directly to either the sling procedure or the retropubic urethropexy. These indications are enumerated in the foregoing section on the plication procedure. We have reserved the use of the technically more complicated yet dependable procedures to the minority of cases which have had previous operative failures by other techniques or in those cases of primary tissue failure. This means that one must choose an operation for the ultimate effort to correct

the failures of previous procedures or in those cases in which plication is impossible.

Historical Development of the Sling Procedure

It is to be noted that gynecologists for a century have been aware of the fact that poor support of the anterior vaginal wall has the frequently coexisting condition of stress urinary incontinence to varying degrees (12, 13). In truth this condition has always been the most common presenting complaint of the woman with incompetent vaginal support. Although not all cases of anterior vaginal relaxation have stress urinary incontinence, the symptom, when troublesome, demands a corrective effort. In 1907 Giordano (14) used a part of the gracilis muscle transposed beneath the bladder neck to give the needed support. Thus one sees that the gynecologists of another era appreciated the importance of reconstruction of the support of the bladder neck with re-establishment of the posterior urethrovesical angle and the correction angle of inclination of the urethra to the vertical axis of the symphysis. In light of our present knowledge and better understanding of this phenomenon of stress urinary incontinence, it is clear that the gynecologists of the earlier era were correcting the condition empirically without the full understanding that we have today. It may be projected further that as time passes future gynecologists who will have an increasingly better knowledge of stress urinary incontinence will marvel at the fact that we get the favorable results we do at the present time. It is obviously to be concluded that no one operation is so successful as to exclude all others.

In 1910 Goebell (15) described an operation in which he went above to the anterior abdominal wall, dissected free the pyramidalis muscles and brought them down posterior to the symphysis through the space of Retzius to form a sling beneath the urethra near the bladder neck. He reported two successful cases in which no other type of procedure would have been feasible, and continence was established. An obvious shortcoming of this technique was the inconsistency or even congenital absence of the pyramidalis muscles.

In 1914 Frangenheim (16) utilized what pyramidalis muscles were existent but with a

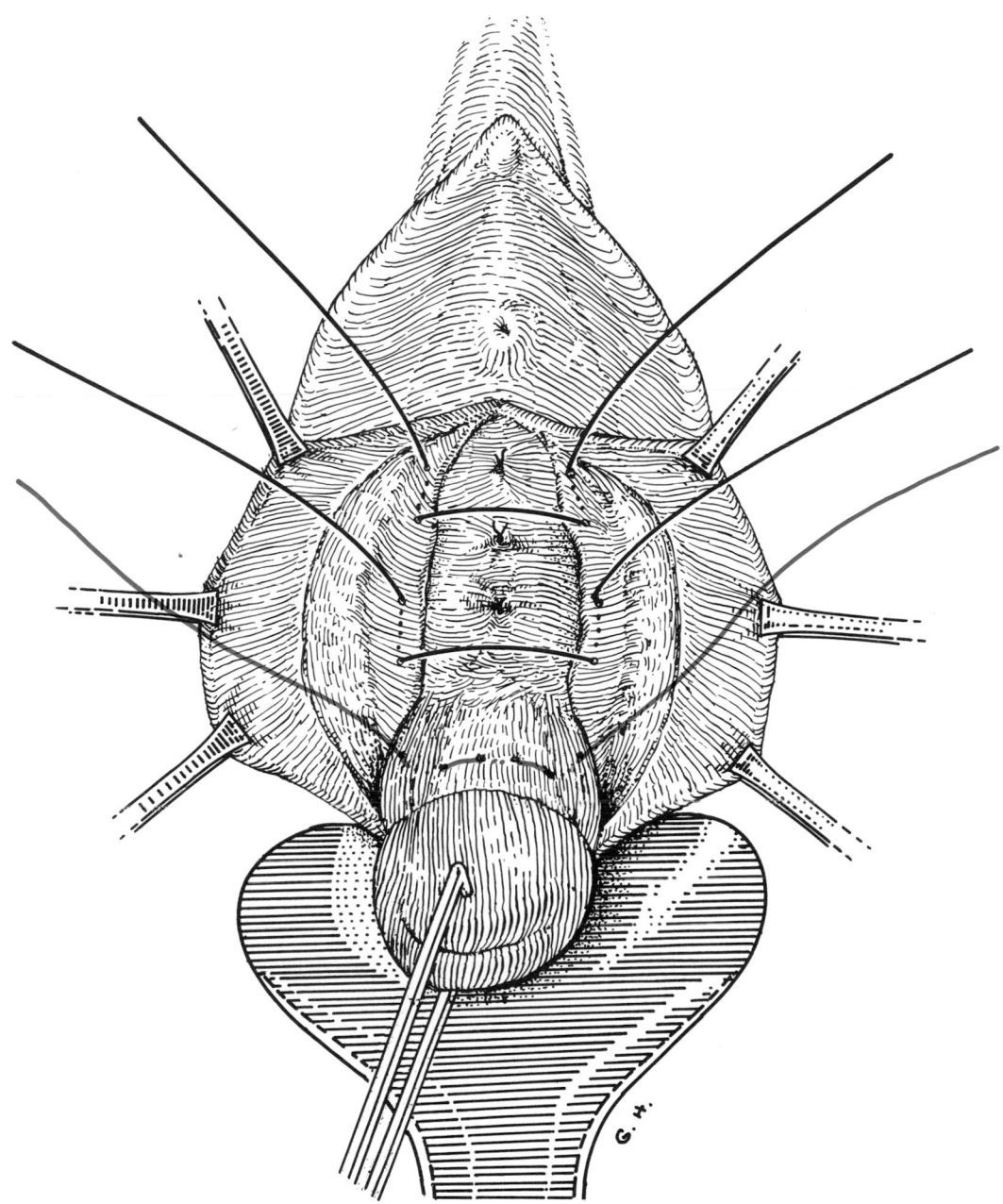

Fig. 4.10. The second layer of plicating sutures is being placed in the pubovesicocervical fascia which has been dissected from the overlying vaginal mucosa. An important suture is the lowest one (red), being placed in such a way as to approximate the pillars of the bladder and advance and anchor the bladder base to the anterior aspect of the cervix, making recurrence of the cystocele less likely.

strip of the anterior abdominal fascia attached. He reported a successful operation performed on the male. The strap thus formed a continuous sling and was attached to itself after the loop had been made beneath the urethra.

In 1917 Stoeckel (17) combined the use of the pyramidalis muscle and the strip of fascia from the anterior abdominal aponeurosis, thus

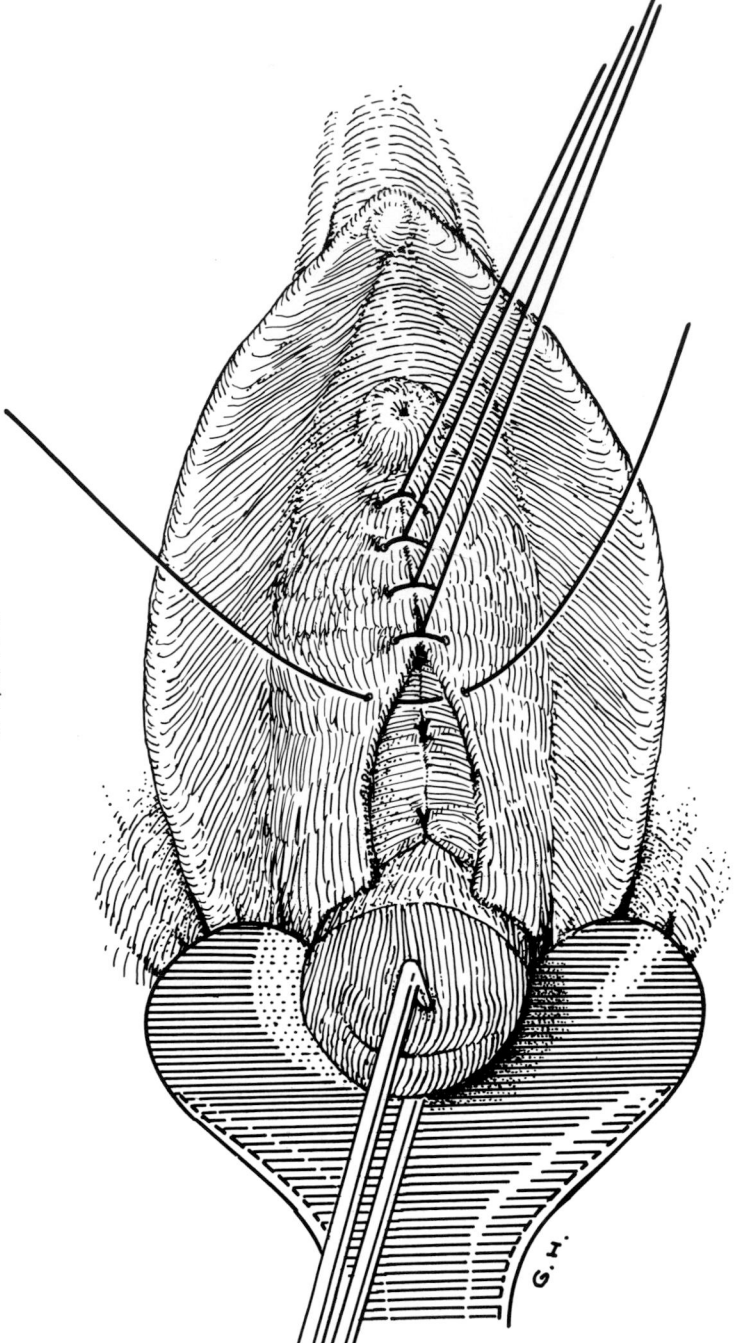

Fig. 4.11. The redundant vaginal mucosa has been trimmed away and the new edges are being approximated as the third layer of the repair with 0 chromic catgut interrupted sutures.

not completely depending on the inconsistent muscle. The superior end of the fascia was split, passed retropubically, and plicated beneath the urethra with the appropriate tension. He reported success in two difficult cases, one with previous successful repair of a vesicovaginal fistula, and the other with a large cystourethrocele.

In 1932 Norman Miller (18) modified the technique of the now called Goebell-Frangenheim-Stoeckel operation by bringing the developed musculofascial sling of the pyramidalis and anterior abdominal aponeurosis anterior to the symphysis, then beneath the urethra. The idea was to avoid the danger and likelihood of hemorrhage that might be encountered in the retropubic space, particularly from the venous sinuses about the bladder neck. The bleeding encountered, however, at the clitoris was most troublesome. Also the fascia sling would not give the proper angle of support at the posterior third of the urethra, where it must be placed; it had rather a stripping action on the urethra. The procedure therefore did not gain wide acceptance.

In 1933 Price (19) reported a modification of the Goebell-Frangenheim-Stoeckel, in which he obtained a cure of urinary incontinence in a young girl who had no bladder sphincter control because of congenital deformity of the lower spinal cord, sacrum and coccyx. He used a sling of the patient's fascia lata, which he brought retropubically and beneath the urethra to form a continuous supporting sling, attaching both ends with proper tension to the anterior rectus fascia just to either side of the suprapubic midline. She was cured. The basic principles of this technique with subsequent modifications have been used as a most dependable operation and will be discussed more fully.

In 1942 Aldridge (20) devised a modification in which he combined some of the points of other sling procedures. Making a transverse abdominal incision, he developed strips of the anterior abdominal aponeurosis about 1 cm wide and parallel to Poupart's ligament. The medial ends were left attached, and the distal end of the strap was passed retropubically around or through the lower muscle bellies of the anterior rectus abdominus muscle and beneath the urethra at the posterior urethrovesical angle. The two ends were plicated in the midline with silk to form the sling. This is a dependable procedure, but great care must be used to approximate the edges of the incised abdominal aponeurosis to avoid the danger of an incisional hernia in this vulnerable area, particularly if one is so unfortunate as to get a postoperative infection.

In 1949 Shaw (21) devised a further modification of the sling procedure by passing autogenous fascia beneath the urethra, but fastening the free ends to holes drilled in the symphysis pubis. In 51 cases he reported 35 successes and 1 death.

In 1947 Millen and Read (22, 23, 25) reported a further modification of the basic sling procedure by a rather complicated maneuver of passing two straps completely beneath the bladder neck retropubically up to the anterior abdominal fascia as a continuous support. The strips of fascia had been developed from two complete transverse incisions across the lower abdominal fascia, leaving one attached on the left lateral end and the other on the right lateral end of the incision of the abdominal fascia. This procedure, although reported as dependable, has never gained wide popularity in this country.

Ball and Hoffman in 1963 (24) reported an operation combining with the retropubic and vaginal approach a plication of the bladder and suspending procedure.

More recently in 1967, Pereyra and Lebhertz (26) have used a particular type of ligature carrier to pass a suspending suture retropubically on either side of the urethra. The type of material for this suture varies with the individual surgeon, but it has been found by us that the absorbable material is more dependable, being less likely to cut through the suspended tissues and less likely to form a wick for postoperative drainage. Although there is no doubt that this type of urethral suspension will find a place in our armamentarium for correction of stress urinary incontinence, it has nevertheless thus far shown a disappointing incidence of late failures (27, 28). Despite its relative simplicity, it has nevertheless the same danger of operative and postoperative complications, such as hemorrhage and infection, that is seen in the other retropubic procedures.

Other means of suspension of the posterior urethrovesical angle have been used and although none has been adopted for widespread use to the exclusion of others, these procedures are mentioned for historical interest. More recently, Moir (29), of the Oxford Clinic, has used a Mersilene gauge hammock fixed beneath the urethra and bladder neck, sutured in a fashion as to prevent the material from wrinkling in its final position.

Other more recent procedures that are well worth mentioning are those of Ingelman-Sundberg (30) using contiguous muscles and fascia of the pelvic floor; Hodgkinson (31) using the round ligaments to suspend the bladder neck; and Zacharin (32) which combines the structures of the pelvic floor and perineum to reconstruct the needed support.

The history of the development of the retropubic urethropexy, or the so-called Marshall-Marchetti-Krantz procedure, is more recent. Marshall had noted that a loss of support at the bladder neck contributed to incontinence in both the male and female. In 1949 (33) publication of the procedure was made applying the principle of creating again this support and improving the posterior urethrovesical angle. Marshall, Marchetti, and Krantz (33) mutually revived and improved this procedure which has proven to be so dependable and comparably successful to any other type of operation for correction of a stress urinary incontinence.

Choice of Operation

The gynecologist must be capable of calling upon any one of the numerous basic procedures that can be used to correct stress urinary incontinence. In addition he must be familiar with the various modifications that may be applicable to the patient's particular problem. Finally, he must be ingenious enough to improvise during any procedure in order to fit an operation to the patient's problem, not only to gain success but to avoid errors which may be committed in the procedure.

Generally speaking, we feel that the simple plication procedure is the first choice in the great majority of cases. Already stated is that this procedure, when carefully done, affords a cure rate of from 75 to 90 per cent. Various clinics have reported varying amounts of success, but the overall average for me and in the ward service of the Grady Memorial Hospital of Atlanta, has been 87 percent cured, 7 per cent improved, 6 per cent failure (35). Oddly enough, this figure of approximately 85 per cent cure rate is generally applicable to the results of most operations for stress urinary incontinence, considering the fact that the cases

have been wisely chosen for the particular procedure. Also true is an irreducible number, although relatively few, of cases which defy all efforts at surgical cure. These cases finally must be evaluated as to whether urinary diversion might be necessary to relieve the patient of an intolerable situation, but such an ultimate effort is rare indeed.

The Technique of the Goebell-Stoeckel-Frangenheim Sling Procedure

In the past 25 years we have used the fascia lata strap in the great majority of cases, having been satisfied that it is dependable, safe, relatively easy, and has a very low percentage of late recurrences of stress urinary incontinence. Thus far this autogenous fascia, easily obtained from the lateral thigh of any age patient whether thin or obese, has proven to be easily workable, causing the rarest postoperative complications. However, our search goes on in the effort to find the most perfect material for the sling. It must be easily available, easily workable, and cause no tissue reaction or rejection. Numerous heterogenous materials have been tried, but with generally disappointing results; dacron polyester (Mersilene) strap was used (34) but condemned because of a rather high incidence of local reaction in this area of the body, necessitating the subsequent surgical removal or transection of the sling (35). Other materials, both absorbable and nonabsorbable, have been tried but none has worked to any comparable success of the autogenous materials.

The patient is placed in the supine position on the operating table with exposure of one or the other thigh, depending on the gynecologist's choice. The entire thigh, having been shaved, is prepared with the skin antiseptic of choice. The location of the incision may vary depending on the patient's sensitivity to an exposed scar, small as it will be, or the facility with which the gynecologist can work. Figure 4.12 shows the sites for the making of an incision on this iliotibial band. The incision "a" is recommended for several reasons: the overlying fat is usually minimal at this site; the fibers of the fascia lata are condensed and very easily demonstrated here; and these fibers radiate or fan outward in the superior aspect making it easier to procure a satisfactory strap of uniform width (Fig. 4.13). The fascia in either location is cleaned with the gauze-tipped finger and bleeding is easily controlled. Two incisions are made, parallel to the fibers and approximately 1 cm apart—the width of the strap to be taken. It is transected just above its attachment into the lateral condyle of the femur, thus mobilizing the distal 5 or 6 cm (Fig. 4.14). The free end of the strap is now threaded through the eye of the Masson fascia stripper (Fig. 4.15), and held firmly with a toothed clamp such as a straight Oschner forceps, applied at its very tip.

Other fascia strippers may be used with equal ease, or in a rare instance the operator may choose to make an incision over the entire length of the fascia strip to be removed. The fascia stripper is now thrust firmly and evenly cephalad (Fig. 4.16), paralleling the fibers of the fascia and just beneath the skin to the full depth possible, usually bout 30 cm. The outer tube of the Masson stripper is now slipped toward its tip and over the eye of the inner tube through which the tip of the fascia has been threaded. Thus the strap is transected at the superior end. If the operator is not satisfied with either the length or breadth of the procured fascia, he may at this time cut an extra section with very little additional trouble, realizing that an excess of the fascia is better than a deficiency. The visible defect in the iliotibial band is approximated with three or four interrupted sutures of chromic 0 catgut to

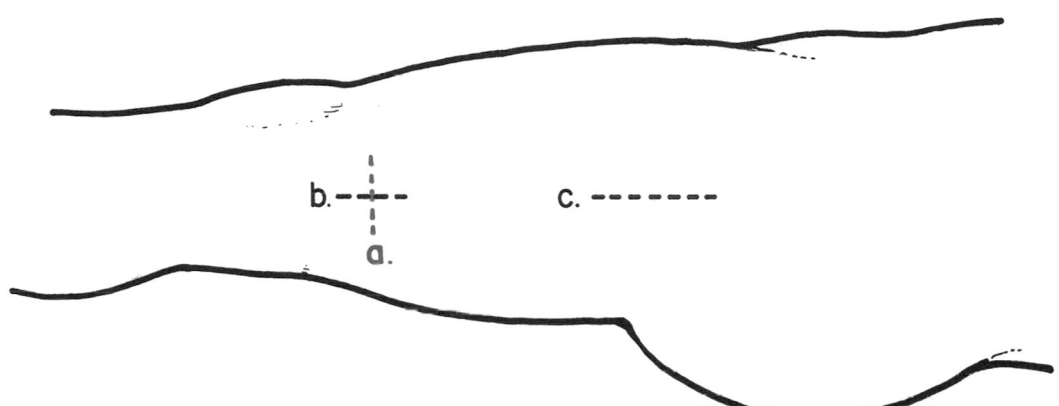

Fig. 4.12. Various sites (a, b, c) for incision for procurement of a strap of the fascia lata. Incision "a" is the most commonly chosen, giving access to the fascia lata near its attachment and at a point of the closest condensation of the longitudinal fibers. This location also offers less of an overlying adipose layer than incision "c" in an obese individual.

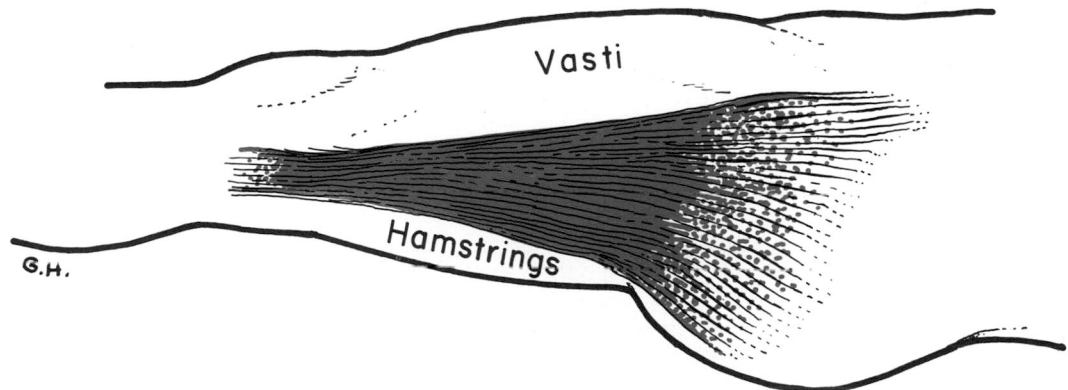

Fig. 4.13. Lateral aspect of left thigh showing position of the fascia lata (iliotibial fan). Note that the fibers of the fascia diverge from the knee toward the hip.

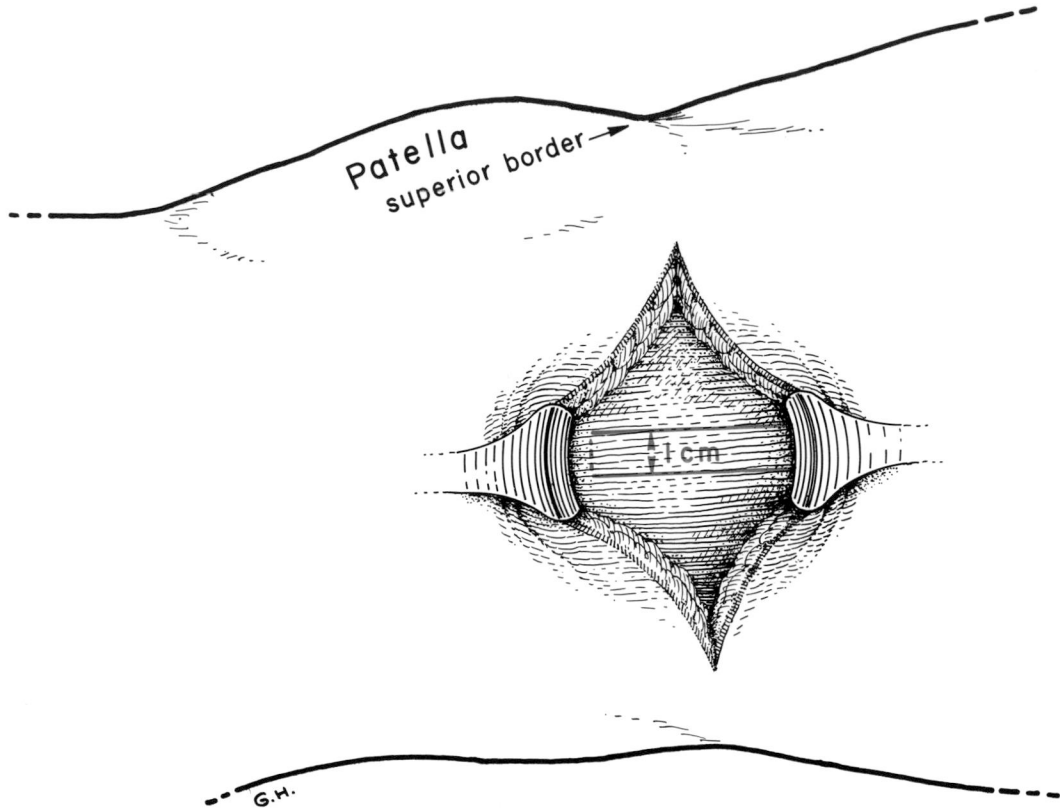

Fig. 4.14. The fascia lata has been exposed and incisions made parallel to direction of the fibers. The width of the strap can be selected and its inferior end detached near its insertion into the lateral condyle of the femur. An additional width or even a second strap may be obtained here with no difficulty.

control any chance for bleeding at the lower attachment. The subcutaneous tissues and skin are closed per routine. It is not thought necessary to wrap the thigh, unless there is evidence of bleeding, which is an exceedingly rare occurrence. The procured strap is wrapped in moist saline gauze and safely put aside for use subsequently in the procedure.

Obviously procurement of the fascia lata strap is very easy and safe, taking not much longer to perform than to write this description. This autogenous material is uniform, easily workable, and trouble-free. We have had no bothersome complications from this simple procedure other than a soreness of a few days. It is well to mention here that procurement of the supporting sling from the abdominal fascia in the Aldridge or Studdiford modification has a chance, even though small, of developing a postoperative hernia, particularly if any infec-

tion is encountered, a possibility in any combined abdominovaginal procedure. Also, the use of the thigh permits much earlier ambulation which is important in postoperative bladder care.

The patient is changed to a dorsolithotomy position, cleaned, and draped in a manner to expose both the lower abdomen and the perineal area for simultaneous accessibility. A suprapubic cystotomy is routinely done. The bladder is filled by an indwelling #18F 5-cc bag Foley catheter with 500 to 600 cc normal saline. A small #10F or #12F trochar with cannula is thrust firmly but under careful control into the dome of the bladder. The site of this puncture is approximately 4 cm above the symphysis pubis, thus staying extraperitoneally in the midline for the bladder tap. A polyethylene or Silastic straight catheter, #10F, or the largest that can be threaded through the

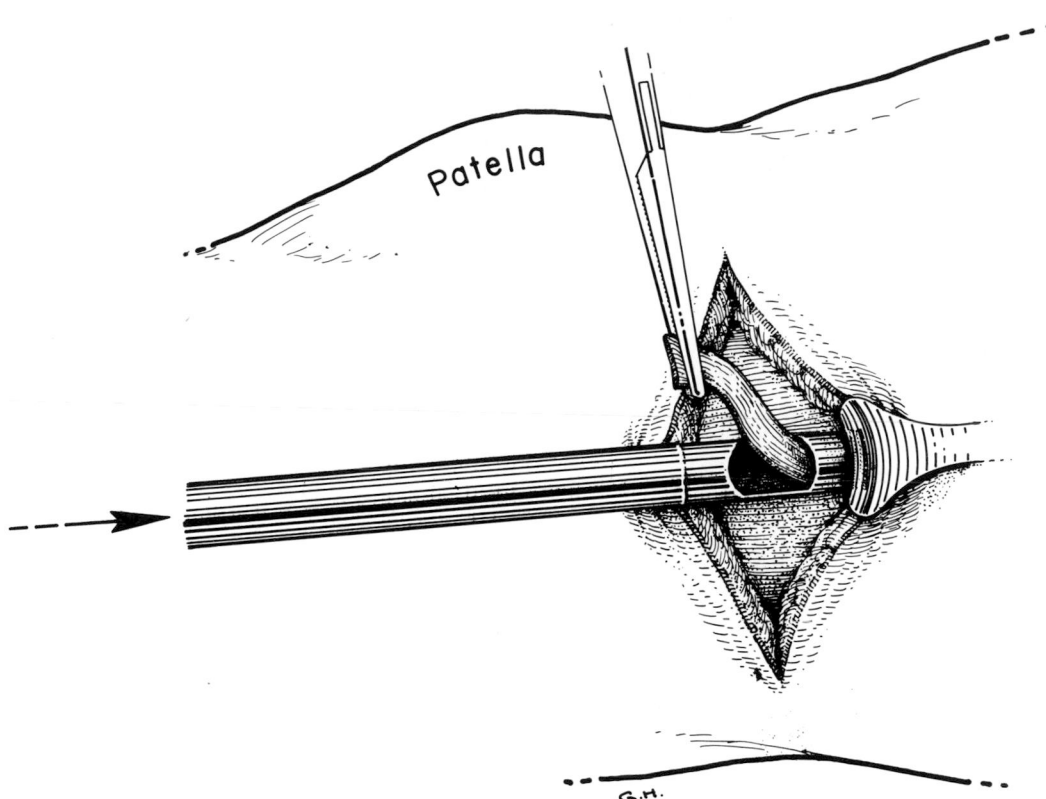

Fig. 4.15. The inferior end of the fascia lata strap has been threaded through the tip and eye of the Masson fascia stripper preparatory to procuring the strap. The tip of this fascia is firmly held with a strong clamp as the instrument is thrust cephalad.

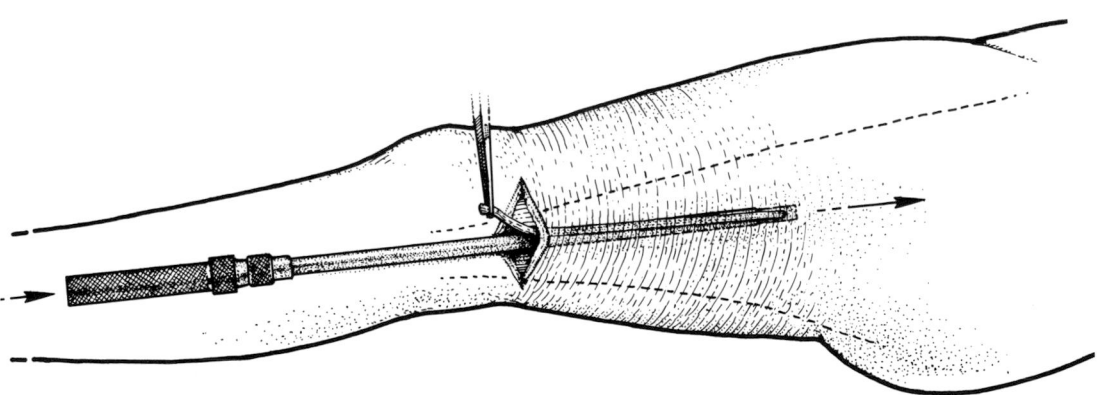

Fig. 4.16. The Masson fascia stripper is about half way to its full depth being thrust cephalad along the nearly parallel fibers of the fascia lata. When the full depth has been attained, the outer sleeve of the instrument is loosened and slipped over the eye and tip of the inner tube to cut the fascia strap at its superior end.

cannula, is placed into the cystostomy and fastened securely to the skin after the cannula is slid off (Fig. 4.17). Our choice is to perform this suprapubic cystostomy preoperatively in order to watch for any troublesome bleeding or failure of the catheter to function. Also, to perform it after the main part of the operation has been done increases the chance for infec-

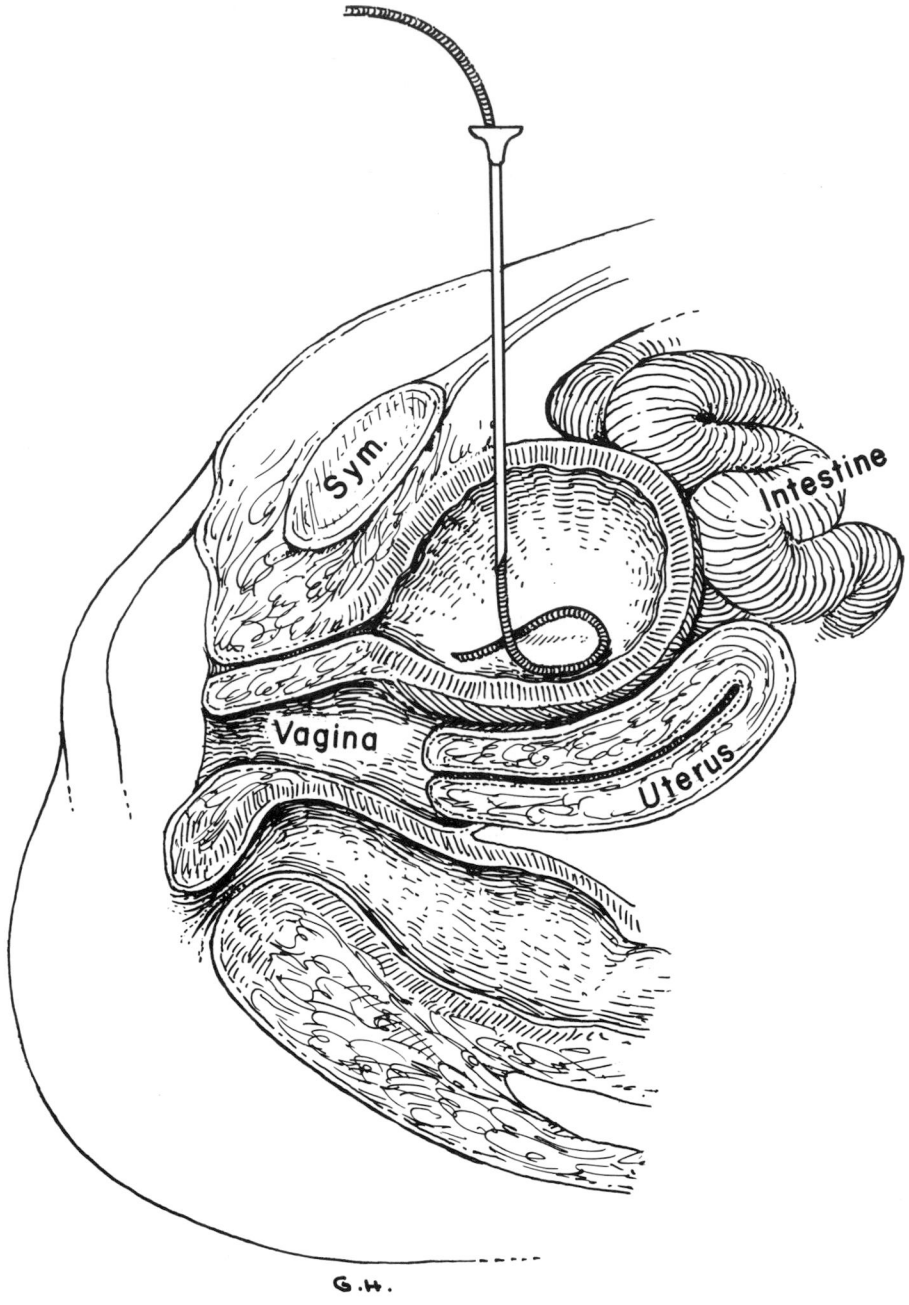

G.H.

Fig. 4.17. Trochar-cannula suprapubic cystotomy performed preliminary to principal part of operation. A #10F silastic tube is left in place for postoperative bladder care, until patient is voiding satisfactorily per urethrum.

tion. The numerous descriptions of technique of performing this valuable bladder drainage are available in periodicals (36) and textbooks.

After the suprapubic drainage of the bladder has been established, an 8- to 10-cm transverse incision is made just inferior to or at the level of the puncture site, being careful not to transect the indwelling Silastic tube as the anterior abdominal aponeurosis is exposed (Fig. 4.18a). This is cleaned with a gauzed finger and

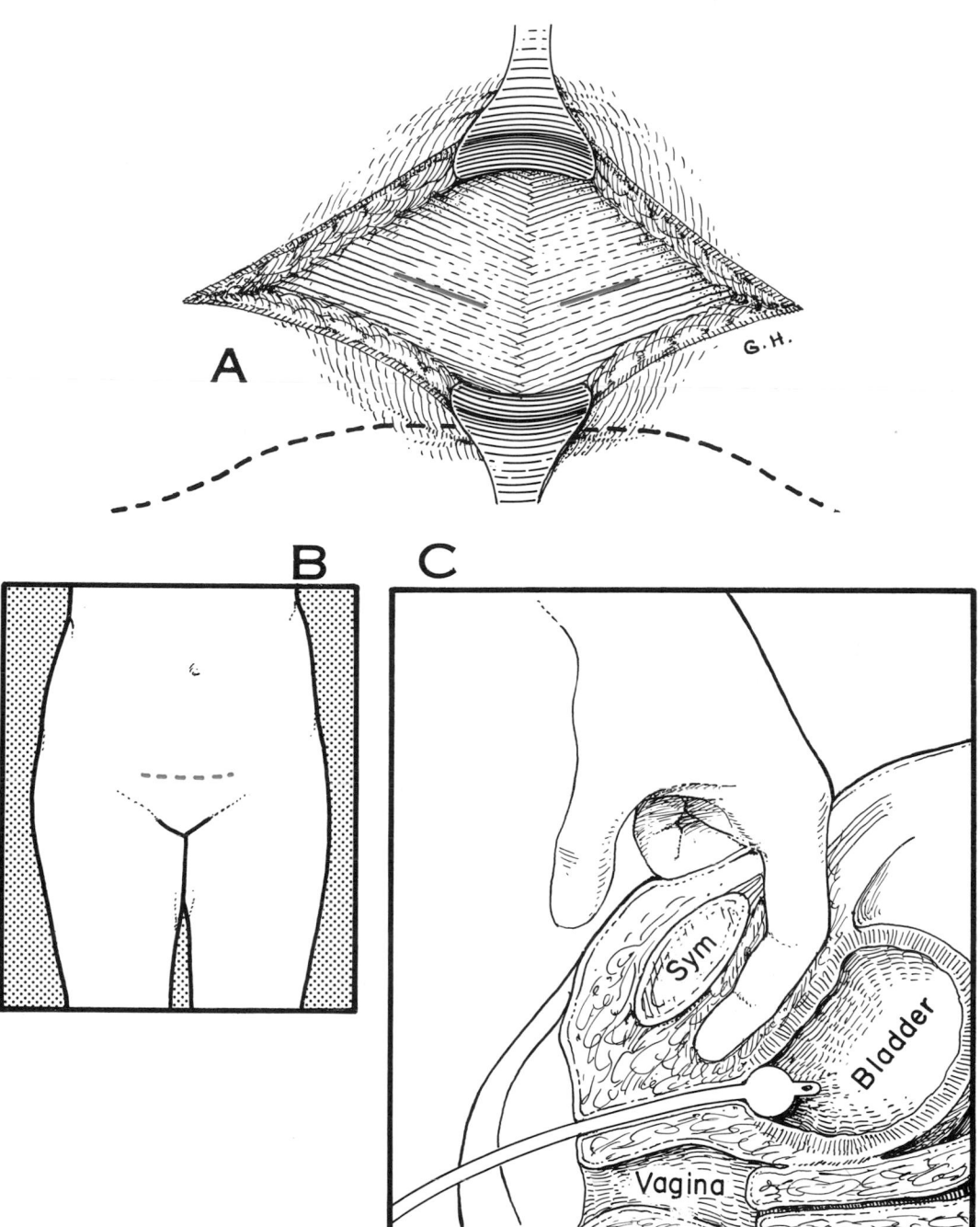

Fig. 4.18. (A) The site of the small suprapubic incision.

(B) The anterior abdominal aponeurosis has been exposed and two 2.0-cm incisions made therein, parallel to the fibers of this fascia, 3 cm superior to level of Poupart's ligament.

(C) Gentle finger dissection is done retropubically through the space of Retzius down to the level of the urogenital diaphragm and inferior aspect of the ramus of the pubic bone on either side. If the space of Retzius has been scarred by previous surgery, dissection may be performed with blunt tip of uterine dressing forceps.

all bleeding controlled. Two small incisions are made, one on each side of the midline, paralleling the fibers of the anterior aponeurosis, 2 cm in length, 2 cm above the superior aspect of the pubic ramus, and 2 cm from the midline (Fig. 4.18b). Beneath the incised fascia may be seen the bellics of the rectus abdominis muscle, the fibers of which are divided by blunt dissection, either by finger or blunt scissors. The space of Retzius is entered with the index finger, which is thrust downward toward the bladder neck and the inferior aspect of the pubic rami (Fig. 4.18c). The indwelling catheter is felt. The error of causing retropubic bleeding can be minimized here if the finger is kept close to the posterior surface of the symphysis, and the bladder gently thrust backward.

In instances where previous operative procedures have left severe scarring in the space of Retzius, this retropubic dissection must be performed carefully with a blunt instrument with the point directed toward the bone. for this more difficult dissection, moderately blunt-pointed uterine dressing forceps or a curved staphylorrhaphy spatula is ideal. When this retropubic dissection has been accomplished bilaterally, the abdominal wound is temporarily packed with gauze and the operative site changed to the vaginal area.

The vaginal retractor with as long a blade as needed is placed in the vagina to expose the entire length of the anterior vaginal wall, which may vary markedly depending on the amount of previous surgery. It is usually scarred and the cervix may be absent because this sling procedure is, as a general rule, reserved for those cases in which previous operations have failed. A midline incision is made from 1 cm of the external urethral meatus over the entire length of the anterior vaginal wall and through the depth of the subjacent fascia and scar tissue. An error can be made here in injuring the urethra, but with care and the presence of the indwelling catheter, this can usually be avoided. However, if at anytime the urethra or bladder is entered or stripped, the defect must be immediately closed in three layers, the first layer inverting the mucosa. This misfortune does not preclude proceeding with the planned operation. At times one must rely entirely on sharp dissection to develop the identity of the fascia and the approach to the space beneath the rami

of the pubic bone on each side of the urethra. However, to minimize the chance for injury or hemorrhage, one must use finger dissection to develop these shallow "tunnels" towards the space of Retzius above. This can be done to the depth of the triangular ligament or the urogenital diaphragm, which has been approached from above via the abdominal incision. With the use of the index finger—the most valuable dissecting instrument the operator can employ—error of causing unnecessary bleeding or injury can be minimized.

After this portion of the vaginal procedure is completed, the simultaneous use of the abdominal and vaginal procedures is done. A long curved, blunt-tipped instrument (the uterine dressing forceps is ideal for this) is passed through first one incision through the rectus abdominis fascia and muscle, then the other, traversing the space of Retzius again to impinge on the tip of the index finger placed on that side of the urethra.

A serious error can be made by mistakenly crossing over the midline from above downward, thus injuring the bladder neck. However, with care and the constant awareness of the indwelling catheter, one may safely stay in the proper channel for the placement of the sling. As the tip of the clamp, which has been passed from above downward, is felt on each side of the urethra, it may be then presented vaginally with a gentle thrust through the triangular ligament. At times a small incision over the presenting tip of the clamp is made to facilitate its passage into the vaginal paraurethral space. The clamp tip is spread just wide enough to grasp the tip of the fascia lata strap. With gentle traction the strap is drawn upward retropubically, without twisting, and fastened securely with several sutures of 3-0 silk to the anterior abdominal aponeurosis. As this is then done on the other side of the urethra, a continuous sling is thus formed beneath the urethra (Fig. 4.19).

Proper tension is applied to the sling for support of the bladder neck under which the strap has been placed. The "proper tension" placed on the sling is very important. The bladder neck and the posterior third of the urethra under which the sling naturally will fall is supported, not obstructed. The chief error of this operation is the use of too much tension on this sling. Conversely, paradoxically one can use

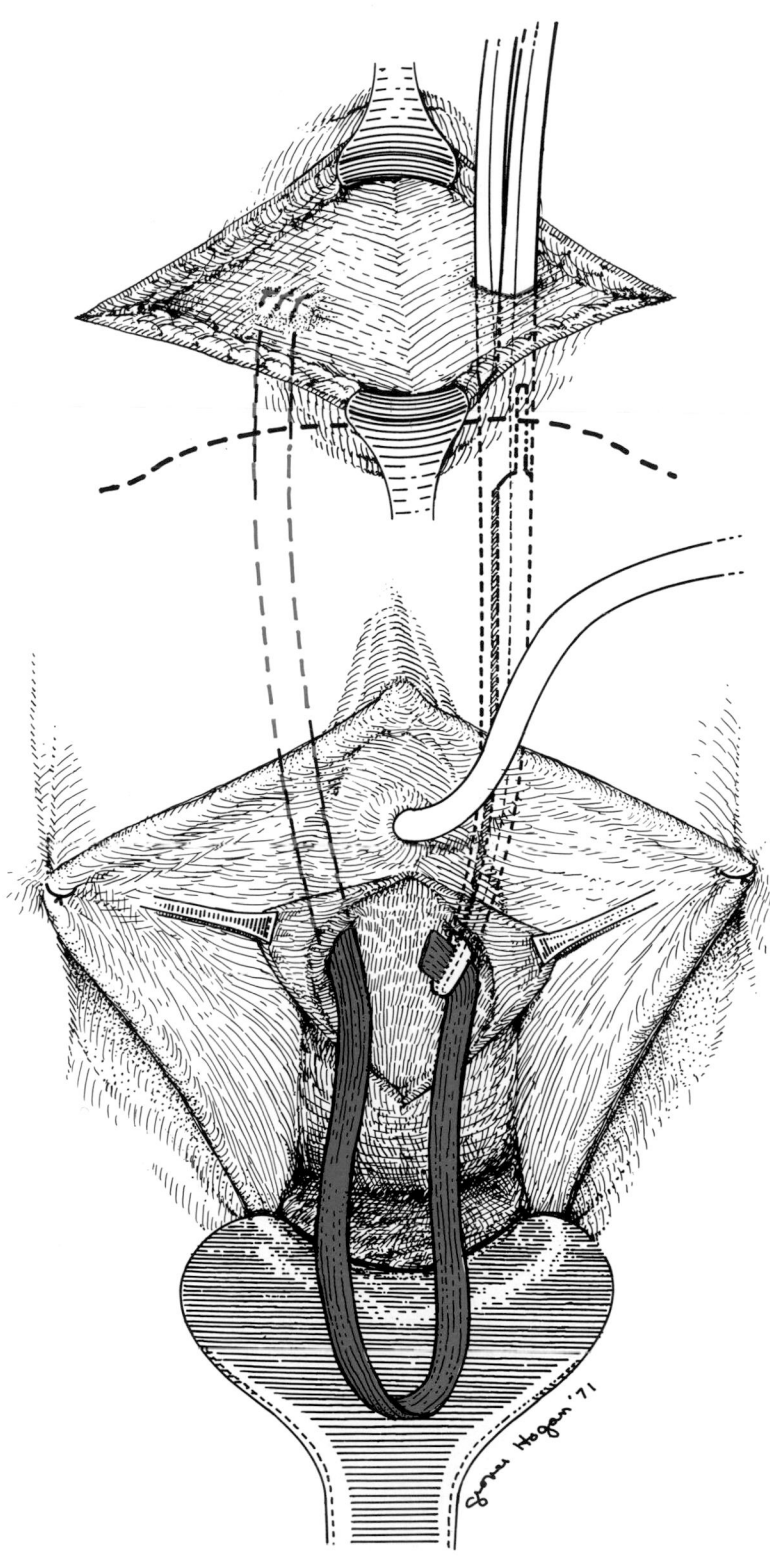

Fig. 4.19. Showing the passage of the fascia lata strap beneath the urethra and retropubically. The strap has been anchored to the anterior abdominal fascia on the patient's right side and drawn into the vagina. It is now being grasped by the uterine dressing forceps to be drawn up on the left side and anchored with proper tension at the other slit-like incision in the fascia. Thus a sling is formed beneath the urethea at the bladder neck. The retention catheter remains in place during the entire sling procedure.

scarcely too little tension. If the operator will recall what the position and inclination of this urethra was by his preoperative examination under anesthesia, to alter this angle and inclination appropriately is then an easier matter. The use of a straight metal catheter, temporarily replacing the indwelling balloon catheter, will show the changed angle of the urethra as was described previously in this chapter. The curved tip of the gallbladder type clamp is easily used to pass between the sling and the urethra to adjust the tension. Remembering that it is difficult to place a sling too loosely, the tension is applied and the second tip of the fascia lata strap is secured to the anterior abdominal aponeurosis with interrupted sutures of 3-0 silk. These small defects in the aponeurosis are completely closed at the same time, and the abdominal incision is closed in layers usually without drainage. If any troublesome bleeding has been encountered or if the urethra or bladder has possibly been injured, the wound is drained through the suprapubic incision.

Before the operator closes the vaginal portion of the incision, he must be positive that the sling is placed beneath the urethra from side to side and that the force that has been applied to the supporting sling is just that, and not an obstructing force. Little or no resistance need be felt as the tip of the metal or rubber catheter is passed into the urethra, but the angle will have been changed. One must remember that the patient will assume, postoperatively, the erect standing or sitting position; and since the sling is relatively inflexible, the bladder with the other pelvic structures will change position downward with the pull of gravity, thus augmenting the supporting action of the sling (Fig. 4.20).

As the operator prepares to close the vaginal portion of the operation, he considers the necessity of performing the frequently needed anterior colporrhaphy. This is another one of the advantages of the Goebell-Frangenheim-Stoeckel: the anterior vaginal support can be repaired simultaneously with the remainder of the procedure (37). This is particularly desirable if there is a cystocele giving the patient residual urine and likely a chronic urinary infection. Elimination of the residual urine is most important before one can hope to clear up a concomitant infection in the bladder.

Unless one resorts to a combined approach, the inability to correct the cystocele or the cystourethrocele at the time of a Marshall-Marchetti-Krantz procedure is one of the shortcomings of this operation. The vaginal portion is closed with the proper placement of any augmenting plication sutures of the paraurethral tissues, not interfering with the sling in its place. The vaginal fascia is plicated, and the edges of the vaginal mucosa are reapproximated in the midline with interrupted sutures of chromic 0 catgut. The redundant vaginal mucosa has been trimmed away.

Any other vaginal repair needed, such as an enterocele, rectocele, or vaginal stenosis, can now be done as this operation is terminated. The #18F Foley urethral catheter and the suprapubic tube are checked to see if there is any evidence of hematuria. An iodoform pack is placed in the vagina temporarily to provide a moderate tamponade and to cleanse the vagina of any blood clots when this pack is removed 24 hours postoperatively.

Technique of the Aldridge Modification of the Sling Technique

The Aldridge (20) modification of the sling procedure employs the same fundamental principles, but for various reasons the operator, or the patient, prefers that the straps of fascia be procured from the abdominal aponeurosis. This choice of site for obtaining the fascia may be necessary if there has been some injury to the thighs or hips, or some history of vascular disease of the extremities. In rare instances, if the patient has a preference, she may not wish to have a scar on her thigh, a request not found in this series of cases. On the other hand, the gynecologist may feel that procurement of the fascia from the anterior abdominal aponeurosis is easier and does not require an additional operative field, simple as it may be.

The preoperative evaluation of the patient has been completely performed, as mentioned previously in this chapter. The patient is placed in the dorsolithotomy position with the lower abdomen and perineal areas simultaneously draped and properly exposed. If the gynecologist prefers, as is sometimes the case, the procurement of the abdominal fascia can be done with the patient first in the supine

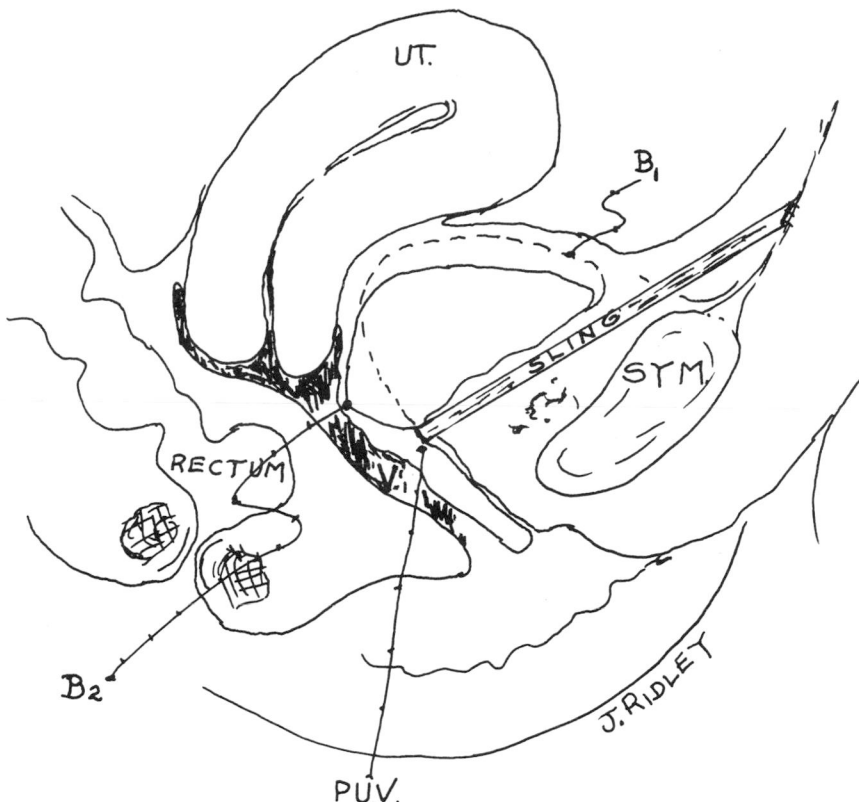

Fig. 4.20. A composite illustration to show difference in the posterior urethrovesical angle (P.U.V.) with patient in lithotomy position B_1 (dotted line), and patient in upright position, B_2 (solid line). The effect of gravity exaggerates and augments the effect of the sling.

position, and then in the lithotomy position for the placement of the sling. This, however, will mean the additional work of redraping the patient when she is changed to the lithotomy position.

A low transverse crescentic incision is made between the anterior superior spines of the ilia and approximately 3 cm above the level of the symphysis. The suprapubic cystostomy tube is avoided without difficulty. After exposing the anterior fascia by blunt and gauzed finger dissection, the two portions of the sling are mobilized. Parallel incisions are made 1 cm apart—the desired width of the strap—lateralward to near proximity of the anterior superior spines of the ilia. This is done parallel to and a few millimeters above, but not including Poupart's ligament. The medial portion of this strap is left attached to within 2 cm of the midline (Fig. 4.21). In those cases in which previous attempts to correct stress urinary incontinence

or other pathology, there may be a varying amount of scar tissue formation. Procurement of this strap may necessitate more sharp dissection, but it can usually be done without too much difficulty.

Just beneath the proximal attachments of this developed strap, the fibers of the belly of one rectus abdominus muscle are separated by blunt dissection and the space of Retzius entered either with the finger or with blunt scissors. The finger is passed retropubically, dissecting the bladder posteriorly. This is easily accomplished if previous surgery has not been performed here; however, if scarring is present, this passage retropubically must be done with a blunt instrument, such as uterine dressing forceps or long Mayo, curved scissors. The point of the clamp, as it is passed inferiorly, is kept directed toward the periosteum of the pubic ramus, thus minimizing or usually avoiding troublesome bleeding. If the error is made

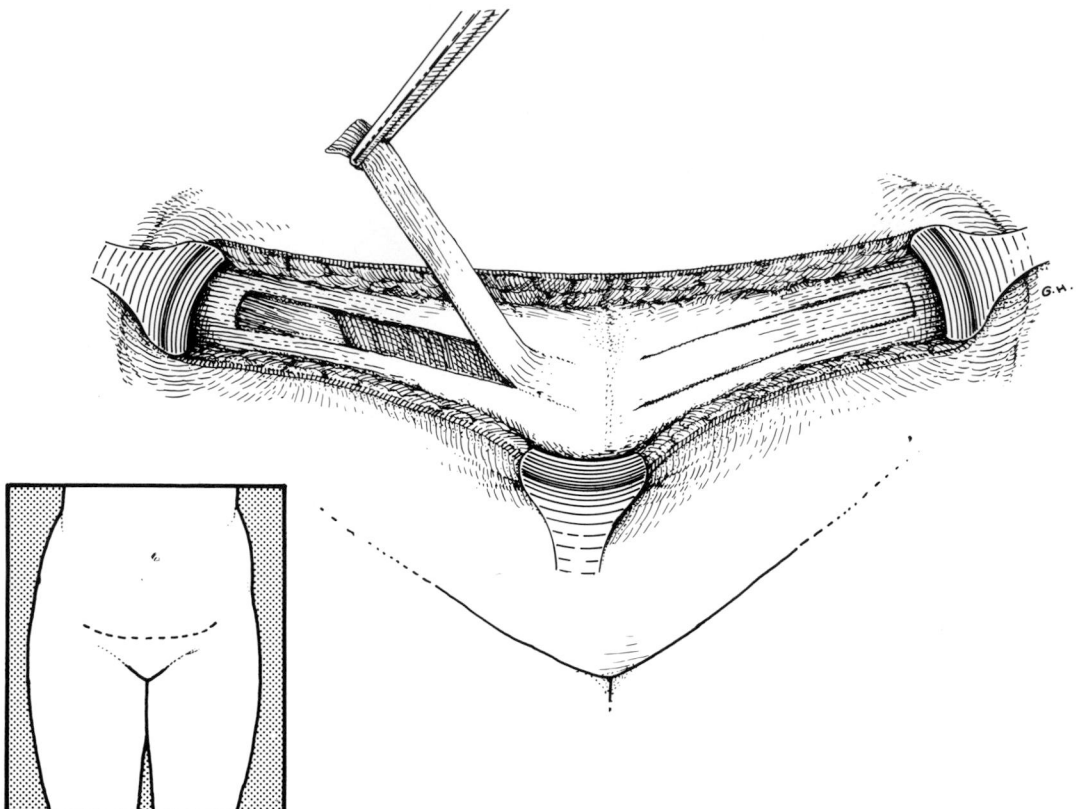

Fig. 4.21. Aldridge modification of sling procedure. Lower abdominal transverse skin incision down to anterior abdominal aponeurosis. Paired fascial straps are developed parallel to and 2.0 cm above Poupart's ligament. These straps are allowed to remain attached near midline, and free ends are turned downward retropubically to be joined beneath the urethra to form the sling. The defects of the abdominal fascia must be closed carefully to avoid risk of postoperative hernia.

of opening the venous sinuses about the bladder neck, pressure must be temporarily applied either from above or below, or in combination, to control this bleeding. Since this is usually venous, this digital pressure will suffice. If the bleeding is too brisk, which is indeed a rare occurrence, the entry into the space of Retzius must be widened so that control of the hemorrhage can be accomplished under direct vision.

After the dissection retropubically has been carried down to each side of the urethra, the site of operation is shifted to the vaginal field as described in the foregoing section using the fascia lata strap. After the midline of the vaginal mucosa has been opened and the subjacent fascia developed as well as possible, a shallow tunnel on each side of the urethra is

developed by blunt finger dissection up to and just behind the inferior surface of the pubic ramus. A blunt clamp, either uterine dressing forceps or a long Kelly forcep, is passed through the space of Retzius along the path which had been developed previously. As the tip of the clamp, having been passed from above downward, is felt just lateral to the urethra, a gentle punch passes it further downward into the vagina through the triangular ligament or urogenital diaphragm. A small incision over the tip of the clamp may be necessary to facilitate its passage. The tip of a similar clamp is grasped vaginally and the lower clamp carefully drawn upward through the space of Retzius. Now the free end of the strap of the anterior aponeurosis is grasped and drawn downward retropubically to present in the vaginal field. This is performed on each side and the two free ends of the abdominal fascia are joined beneath the urethra in which the indwelling catheter has remained. The two ends are joined with three or four interrupted sutures of 3-0 silk as the proper tension is applied. The amount of tension must not be excessive; it must merely support the bladder neck without causing any obstruction, more fully explained in the foregoing description using the fascia lata sling. In our experience the tension is more accurately adjusted beneath the urethra when the continuous fascia lata sling has been used than when the two ends of the abdominal strap are joined in this currently described technique. Nonetheless, the end results are the same.

The vaginal portion of the operation allows the gynecologist to further correct any concomitant cystocele, rectocele, or enterocele, whether recurrent or primary. After this is done, the vaginal portion is completed in the routine manner. As the operator closes the abdominal incision, he must carefully close the large fascial defects which have resulted from procurement of the fascia straps. Drainage is optional and usually not employed.

Technique of the Transected Sling Procedure

Ridley (35, 38, 41) has described a modification of the fascia lata strap technique of Goebell-Frangenheim-Stoeckel that can be used under certain conditions where other techniques are not feasible. In relatively rare cases the operator finds that the urethra is really abnormal or unworkable, with the following examples. (a) Absence of the urethra either congenitally, surgically, or by disease in which a mucosal tube has been fashioned by a previous procedure but with no control of the urine. Although this membranous tube has been successfully created, the intolerable situation of urinary incontinence persists. (b) Previous successful closure of a urethrovaginal or a urethrovesicovaginal fistula resulting in a thin unworkable membrane but no urinary control.

Although either the fascia lata strap or the Aldridge technique may be used, we have preferred the fascia lata because of its workability and less trauma to the abdominal wall. The approach retropubically in this Ridley modification is identical to that described just

previously in the fascia lata technique; however, the vaginal portion of the operation is necessarily changed.

The patient is in the lithotomy position, and the retropubic dissection has been accomplished from above through the two slit-like incisions in the anterior abdominal aponeurosis. This abdominal wound is temporarily packed with a moist saline sponge. The anterior vaginal wall is exposed and the bladder neck or what would ordinarily be the posterior urethrovesical angle has been identified by an indwelling #16F 5-cc Foley bag catheter. Because of the unworkability of the urethral tube, for reasons enumerated above, two 2-cm slit-like incisions are made parallel to the axis of the urethra and 1 cm to each side of the midline in the area identified as the bladder neck (Fig. 4.22). By blunt or sharp dissection as the case may be, a tunnel is created paraurethrally up to the inferior aspect of the pubic ramus. The vaginal mucosa overlying the urethra in the midline has not and will not be disturbed. A curved clamp is passed from above downward retropubically and the tip presented first in one vaginal slit incision and then in the other. The fascia lata strap is drawn upward on each side, forming a sling beneath the urethra. Proper tension and support is applied without obstructing the urethral tube, and the free ends of the fascia lata strap are secured abdominally as previously described.

The important part of this modification is fastening the fascia lata to the paraurethral tissues without injuring the urethra. This is done in the following manner: after the proper supporting tension has been applied to the sling, the paraurethral tissue or fascia is securely sutured to the sling at the point of the two small vaginal slit-like incisions. This is done with 3-0 silk interrupted sutures. The yet exposed portion of the sling subtending the urethra is excised, and the two small incisions are closed with 0 chromic catgut, further anchoring the transected ends of the supporting sling on each side. In this manner the bladder neck is given support without injury to the previously injured or reconstructed urethra. Six cases have been done in this manner with five satisfactory results and one failure.

The overall versatility and dependability of the sling procedure has led this operator to use

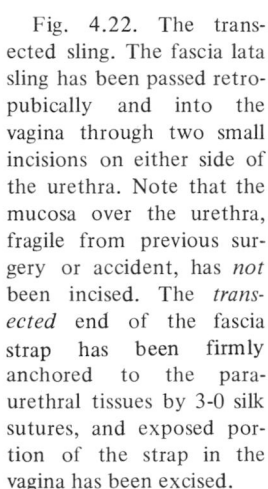

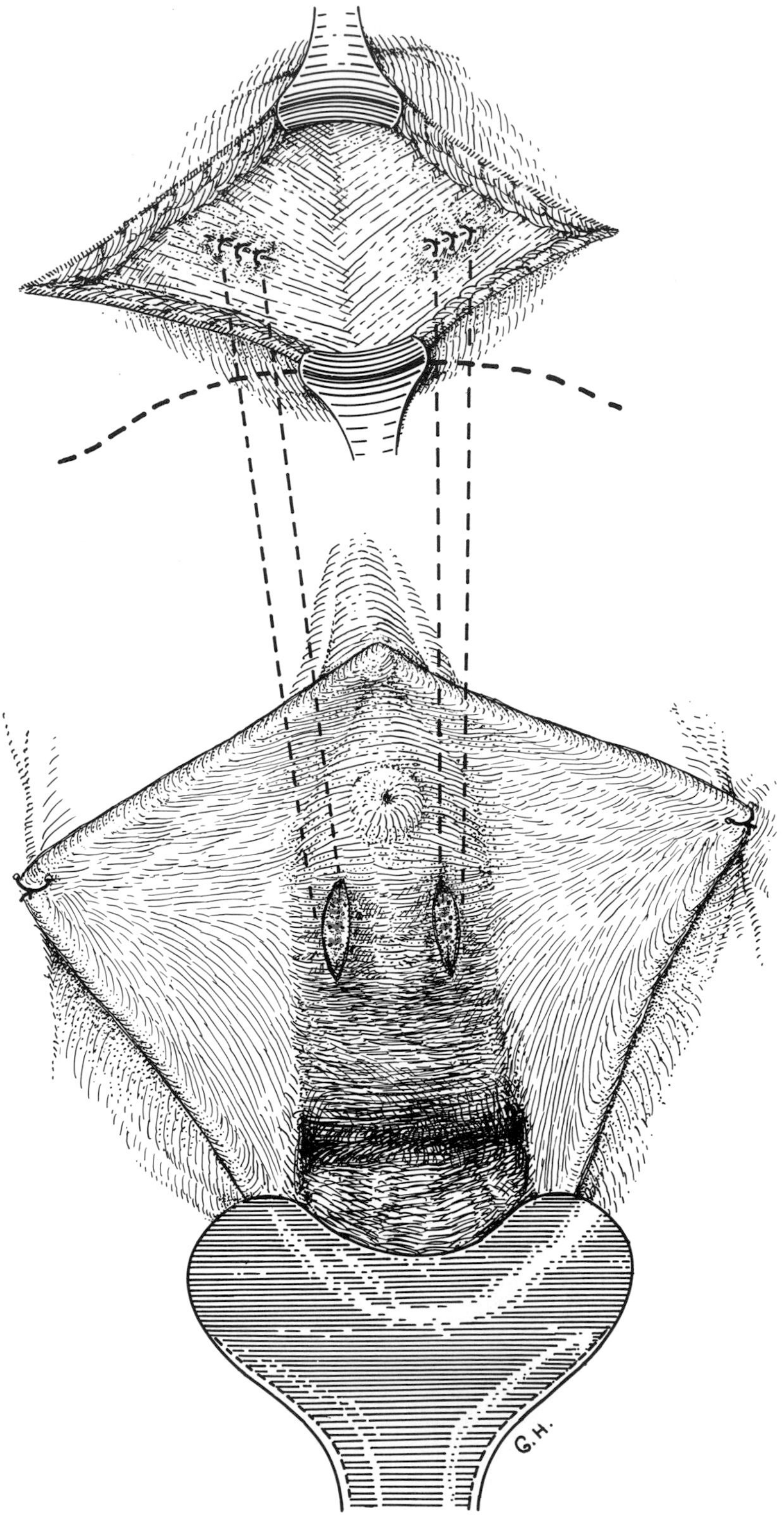

Fig. 4.22. The transected sling. The fascia lata sling has been passed retropubically and into the vagina through two small incisions on either side of the urethra. Note that the mucosa over the urethra, fragile from previous surgery or accident, has *not* been incised. The *transected* end of the fascia strap has been firmly anchored to the paraurethral tissues by 3-0 silk sutures, and exposed portion of the strap in the vagina has been excised.

In the event that the paraurethral tissue is too weakened to be identified for anchoring the fascia, the strap is left uninterrupted beneath the urethra *exteriorized* in the vagina but giving support to the bladder neck. This vaginally exteriorized portion of the strap is anchored to the subjacent intact vaginal mucosa of the midline and will shortly become covered by new epithelium.

it by choice in most of the very difficult situations in which other procedures have failed or where the anatomy and tissues are virtually unworkable by any other approach. A recent case, successfully operated upon, had previous failures of the anterior colporrhaphy with plication, the Marshall-Marchetti-Krantz, and the Pereyra needle suspension. Despite extensive cicatrix of the vagina and retropubic space, the Goebell-Frangenheim-Stoeckel sling procedure was done and the patient was made continent.

Case Report #1. B.C. WF grav. T para T (Hosp#-P.H.360-297), age 68. Chief complaint: recurrent marked stress urinary incontinence existent for 35 years, since birth of only child. Menopause occurred at 50 years of age without complications. Previous surgical attempts consisted of abdominal hysterectomy with vaginal repair with plication; Marshall-Marchetti-Krantz, 1966; Pereyra needle suspension and Y-plasty of bladder neck, 1969. It had now become necessary to wear indwelling catheter to have any urinary control. The resulting scarring of the bladder base and lower abdomen and loss by necrosis of the distal two-thirds of the urethra left tissues practically unworkable. The patient's general health had been good but she had become practically a recluse because of the nearly constant urine leakage.

Physical Examination. Her general physical condition was good. The abdomen was moderately obese with two well healed lower abdominal surgical scars.

Pelvic Examination. External genitalia were macerated due to nearly constant urinary drainage. The anterior vaginal wall was inelastic and shortened due to scarring. No recurrent cystocele was present. The external urethral meatus was patulous and now located well within the vagina. The urethra was 1.2 cm long and of 30F caliber. Cystoscopy showed normal trigone and ureteral orifices. Cystometrogram tracing was within normal limits. Any physical movement increasing the intra-abdominal pressure caused a spurt of urine from the urethra. No fistula was present.

Operation. On September 12, 1969, a Goebell-Frangenheim-Stoeckel was performed using fascia lata sling. This was transected and fixed to the paraurethral tissues and vaginal mucosa

lateral to the midline without disturbing the thinned vaginal and urethral membranes at the midline.

Postoperative Course. The urethral catheter was removed on the third postoperative day after the suprapubic cystostomy tube was functioning properly and giving adeqaute drainage. The patient was able to void per urethrum in increasing amounts, and on the ninth postoperative day the suprapubic tube, no longer necessary, was removed.

Six months postoperatively the patient was continent and running about 30 cc residual. Twenty months postoperatively she was continent and well.

Another three cases in which the complete colpocleisis had been performed with an effort to plicate the bladder neck had failed but were finally operated upon secondarily by the sling procedure and were cured of incontinence.

Recently another variation of application of the fascia lata sling has been created with successful results. A newly constructed urethra, constructed because of postoperative slough of the original urethra, was a patent musosal tube but completely incontinent. The fascia lata strap was not transected as described above because the attachment of the paraurethral ends would be insecure, it was thought. The end of the fascia lata was brought out through the paraurethral slit-like incisions, passed beneath the urethra and back into the slit on the opposite side, then retropubically attached on the anterior abdominal aponeurosis as previously described. The exposed portion of the fascia lata in the vagina beneath the urethra was not transected but left exteriorized and fixed lightly but securely to the underlying vaginal mucosa with interrupted 3-0 black silk sutures. The slit-like incisions were closed on each side of the urethra. Five weeks later the fascia lata was covered by new epithelium overgrown from the vagina, and the patient has remained continent. Where an ultimate effort is to be made, Green, Marchetti (38), and other authorities have resorted to the sling procedure for most cases where previous failures have been encountered.

To date this operator has performed or had direct supervision of 146 cases in which the sling procedure has been used for the following indications and with these results.

Goebell-Stoeckel Sling Procedure

1948-1973

Total number of cases	146
With fascia lata strap	127
With Aldridge strap	2
With Mersilene strap	17
Previous surgical procedures	
None	14
Vaginal repair alone (one or more)	68
Combination of procedures (vaginal repair,	64
Marshall-Marchetti-Krantz, sling,	
fistula repair)	
Complications of sling material	
Fascia	0
Mersilene (of 17 case) (23%)	4
Postoperative complications	
Chronic urinary tract incontinence	18
Residual urine (30 cc or more after 6	32
months)	
Final results	
Cured	127 (87%)
Improved	11 (7%)
Failed	8 (6%)

Technique of the Marshall-Marchetti-Krantz Operation

This is the third basic procedure available to the gynecologist for correction of stress urinary incontinence. Retropubic urethropexy had been used previously, but in 1949 Marshall, Marchetti, and Krantz (33) published a description of the procedure with very favorable results in 45 cases. Since that time the basic operation has remained virtually unchanged except for some modifications of the suture material, the placement thereof, and the preoperative and postoperative care (39, 42). An effort is made in this text to point out the fundamentals of the procedure, the errors which may be encountered, and safeguards against these errors and ultimate failure (45).

The patient under satisfactory anesthesia is given a pelvic examination routinely to check the exact nature of the pelvic pathology. Coexisting intra-abdominal pathology can be treated in conjunction with the Marshall-Marchetti-Krantz procedure in most circumstances except where active pelvic infection or extensive malignancy is present.

Foregone is the conclusion that the routine preoperative evaluation of the bladder, mentioned earlier in this chapter, has been done including history, general physical examination, and a comprehensive study of the urinary tract. The Marchetti or coughing test, in which the bladder neck is supported without compression, is very helpful in prognosticating what surgical results may be anticipated. The cystometrogram is done routinely to rule out urge incontinence or bladder atony. Chain cystourethrography may be used as an adjunct, but not always routinely in the preoperative evaluation of the bladder function. The techniques of these two simple and valuable procedures have been discussed elsewhere in this chapter.

The patient is placed in the supine position with an indwelling #20F Foley catheter with an inflated 5-cc bag. We formerly had used a slightly larger catheter but with a 30-cc balloon; however, the larger balloon actually got in the way of proper placement of the suspending sutures. The vagina may or may not be packed depending on what other procedure is to be done in conjunction with the retropubic suspension. If abdominal hysterectomy is to be performed, it is preferred not to pack the vagina; but if the vagina is not to be opened, a vaginal pack is placed within to help delineate the vault and urethra. An even more satisfactory maneuver is to have an assistant elevate the vaginal vault with two examining fingers in the vagina while the suspending paraurethral sutures are actually being placed.

In the case where the Marshall-Marchetti-Krantz procedure is being done primarily, a tranverse incision is made down to but not into the peritoneal cavity. If intra-abdominal work is to be done, this portion of the operation is dispatched and the peritoneal cavity is securely closed. An error can be made by not securely closing the peritoneum or by unavoidably tearing into it, allowing the possibility of urinary leakage into the peritoneal cavity itself. Although not a frequent error, the bladder neck or urethra can be pierced with the needle point at times, unknown to the operator, thus allowing urine seepage into the space of Retzius. For this reason many operators routinely drain the Marshall-Marchetti-Krantz procedure through the suprapubic incision. We routinely drain the operative site only in cases in which troublesome bleeding has been controlled or obvious urinary tract injury has taken place. However, great care is used to be sure that the peritoneum is either uninjured or securely closed at the end of the operation.

The space of Retzius is developed by blunt dissection after the rectus muscles have been divided in the midline. If previous retropubic surgery has been performed, some sharp dissection may be necessary in the approach to the urethra and the bladder neck. One must safeguard as well as possible against the chance of causing brisk, troublesome bleeding. If this occurs, it may be difficult to control except by pressure. Ligating torn venous sinus is usually unsatisfactory, as is fulguration. When troublesome bleeding, which is really relatively rare, has been controlled, the suspending sutures are properly placed.

The #1 chromic catgut suture proves to be the most satisfactory material. Various operators through the years have experimented with different suture materials both absorbable and nonabsorbable with no such consistently dependable results as to exclude all others. Nonabsorbable materials in this location of the body have generally proven unsatisfactory. The #4 Mayo taper point needle is satisfactory as opposed to a cutting needle which will cut out of the periosteum of the pubic bones.

The lowermost pair of sutures are placed under direct vision, taking a firm bite into the paraurethral tissues without piercing into the vaginal vault, then a light bite into the periurethral tissue just lateral to the midline as marked by the indwelling catheter, and finally a firm bite into the periosteum of the pubic bone. The latter portion of this important three-phase suture is placed carefully by following the curve of the needle with pressure to drive the point beneath the periosteum. If an error is made by the needle tearing or cutting out of the tissue, another bite must be taken as closely as possible to fix the suture. Either two or three pairs of sutures are placed, depending on the depth of the symphysis. Each pair of sutures is tied when placed, to facilitate the placement and tying of the following pairs of sutures. A final one or two sutures are taken to fix the anterior aspect of the bladder to the superior aspect of the symphysis. The suture is passed from Cooper's ligament on the one side, into the bladder wall in the midline, and to the Cooper's ligament on the other side (Fig. 4.23).

Careful inspection is made of the retropubic space, checking for any evidence of thus far undetected bleeding or bladder or urethral injury. It is up to the judgment of the operator whether the wound is to be drained. We hardly ever do so unless there has been evidence of oozing or of urinary tract injury. The abdominal wall is then closed in routine layer-for-layer manner. A final check is made to ascertain that the urethral catheter and suprapubic cystostomy are draining well.

In the unfortunate event of delayed bleeding in the retropubic space or of a previously undetected urinary tract injury, the patient will begin to show an unexpected amount of suprapubic pain, possibly hematuria, and a palpable mass forming that can be felt on careful abdominovaginal examination. If drainage of the wound has not been done at time of surgery, drainage must be considered now. If the signs and symptoms of such trouble worsen, then immediate suprapubic drainage must be done. It is usually possible to accomplish this by gently separating the sutured layers of the abdominal wall with a blunt instrument and placing a Penrose drain into the retropubic space to each side of the midline. Broad spectrum antibiotics of choice are given. Cephalin, intravenously or intramuscularly, has been a drug of current choice, but sulfonamide or tetracycline therapy can be used depending on culture and sensitivity tests taken at the time of the postoperative drainage. In two cases out of 120 having such postoperative complications, the recovery was otherwise uneventful, and fortunately both patients were cured of their stress incontinence. No doubt the retropubic scarring resulting from the complication properly positioned the bladder neck retropubically.

The overall success rate of the Marshall-Marchetti-Krantz procedure, when this operation has been performed in those cases in which plication had failed or previous complications had been encountered, is quoted as being between 80 to 90 per cent cured. We have rarely used the Marshall-Marchetti-Krantz procedure primarily to correct stress urinary incontinence without first considering simple plication. Burch (43) had reported a 96 per cent cure rate, but analysis will show that 96 per cent of these cases were primarily operated upon by a modification of the Marshall-Marchetti-Krantz.

In the event of failure of the Marshall-Marchetti-Krantz procedure, success may yet be salvaged in about 80 per cent of these cases by

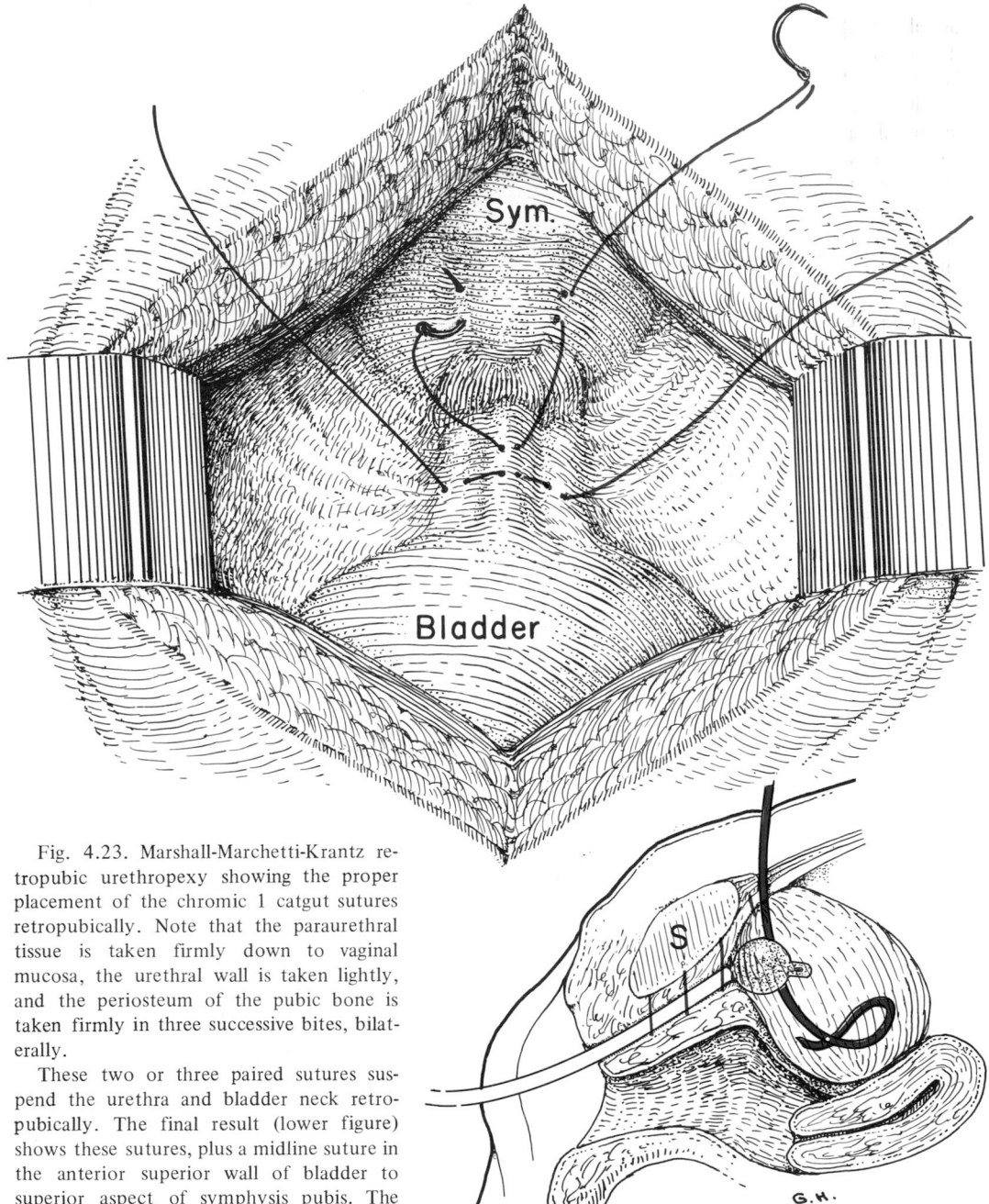

Fig. 4.23. Marshall-Marchetti-Krantz retropubic urethropexy showing the proper placement of the chromic 1 catgut sutures retropubically. Note that the paraurethral tissue is taken firmly down to vaginal mucosa, the urethral wall is taken lightly, and the periosteum of the pubic bone is taken firmly in three successive bites, bilaterally.

These two or three paired sutures suspend the urethra and bladder neck retropubically. The final result (lower figure) shows these sutures, plus a midline suture in the anterior superior wall of bladder to superior aspect of symphysis pubis. The suprapubic cystostomy tube is in place.

the use of the Goebell-Frangenheim-Stoeckel sling procedure. Although a second Marshall-Marchetti-Krantz may be attempted, the operator will usually find that the retropubic dissection, sufficiently wide to permit replacing the suspending sutures, may be unsatisfactory or impossible because of scar tissue from previous surgery. The passage of the fascia sling retropubically demands less dissection and may be more safely done. For this reason the

Goebell-Frangenheim-Stoeckel sling procedure is the operation to choose in the final effort to salvage an otherwise unsatisfactory result. Its versatility has been proven not only as an occasional primary procedure, but most importantly as a salvage procedure, not only where other procedures have failed but also when antecedent procedures such as colpocleisis, irradiation, fistula repair, or construction of a urethra have been done.

Postoperative Care

Improper postoperative care, a most serious error, can jeopardize or cause failure of the most perfectly planned and executed pelvic operation. Every effort must be made to (a) insure proper drainage to protect the recently operated tissues from overdistension; (b) prevent, control, or eradicate urinary tract infection; and (c) detect and control delayed hemorrhage by judicious observation, pressure, or by actual reoperation.

Establishment and maintenance of proper drainage are most important. One must select the proper sized catheter for retention in the bladder either by balloon, catheter shape, or suture. The #16F to #20F Foley catheter with the 5-cc bag is most commonly employed, but under certain circumstances one may use the Malecot, Pezzar, or other specially shaped catheters that are available, allowing two-way drainage for constant or intermittent irrigation, particularly if the patient has shown postoperative hematuria or encrustations. The time that the catheter is allowed to remain in the bladder varies, depending on many factors. However, for the routine uncomplicated care of surgical correction for stress urinary incontinence, the catheter is left in place for about 2 to 4 days.

Early ambulation is most important; where once the patient was kept in bed and the indwelling catheter in place for 10 days to 3 weeks, particularly if vaginal or abdominal hysterectomy had also been done, we now ambulate as early as possible. If there is no evidence of postoperative hematuria, the indwelling catheter is clamped intermittently for 2 hours or less for 24 hours prior to the time of anticipated removal. The catheter is then removed, freeing the patient at least enough to sit upright on the bed pan placed on a bedside chair or commode, or allowing her to go to the nearby toilet. It is important whenever practicable to promote early natural physiologic micturition. The voided amount is measured, and the interval between voidings is noted. If the patient is passing 150 to 200 cc per voiding every 2 hours or so, and is comfortable, the suprapubic catheter is clamped off. However, if she is obviously voiding inadequately in frequent small amounts, *i.e.,* 30 cc every 30 to 60 minutes, distention is likely present with simple overflow voiding. Good and alert nursing care will detect and remedy this by prompt release of the suprapubic tube or even catheterization. If the residual urine is more than 150 cc, the suprapubic tube is left open for adequate drainage. This is clamped intermittently to test if the patient is voiding more effectively. This small "safety valve" tube must be irrigated intermittently to guarantee against its occlusion. It is not withdrawn until the patient is emptying her bladder satisfactorily. This may take as long as 10 days in unusual circumstances, but it is obviously of great value in obviating repeated catheterizations.

It has been shown by Kass and Schneiderman (2) that the bacterial count of the urine soars geometrically if the indwelling catheter is left in place more than 48 hours. The infection ascends particularly along the outside of the catheter but also within its lumen. Despite all efforts to prevent unwanted in and out mobility of the catheter, it is practically impossible as the patient turns or sits up. Any preoperative urinary tract infection is noted, establishing what organism is present and to what drugs it is sensitive. Postoperatively the culture is repeated, often showing a newly introduced organism and a mixed infection. Sensitivity tests are again done and appropriate therapy instituted, using chemotherapy or antibiotic as selected. This therapy is preferably continued until the patient is emptying her bladder satisfactorily, and ideally until the urine is sterile.

Sterilizing the urine may be impossible in some cases in which well established upper urinary tract pathology exists, such as chronic pyelonephritis or lithiasis. Nevertheless, the effort must be made for at least 10 days to bring the infection under control. Even with the essentially satisfactorily performed operation for stress urinary incontinence, regardless of the type, there is a certain small percentage of cases that will carry a residual urine, either due to the errors of an uncorrected cystocele, overcorrected posterior urethrovesical angle, or excessive tension on a sling beneath the bladder neck.

Hematuria, postoperatively, is very frequently seen, likely due to catheter or instrument trauma without actual bladder perforation. Regardless of how frequently it is seen, it must nevertheless be observed carefully and treated expectantly. In the great majority of instances the hematuria is self-limiting and clears up promptly within a few hours. One must watch for any clots or diminution of catheter flow to prevent overdistention. Regardless of the amount of bleeding, the bladder drainage—whether it be by urethral catheter alone or by the preferable combination of the suprapubic cystostomy tube and urethral catheter—must be unimpaired; irrigation of the catheters is done every 30 to 60 minutes until the urine has cleared or appropriate measures instituted to stop the bleeding. If clots are forming, signifying significant bleeding, these clots must be removed either by repeated irrigations or by the use of the clot evacuator. The collapsed bladder is more likely to stop bleeding than the overdistended, clot-filled organ.

A Foley catheter with a tamponade balloon is helpful in controlling bleeding about the bladder neck, where it is most likely to occur. Firm but not vigorous vaginal packing is helpful. Pressure over the lower abdomen by suprapubic placement of a 5-pound sandbag is used at times. Finally and fortunately unusual, the site must be actually investigated either by cystoscopy, to look for obvious bleeding points, or by reopening the wounds to check for the point of hemorrhage. This may necessitate exploration of the space of Retzius and a cystotomy. If the actual bleeding points are not identifiable, firm pressure over specific bleeding areas can be used, or carefully placed mass ligature taken. Before any mass ligature is taken, gentle trial pressure with ring forceps or sponge clamp without sponge and without clamping the ratchet, is applied over the suspected area here and there (Fig. 4.24).

When bleeding is controlled, the gently clamped tissue is carefully inspected to determine whether a vital structure such as the ureter has been included. If so, reapplication of the trial forceps is done until bleeding is controlled without injury to this structure, and the ligature then carefully placed. This technique is useful anywhere in the pelvis when a disturbing hemorrhage has occurred.

The postoperative bladder frequently will have a variable amount of atony, particularly in cases in which a cystocele has been concomitantly repaired. In these cases it is of value to use sympathicomimetic, bladder-stimulating medications to stimulate muscle contractions and to increase muscle tone; Urecholine given in 10- to 20-mg doses by mouth every 6 to 8 hours has been found to be a valuable adjunct in promoting adequate bladder drainage.

Salvage

Failure of any surgical procedure must be anticipated, although failure is relatively rare in these operations for the correction of stress urinary incontinence. Even the most basic procedure, the plication operation, has a percentage of failures or at least less-than-satisfactory results. This percentage of failures is variously quoted by different clinics and authors. Study of the author's cases during the past 25 years while using primarily the plication procedure shows 86 per cent cured, 8 per cent improved, and 6 per cent failures. The Mayo Clinic has reported slightly less success and a certain number of "late" failures (40). The Johns Hopkins Hospital Gynecologic Service in its more recent reappraisal of the Kelly procedure quotes 92 per cent cured with only 5 per cent failures. The so-called late or delayed failures occur in a few plication procedures, but if this occurs later than 3 years after the primary operation, it is thought that tissue failure has again been the main factor. Late failures are very uncommon in those cases in which the sling procedure has been used, and relatively rare for the Marshall-Marchetti-Krantz procedure. The overall value of any operative procedure for the correction of stress urinary incontinence must not be judged until the chance of these late failures can be evaluated. The more recent procedure for urethral suspension, the Pereyra needle operation, has shown a

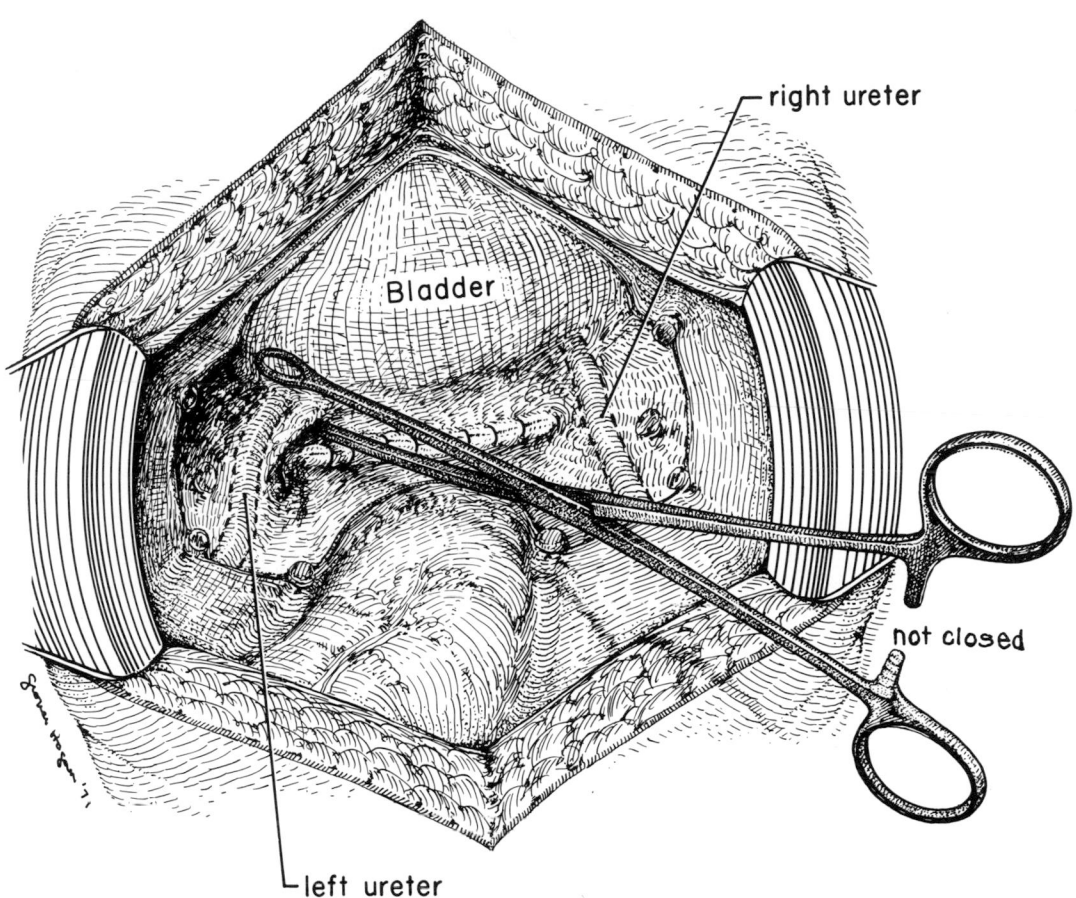

Fig. 4.24. A very practical maneuver if brisk, uncontrollable bleeding is encountered in vital area of the base of the broad ligament. This can occur with any type of pelvic procedure. The empty sponge clamp is placed gently in the area of hemorrhage and the tissues compressed but *without* closure of the clamp. In this way the bleeding can be slowed or stopped long enough to pinpoint the source without injuring the ureter or bladder by blind clamping with a powerful instrument, or by a deep blind ligature.

discouraging number of delayed failures (28), albeit a relatively easily performed operation.

Regardless of what technique is used and with what skill the surgeon performs the operation, whether it be of primary or secondary nature, there will occur a certain irreducible number of failures. The surgeon must then strive to salvage what can be done from these cases.

Failure of the plication procedure leaves the operator with several alternatives. It is possible to perform another plication procedure, but usually this is inadvisable unless the patient's physical condition prevents a more extensive approach, or if the patient shows a distinct recurrence of the cystocele and Type I configu-

ration of the posterior urethrovesical angle. If the patient has shown a Type II change of the urethral relationship to the symphysis and bladder base, the plication procedure probably should not have been chosen in the first place. The operator may choose the Marshall-Marchetti-Krantz procedure as salvage when previous attempt by the plication procedure has failed, and there has been no recurrence of a troublesome cystocele. If the space of Retzius has not been scarred by previous surgery, the retropubic urethropexy will usually offer no problem. However, if the space of Retzius has been obliterated previously, dissection here may be difficult, but not usually impossible. Inasmuch as the dissection here must be more extensive for the Marshall-Marchetti-Krantz than for the sling procedure, bleeding and injury to the bladder and urethra may be more likely. Regardless of this, the Marshall-Marchetti-Krantz procedure has been used successfully in experienced hands as a salvage procedure for operative failures by a previous Marshall-Marchetti-Krantz procedure and even a sling procedure.

The sling procedure, however, using the fascia lata, is felt to be the ultimate operation for the salvage of previous failure by any other procedure. Even in the event of extensive scarring of the anterior vaginal wall and in the space of Retzius, the operator will find that these tissues can be worked when using the sling. It may be necessary to use sharp dissection to mobilize the urethra and its posterior angle, and great care must be used while passing the sling retropubically, but it can be safely and effectively performed.

The error of putting too much tension on the sling beneath the urethra or with the suture of the retropubic urethropexy both can cause obstruction of the urethra of a varying degree. Although experience will guide the determination of the amount of correction to be used, this error of overcorrection must be remembered. To the less experienced operator, the main error is that of applying too much tension in any of these procedures.

In the event that the urethra or bladder neck has been suspended too snugly retropubically by the Marshall-Marchetti-Krantz procedure, preventing the patient from initiating micturition or completely emptying her bladder, correction may be difficult. Although complete obstruction in this procedure is possible by an inaccurately placed suture, it is indeed rare. If this misfortune occurs, the surgeon must, by necessity, re-enter the operative area as soon as feasible to remove the obstructing suture, while maintaining adequate bladder drainage until such corrective measures can be taken. One should remember that more than one erroneous suture may be present. However, in the event that only partial obstruction exists, which is a more likely occurrence, the urethra may be dilated cautiously and gently to a #34F with either the Hegar or Hank's dilators. This can usually be done with local anesthesia or without any anesthesia at all.

If the fascial sling, whether it be from the fascia lata or from the anterior abdominal aponeurosis, is causing partial or even complete obstruction, the tension on this sling can be lessened by one of the following techniques.

If the patient has not been able to void, even partially, after 7 days postoperatively, the urethra is gently sounded and dilated to #27F or #30F. The suprapubic cystostomy tube has not been removed and its patency is guarded. If after 7 more days, the 14 postoperative day, the patient has not voided satisfactorily, she is sent home to be readmitted 6 weeks postoperatively for manipulation or transection of the strap. This amount of time is allowed for scar tissue to form about the strap in its course retropubically. Now when the strap is manipulated and transected, there will be a good chance that enough support by scar tissue will have formed to salvage a satisfactory result. The operator must not allow himself to be pressured into a corrective procedure unwisely too soon, or at an inappropriate time. He must be prepared for this coercion by the patient, the family, or his sense of guilt and failure, but must act only according to the dictates of sound surgical principles and judgment.

The patient is anesthetized and the urethra calibrated to see if the lumen is #27F or larger and without actual obstruction. A firm downward but well controlled thrust at right angles against the strap can first be tried. It can be felt to "give" a slight amount when the fascia straps have overlapped beneath the urethra in the Aldridge type procedure. Although this is not an exact corrective procedure, it nevertheless has worked satisfactorily in two cases in which release of some tension of the sling was necessary. The fascia itself will not stretch.

In the event that this simple maneuver has not released any tension on the sling, the strap must be transected either by a small slit-like incision to one side of the midline through the vaginal mucosa, being very careful not to injure the urethra. It is usually not difficult to identify the strap when gentle tension is applied downward on the urethra. After the strap has been cut, the small mucosal incision is closed. In one case the strap was necessarily cut transureterally where slight erosion had taken place through the inferior aspect of the urethral mucosa. Care was used to only transect the fascial band and not open the vaginal mucosa, thus running the risk of creating a urethrovaginal fistula.

In all five of these cases in which the fascia was either manipulated or transected, the results were satisfactory because enough time had elapsed for scar tissue to form. In the course of time when the Mersilene strap was being tried, it became necessary to remove as completely as possible this synthetic material in four cases because it had either caused tissue reaction or low grade infection, thus acting as a wick, or had apparently shrunk enough to create an obstructive problem (35). Even though the second procedure had been necessary to remove the material, three of the four cases involved had satisfactory results, very likely because enough cicatrix had formed along the course of the Mersilene strap to give a desirable support. Nevertheless the use of this material in this type of operation has been condemned and discontinued.

Inevitably, a certain irreducible number of cases of urinary incontinence per urethra is incurable by any of the aforementioned operations. Perhaps the tissues are truly unworkable due to changes by irradiation or surgical scarring, or by altered bladder dynamics which would prohibit normal micturition under any circumstances. In these distressing cases, one must use urinary diversion into an ileal or sigmoid colon conduit but only after the patient has come to consider that the urinary incontinence is intolerable to an extent to warrant employing this rather radical and sometimes dangerous operation. Nevertheless, in rare instances this measure is chosen, which gives her continence but saddles her with the aftercare of this altered anatomy and physiology. A detailed description of the operations for diversion of the urinary stream is given in Chapter 9.

Recapitulation of Common Errors

1. Improper and misunderstood initial confrontation of patient and her problem.

2. Inadequate history of nature of chief complaint; its onset, severity, and intolerability.

3. Inaccurate evaluation of what previous surgical effort or treatment has been attempted.

4. Failure to clearly test for and define exact physical nature of complaint, *i.e.,* true stress incontinence, urge incontinence, fistula, neurogenic cause, or combination of any of these.

5. Inappropriate selection of the type of surgical approach or in rare instances, the conservative effort.

6. Selection of wrong, poor, or inadequate surgical instruments.

7. Direct operative injury to the urethra, bladder, or adjacent structures.

8. Failure to detect this operative injury at the time it occurs or at least before the surgical procedure is completed.

9. Inadequate drainage of bladder.

10. Postoperative dehydration and electrolyte imbalance.

11. Failure to anticipate and properly treat urinary tract and/or wound infection.

12. Overcorrection or partial obstruction of urethra by plication.

13. Overcorrection or posterior urethrovesical angle by sling or by retropubic fixation.

14. Undercorrection of the urethral and bladder weakness by insufficient plication, tension on sling, or retropubic fixation.

These are some of the more common errors which one may commit in the course of this type of surgery. This list is, of course, a generalization without being able to encompass all the minute mistakes one may make. However, a review will alert the operator so that he may possibly avoid these and other errors.

The most important safeguard against operative errors is to be forewarned of their possible occurrence and take proper precautions at the very outset of the surgical procedure beginning with the initial meeting with the patient. Constant awareness of the possibility of the occurrence of these errors comes through training, concern, and experience.

References

1. Everett, H. S.: A condemnation of resectoscopic procedures upon the female vesical neck. Urol. Cutan. Rev. 52: 121, 1948.
2. Kass, E. H., and Schneiderman, L. S.: Entry of bacteria into the urinary tracts of patients with inlying catheter. N. Engl. J. Med. 256: 536, 1957.
3. Beeson, P. B.: Case against the catheter. Am. J. Med. 24: 1, 1958.
4. McDonald, R. A., Levitin, H., Mallory, G. K., and Kass, E. H.: Relation between pyelonephritis and bacterial counts in the urine. N. Engl. J. Med. 257: 915, 1957.
5. Green, T. H., Jr.: Development of a plan for the diagnosis and treatment of urinary stress incontinence. Am. J. Obstet. Gynecol. 83: 532, 1962.

6. Kegel, A. H.: Progressive resistance exercise in functional restoration of the perineal muscle. Am. J. Obstet. Gynecol. 56: 238, 1948.

7. Ridley, J. H.: Surgical treatment of stress urinary incontinence in women. J. Med. Assoc. Georgia 44: 135, 1955.

8. Kelly, H. A.: Incontinence of urine in women. Urol. Cutan. Rev. 17: 291, 1913.

9. Kennedy, W. T.: Incontinence of urine in the female. Amer. J. Obstet. Gynecol. 33: 19, 1937.

10. Symmonds, R. E.: Loss of urethral floor with total urinary incontinence. Am. J. Obstet. Gynecol. 103: 665, 1969.

11. Krantz, K. E.: Anatomy of the urethra and anterior vaginal wall. Trans. Am. Assoc. Obstet. Gynecol. Abd. Surg. 61: 31, 1950.

12. Schultze, B. S.: The Pathology and Treatment of Displacements of the Uterus. Trans. from German by J. J. Macan. D. Appleton, New York, 1888.

13. Jeffcoate, T. N. A.: Principles governing the treatment of S.U.I. in the female. Brit. J. Urol. 37: 641, 1965.

14. Giordano, D.: 20 ieme Congres. Franc de Chirug., p. 506, 1907.

15. Goebell, R.: Fur Operativen Beseltigung der Angeborenen Incontinentia Vesicae. Z. Gynaku. Urol. 2: 187, 1910.

16. Frangenheim, P.: Zur Operativen Behandlung der Inkontinenz der Mannlichen Harnrohre. Verh. Dtsch. Ges. Chir. 43: 149, 1914.

17. Stoeckel, W.: Veber die Vermendung der Musculi Pyramidales bel der Operativen Behandlung der Incontinentia Urinae. Zentrabl. Gynaekol. 41: 11, 1917.

18. Miller, N. F.: The surgical treatment of urinary incontinence in the female. JAMA 98: 628, 1932.

19. Price, P. B.: Plastic operations for incontinence of urine and of feces. Arch. Surg. 26: 1043, 1933.

20. Aldridge, A. H.: Transplantation of fascia for relief of urinary stress incontinence. Am. J. Obstet. Gynecol. 44: 398, 1942.

21. Shaw, W.: Vaginal operations for cystocele prolapse of the uterus and S.U.I. Surg. Gynecol. Obstet. 88: 11, 1949.

22. Millin, T.: Discussion on stress urinary incontinence in micturition. Proc. Roy. Soc. Med. 40: 361, 1947.

23. Reed, C. D.: Stress incontinence of urine with specific reference to failure of cure following vaginal operative procedures. Am. J. Obstet. Gynecol. 59: 1260, 1950.

24. Ball, T. N., and Hoffman, C., Jr.: Urinary stress incontinence. Eight year appraisal of a combined operation without periosteal suspension. Am. J. Obstet. Gynecol. 85: 96, 1963.

25. Ullery, J. C.: Stress Urinary Incontinence in the Female. Grune and Stratton, New York, 1953.

26. Pereyra, A. J., and Lebhertz, T. B.: Combined urethrovesical suspension and vaginourethroplasty for correction of urinary stress incontinence. Obstet. Gynecol. 30: 537, 1967.

27. Greenwald, S. W., Thornberg, I. R., and Dunn, L. J.: Cystourethrography as a diagnostic aid in evaluating stress incontinence. Obstet. Gynecol.

29: 324, 1967.

28. Crist, T., Shingleton, H. M., and Roberson, W. E.: Urethrovesical needle suspension; postoperative loss of vesical neck support demonstrated by chain cystography. Obstet. Gynecol. 34: 489, 1969.

29. Moir, J. C. The Gauze-Hammock operation. J. Obstet. Gynaecol. Br. Commonw. 75: 1, 1968.

30. Ingelman-Sundberg, A.: Urinary incontinence in women excluding fistulae. Acta Obstet. Gynecol. Scand. 31: 266, 1951-52.

31. Hodgkinson, C. P.: Stress urinary incontinence in the female. Surg. Gynecol. Obstet. 120: 595, 1965.

32. Zacharin, R. J.: Anatomic supports of the female urethra. Obstet. Gynecol. 32: 754, 1968.

33. Marshall, V. F., Marchetti, A. A., and Krantz, K. E.: The correction of S.U.I. by simple vesicourethral suspension. Surg. Gynecol. Obstet. 88: 509, 1949.

34. Williams, T. J., and Te Linde, R. W.: The sling operation for S.U.I. using Mersilene ribbon. Obstet. Gynecol. 19: 241, 1962.

35. Ridley, J. H.: Appraisal of the Goebell-Frangenheim-Stoeckel sling procedure. Am. J. Obstet. Gynecol. 33: 680, 1969.

36. Hodgkinson, C. P., and Hodari, A. A.: Trocar suprapubic cystostomy for postoperative bladder drainage in the female. Am. J. Obstet. Gynecol. 96: 773, 1966.

37. Low, J. A.: Management of severe anatomic deficiencies of the urethral sphincter function by a combined procedure with a fascia lata sling. Am. J. Obstet. Gynecol. 105: 149, 1969. Management of anatomic urinary incontinence by vaginal repair. Am. J. Obstet. Gynecol. 97: 301, 1967.

38. Ridley, J. H.: The Goebell-Frangenheim-Stoeckel procedure using a transected fascia lata sling. In Operative Gynecology, edited by R. W. Te Linde and R. F. Mattingly, 4th ed., p. 563. Lippincott, Philadelphia, 1969.

39. Marchetti, A. A., Marshall, V. F., and Shultis, L. D.: Simple vesicourethral suspension for S.U.I. Am. J. Obstet. Gynecol. 74: 57, 1957.

40. Counseller, V. S.: Surgical connection of S.U.I. methods and technique. J. Int. Coll. Surg. 24: 330, 1960.

41. Ridley, J. H.: The use of the transected sling for urethral incontinence (discussion). Am. J. Obstet. Gynecol. 103: 678, 1969.

42. Lapides, J.: Simplified operation for stress urinary incontinence. J. Urol. 105: 262, 1971.

43. Burch, J. C.: Cooper's ligament suspension for S.U.I. Am. J. Obstet. Gynecol. 100: 764, 1968.

44. Noll, E. N., and Hutch, J. A.: The SCIPP Line—an aid in interpreting the voiding lateral cystourethrogram. Obstet. Gynecol. 33: 680, 1969.

45. Benson, R. C.: Retropubic vesicourethropexy—success or failure? Obstet. Gynecol. 35: 665, 1970.

46. Moolgaoker, A. S., Adrian, G. M., Smith, J. C., and Stallworthy, J. A.: Diagnosis and management of urinary incontinence in the female. J. Ob. Gyn. Br. Comm. 79: 481, 1972.

CHAPTER FIVE

JOHN H. RIDLEY, M.D.

SURGERY FOR
VAGINAL FISTULAE

The vaginal fistula has always been the most intriguing and demanding problem to the gynecologist. It has also been the most stringent test of his diagnostic acumen, patience, and, above all, his surgical skill. These fistulae include both urinary and fecal. Urinary fistulae have proven to be the most challenging; they are more common and because of the constancy of the leakage are more distressing, if that can be possible, to the patient.

Types of Urinary Fistulae

A. Vesicovaginal
B. Urethrovaginal
C. Ureterovaginal
D. Miscellaneous
    1. Vesicocervicovaginal
    2. Ureterocoliovaginal

Types of Fecal Fistulae

A. Rectovaginal
B. Enterovaginal
    1. Colon
    2. Small bowel

There may be a combination of two or more of these various types of fistulae depending on the nature of injury (Fig. 5.1). It is to be noted that in a case where coexisting fistulae exists, the operator may at first overlook the less obvious one and have a failed operation from the very beginning of his effort.

HISTORY

Detailed historical comments are to be limited in this type of text, although a few events are noteworthy to emphasize the development of techniques and avoidance of errors. When one speaks of the history of the repair of vesicovaginal fistulae, the name of Marion Sims (1) is always suggested. However, Sims was not the first surgeon to successfully repair a fistula, or even have a successful series to report, but he is certainly to be credited with being the surgeon who developed not only ingenious techniques and instruments but also sound and systematic application of the surgical principles then in use. Even today we still use these basic techniques: nonabsorbable sutures, such as silver wire as Sims recommended, and meticulous dissection. A few other surgeons, among the very many who have made significant contributions to the successful repair of the vaginal fistulae, deserve special mention. Probably the first to have recorded notable success was H. Van Roonhuyse (2) in 1672. Gossett (3) of London in 1834 is now credited with noteworthy skill and success, but his teachings were not widely published and didn't persist.

Since the J. Marion Sims era, the degree of success of the repair of the vesicovaginal fistula has greatly increased within the framework of his basic teachings: proper preoperative evaluation and preparation; adequate exposure; mobilization of the bladder and vaginal mucosa; preservation or enhancement of blood supply; closure without tension with non-absorable sutures; proper postoperative drainage; control of infection; and protection of the healing areas.

Until 50 years ago, the chief cause of vaginal fistulae was obstetrical, followed next by surgical, with a scant few resulting from neoplasm. However, irradiation therapy chiefly by radium element was becoming more popular, and an increasing number of these fistulae were being seen (4).

Etiology of Vaginal Fistulae in 1920

Obstetrical	60%
Surgical	30%

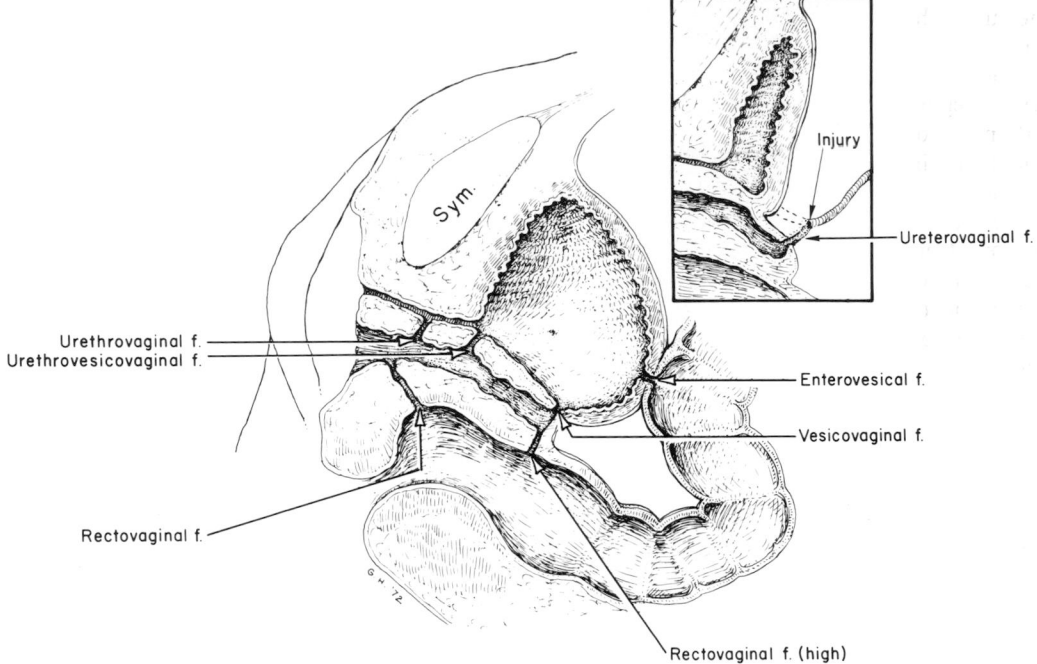

Fig. 5.1. A composite drawing of the many locations of the more common urinary and fecal fistulae. Fortunately, these fistulae usually occur solitarily; however, depending on the etiologic factors, there may be a coexistence of two or more. Awareness of this possibility is most important and is outlined more fully in the text. The inset shows the channelization of the fistulous tract into the vaginal vault from the site of the ureteral injury in the region of the broad ligament.

Neoplasm	5%
Irradiation	5%

As years have passed these statistics have been practically reversed.

Etiology of Vaginal Fistulae in 1970

Surgical	60%
Obstetrical	20%
Postirradiation	15%
Neoplasm	5% or less

This indicates the vast improvement in obstetrical practices, both by the obstetrician and the trained midwife. It also reflects the bolder and more radical use of surgery in treating malignancies and very difficult benign problems. It is not surprising that there is the increasing incidence of postirradiation fistulae because this method of the treatment of malignancies has increased tremendously not only in the number of cases treated but also by the use of supervoltage sources.

Since the majority of the number of vaginal fistulae are now resulting from surgery and irradiation, the problem for the gynecologist has grown harder because these types of fistulae present the most difficult problems of repair and invite more errors and complications. This must be realized by the operating surgeon, the patient, and the courts of law.

Preoperative Evaluation and Preparation

The existence of a vaginal fistula, whether it be urinary or fecal, is very obvious to the patient in most cases. There is usually some momentous event that causes the fistulae whether it be by surgery, irradiation treatment, or childbirth trauma. The presence may become known immediately postoperatively or it may be delayed for a variable time, depending on failure to heal or by tissue necrosis. The patient, as well as the responsible doctor, are psychologically upset: the patient with disappointment and inconvenience, and the doctor with feelings of guilt, incompetence, and fear of the ugly threat of a malpractice suit against him.

The avoidance of this mutually distressing error begins with the first meeting of the patient and surgeon and with his thorough understanding of the problem.

The careful history is, as always, important to determine the nature of the previous trauma or condition which led to the fistulous formation. The questioning surgeon must be most circumspect in his approach because it will have been the obvious feeling of the patient that this fistula has resulted from neglect, incompetence, or indifference on the part of the operator because here is a fertile field for accusations leading to litigation. It should be explained patiently that these unfortunate results can occur and are even to be anticipated in a certain percentage of cases. It takes only one inappropriate word or opinion from the present surgeon to start the unhappy and usually unnecessary legal steps against the unfortunate original surgeon.

The patient is usually acutely distraught not only by physical discomfort and social embarrassment but also by the dread of the obviously needed secondary operation. She must be made as comfortable as possible by treating the excoriated macerated skin and odor. At times a makeshift apparatus may be devised to at least temporarily contain the leaking urine or bowel contents. Various apparatus, sometimes products of ingenuity, can be fashioned to give the patient some respite while further preparations are being made for surgical correction. Although these makeshift measures very rarely will allow the fistula to close spontaneously, it can be given even that slight chance. There are cases reported of small vesicovaginal fistulae finally closing spontaneously if proper drainage and local treatment are applied. Balloon vaginal tampons may lessen the amount of fistulous drainage so that the perineal tissues may be brought back to a more healthy state. These temporary efforts will also give the patient some hope and encouragement in the waiting period that must elapse before the optimal time for surgical repair comes.

It is absolutely necessary to completely delineate the fistula. The operator must rule out the possible presence of one or more other fistulae; he must be sure of the extent of injury to adjacent structures such as the ureter, loops of bowel, vital vessels, and nerves. A grave error is committed if the gynecologist overlooks coexisting fistulae and contiguous injury. In the first place, the success of his operation is doomed before he starts, and secondly he may be unjustly accused of an injury which actually has been incurred by previous accident or surgery.

The adjacent tissues to the fistula margins are inspected visually, manually, by contrast media, and by transillumination when possible. The persistence of malignancy must be ruled out by actual tissue study. Although at first the fistula may seem to be an uncomplicated case requiring the simplest repair, no vaginal fistula is uncomplicated until the operating surgeon has satisfied himself that it is, in fact, a routine surgical approach.

To avoid error in diagnosis and surgical plan, these basic studies should be done:

a. Complete history and physical exam
b. Intravenous pyelography
c. Cystoscopy and retrograde pyelography wherever feasible
d. Rectovaginal examination with biopsy of fistula margin if history of malignancy is presented
e. Indirect air cystoscopy of all urinary fistulae
f. Methylene blue and phenylsulfophthalein (PSP) excretion tests to rule out possible presence of ureterovaginal fistula
g. Barium enema and proctosigmoidoscopy in cases of fecal vaginal fistulae

All of these tests are immediately available to most gynecologists either in his office or at the hospital. He should feel obligated to become proficient in simple cystoscopic studies, retrograde pyelography, and lower bowel inspection. These are simple, important, and necessary diagnostic procedures for the compleat gynecologist.

The gynecologist may at first be misled by an intermittently leaking fistula, usually small in size, but nonetheless distressing. A small opening into the bladder or bowel may not leak until that organ is distended by urine or gas with feces as the case may be. On the other hand, leakage may only occur when the patient is at rest with a nearly empty affected organ, because the fistulous tract may be oblique through the vaginal wall, and any compression will close it temporarily, at least. Intermittent urine leakage is nearly pathognomic of the urethrovaginal fistula when the bladder sphincter is competent. After the patient has finished voiding, there may be an accumulation of urine in the vagina and trickle from the yet full urethra into the vagina.

Excretory urography, with special technical effort to visualize the entire ureter is very valuable. The operator may find a distorted or dilated ureter on either or both sides, or one may even find an impaired or functionless kidney. This helps to locate the fistula; it also makes note of the pre-existence of this condition not only for legal reasons but also to warn the surgeon to use particular care to protect the unaffected side. Even the affected kidney after proper study may yet be salvagable to a varying extent for several weeks after the initial injury.

Cystoscopy and retrograde pyelography are indicated in most cases because there may always be additional injury to the urinary tract whether it be an additional fistula or some adjacent tissue injury that could compromise the surgical effort. Direct air cystoscopy and urethroscopy have been used in the past but to a diminishing amount now. Catheterization of the ureters by air cystoscopy with the patient in the knee-chest position is usually too difficult except for experienced hands to be of practical value. However, good visualization of the trigone and urethra may be obtained by this direct method.

The examination by indirect air cystoscopy, first described by Ridley (5) in 1951, has proven to be the most satisfactory technique for examination of the entire bladder and urethra in cases of fistula. Retrograde study by this technique is easily performed when indicated by a suspected ureteral obstruction. Where water cystoscopy may be actually impossible because of the size of the fistula and inability to distend the bladder satisfactorily because of the reflux of the water and distortion of the trigone (Fig. 5.2), indirect air cystoscopy with the patient in knee-chest position is usually completely satisfactory (Fig. 5.3). No anesthesia is needed and the bladder and vagina distend adequately with the negative intra-abdominal pressure thus created. The cystoscopic telescope, as used with water as the medium, is passed into the urethra and bladder. It has been found that for simple inspection, the culdoscopic or laparoscopic telescope is very satisfactory, is nearly always available to the gynecologist, and has excellent optical qualities. The entire trigone and ureteral orifices are inspected and a note made of the spurts of urine from the ureteral orifices. The entire bladder mucosa is inspected. Particular note is made of the fistula margin and what

Fig. 5.2. Satisfactory cystoscopic examination of the fistula area using water as the medium is practically impossible because of reflux of water through the fistula opening. This is particularly true if the defect is not of very small size. (From J. H. Ridley: Indirect air cystoscopy. South. Med. J. 44: 114, 1951.)

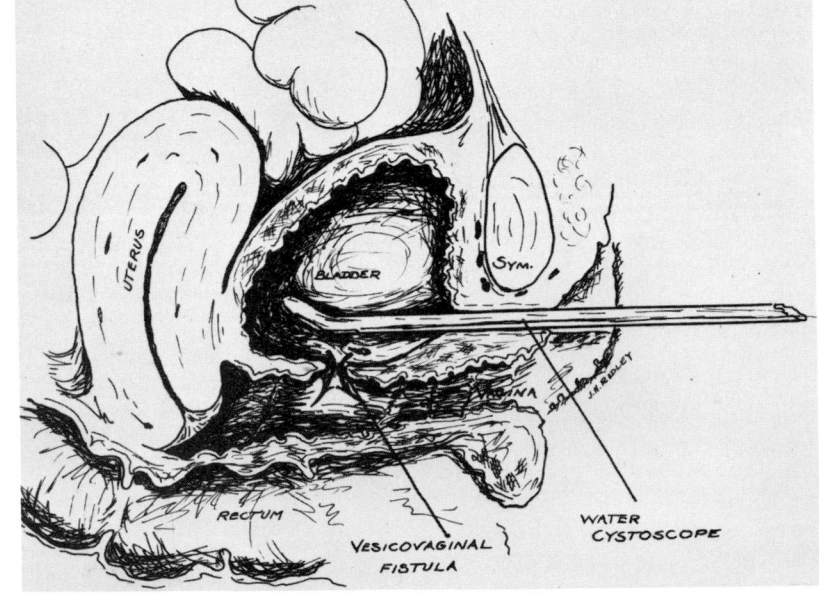

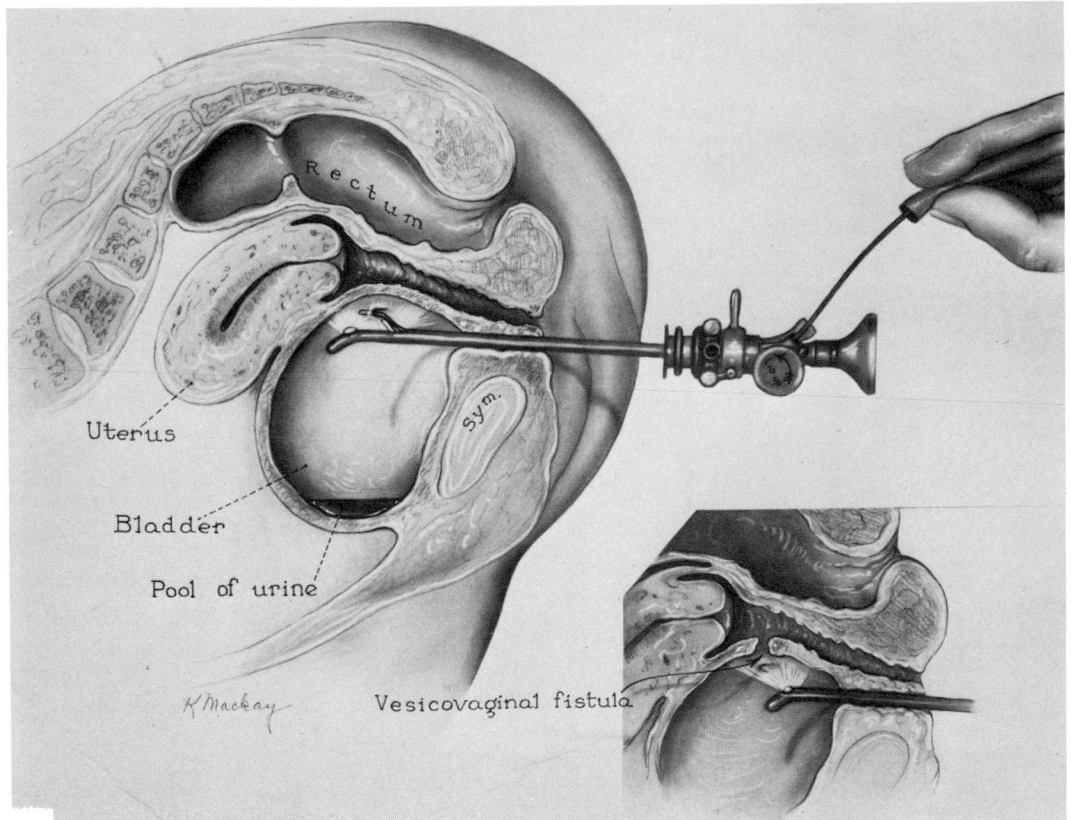

Fig. 5.3. Indirect air cystoscopy with the patient in the knee-chest position. The bladder distends with negative intra-abdominal pressure whether fistula is present or not. The inset shows the case of inspection of the fistula, its relationship to the trigone and ureteral orifices, and by transillumination, the condition and vascularity of the surrounding tissues. The ureters may be probed or catheterized if indicated. (From J. H. Ridley: Indirect air cystoscopy. South. Med. J. 44: 114, 1951.)

proximity it has to the ureters, thus more clearly warning the operator of what danger lies there. The coexistence of another fistula is looked for at the same time, noting the actual distortion of the trigone.

One of the most satisfactory advantages of the use of indirect air cystoscopy is transillumination of the base of the bladder and the entire urethra. The light of the telescope will usually shine through even the smallest fistula. The amount of light that passes through the tissues adjacent to the fistula gives an accurate index of the tissue vascularity and health. It may be found that the immediately adjacent tissues are parchment-thin either by necrosis or by irradiation scarring, thus forewarning the operator of more difficulty in repair than expected. The technique of indirect air cystoscopy is an office procedure, requiring no anesthesia, minimal aseptic technique, and minimal outlay of instruments. More complete details may be found in the original article (5).

The presence of a ureterovaginal fistula may be suspected first if the patient voids normally but despite this has a constant urinary leakage. Further study by contrast media and catheterization of the suspected side may clinch the diagnosis. In rare instances there may be coexistence of a ureterovaginal and vesicovaginal fistulae. The vaginal vault must be watched carefully to detect any spurt of urine not coming from the bladder which has been partially filled with a dilute solution of methylene blue. Even more contrast may be detected by giving the patient an ampoule of phenylsufophthalein intravenously and packing the vaginal vault firmly with a cotton tampon alkalinized by a weak base solution such as sodium bicarbonate. A pink color may be seen on this tampon in the vault whereas the methylene blue stain will be detected in proximity of the bladder fistula. Even all of these specific tests, carefully done, may fail to accurately define the complete problem. The operator must always be suspicious of the presence of this peculiar and difficult condition where there may be a combination of fistulae (Fig. 5.4). Peculiarities of the fistula tracts, whether they be of urinary or of fecal origin, may reveal a double fistula with a single vaginal opening (Fig. 5.5) or a tract that burrows between the adjacent membranes.

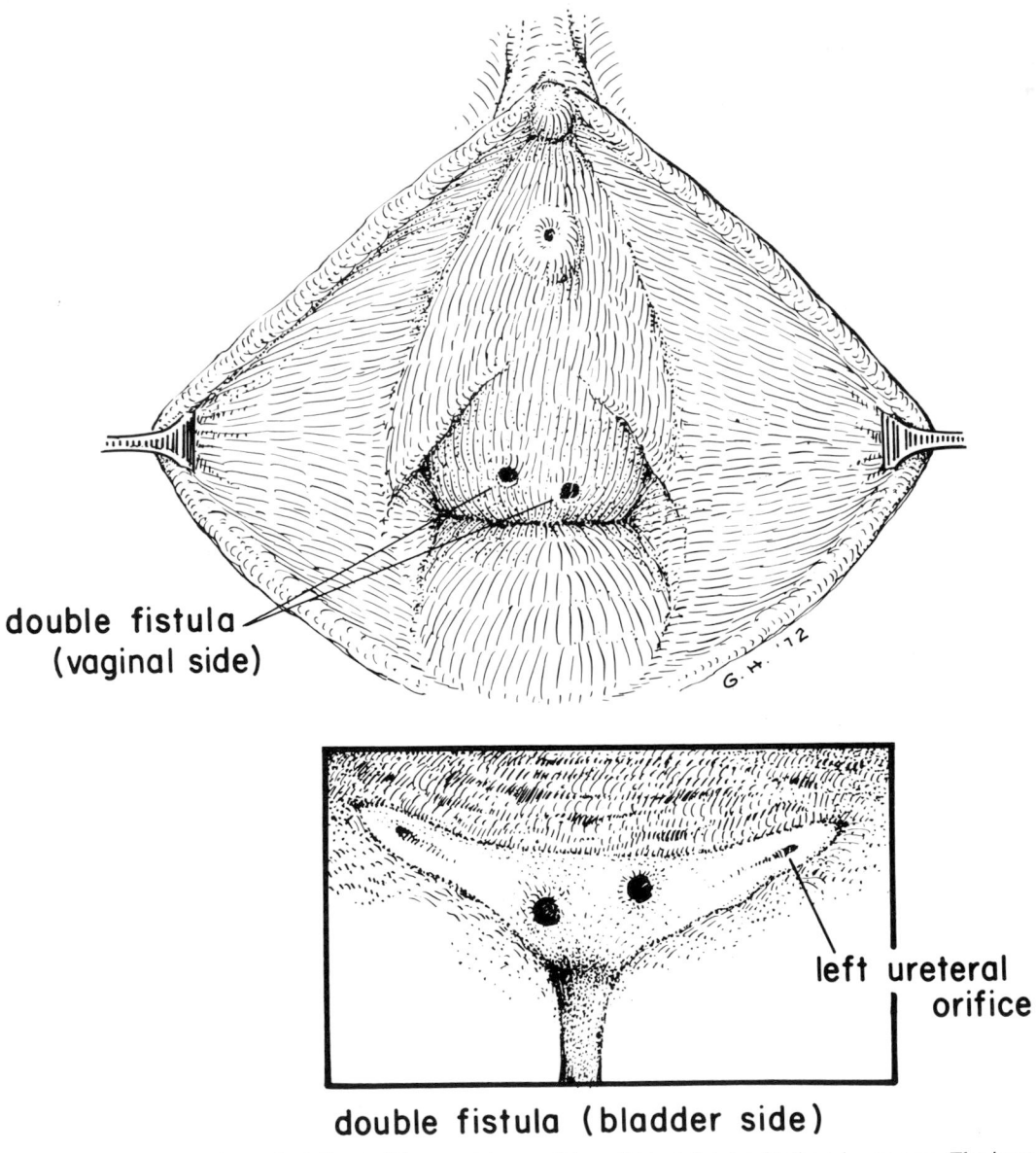

double fistula (vaginal side)

left ureteral orifice

double fistula (bladder side)

Fig. 5.4. Double vesicovaginal fistula. The coexistence of two distinct fistulae in the trigone area. The inset shows relationships of the fistula to the trigone, ureteral orifices, and interureteric ridge. The decision must be made as to whether the fistulae will best be reparied individually or compounded to be repaired as one. The latter choice is most frequently taken when the operator knows that the ureters are safely remote.

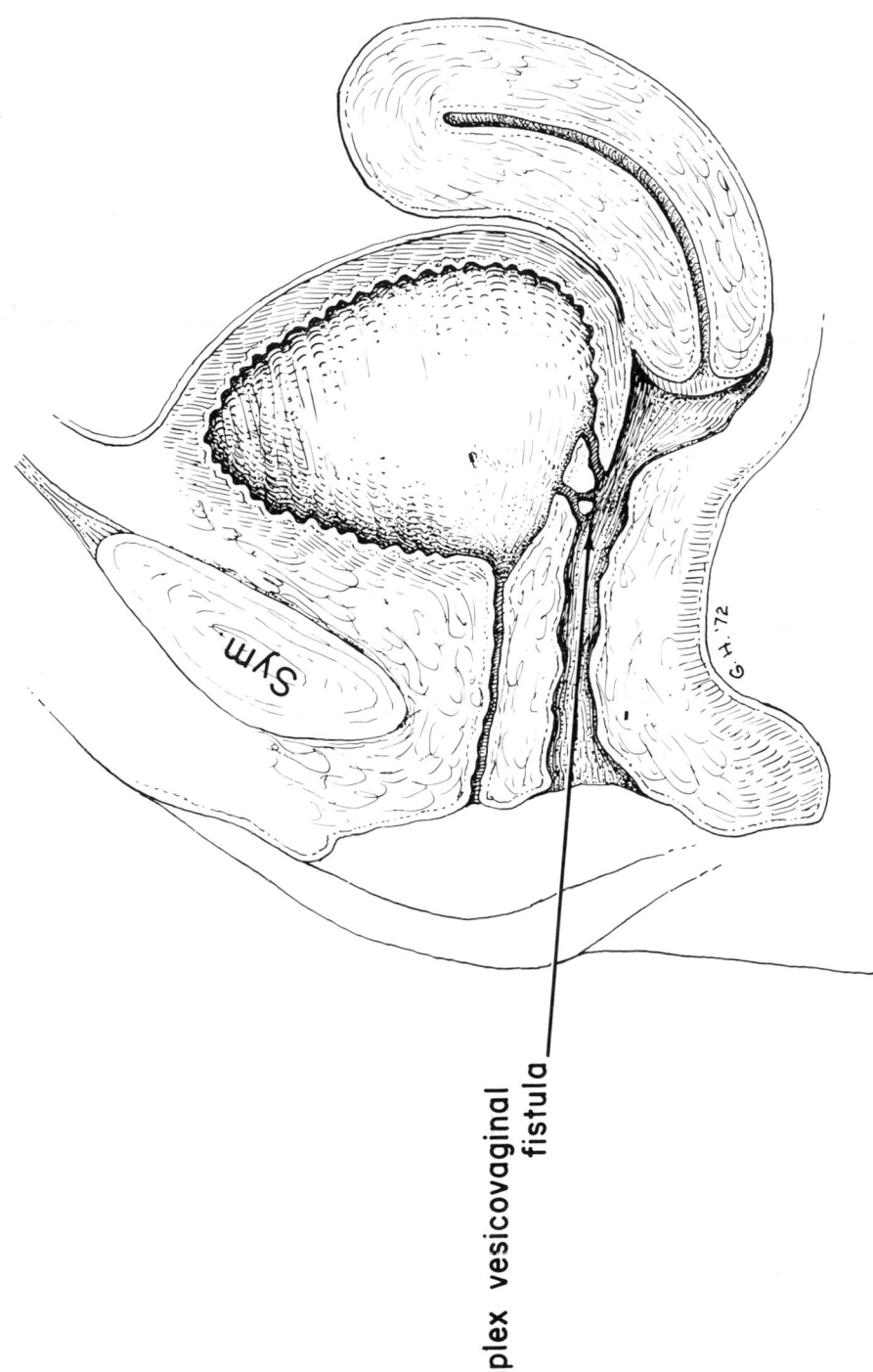

Fig. 5.5. The complex vesicovaginal fistula. Unless recognized, this type of fistula, occurring not infrequently, can lead to failure of the attempted repair. One should always suspect that more than one vaginal and/or vesical ostium can coexist. This puzzling condition results more frequently following previous surgery than from obstetrical trauma.

The existence of a rectovaginal fistula may be confounding to the examiner because of the sometimes intermittent leakage per vaginum. If the fistula is small and the patient remains constipated for long periods of time, there may be no evidence of the defect. However, if the stools become softer and with much flatus, the soilage may become nearly constant and distressing. It is to be remembered that some fecal material may be found in the vagina of women at times when no fistula exists. This can be the case of the obese multipara with a poor perineal body and poor anal sphincter tone and with poor hygienic habits.

If the fistula is not found on careful vaginal examination, the gynecologist may use methylene blue per rectum as the contrast medium. A tampon placed in the vagina may show the leaking rectal contents escaping through the small fistula. Transillumination again is of great value and can be easily done with a lighted lucite probe or some other light source as a fiberoptic sheath or telescope with an exposed light at the tip. Careful proctoscopy and sigmoidoscopy is always done to more clearly define the ostium or ostia in the bowel mucosa. Here again, the operator must always suspect the slight possibility of coexisting fistulae. *It is axiomatic to say that no fistula can be successfully closed unless the antivaginal ostium in the bowel or urinary tract mucosa is securely obliterated by reapproximation.*

General Principles of Fistula Repair

There are a few principles, of long proven value, that must be observed in the repair of vaginal fistulae. To violate these, the gynecologist runs a much greater risk of failure. However, he must be able to improvise within the realm of good surgical practices, to care for all of the vagaries that may present themselves as the operative problem unfolds.

The general physical condition of the patient and the tissue itself must be optimal—even if this must mean postponement of the repair. Although the surgeon may be anxious to get on with the task particularly if he has had pressure put on him by the patient and her family, he must realize that the chance for success is greatly enhanced by choosing the proper time to operate. If the fistula has not been detected at the time of the error and repaired immedi-

ately, postponement of the repair for the proper length of time is of paramount importance. The length of this time varies in the opinions of many experienced surgeons. Te Linde (2) advocates waiting for as long as 6 months before the attempt at repair is made. Moir (6) suggests that at least 3 months be allowed to elapse and Counseller (7) had also suggested this same length of time. Collins, Rent, and Jones (8), however, have used preparation of cortisone to hasten the healing process and condition the tissues sooner for repair. This type of preparation, although favorable in some cases, has not met with universal approval.

The skin of the vulva and perineum is usually macerated, excoriated, or encrusted. There is usually present a secondary infection in the skin glands and hair follicles with concomitant edema and pain. These conditions must be dealt with by sitz baths, antibiotics as needed, and scrupulous cleanliness.

It is remarkably infrequent that we see cystitis with a vesicovaginal fistula even though the bladder may be constantly invaded by organisms from the vagina. It is due to the unobstructed urine drainage which is without residual. However, an infected urine may be found in cases in which an upper urinary tract infection exists either prior to or along with the development of the fistula. This pyelonephritis is wisely treated immediately and vigorously after studies have been completed evaluating kidney function and sensitivity of the existing organisms to drugs. The presence of urinary calculi either in the kidney parenchyma, in the collecting systems, or in the fistulous tract must be suspected and eliminated because infection can hardly be eliminated if calculi are present anywhere.

Finally, an error may be made by improper psychologic preparation of the patient. Realizing the capriciousness of a repair of a vaginal fistula, the gynecologist should clearly explain the odds for and against chances of success with the first attempt at repair. The patient must not be given false hopes of sure success nor should she be deprived of what hope for success does exist.

Selection of Instruments

Although the most complicated vesicovaginal fistula may be repaired with very few instruments, these must be the exact type needed for this particular type of operation and may be unsuitable for another type of fistula. Therefore the gynecologist must have at hand not only a basic set of tools but also a variety of other instruments from which he may choose for a specific task. At times the most important single suture depends on the exact placement made possible by the appropriate instrument and suture material. The success of the procedure may depend on this pivotal maneuver, and all may be lost if the operator does not have proper equipment at hand. The basic instruments must be light, delicate, and accurate. It is well for the gynecologist to have available a special set of fistula repair instruments (Fig. 5.6). However, if this is not practicable he should find many of the desired types of instruments in the cabinet of the neurosurgeon. He may borrow the toothed long offset or bayonet tissue forceps, delicate sharp curved nerve retractors, small curved or offset scissors,

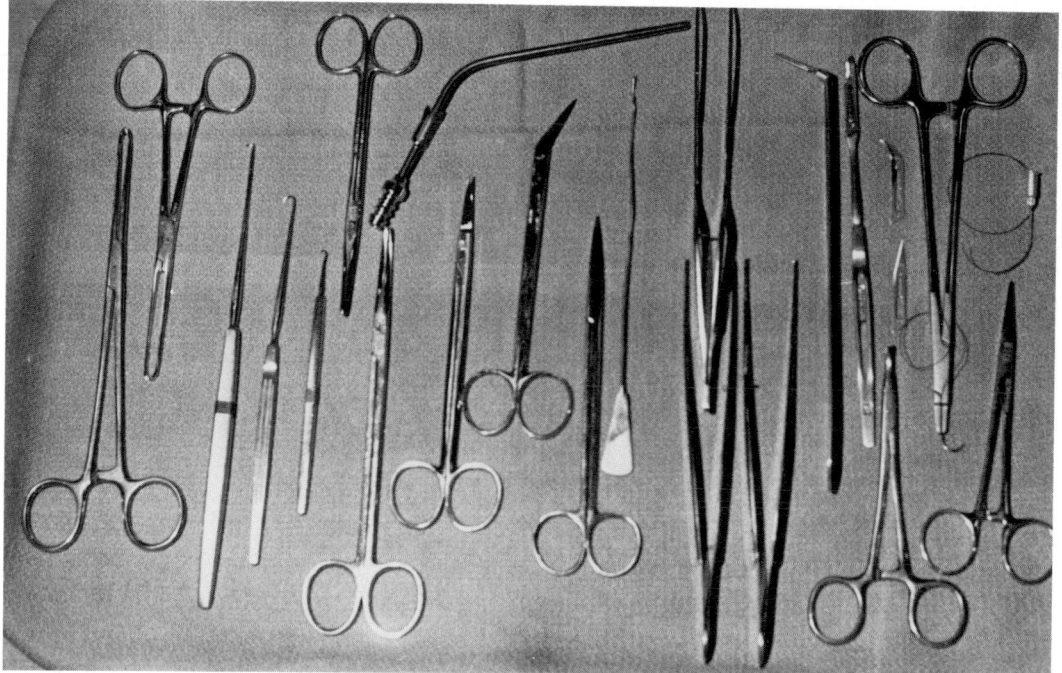

Fig. 5.6. An assortment of basic instruments which facilitates the effort for fistula closure. From left to right:

Long and medium length Allis clamps

Three nerve hooks very useful for delicate traction about fistula margins

Two pairs of Metzenbaum curved scissors—a long and medium pair

Delicate neurosurgical suction tip

An assortment of three fistula scissors:
  curved pointed
  straight offset
  straight pointed

A malleable silver probe

An assortment of three delicate tissue forceps:
  straight without teeth

bayonet without teeth
straight mouse toothed

An assortment of knife handles and blades:
  long offset handle (3-L)
  Delicate dissecting handle (#7) fitted with #15 blade
  #12 curved hawk bill blade
  #11 straight blade

Curved mosquito hemostat

Long delicate needle holder, grasping a threaded fish-hook needle

#20 gauge hypodermic needle through which is threaded 3-0 chromic catgut

Straight mosquito hemostat used as needle holder

and various shaped malleable or rigid spatula retractors.

Retractors. There should be available at least three types of retractors. The weighted vaginal speculum will often suffice as the primary instrument. The blade must not be too long or broad because it will deprive the operator of much needed maneuvering space. Lateral vaginal wall retractors such as the Wertheim instrument, and the basic Sims double ended speculum must be at hand.

Beyond these fundamental instruments, the operator must improvise in any way that is necessary and with whatever instrument is available to make the fistula accessible. The long curved Allis tenaculum forceps are frequently used not only to help exposure but also to immobilize the tissue for the tedious dissection. The operator may also use appropriately placed traction sutures about the fistula margins to aid exposure. At the time that the bladder or rectal mucosa is being identified and accurately mobilized from the scar tissue, the delicate curved hook (nerve) tenaculum is of value. Some probing instruments of practical value may even be obtained from the cabinet of the dentist. The gynecologic surgeon can at times bring the fistula into a more accessible range and at the same time more easily identify the mucosal margins by inserting an appropriately sized balloon catheter, inflating the balloon within the bladder or rectum, and drawing the catheter gently outward. A glass bead, small enough to be drawn through the urethra or anus, but large enough not to go through the fistula may also be used. Thus with careful dissection the bladder or rectal mucosal margin may be circumcised and the vaginal mucosa mobilized. It has been found that a Young's prostate retractor may be similarly used by passage through the fistula and opened to give more accessibility; of course, the size and location of the fistula will dictate the choice of such helpful paraphernalia. Further exposure may be obtained to high fistulae or through a scarred vagina by cutting an adequate Schuchardt vaginal incision.

Hemostasis

Although adequate vascularity is the most desirable condition about the fistula margin, bleeding by ooze may be very troublesome at times of the necessary tedious dissection. This may be particularly true in those fistulae resulting from surgery and obstetrical trauma, but, of course, not in the case of postirradiation scarring. A dilute solution of a vasoconstricting agent such as Neo-Synephrine (1 ampoule in 50 cc normal saline) (Fig. 5.7) is injected by a small needle and in small amounts about the circumference of the fistula. If done properly, this does not distort the tissues but will help delineate the layers and control temporarily the troublesome ooze which may obscure the tissues and planes to be worked with. This will not permanently affect the desired vascularity for healing.

An error may be made by not having at hand all necessary types of cutting instruments of suitable weight and keenness. It has been found that the #7 Bard-Parker handle with #15 blade is indispensable. In addition one must have the #11 straight blade and #12 curved hook blade. An offset handle is needed at times and the Beaver or B-P instrument is acceptable. A variety of delicate, accurate scissors is needed; basically one must have the straight, slightly curved, offset, and deeply curved instruments. These special instruments should be stored and guarded against general use because of dulling by heavier types of work and careless handling.

Although it may seem too elementary to include a description of lighting during the operation and positioning of the patient, it is nonetheless most important and can avoid basic technical errors. Most modern operating rooms have adequate light sources for ordinary procedures, but additional lighting is always needed, particularly for the high vaginal fistula with either a commodious or scarred vagina. We have found one or two easily maneuverable spotlights in addition to the main light will suffice. The use of a headlamp is a question of the surgeon's individual choice, but for the most part these are found to be cumbersome and not so well suited for fistula work. An important simple technique is the use of transillumination as needed during the procedure; as described previously in this chapter, the light source can be a lucite probe, or the fiberoptic or ordinarily lighted cystoscopic telescope. By this means the operator may further test for integrity of his suture line or the condition and vascularity of the surrounding tissues. The cystoscope should be kept at hand by the gynecologist so that he

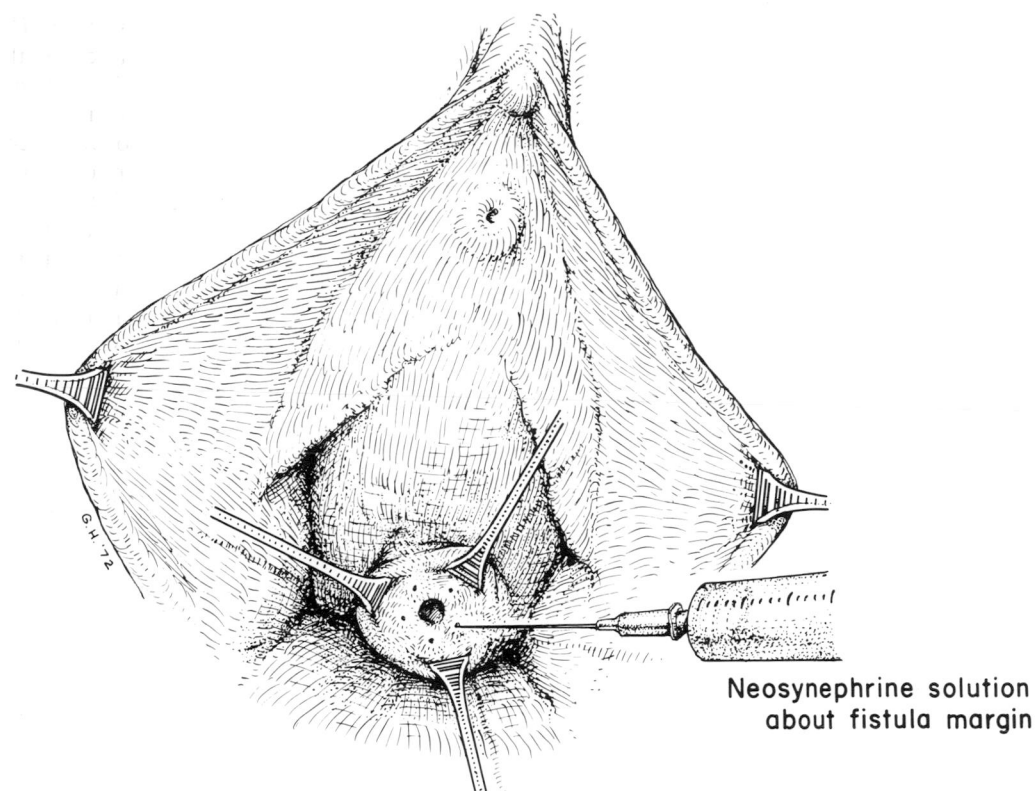

**Neosynephrine solution
about fistula margin**

Fig. 5.7. A dilute solution of Neo-Synephrine is injected with a small needle into the vaginal mucosa about the fistula margin before any incision is made. This temporary hemostasis facilitates undercutting and mobilizing both the vaginal and bladder mucosa, but does not retard healing.

may inspect, if necessary, the bladder side of his repair. In this way he may be able to detect the error of having passed a suture into the bladder lumen, or to see accurately the repaired ostium and the proximity of the ureteral orifices. To do this simple cystoscopic exam, if it is needed, one does not have to distend the bladder beyond 75 to 100 cc thus causing no dangerous strain on the suture line.

Positioning the patient is a basic part of the procedure, and if done properly can make a most difficult operation less so. Traditionally and also for good reason, the gynecologist has used the approach with the patient in the dorsolithotomy position. This may be accentuated by lowering the patient's head in Trendelenburg position and exaggerating the flexion and abduction of the thighs on the abdomen. The gynecologist is usually better oriented to the pelvic anatomic relationships with the patient in this position and will find that blood, urine, and testing fluids gravitate away from the operative site. This is particularly true when the repair is that of a urinary tract fistula. In the case of the rectovaginal fistula, this dorsolithotomy position is the only practical approach.

The transabdominal approach is seldom used by the gynecologist, but is more frequently used by the general urologist or general surgeon. This is probably true because of the orientation of the latter concerning the pelvic anatomy from above. It has been found that the Latzko vaginal procedure has proven dependable for a high degree of success for repair of the fistula near the apex which was formerly approached transabdominally and transvesically. However, certain cases demand approach from above. In the case where there is such vaginal scarring as to make the fistula practically inaccessible from below, it may be feasible to go from above. This technique will be described more fully below under the section on "Transabdominal Approach of the Vesicovaginal or Colovaginal Fistula."

Sutures and Needles

The choice of sutures and needles is important in safeguarding against errors and possible dehiscence of the suture line. The quality of catgut, including all types of absorbable materials, has steadily improved through the years. We must choose the finest caliber strand that can be depended upon for closure of the bladder or rectal membrane opening. This allows the least trauma in this most delicate phase of the procedure. Unless the opening on the bladder or rectal side of the fistula is securely closed, practically no hope for the success of the operation can be held. The second layer of closure whenever possible is done with similar catgut or one of slightly heavier caliber. It has been found that 3-0 chromic catgut swaged on a small taper point needle serves admirably in these first two layers of closure. The vaginal mucosa is best closed in most cases with the nonabsorbable, nonreactive suture material. The most important contribution of Sims was the use of silver wire which is still in wide use. However, newer synthetic materials have been tried and found to be just as satisfactory, and in some cases more so. The gauge of malleable silver wire more frequently used is #26. This is twisted or tied for security. It is usually not readily available as a swaged-on-ready-to-use suture. The following materials have been used successfully: stainless steel wire, braided or monofilament; monofilament nylon; dacron; and similar nonreactive synthetic products. These materials are left in place for the same length of time as would be silver, *i.e.*, about 15 to 21 days.

The proper caliber and shape of needles are most important. Usually the half circle taper point Ferguson or Mayo type is used. The trocar needle with cutting edge is practically never used for fear of cutting already placed sutures or cutting the soft tissues beyond what is needed to simply pass the suture material. Small caliber, semi-malleable, round needles with swaged on suture material are the choice. It is found to be helpful to be able to bend the contour of the needle, without fear of breaking it, to fit the confines of rather limited space. The use of a hollow needle is helpful when the operator finds that it is impossible to fully swing his needle holder. The 3-0 chromic catgut is threaded into a #20-gauge hypodermic or tonsil needle until the suture tip is just within the needle point (Fig. 5.8). The thrust of the needle may be straight forward, or the needle may be carefully bent to a desired curve or even held at an appropriate angle with a Kelly or gallbladder clamp. As the needle is passed through the desired submucosal layers, the 3-0 catgut is thrust beyond the needle tip, grasped, and the needle withdrawn, leaving the suture in place. This technique can give a quickly available atraumatic type of suture placement when other methods may not be feasible.

The use of a fish-hook type needle may allow the placement of a difficult suture high in the vagina (Fig. 5.9). The needle is held in line of the axis of the holder and a pull back movement may drive the needle in just the right layer desired.

In essence, it can be seen that the gynecologist needs these basic tools with which he can work. Even though just one type of needle and suture material and one set of instruments may prove to be all that is needed for a particular fistula repair, the operator must nevertheless have other instruments and materials at hand which he can ingeniously use.

Basic Repair of the Simple Vesicovaginal Fistula

Most commonly, the gynecologist will see the simple solitary vesicovaginal fistula occurring following surgical error, tissue failure, or obstetrical trauma, these being the most frequent causes of vaginal fistula. The chance of success in this repair is very good if the operator will conscientiously adhere to the well established and time-proven precepts of surgical technique and postoperative care. The margin for error is small and critical; mostly he is dealing with a situation that will be either completely successful or a complete failure. We can hardly convince a patient that the fistula is improved if she still leaks, even though through a tract of somewhat smaller caliber.

The history and complete physical examination have been completed. The genitourinary tract has been studied in detail as outlined previously in this chapter, and the patient now comes to operation. Her physical condition is optimal for the planned operation.

Position of the Patient

With rare exceptions the gynecologist prefers the vaginal approach with the patient in a

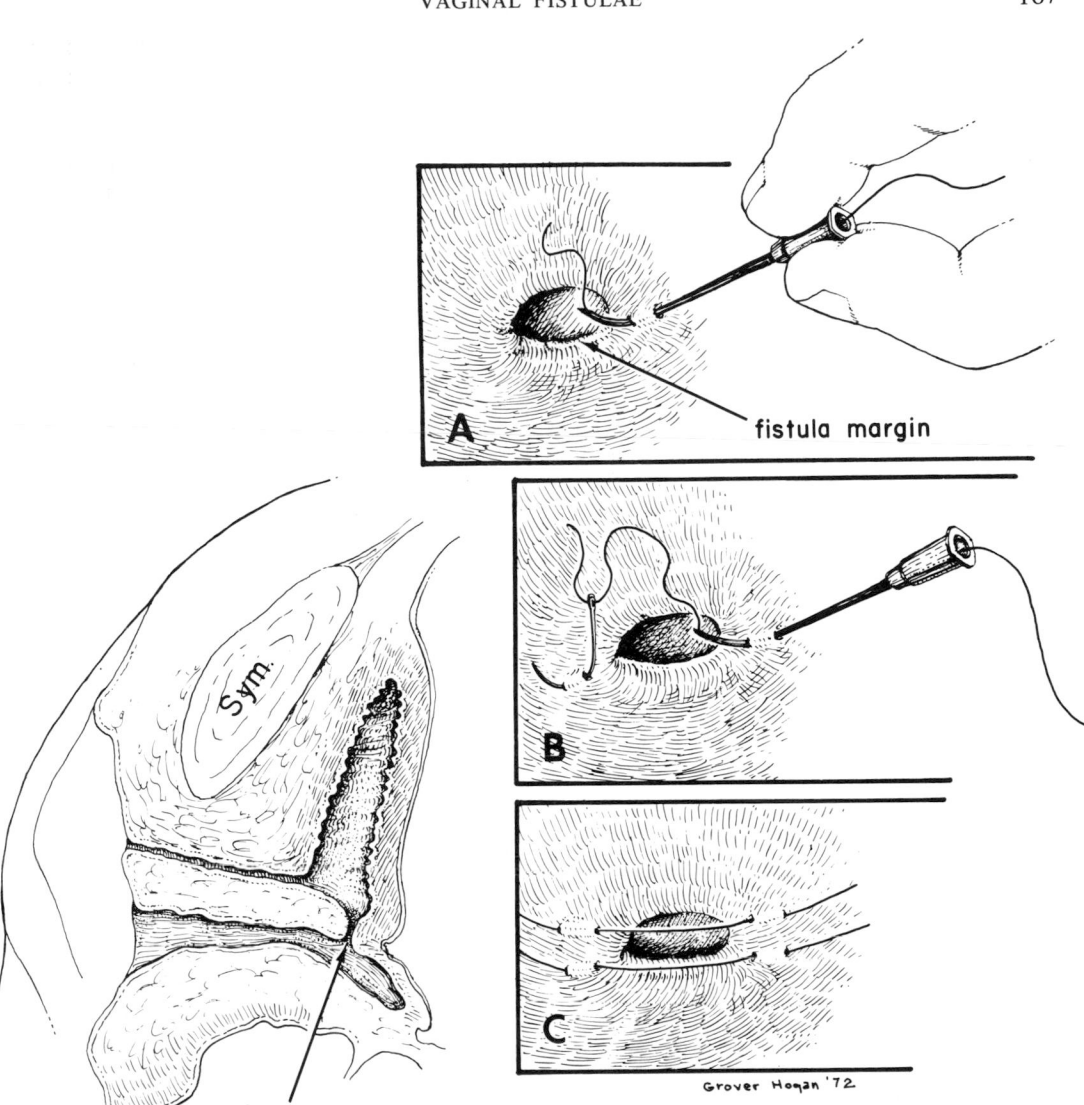

fistula margin

Sym.

fistula

Grover Hogan '72

Fig. 5.8. A high and less accessible vesicovaginal fistula resulting from necrosis of bladder base following hysterectomy. Detailed illustrations show a method of placement of the first layer of sutures of catgut for closure of the fistula. A #20 gauge 2-inch hypodermic needle bent appropriately is threaded with 3-0 chromic catgut but leaves the point free. (A) This is passed through the bladder submucosa and muscularis layer, and the catgut is then thrust past the point and grasped as the needle is withdrawn. This suture is now in turn threaded onto a fish-hook shaped needle (B) fashioned from a small malleable Ferguson type and placed delicately through the bladder submucosal and muscularis layer on the opposing side of the fistula. This is repeated (C) as frequently as needed to completely close, reapproximate, and invert the fistula margins.

dorsolithotomy position with thighs well flexed and abducted. A moderate head-down Trendelenburg position may be added to aid exposure. In rare instances the knee-chest, prone, or jack-knife position may be used. In fact, Kelly did many of his more difficult cases with the patient in this position. However, the advantages are not so great that the disadvantages can be overlooked. The patient and the anesthesiologist suffer through the procedure, particularly if the patient is obese and the anesthesiologist has difficulty in maintaining the adequate airway. It is also to be mentioned that the transvesical or transperitoneal approach with

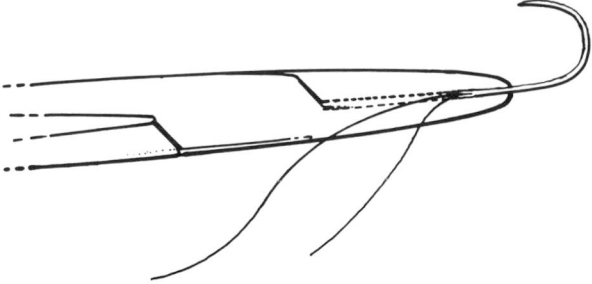

Fig. 5.9. Detail of small, round taper point needle bent to fashion a fish-hook type. This has been threaded with 3-0 chromic catgut and grasped endwise to facilitate passage of a suture in less accessible locations.

the patient in the supine position has certain advantages, to be discussed later, particularly if the vault and vaginal scarring are so great as to prohibit adequate exposure and mobilization below. However, the gynecologist will finally choose for his particular case that position which serves its purpose best. The vaginal approach remains the much more frequently used.

In this given case of a typical and frequently seen fistula, the patient is placed in dorsolithotomy position and exposure obtained by proper specula. The labia minora are sutured lateralward temporarily, and an episiotomy (Schuchardt) incision made if necessary. Three or four long, curved Allis clamps are placed about the periphery of the fistula well away from the line of incision and dissection. If the space available limits the use of clamps, traction sutures are used to draw the fistula toward the operator. In applying the traction the surgeon must remember that the fistula tract, albeit very short, is "funnelled" so that the bladder (or rectal) mucosa is also drawn downward under some tension (Fig. 5.10). As the dissection is done and the mucosal margin of the bladder mucosa is freed, it tends to retract into the bladder. However, with proper alertness and application of hooks or sutures, this most important membrane and step of the procedure can be managed effectively. In rare instances, the operator may choose to use indwelling small ureteral catheters; #4 ureteral catheters may be used, but even with these small and pliable catheters, they usually interfere with the limited operating space. Careful preoperative appraisal by indirect air cystoscopy of the interrelationship between the fistula margins

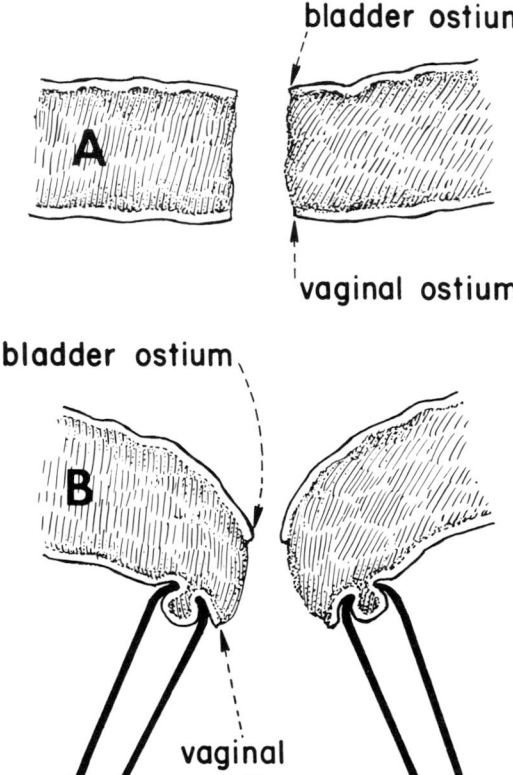

Fig. 5.10. These diagrams illustrate a cause of a common error in dissection and reapproximation of the fistula margins (A). As traction is applied (B) the mucosal margins of the bladder ostium are also drawn downward or funneled outward, and as dissection proceeds the fistula may be inadvertently greatly enlarged. The operator may safeguard against this by careful hemostasis and an acute awareness of the appearance of the bladder mucosa.

and ureteral orifices will usually give the operator accurate enough detail of what safety margin he has and thus an error can be avoided.

As proper exposure of the fistula is obtained, it is wise for the operator to pause and take inventory of what he now thinks he will need in this particular repair. It is better, at this moment, to request the desired lighting adjustment, instrument, or suture than to get well into the repair and then have to wait for the important item. Of course, not all of these things can be foreseen, but proper preoperative planning will have made available the other instruments and paraphernalia which might be needed. Using a fine #25 hypodermic needle, the margins of the fistula are carefully infiltrated with dilute Neo-Synephrine solution—just enough to control oozing and make dissection of the various layers much easier. The vaginal membrane about the fistula is circumcised as widely as possible without giving undue tension to the subsequent closure. This mucosa is now dissected off in its full thickness exposing the subjacent vaginal fascia and bladder muscularis (Fig. 5.11A). Very careful circumcision of the bladder mucosa is done in a way to remove the length of the fistulous tract, however small or large. A serious error can be committed here if the bladder mucosal margins are lost sight of, retract away, and make the all important reapproximation impossible. Now with use of the small traction hook or delicate forceps, the first suture of 3-0 chromic is placed in such a way as to invert the bladder, thus not exposing the suture material itself to the urine stream (Fig. 5.11B). The operator has a choice here of using a continuous locking suture which gives good control of the margins of the mucosa; but if it fails, all may be lost. On the other hand, he may use interrupted sutures placed close enough together for hemostasis and give a water-tight closure. In some instances the use of the interrupted sutures gives better control by gentle traction for placement of subsequent sutures. The line of suture is now tested by instilling into the bladder a contrast medium such as dilute methylene blue or sterile milk. The latter serves the purpose well and doesn't give troublesome staining of the tissues.

In placing this all important first line of sutures, the operator must use any of the numerous types of needles and needle holder that have been described previously in this chapter. It is not unusual to find that different needles or needle carriers must be used first on one side of the closure, and then to change to facilitate the passage of the suture into the other side. This would preclude the use of a continuous suture in this circumstance.

Although it is not always possible, it is always desirable, if feasible, to employ a second layer of sutures to protect this first line. If the bladder has been properly mobilized, this second layer of 3-0 chromic catgut sutures can be used without too much trouble. If it can be done in another axis, it is wise to do so in order to strengthen the innermost line and obliterate any dead space by this grid effect (Fig. 5.11C). Finally, the third layer closing the vaginal mucosa is done. The nonabsorbable, nonreactive suture is used here in full thickness of the vaginal membrane and taken in a mattress fashion (Fig. 5.11D). The choice of this suture material may vary from silver, stainless steel, or monofilament synthetic fiber such as nylon or dacron. Nevertheless a serious error can be committed here, as has been proven by years of experience, if improper suture such as catgut, silk, or other materials which cause tissue reaction are used. It is possible that these latter materials may be employed, but it has been found since the teachings of Sims that nonreactive suture left in place for an extended period of time gives the best chance for success.

Care must be used to insure that the vaginal membrane sutures are not disturbed subsequently by vaginal packing, improper douches, or manipulations.

Ordinarily adequate drainage per urethral catheter will suffice *if* everyone in attendance of the patient is made aware of the necessity to prevent blockage of the flow. When the patient is fully reacted from the anesthesia, she is also enlisted to be aware of proper catheter drainage. The catheter must be irrigated frequently if there is any tinge of blood to insure no clot obstructs the flow. If more than the expected or usual amount of bleeding is noted at the completion of the procedure, then the operator must make the decision about the advisability of creating a temporary additional bladder drainage either by vaginal or suprapubic cystostomy. For adequate urethral drainage the #22 or #24 5-cc Foley bag catheter is employed. We

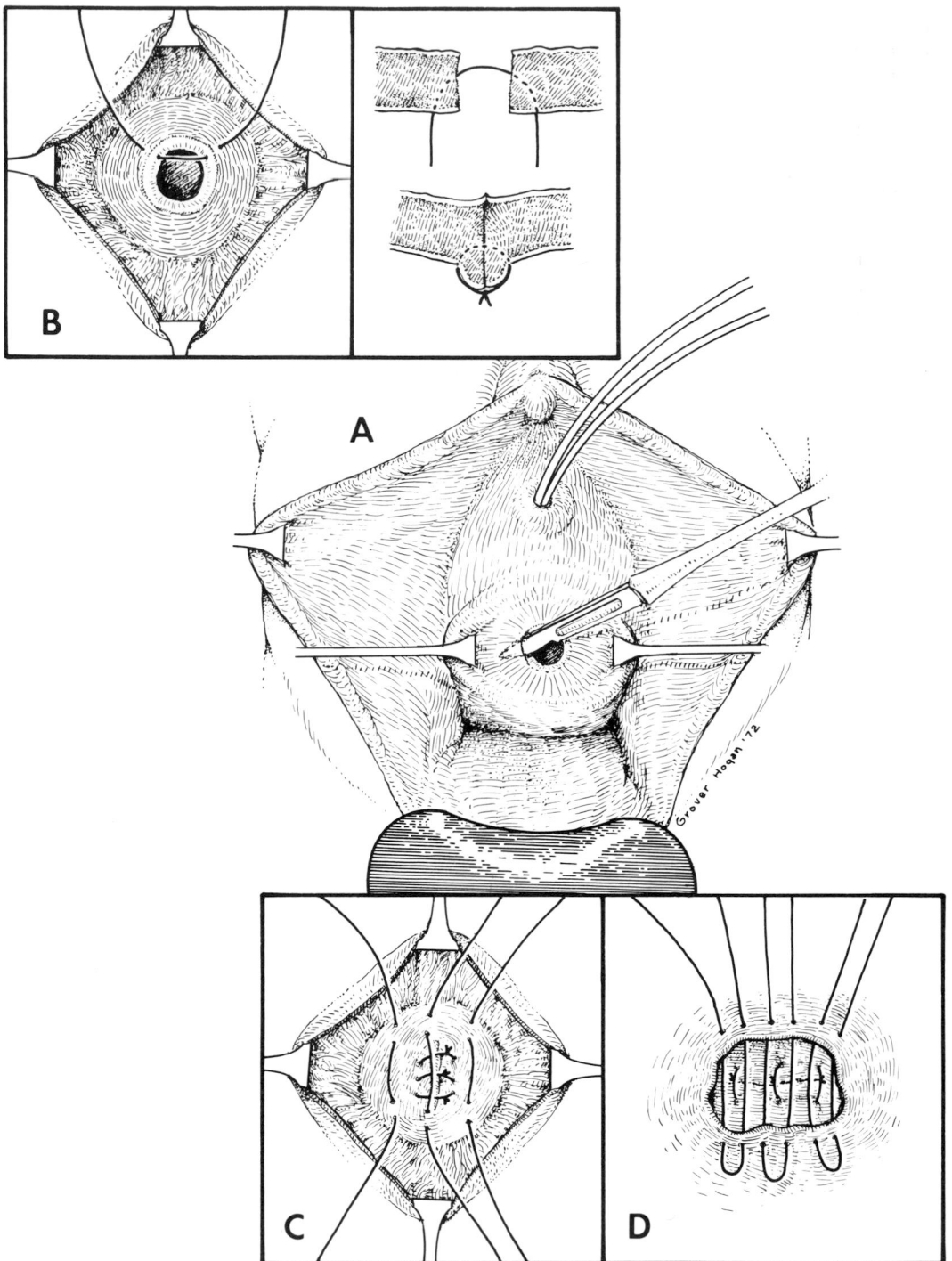

Fig. 5.11. The basic steps of repair of the simple vesicovaginal fistula.

(A) The vaginal mucosa has been infiltrated and immobilized. A delicate scalpel blade is undercutting and mobilizing the vaginal mucosa. Indwelling ureteral catheters may be used temporarily as a safeguard during the dissection, particularly if the operator is concerned about the proximity of the ureteral orifices to the fistula margin.

have used a combination of #20F Foley 5-cc bag catheter with an accompanying #8F French catheter lying alongside extending into the bladder. It is less likely that both catheters would simultaneously fail.

Vaginal Cystostomy

Although this may be a desirable means of giving extra bladder drainage because of its accessibility at the time of operation, it nonetheless may be difficult to perform without injury to the newly repaired fistula. This is particularly true in instances when the anterior vaginal wall has been shortened and scarred by previous surgery or irradiation. Creation of a fistula through the trigone with the close proximity of the ureters and the internal urethral sphincter invites permanent injury to these structures. However, if the fistula has been repaired in the trigonal area, and the upper vagina is voluminous, a cystostomy may be created posterior to the interureteric line. A small Kelly clamp is inserted into the bladder per urethra and the tip directed downward toward the vagina but posterior to the trigone and fistula repair area. The tip is spread slightly and presented against the vaginal wall which is exposed properly. A small stab wound is made to the clamp tip. Bleeding is usually not a problem as the tip is spread slightly and passed into the vagina. The tip of a mushroom or small caliber Foley catheter with a 5-cc balloon is drawn into the bladder and fixed in place. In this way minimal trauma is done to the bladder. The tip of the Foley catheter beyond the balloon may be cut off smoothly so as not to "tent" into bladder mucosa causing unnecessary trauma and possible bleeding. This catheter may be left in place as long as drainage must be assured.

The suprapubic cystostomy is another means of assuring adequate bladder drainage postoperatively. In fact, this may be the method of choice when drainage in addition to the urethral catheter must be employed. In the thin individual, a maneuver similar to that described for the vaginal cystostomy may be done. A long, thin, curved Kelly clamp or uterine sound is passed into the bladder and presented toward the abdominal wall 1 inch above the superior surface of the symphysis pubis. Using a pointed scalpel blade, an incision less than 10 mm in size is made through the skin and down to the clamp point. If one stays in the midline, one is unlikely to cause any troublesome bleeding or enter the peritoneal cavity. As the clamp tip is presented abdominally, a small caliber Foley catheter or mushroom catheter is drawn into the bladder and fixed in place. However, if the patient is obese or if there has been previous surgery through a lower abdominal incision, this suprapubic cystotomy may be inadvisable or impossible. We have used the suprapubic trocar punch placement of the suprapubic tube in one case in which the fistulous opening was small and could be occluded enough preoperatively to allow for the necessary distention to 55 cc of the bladder. It is thought erroneous to distend the bladder after the repair has been done for fear of disrupting the suture lines; therefore the trocar suprapubic punch cystotomy has found limited use thus far.

In the event that entry is mistakenly made into the peritoneal cavity by the suprapubic cystotomy, it is usually not discovered until later when the patient may show peritoneal irritation from either urine or blood. Urine ascites can be a most serious complication and must be corrected forthwith. It is possible to withdraw the suprapubic catheter, keep the bladder deflated, and get spontaneous closure. However, if the patient's condition worsens, exploratory laparotomy must be done for salvage.

Fig. 5.11 *continued*

The vaginal mucosa (B) has been reflected by full thickness mobilizing away from the fistula margin. Inset shows diagrammatically the proper placement of the most important suture in the repair. The catgut does not go completely through the bladder membrane but is placed in such a way as to reapproximate the fistula margins and invert the margins into the bladder lumen. The error of placing suture material into the urine stream is always avoided.

The second layer (C) of closure places the catgut sutures in the mobilized bladder muscularis in another axis, if possible, to the line of closure of the first layer.

The third and final layer of the fistula closure (D) is taken with mattress fashion sutures, using nonabsorbable, nonreactive suture material (monofilament nylon, silver wire, or stainless steel). This line of the closure is in whatever direction provides the least tension.

Immediate Postoperative Care

Important steps of adequate postoperative care begin at the very time the last suture is placed in the repair. The operator must at that time satisfy himself that a water-tight repair has been accomplished thus far. This is done by gently distending the bladder with about 50 cc of contrast media, either dilute methylene blue or sterile milk. He must at this time be sure that no undetected bleeding is occurring and that adequate bladder drainage is assured, even if cystostomy must be employed. The patient is kept flat in bed for 14 days but may roll from side to side being careful not to kink the drainage catheter or tubes. We have not employed the face-down position or the Bradford frame because of the acute discomforture of the patient and no more of a guarantee that the suture line is protected from distention.

It has been advocated by some authors that mobilization and ambulation may be more rapidly accomplished in some patients with "small" fistula. Even though this may be done without undue risk, there is always a chance for failure if the error is made of departing from the well established axioms of care. Success or failure hinges on many little details of common sense care, and since the healing of the vaginal fistula is a capricious thing, it is advised that every opportunity to heal be given because subsequent procedures get geometrically harder to do successfully.

At the end of approximately 2 weeks, the drainage of the bladder is intermittently stopped before the catheters are actually removed. It is a good idea to allow the bladder to fill for 30 minutes at the time for a day before all catheters are removed. Even then the patient is cautioned to void frequently, every 2 hours night and day for a week to avoid overdistention. She is warned against the use of a douche nozzle being thrust into the vagina, but may take low pressure vaginal douches with the introduction of a small nozzle tip just within the vaginal introitus. The patient must be specifically warned about coitus in the postoperative era; this is prohibited for 2 months postoperatively. The author had one apparently successful repair of a particularly difficult vesicovaginal fistula destroyed when the patient had intercourse on the 17th postoperative day. There was necessarily another delay for tissue healing and two more efforts were needed before it was finally successfully closed.

Removal of Sutures

The proper removal of the nonabsorbable sutures from the vaginal mucosa is most important. It will have been noted that these sutures while in place cause moderate vaginal discharge. This can be made more tolerable by low pressure shallow vaginal douching and sitz baths after the 14th postoperative day. The time of removal of these sutures is important although various operators will choose their own time interval postoperatively (9). The chief error here would certainly be removing the sutures too early. The elapsed time should be at least 21 days (10), because before this time, healing has usually not progressed safely enough, and there is always postoperative edema about the repair making the exposure of the sutures difficult. In fact, there is no harm to be done in allowing the nonabsorbable suture to remain in place for 30 days. If the more pliable sutures (and therefore less traumatic) such as monofilament nylon have been used, there is practically no danger of erosion into the bladder. On the other hand, it is likely that these sutures may come out automatically in this waiting period. It is not unusual to find that one or all nonabsorbable sutures may lie free in the vaginal vault or have been irrigated from the vagina. We have seen no instances where erosion has taken place back into the bladder, urethra, or rectum.

When the time comes for the inspection and removal of the sutures, a safeguard against error is good exposure and good illumination of the operative area. The patient will usually have the right to complain of vaginal pain, particularly if an episiotomy or the larger Schuchardt incisions have been utilized at the time of the original operation. It is all right to make the effort to remove these sutures using no anesthetic, but very often this is completely unsatisfactory. This will surely lead to a possible error by not having the best possible exposure and improper removal or "tearing-out" of the suture. The patient has been forewarned before she leaves the hospital or at least at the time of her complete ambulation that she may have to undergo a second and usually very short anesthesia for the suture removal. Usually there is no objection on the patient's part even though there must be another expense of the hospitalization and anesthesia.

With the operative area well lighted and exposed, gentle traction is applied on each suture. When that portion of the suture within the tissue is exposed, it is carefully hooked with a delicate but blunt and angled nerve hook. The suture material is cut and carefully withdrawn allowing the suture to come out by itself. A small amount of bleeding may occur at this time, but this is of no consequence. It has been found that the removal of silver wire presents more of a problem because it has been bent in the form of the mattress suture and will, at times, form a hook which could cause great trauma if dragged through the healing tissues. Therefore a small stabilizing clamp is needed to immobilize the silver wire while the cut is made with small pointed wire clippers or scissors especially reserved for this. The wire is then straightened of any hooked ends or kinks, and gently withdrawn. The operator, having carefully counted and recorded the number of nonabsorbable sutures that he applied at the time of repair, now counts these as he removes them. If all are not found, either by sight or palpation, it usually means that the suture has come out of its own accord. It is possible, however, that a fragment of a suture may be missed and remained buried in the healing and yet slightly edematous tissue. This possibility should be explained to the patient, stating that subsequent inspection is always made just for this eventuality. In this way the patient is not likely to feel that "something has been left in" and invite consideration of a law suit. It is disquieting to the surgeon to have a call from the irate husband who has "found" the suture fragment 1 or 2 months later.

After these sutures are removed, the patient is again cautioned to void every 1 or 2 hours for 2 days to again avoid overdistention. After that, her routine is unrestricted except for coitus and ordinary douching for the 2 months postoperatively. The operator must be alert for the possibility of a urinary tract infection which might have gained foothold postoperatively during the prolonged bladder drainage (11). If this infection exists, he must determine the identity of the offending organisms and find to

what drugs they are sensitive. The patient is kept on this appropriate drug routine for 2 weeks or until the infection clears.

In the remote postoperative care, in the event the woman gets pregnant, it is felt that cesarean section is clearly indicated to avoid distention of the vagina in parturition, inviting reopening of the scarred but healed fistula area whether this successful repair has been of the bladder, urethra, or rectum.

Repair of Other Types of Fistulae

In the foregoing discussion, an effort has been made to describe in detail the general principles and practices of the most common type of vaginal fistula—the usually uncomplicated vesicovaginal fistula. Unfortunately no two fistulae are alike and although the broad principles of technique and care must be applied as outlined, wide variation, individualization, and ingenuity must be used. The vesicovaginal fistula at the vault seen following total hysterectomy whether abdominal or vaginal, is increasingly common (12). Also we see this type of fistula presenting even more of a problem of repair and postoperative healing if irradiation has been used in cancericidal dosages (13). The demands for satisfactory exposure, meticulous dissection, and tissue management are greater because these tissues have changed more markedly due to postsurgical or postirradiation cicatrix and devascularization. This is also true of those fistulae in which previous failure has been the case. Revascularization is most important and can be helped by the relatively simple technique of gracilis muscle transplant of Martius (14) or fat pad transplant described by Betson (15).

The Latzko Closure of the Vault Vesicovaginal Fistula

In the Latzko procedure (16), the patient has been carried through the comprehensive preoperative survey and tests to determine the existing kidney function, ureteral anatomy, and presence of any more than the one fistula in question. A serious error may be made if it has not been determined that no malignancy yet exists in those patients in whom treatment of cancer has been contributory to the formation of the fistula. Cytologic smears are made and tissue biopsies are taken as widely or as deeply as possible without enlarging the fistula beyond repair.

The first consideration of exposure of the fistula is with the patient in the dorsolithotomy position, although in some instances the operator can choose to put the patient in the jack-knife or knee-chest position. It is frequently necessary to cut a moderate midline episiotomy to enhance exposure. Traction about the fistula is applied and the opening circumcised at least 1 cm from the margins, and this area denuded. Usually this will be both the anterior and posterior vaginal walls just at the vault seam. More extensive denudement can be done and is more desirable in properly mobilizing the bladder up and away from the vagina.

The bladder mucosal margins are carefully identified and an error of getting into the peritoneal cavity is avoided if dissection is done meticulously. However, if entry is made into the peritoneal cavity, it must be recognized then because subsequent leakage of urine could occur forming the fearful urine ascites. This opening is first closed before the operation proceeds to the closure of the bladder mucosa. It is axiomatic to say that the more mobilization of the bladder wall with preservation of its blood supply, the better the chance for successful invagination of the bladder mucosa and closure of the fistula opening (Fig. 5.12). If the second layer of closure using again the 3-0 chromic catgut on the appropriate needle can be "rolled inward" toward the first line of closure, the chance for success is greater. Finally, the widely denuded area of the vaginal vault seam is reapproximated with interrupted mattress sutures of nonabsorbable material whether it be monofilament nylon, stainless steel, or silver wire. The patient has been made to understand that there may necessarily be some shortening of the vagina to get a successful cure of the fistula, but this is a small price to pay to cure the incontinence. This upper partial colpocleisis of Latzko (16) has proven to be a very satisfactory and dependable procedure. What we are really trying to do in the repair of any vaginal fistula is to re-establish as nearly as possible the normal conditions of blood supply, tissue approximation, and tissue tension, because one remembers that an opening into the bladder, when discovered at the time it is done, rarely ever fails to close if the layers are reapproximated while the tissues are fresh. It is also noted that the cystostomy used for therapeutic drainage of the bladder never fails to close if adequate drainage is maintained for 1 week after the cystostomy tube is removed.

It is impossible in a given text to fully describe all the different types of fistulae which can occur, or to detail the techniques of the closure of these types of fistulae. The variations of anatomy and fistulous tracts are legion, but it is to be emphasized that the general principles outlined in these foregoing pages should incorporate the proper guide for application to any type of fistula.

The Urethrovaginal Fistula

The urethrovaginal fistula is usually not so frequently seen, comprising 15 per cent of the urinary tract fistulae into the vagina. Inasmuch as it is a cause of incontinence, it is distressing. However, the leakage of the urethrovaginal fistula is somewhat different from the vesicovaginal and ureterovaginal fistulae, in that it may be intermittent, giving the patient some periods of remaining dry. Since the defect is beyond the sphincter action at the internal urethral meatus, it will not leak unless the sphincter is incompetent allowing the urethra to fill with urine. With the competent sphincter, the leakage through the urethrovaginal fistula is at the time the patient is actually voiding. However, the urine will accumulate in the vagina and then leak out as the patient has finished voiding and left the commode. Some patients having a relatively small urethrovaginal fistula will find that the incontinence can be fairly well controlled by wearing a large sized vaginal tampon to absorb the leakage. However, there is always maceration and bad odor that sooner or later becomes intolerable.

The fistula may be anywhere along the course of the urethra, but with a closer proximity to the bladder neck the problem of repair gets more challenging. In particular, if there exists the urethrovesicovaginal fistula, the problem of repair becomes comparably enormous. This will be discussed more fully under a separate heading.

Etiology of the Urethrovaginal Fistula

The etiology of the urethrovaginal fistula is usually a surgical error; however, obstetrical

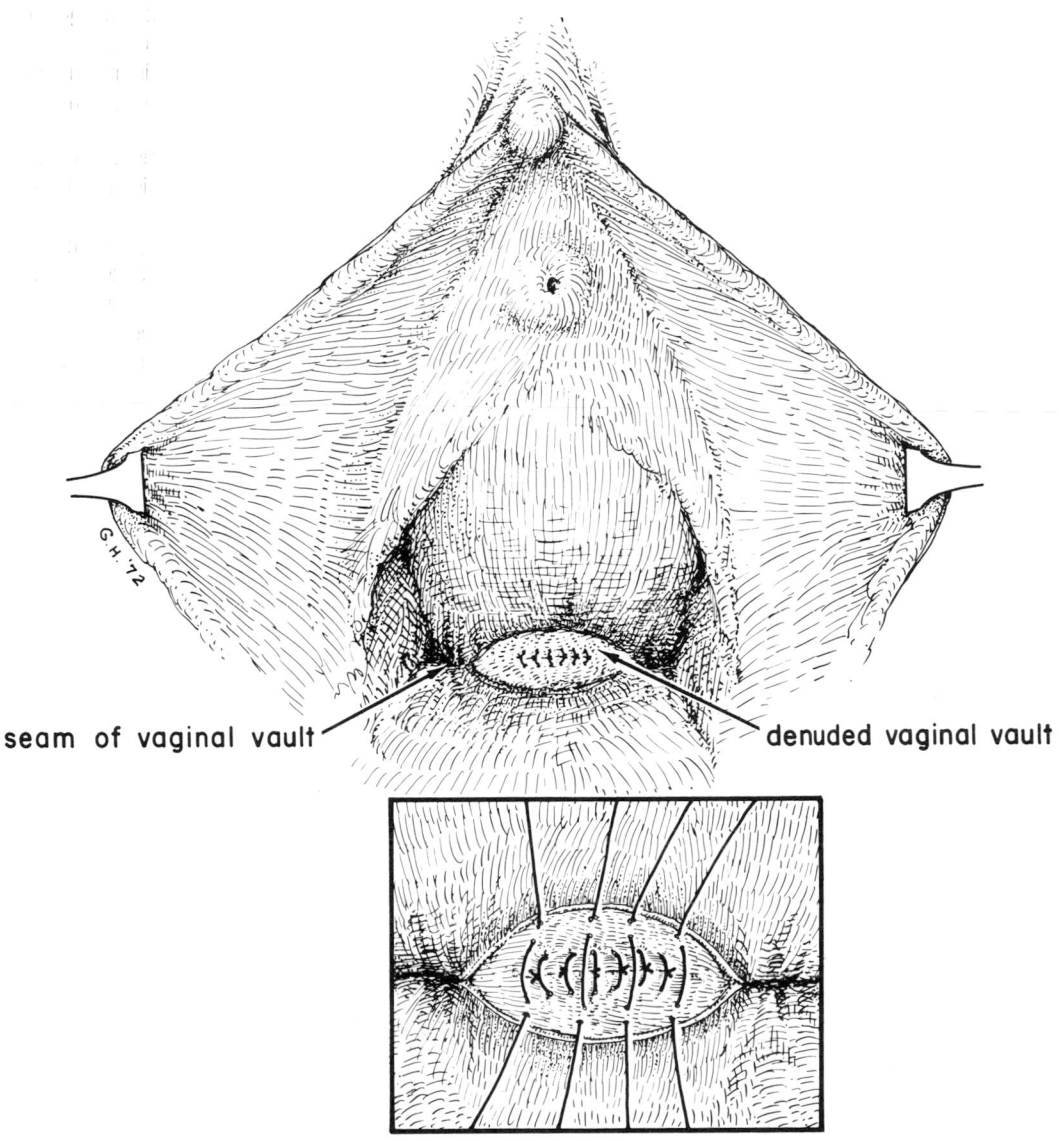

seam of vaginal vault   **denuded vaginal vault**

Fig. 5.12. The dependable Latzko procedure for closure of the high fistula in the vaginal vault along the seam of closure of a previous operation. This type of repair, usually elected for the vesicovaginal fistula resulting from total hysterectomy, can also be used for the closure of a similarly located rectovaginal fistula. This illustrates the first layer of closure inverting the bladder mucosa into the bladder. Denudement of opposing vaginal mucosal areas on the anterior and posterior vaginal walls allows mobilization of the subjacent bladder (or bowel) wall beneath the vault seam. Inset shows placement of the second layer of catgut sutures further inverting the bladder wall. A final layer by monofilament nylon or silver wire closes the juxtaposed vaginal walls, effecting a small upper colpocleisis.

trauma particularly with misapplication of forceps plays a part. A few fistulae are seen resulting from malignancy, treatment thereof, or residual of a granulomatous venereal disease. These causes, listed in the order of their frequency, are:

1. Surgery
2. Obstetrical trauma
3. Malignancy
4. Irradiation
5. Granulomatous lesions
6. Miscellaneous

a. Erosion by pessary
b. Spontaneous rupture of urethral diverticulum
c. Self-inflicted
d. False passage of catheter or sound

Surgical error must be guarded against while operating about the bladder neck and urethra. The most frequent error is the too vigorous dissection of the pubovesicocervical fascia in the anterior colporrhaphy. As the curved scissors are thrust beneath the vaginal mucosa and this vaginal fascia, the dissection may be deep enough to pierce the urethra against the indwelling catheter that is so frequently used in this anterior repair. Or the blood supply may be so compromised that an actual slough will take place. The operator must be aware of the blood supply of the urethra; although it is generous it can nevertheless be impaired if dissection is either too vigorous directly onto the urethra or just as importantly, if dissection of the paraurethral tissues is taken too far about the lateral circumference of this structure. When performing the Kennedy modification of the basic Kelly plication of the urethra, the lateral and posterior dissection can easily be overdone, and instead of correcting the stress urinary incontinence, the surgeon has created a fistula. The safeguard is to dissect just to a point lateralward on either side of the urethra so that no more than 180° of the circumference is skeletonized (see Fig. 4.7a, b).

A fistula, although small, may be created by improper placement of the plicating needle. If the point is thrust into the urethra inadvertently but withdrawn without passage of the black silk suture, this opening will close spontaneously if the indwelling catheter is allowed to remain in place for 7 days. However, if the suture is passed into and remains in the urethra, it is likely to allow a fistula or calculus to form.

The entire urethra has been avulsed in cases of ordinary anterior colporrhaphy. It is difficult to understand how the entire urethra could be dissected off without the operator being aware of this error. However, if the colporrhaphy is being done without a small indwelling bladder catheter, the initial thrust of the dissecting scissors can go into the lumen of the urethra and the entire structure opened or dissected away. A safeguard against this is the indwelling catheter, but the salvage may be a most

difficult job as will be discussed more fully in connection with the vesicourethrovaginal fistula.

Incision and drainage of a suburethral abscess, usually arising from a diverticulum, can allow a urethrovaginal fistula to form. This is particularly true if the ostium of the abscessed diverticulum has not closed into the lumen of the urethra. The gynecologist may make the error of either overlooking this ostium or recreating one when he is dissecting out a urethral diverticulum. The distention of the urethral diverticulum either by pus or stone actually will be an aid to the operator in identifying the sac and the urethral ostium (Fig. 5.13). A careful search is always made because if this is overlooked the chance for the formation of a urethrovaginal fistula is good indeed. The operator must also be aware of the possibility of other diverticuli nearby or that this one upon which he is operating may burrow proximally or distally. If a portion of the diverticulum burrows into the bladder neck, a more delicate problem of dissection arises. If the dissection is too traumatic, the sphincter of the bladder may be impaired or there may be created a formidable urethrovesicovaginal fistula. A safeguard to be used here after the diverticulum has been identified and traced into the bladder neck, is (a) to be sure that no ostium exists into the lumen of the bladder or urethra and then (b) to destroy this portion of the diverticulum mucosa with careful electrocoagulation or cauterization with phenol or some other controllable caustic agent.

Obstetrical trauma plays a part in the etiology of the urethrovaginal fistula. Misapplication of forceps allowing the urethra to become impinged between the blade and the symphysis will either tear the urethra or so embarrass the blood supply that a fistula can soon form by necrosis. A fistula may also form, usually including the urethra and bladder base, with baby's head impinging for a long period of time against the symphysis pubis. This can occur with a deep pelvic arrest in the first stage of labor, leading to necrosis and later formation of a most difficult "circumferential" urinary fistula for which extensive reconstruction is needed. It is advisable to always suspect the possibility of urethral injury with any difficult forceps application. It takes practically no time and is of no danger to gingerly pass a small

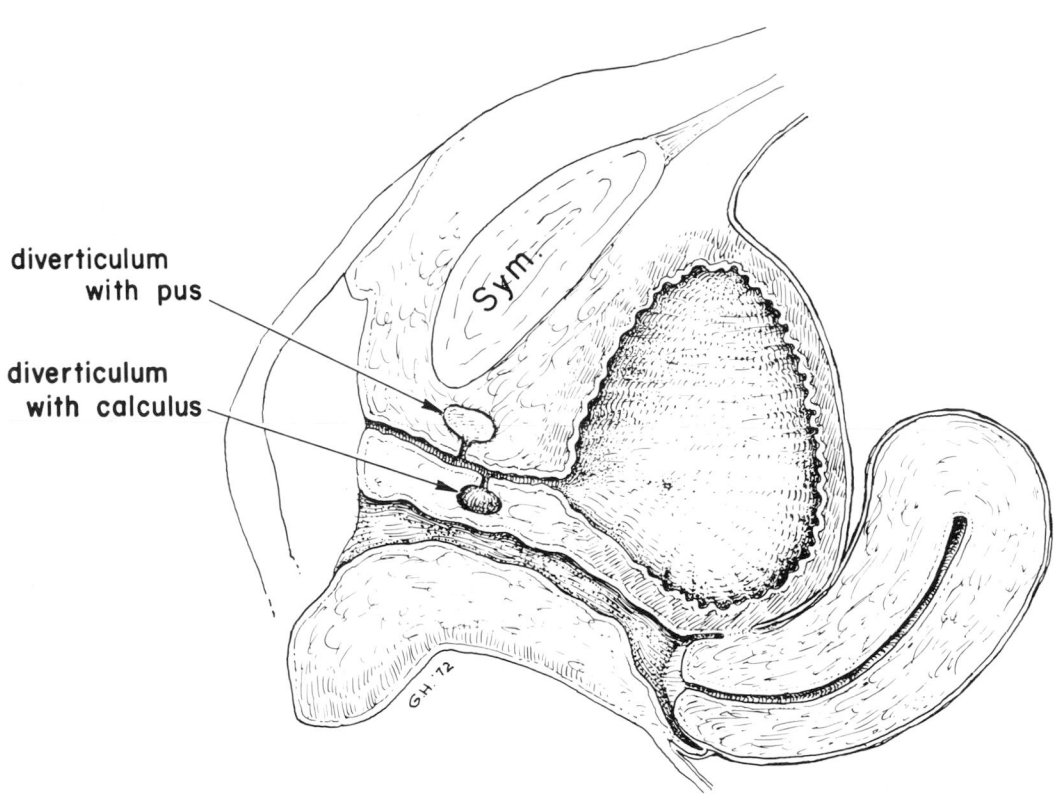

diverticulum
with pus

diverticulum
with calculus

Fig. 5.13. Demonstration of the more common suburethral diverticulum with stone formation and also the elusive subpublic diverticulum which may escape detection unless the examiner always suspects the capriciousness of this troublesome condition. Two or more diverticuli of various locations may coexist. In any case the ureteral ostium must be closed and the sac extirpated.

metal catheter or sound to explore the urethra before the patient leaves the table. It is now a simple matter to repair the fresh injury, and with proper splinting and drainage one expects prompt closure. One patient had her urethra completely transected by the forceps blade. The severed segments of the urethra were difficult to identify in the edematous tissue and blood of parturition; however, the urethral continuity was re-established by interrupted sutures of 3-0 chromic catgut. An indwelling catheter was left in place for 14 days and healing was satisfactory without fistula formation. However, it was necessary to dilate this portion of the urethra several times in the following year to finally re-establish adequate caliber.

Carcinoma of the urethra, either transitional cell or squamous, may cause fistula formation. However, if an undiscovered or untreated carcinoma of the urethra or anterior vaginal wall has progressed far enough for fistula formation, the prognosis is usually grave. Wide excision is usually necessary including the urethra, portions of the vagina, and the bladder itself. Urinary diversion must be resorted to in most instances in which such an extensive procedure is needed. However, irradiation necrosis, resulting from treatment of cancer of the cervix, vagina, or lower urinary tract, can result in a fistula formation of the urethra. As soon as the slough has occurred and edema subsided, careful biopsies are taken locally to exclude the possible presence of persistent malignancy. Repair can then be undertaken.

Granulomatous lesions of all types including granuloma inguinale, lymphopathia venereum, syphilis, and tuberculosis can cause tissue loss enough to establish a urethrovaginal fistula or even the loss of the entire urethra. These lesions can be treated usually successfully with appropriate antibiotics. As the tissues recover and the reaction subsides, the actual tissue loss can be determined. Then the necessary repair can be decided upon depending upon what deformity has occurred.

The task of the repair of a urethrovaginal or other type of vaginal fistula resulting from irradiation and treated granulomatous lesions can be a challenging one. This is chiefly due to the diminished blood supply and scar tissue.

The urethra may be damaged by bizarre miscellaneous means, resulting in fistula formation, stricture formation, or total loss. If the urethral injury is due to trauma whether it be accidental or even self-inflicted, and the loss of blood supply or tissue loss is not too great, repair can be less difficult. Rare instances of rupture or perforation of the urethra are seen in attempts at masturbation with a rigid or sharp object. In most of these instances if the defect is detected within 48 hours, repair can be done successfully. Unattended vaginal pessaries of various sorts, causing compression on the urethra against the symphysis, may erode into the lumen of the urethra forming a troublesome fistula. Although the error of leaving the pessary in too long may be actually the patient's fault, it nonetheless is the responsibility of the gynecologist who inserted it. Rare instances of fistula formation with the spontaneous drainage of a urethral diverticulum into the vagina can cause a fistula to form. This type of case is cared for in the similar manner of incision and drainage of the urethral diverticulum abscess or suburethral abscess.

Technique of Repair of Urethrovaginal Fistula

The repair of the urethrovaginal fistula may be tedious but usually not so difficult as the high vesicovaginal fistula. The principal error that can be made in the urethra repair is improper closure of the urethral ostium, and excessively wide mobilization of the urethra prior to this closure. It must be remembered that since the urethral circumference is rather limited, wide mobilization may lead to necrosis or actual mechanical obstruction. A safeguard against this is the use of a #20F indwelling urethral catheter during and following the repair. This is not too large to distend the urethra excessively but large enough to show the defect and also to allow adequate postoperative drainage.

The urethra may be transilluminated easily with a lighted telescope thus giving the exact location and size of the defect as well as the vascularity of the adjacent tissue, much in the same technique as recommended for study of the vesicovaginal fistula by indirect air cystoscopy. The mucous membrane of the urethra, after proper and not excessive mobilization, is closed with 3-0 chromic catgut on a small atraumatic needle. The edges are inverted into the lumen either by interrupted sutures or a continuous locking stitch. The second layer of closure is desirable if practicable, using the same 3-0 chromic catgut. The final closure of the vaginal membrane is done with interrupted mattress sutures of monofilament #1 nylon or malleable silver wire. These are tied with just enough tension to reapproximate the edges of the vaginal membrane without causing blanching. The use of paraurethral incisions to release tension is wisely employed here if there is any suggestion of unusual tension on the new suture line. These incisions are made far enough away from the repaired area in order not to compromise the blood supply (Fig. 5.14). The splinting catheter is left in place for 14 days. The patient may be allowed to be up and around in 4 days postoperatively and home with instructions for care of the indwelling catheter until it is removed. Antibiotics or sulfonamides of choice are given when an indwelling catheter is in place 72 hours or longer.

The Urethrovesicovaginal Fistula

The urethrovesicovaginal fistula can be a most troublesome and distressing defect. Not only are the two distinct organs involved, but the bladder neck with its sphincter action is incompetent. The etiology of this type of fistula can originate from surgical error, obstetrical error, tissue changes occurring with neoplasm, irradiation, or necrosis (17). Inappropriate transurethral resection of the bladder neck, particularly with the electrosurgical unit, has contributed substantially to the number of urethrovesicovaginal fistulae. Everett (18) cites three cases. These various contributing causes have been fully discussed in the foregoing pages of this chapter, with suggestions for safeguards against their occurrence. The chief problem is, of course, the proper repair and the re-establishment of urinary continence. It must be remem-

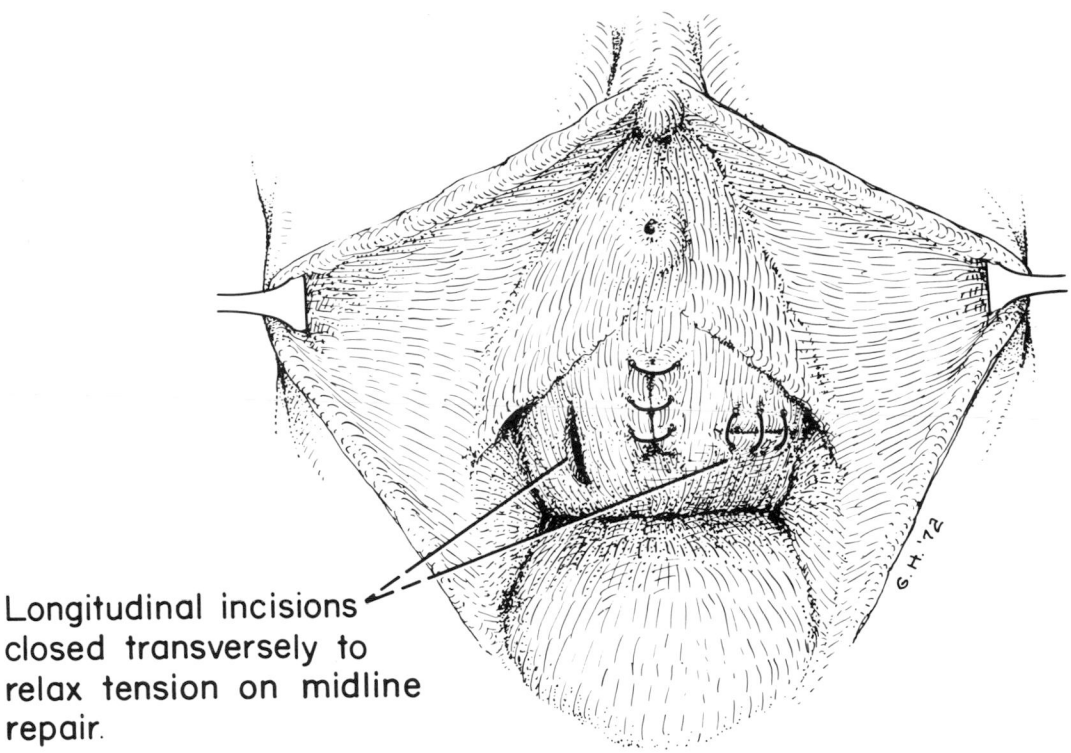

Longitudinal incisions closed transversely to relax tension on midline repair.

Fig. 5.14. Closure of the vaginal mucosa in a fistula repair may necessitate undue strain on the suture line. In this case, the closure of a rather large urethrovaginal fistula can be protected in the mucosa, closed in right angle axis.

bered also that a coexisting fistula may exist besides the large fistula at the bladder neck. Careful preoperative evaluation must be done to rule out the chance of ureteral involvement or occult fistulous tract in the urethra. In the larger urethrovesicovaginal fistula, the trigone is sometimes destroyed and the ureteral orifices may be at the margin or so close to the margin that they are involved in scar tissue. This extent of scarring must be appraised by close inspection by indirect air cystoscopy so that injury can be safeguarded against during the repair. In some instances #4 or #5 ureteral catheters are passed into the ureters to constantly orient the surgeon and help him avoid injury to these vital structures. In one of my cases, the fistula was so large that both ureteral orifices were in the margin of the defect making it impossible to properly close the fistula without injury to the ureters. Bilateral ureteroneocystostomy was performed at the first stage of repair, then the fistula closed later. This was the choice over an ileal pouch because the patient had no history

nor evidence of pelvic malignancy in which case cystectomy might have been considered.

The most extraordinary and difficult vaginal fistula seen is the circumferential fistula (19) in which the entire bladder neck has been lost with or without the loss of the urethra. This type of fistula has been seen only one time in my experience, and eventually had to have urinary diversion into the bowel. Repair from below was finally classified as impossible after three attempts were made. Proper and adequate mobilization of the remnant of the bladder was impossible because of the adherence to the posterior periosteum of the pubic bones.

Technique of Repair of the Urethrovesico-vaginal Fistula

The urethrovesicovaginal fistula is usually in a more accessible situation than the high vesicovaginal or rectovaginal fistula. However, if the vagina is narrowed by scarring, the access to the operative site may be more difficult. We usually can manage this in the lithotomy position with a Schuchardt incision, but in some cases in which mobilization of the bladder is particularly difficult, the knee-chest or jack-knife position may be used. The basic principles of the repair described fully under "Basic Repair of the Simple Vesicovaginal Fistula" above are applicable here. An important point to remember is not to diminish the caliber of the bladder neck and urethra if possible. Because of trauma of the indwelling catheter on this newly reconstructed and sometimes taut tissue, it is recommended that either vaginal cystostomy be used, if feasible, or suprapubic drainage. The technique of this cystotomy with warning of errors has been discussed above. If the operator desires double drainage using some type of urethral tube, a smaller catheter than the #20F used during the repair, can be substituted. A #10F straight catheter without the balloon can be used because the balloon causes unwanted pressure just at the new suture line. It is not uncommon for the patient to have urethral incompetence either by stress or simply by standing after this operation has been otherwise successful. A subsequent plication of the vesical neck and urethra would be inadvisable and in danger of recreating the fistula. It has been found that a sling procedure using the transected or split strap of fascia lata is the most desirable in recovering continence in this situation (see Chap. 4).

The Technique of Repair of Absence of the Urethra

Absence of the urethra can be a congenital deformity as a complete hypospadias or it can result from surgical and obstetrical errors. It is also seen resulting from granulomatous lesion, malignancy, and irradiation necrosis. The absence of the urethra except in rare cases usually results in urinary incontinence and therefore is considered in this category. However, it must be mentioned that even though the urethra may be absent in practically its entirety, there yet may be some urinary control by the sphincter action of the bladder neck. Even though the patient will not leak all the time, she will be troubled by the urine that has been entrapped in the vagina at voiding, leaking out as she stands or walks away from the commode.

To reconstruct a urethra there are basic principles to be observed. The newly constructed urethra must be covered with the vaginal mucosa and lined with epithelium. Before any operative attempt is made, the routine complete general physical and genitourinary tract examinations must be made. There must be enough time elapsed between the time of the injury or cure of the concomitant pathology to allow the tissues to return to their normal and optimal state of health. There are two basic techniques of the reconstruction of the urethra (20). (a) Turn a flap of vaginal mucosa forward forming the tube or (b) construct the tube from the adjacent mucosa if there is enough redundancy of the mucosa to allow this. In most cases in which the absence of the urethra has resulted from disease or irradiation, the scarring will prohibit the use of the latter method.

The Technique of Construction of the Urethra

The anterior vaginal wall is exposed and a U-shaped incision is made in the anterior vaginal mucosa with the upper or anterior arms of the incision 12 to 15 mm beyond the opening into the bladder whether there be any remnant of urethra remaining or not. The posterior extent of the mucosal incision curves across the midline at least 3 cm posterior to the urethral or bladder opening. The full thickness of the mucosa is carefully taken for this flap. An error may be committed here by either taking the flap too thin, depriving it of its vital blood supply, or dissecting too deeply. If the dissection is carried unnecessarily deep, troublesome bleeding may be encountered and worst of all the base of the bladder may be injured. If this is done, immediate repair is done with full awareness of the proximity of the ureteral orifices.

The flap is turned forward and rolled into a tube, fastening the margins of this rolled mucosa to the inner margins of the anterior extension of the U-shaped incision. Interrupted sutures of 2-0 chromic catgut are taken at 1- to 2-mm intervals and in such a manner as to closely approximate the edges, and not allow the suture material to be exposed into the lumen of the new urethra. At this time plicating sutures of 3-0 silk are taken at the bladder neck within the denuded area from where the flap has been dissected. Now the outmost edges of the U-shaped vaginal incision are reapproximated in the midline with interrupted mattress sutures of monofilament nylon.

It is wise to use incisions lateral to this new suture line to relax tension. These are made at least 1 cm from the mucosal closure to avoid circulatory embarrassment. The length of the incisions may be 1 to 3 cm; then either closed in a transverse or 90° axis or left agape after the bleeding points have been stopped by ligature or coagulation. The nonabsorbable monofilament nylon sutures are left in place for 14 days.

Alternate Method of Construction of Urethra

Another method of construction of the urethra is utilizing as much of the remaining wall of the urethra as possible. This may be the operation of choice if such scarring of the anterior vagina exists as to prohibit the chance of developing and turning forward a U-shaped flap of mucosa. This may be the case after the treatment with irradiation of a malignancy or treatment with antibiotics of a granulomatous lesion, revealing a scarred and sloughed membrane.

The incision is made parallel to the original course of the urethra. In some cases there may be a remnant of the external urethral meatus with a few millimeters of the urethra remaining. This can be used in the construction and anastomosis to the tube that is being formed proximal to this remnant. The arms of this U-shaped incision are made wide enough apart to allow suitable circumference of the tube being constructed, and sweep 8 to 10 mm beyond the fistula on the anterior vaginal wall. The mucosa is taken at full thickness to insure proper blood supply, and rolled into a tube over an indwelling #20F catheter. The closure of this tube posteriorly and over the fistula is particularly critical because if breakdown occurs it is most likely to occur at this point. The 3-0 chromic catgut is used within the layers of the vaginal mucosa but not into the newly constructed lumen. Ideally a second layer of reinforcing sutures are used here as in the repair of all fistulae but may be more difficult in this situation because of the lateral spread of the tissues in this area of the urethra. The third or

final layer of closure is performed using nonabsorbable suture material such as monofilament nylon or silver wire taken in a mattress fashion. Small tension-relaxing sutures may be employed 1 cm or more laterally on the anterior vaginal wall, if feasible, to ease the tension on the new suture line. These sutures are left in place for a minimum of 14 days. The healing of this construction of the urethra may be as capricious as that of the vesicovaginal fistula; therefore it is preferred that the patient remain flat in bed for 12 to 14 days to help insure healing. In the postmenopausal patient estrogen by mouth and vagina are given to enhance vascularity and promote healing in this usually hormone-deficient membrane (21).

Per primum healing of the newly constructed urethral tube is not always the case. The most unfortunate thing to happen is a slough of the whole construction. Small areas of nonhealing may also occur amounting to urethrovaginal fistulae. However, these may be closed in due time, allowing at least 2 months to intervene before another effort at repair is made. The patient, however, may have gained continence except for that leakage through the nonhealed defects in the constructed urethra. This then is a step towards cure because the incontinence may not be constant but only intermittent and at least more controllable by vaginal tampons.

Incontinence with the Newly Constructed Urethra

The incontinence which may result after the otherwise very successful construction of the urethra can be as distressing as incontinence from any cause. We have fashioned a mucosal tube which doesn't leak as such, but nevertheless, as a nonmuscular conduit with no sphincter action, it has no control of the flow of urine. It has been found that even though plication of the paraurethral tissues or tissues at the region of the internal urethral meatus has been dutifully performed during the urethral construction, sphincter action is absent. Another postoperative attempt at plication would be unwise and most likely to fail, even causing slough of the new urethra. The retropubic urethropexy, Marshall-Marchetti-Krantz, has been tried, but the chance for success is poor because of the usual inflexibility of the anterior vaginal wall and lack of any sphincter control at all.

However, the use of the Goebell-Stoeckel sling procedure using the fascia lata sling retropubically and fixed into the paraurethral tissues in the posterior third of the new urethra gives a good chance for success. This technique described by Ridley (22) utilizes the fascia lata as a double sling formed by transecting the fascia where it would ordinarily pass beneath the urethra, and fixing these loose ends firmly into the paraurethral tissues with enough tension to elevate and support the bladder neck and to augment the acuity of the posterior urethrovesical angle (see Fig. 4.22). In one case of reconstruction, the final result gave a urethra of only 1.5 cm in length, and the scarring lateralward prohibited accurate and firm attachment of the transected fascia lata. In this case the subtending portion of the fascia was not cut but left exposed and anchored in place by four carefully placed fixing sutures of 2-0 nylon. These sutures were removed on the 14th day and the fascia finally became covered with epithelium. The final result was satisfactory salvage, giving the patient urinary control except for some postvoid leakage which would result from urine collecting in the vagina with the short urethra. The patient learned to allow the vagina to drain by gentle pressure at the fourchette before she left the commode.

The Ureterovaginal Fistula

The ureterovaginal fistula is in the great majority of instances caused by surgical error, usually with the abdominal hysterectomy but also, at times, by the vaginal hysterectomy or repair. In rare instances the fistula may be caused by obstetrical trauma or by direct trauma from external force such as pelvic fracture or vaginal rupture. Of course, the slough caused by malignancy or treatment thereof can cause a vaginal fistula of any type.

Etiology

A. Surgical errors
  1. Abdominal hysterectomy
    a. Radical—Wertheim or exenteration
    b. Routine
B. Obstetrical errors

  1. Broad ligament laceration
    a. Forceps
    b. Spontaneous
C. Miscellaneous
  a. External trauma
  b. Neoplasm

The diagnosis of the presence of the ureterovaginal fistula may at times be perplexing and even overlooked if there is a concomitant vesicovaginal fistula. Its presence should always be suspected, particularly if the patient has had previous pelvic surgery (23). On physical examination one may overlook a pinhole fistulous opening tucked in a fold of the vaginal vault. The leakage may be at times intermittent if the tract from the proximal portion of the ureter to the vagina is devious, allowing temporary closure by pressure from surrounding structures, then discharging a relatively copious amount of urine at one time. The fistula may appear immediately after operation if the ureter has been transected and accidentally "implanted" near or into the vaginal vault. Most frequently, however, it does not appear for several days postoperatively because it has either formed by slough, or gradually dissected into the vagina from its point of injury. Nevertheless, the presence of urine in the vagina is very disturbing, both for the patient and the surgeon, despite the fact that the patient is able to void, and suggests practically without doubt the presence of the ureterovaginal fistula. The presence may be confirmed by the use of a contrast dye, methylene blue, in the bladder and examining the urine collecting in the vagina. If this is clear, a ureterovaginal fistula is present; however, the operator must remember that if the solution is blue, this does not rule out the coexistence of a ureterovaginal fistula and a vesicovaginal fistula. The possibility of the existence of a ureterovaginal fistula is further checked by excretory urography and retrograde catheterization of the ureters. The sooner these diagnostic procedures are done, the better. The injured ureter, within hours of the injury, will show proximal dilatation and frequently the exact point of injury (24).

The care of the injured ureter is dealt with in detail in Chapter 3, but recognition of the fistula by these diagnostic means and simple operative procedures are emphasized here. Retrograde catheterization of the ureters should be tried although this may be relatively difficult because of operative trauma and edema of the trigone; nevertheless it can and should be attempted (Fig. 5.15). This may show the exact point of obstruction, and if the operator is fortunate he may be able to pass a small #5F or #6F catheter past this point of obstruction. If this is possible, the catheter is left in place for at least 10 to 14 days and irrigated frequently, allowing the lumen to re-epithelialize. It is most likely that the fistula will close spontaneously if normal continuity of the ureter has been re-established. This is the case when the ureter has been injured but not completely transected or firmly ligated. It may be possible that the ureter has been torn, allowing escape of urine into a fistula tract but yet not having its lumen completely disrupted. It must be emphasized that an error can be made in the early diagnosis of the ureterovaginal fistula as to which side the injury to the ureter has occurred. Although it is likely that the fistula will show in the vagina on the same side as the injury, there can nevertheless be a contralateral dissection of the fistula to the opposite side (Fig. 5.16). The operative management of the injured ureter, with a fistula or without, is dealt with at length in Chapter 3 in which the abdominal approach is described. It is usually not feasible to correct the ureterovaginal fistula through the vaginal approach, unless the pelvic tissues are in most favorable condition.

The Transabdominal Approach of the Vesicovaginal or Colovaginal Fistula

The transabdominal approach of the vesicovaginal fistula is infrequently chosen by the gynecologist unless the usually easier and more dependable vaginal approach is contraindicated by extraordinary vaginal scarring or some orthopedic condition prohibiting the dorsolithotomy position thus making the vaginal vault inaccessible from below. The choice of the transabdominal (or transvesical) approach is more frequently the choice of the general urologist or general surgeon probably because he is more familiar with the anatomy from above than what we consider easier vaginal operation. The argument will never be settled, but that makes little difference because whatever technique the operator successfully uses, that is the correct technique.

If the abdominal operation is undertaken too soon after the initial injury or a previous

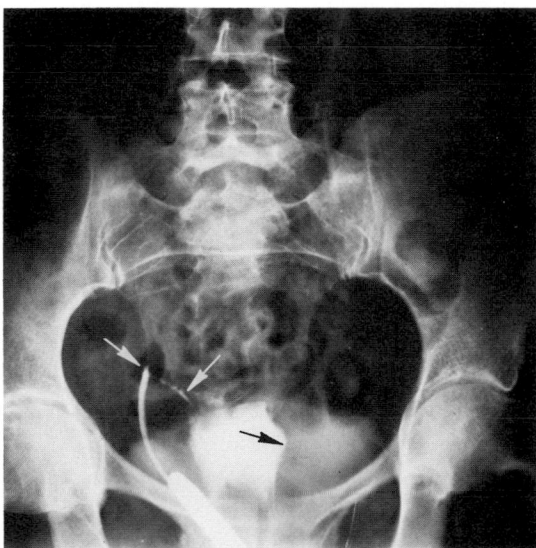 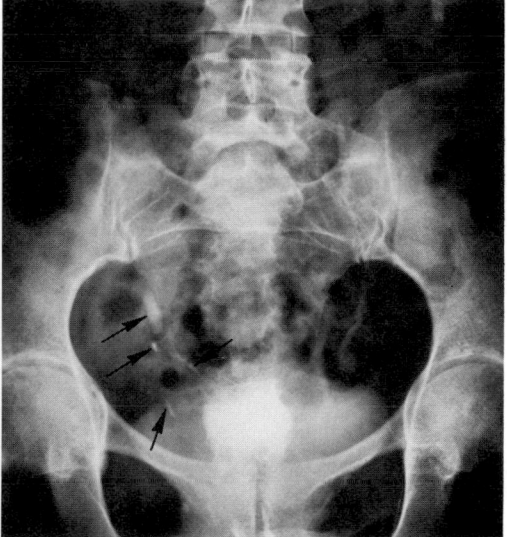

Fig. 5.15. A. Postsurgical ureterovaginal fistula. Ureteral catheter tip at point of obstruction. The fistulous tract to the vaginal vault is well shown between the catheter tip and the vagina. B. Postsurgical ureterovaginal fistula. Combination excretory and retrograde urography shows slightly dilated proximal ureter, the point of obstruction, the distal ureter, and the fistulous tract. This case was repaired successfully by re-establishing ureteral lumen with splinting catheter and without resection.

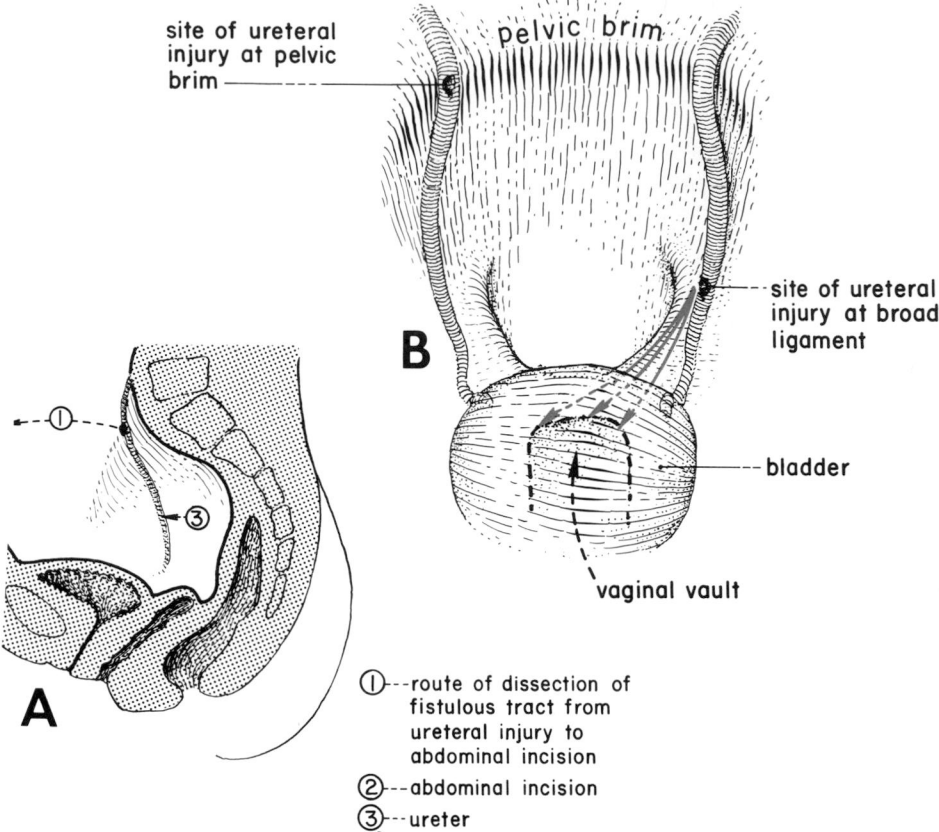

Fig. 5.16. A. The fistulous tract from an ureteral injury at the pelvic brim will usually dissect to the abdominal incision; however, it may follow a path of less resistance into the pelvis and vaginal vault. If the ureter has been occluded by ligature at the pelvic brim, it may result in quiet death of that kidney and may go undetected.

B. A schematic drawing showing possible routes of dissection of the fistulous tract into the vaginal vault from the site of ureteral injury. It is to be noted that a fistulous opening in the right side of the vaginal vault may come from a contralateral injury to the left ureter and *vice versa*.

attempt, the vascularity and edema greatly hamper the effort, if not making it completely impossible. This is particularly true if the previous operation has been necessarily traumatic and extensive due to malignancy, endometriosis, or for the residue of inflammatory disease.

An adequate incision is made even if the original incision scar must be extended. There are really no set rules of dissection, lysis of adhesions, or control of bleeding. The operator must rely on his own skill and experience to gain access to the fistula, which may either be of the vesicovaginal or enterovaginal type. Careful dissection to the vaginal vault is done mobilizing the involved viscus from the vagina.

Brisk bleeding may be encountered about the base of the bladder or bowel involved. This can usually be controlled by individual ligature with fine catgut, by pressure, or by electrocoagulation used judiciously and sparingly. The latter can cause unwanted tissue destruction and necrosis if used too extensively. The vagina, having been packed firmly with gauze, is more easily identifiable, particularly if the patient is obese, deepening the dissection. The fistulous opening into the bladder or bowel as the case may be, after it has been mobilized as well as possible, is closed by an inverting 3-0 chromic suture taken interruptedly or by continuous locking suture (Fig. 5.17). A second layer of closure using the muscularis is done with the same caliber suture. The vaginal opening is now closed with interrupted mattress sutures of monofilament nylon placed in a manner to expose the knots into the vaginal canal if possible. However, this is usually not possible because of limited exposure, and the closure must be with #1 catgut taking interrupted sutures.

Postoperative Care. Adequate drainage is a cardinal rule as in any fistula repair. The site of closure, lest there be urinary or bowel leakage, must be drained either through the abdominal wall by extraperitoneal route or through the vaginal vault 2 cm or more away from the site of closure. A small Penrose drain will suffice and is removed on the sixth postoperative day. Bladder drainage must be insured by urethral catheter. In both the transabdominal and transperitoneal approach, suprapubic bladder drainage is easily established, and wisely used if

there has been an unusual amount of bleeding within the bladder. As in other cases of postoperative fistula care, the bladder drainage is assured for at least 14 days. The nylon sutures, if used in the vaginal closure, are removed on the 21st postoperative day.

The Transvesical Approach to the Vesicovaginal Fistula

The indications for the transvesical approach to the vesicovaginal fistula are similar to those for the transabdominal approach, that is, in most cases in which the vaginal approach is contraindicated for reasons of inaccessibility to the vaginal vault. This may be due to extraordinary vaginal scarring following inradiation treatment for malignancy, previous surgical attempts to close the fistula, or some granulomatous lesion. In rare cases the patient cannot

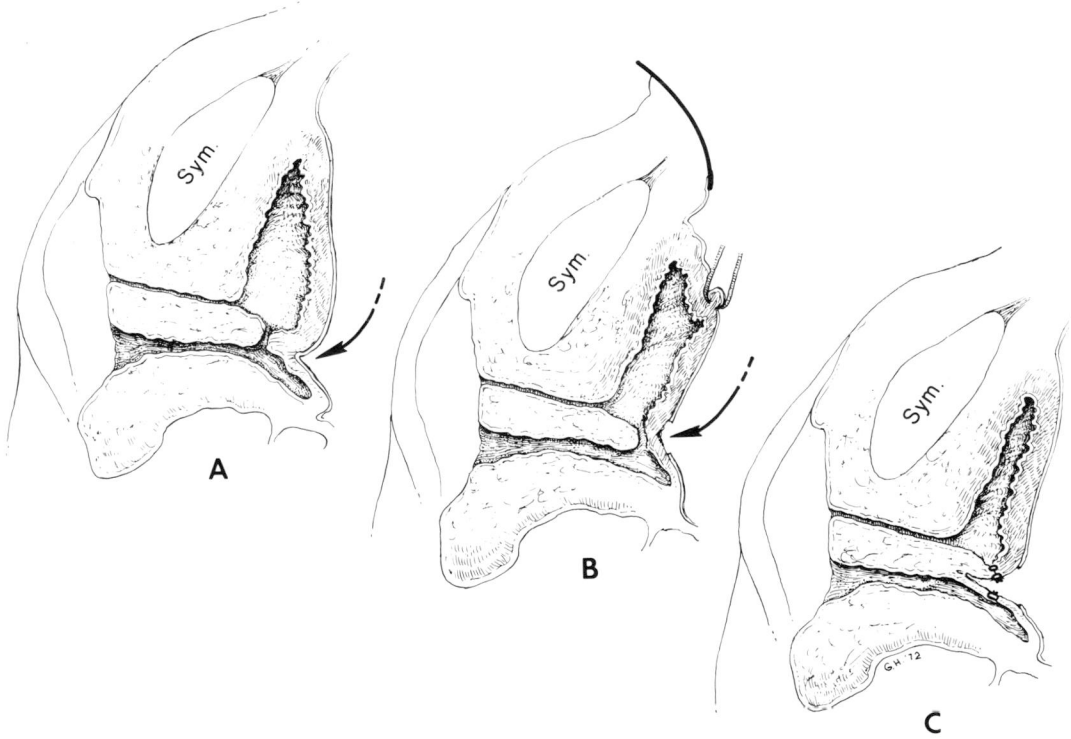

Fig. 5.17. The transperitoneal approach to the vesicovaginal (or enterovaginal) fistula must be relied upon at times when access by vagina is impossible. A, location of fistula between bladder base and vaginal vault, resulting from necrosis following abdominal hysterectomy; B, approach to the fistula after incision through the peritoneum; and C, further mobilization of the bladder wall from the vaginal vault. The bladder opening has been closed in two layers with inversion of the bladder mucosa, and the vaginal wall closed in one layer. Absorbable sutures may necessarily be used here.

be placed in the dorsolithotomy position due to previous hip or back injury or some other orthopedic condition.

The transvesical approach is more direct than the transabdominal approach, and may at times be performed entirely extraperitoneally. This is desirable when possible. The space of Retzius is entered through an adequate lower abdominal incision. For the obese individual with an abdominal panniculus, the incision may be made well along the transverse fold just between the panniculus and mons veneris. This allows more adequate exposure and is through less thickness of anterior abdominal wall fat, as the panniculus is retracted upward. The patient is placed in relatively deep Trendelenburg position. An attempt is made to stay out of the peritoneal cavity, but if entry is impossible or inadvertent, it must be carefully closed before the repair is attempted and double checked as the repair is completed.

The bladder is opened widely in its midline exposing the base where the fistula will be located. Direct visualization of the trigone and ureteral orifices is usually satisfactory and thus injury to the ureters can be avoided (Fig. 5.18). Bilateral ureteral catheterization can be done at this time with #5F ureteral catheters if the operator feels that this will further protect these structures from injury. However, the presence of the catheters in this rather limited space may be more hindrance than help.

The bladder ostium of the fistula is circumcised about 5 mm from the actual opening. A small amount of diluted Neo-Synephrine solution (1:1000) may be infiltrated about this area for dissection with a #25 needle. This will lessen the troublesome ooze and help dissection of the layers of tissue involved. The bladder mucosa is gently undercut and mobilized, exposing the vaginal ostium; this is closed with either interrupted monofilament nylon exposing the ties into the vagina for later removal or by #1 chromic catgut, depending on the accessibility of the opening. The vaginal vault may be drawn upward by inserting through the fistula opening a small Foley catheter, inflating the balloon, and applying gentle traction upward. This is one of the many rather simple but valuable "tricks" the operator may have learned or improvised.

Another type of closure of the fistula by transvesical approach is by opening the bladder

in the midline down to the fistula and excising the fistula in a racket-shaped incision (Fig. 5.19). This defect and incision are closed in three layers as described above. Proper drainage is again emphasized. The bladder is drained both suprapubically and per urethrum. In addition extraperitoneal drainage is done by a small soft Penrose drain either through the vaginal vault or through the lower abdominal incision. This drain is left in for 6 days postoperatively; the bladder drainage is assured for 14 or more days postoperatively; and the vaginal nylon sutures, if used, are removed on the 21st postoperative day.

Condemnation of Transurethral Resection of the Female Bladder Neck

The condemnation of the use of the resectoscope on the bladder neck of women, par-

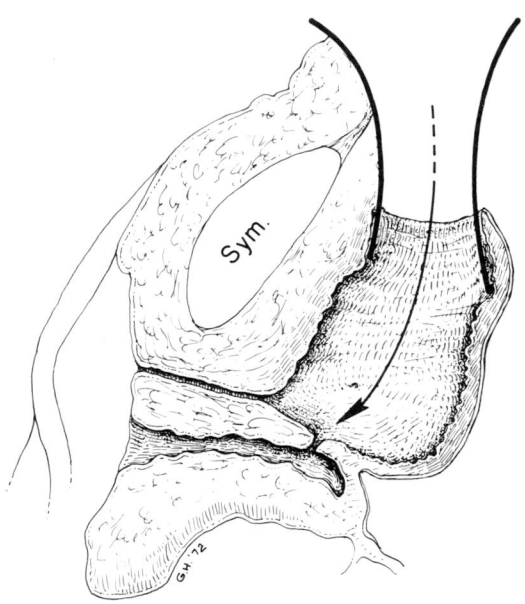

Fig. 5.18. The transvesical approach to the vesicovaginal fistula is usually the secondary choice of the gynecologist where this fistula is inaccessible vaginally because of local scarring or some orthopedic problem obviating proper positioning of the patient. The bladder is opened widely extraperitoneally. The principles of closure by three layers are observed but necessarily performed in reverse order. However, the use of nonabsorbable suture material in the closure of the vaginal ostium from above is questionable in this case where subsequent removal of these sutures is very difficult or impossible.

trigone

right ureteral orifice

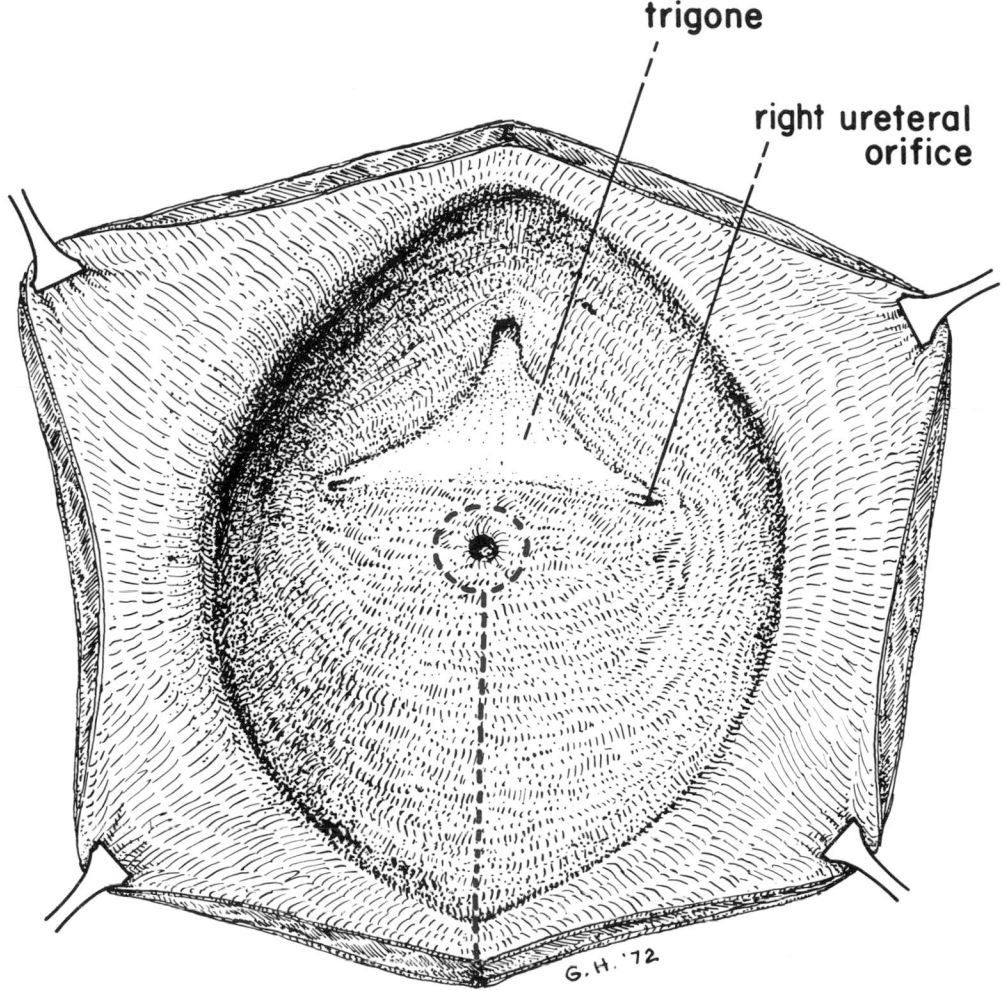

G.H. '72

Fig. 5.19. The transvesical closure of the vesicovaginal fistula may be facilitated by the excision of the scarred fistulous tract allowing closure by reapproximation of more normal tissues. From above, the trigone is easily observed with the relationship of the fistula to the ureteral orifices carefully noted. A racket-shaped incision across the posterior wall of the bladder allows adequate access to the fistula which can be excised and the vaginal and bladder walls mobilized for easier closure. Straight rubber-shod, noncrushing clamps along the incised bladder margins temporarily and satisfactorily control troublesome bleeding.

ticularly in the young girl, must be mentioned. Although it is indicated in rare cases of congenital hypertrophy of the internal urethral meatus, or congenital urethral valves, it must be done only by the experienced and skillful urologist. Every gynecologist will sooner or later see a distressing urethrovesicovaginal fistula in a young girl who has had a transurethral resection. The tissues of the bladder neck and vagina before and at puberty are very delicate and thin, not yet matured by the increasing hormone effect during and after puberty. The

loop of the resectoscope carrying the usual amount of electrical current cuts more deeply than anticipated, and necrosis extends further than wanted. An actual fistula may be cut or a postresection slough may occur in 6 to 10 days. Everett (18) listed three cases coming under his care at the Johns Hopkins Hospital. Moir (6) lists seven (six in young girls) of 268 fistulae reported under his care. This author has seen four cases (two in young girls) resulting from the unwise use of the resectoscope.

The use of the transurethral resectoscope for

the treatment of stress urinary incontinence is also condemned. The condition is practically never improved and in most cases made worse. This author (22) reported five in 105 cases needing secondary surgical correction for severe stress urinary incontinence where transurethral resection has been previously tried and had failed. These cases were salvaged by the Goebel-Stoeckel sling procedure using a fascia lata strap.

The Repair of the Rectovaginal Fistula

The rectovaginal fistula is not so commonly seen and usually doesn't cause the acute discomfort of the urinary fistula; nonetheless the uncontrolled presence of feces in the vagina and on the perineum is a dreadful condition. This is further aggravated by the involuntary passage of flatus per vaginum. The patient may learn to limit this soilage somewhat by keeping her stool constipated and dry as possible by choice of diet and medication. Nevertheless the condition demands correction as soon as would the urinary fistula.

Etiology

A. Postobstetrical
B. Postsurgical
  1. Incomplete repair of complete perineal laceration
  2. Posterior colporrhaphy
  3. Repair of enterocele
  4. Postabdominal hysterectomy
  5. Postvaginal hysterectomy
C. Post-traumatic
  1. Erosion of foreign body into rectum
    a. Pessary
    b. Stint in vaginal construction
  2. Trauma from false passage of recto-sigmoidoscope
D. Postirradiation necrosis
E. Extension of pelvic malignancy with necrosis
F. Rupture vaginally of perirectal abscess

As it will be seen from the above list, the causes of the rectovaginal fistula are numerous. The great majority of fistula occurring between the intestinal tract and the vagina are from the rectum. However, other fistulae may form even under rather bizarre conditions from other bowel segments such as the sigmoid colon, ileum, or actually any loop which may become involved with the pelvic viscera by virtue of malignant or benign disease, irradiation, or operative errors. Our chief concern at the moment is the diagnosis and treatment of the fistula which occurs in the vast majority of instances, the rectovaginal fistula.

Diagnosis of the Rectovaginal Fistula

The diagnosis of the rectovaginal fistula is usually easy. The patient can usually diagnose the condition herself or she will complain of a fetid vaginal discharge present in varying amounts. A sure diagnostic sign is the frequency of passage of a malodorous flatus per vaginum. This will lead to sexual disharmony, pelvic pain, and perineal maceration. Frequent douching is found to be necessary. Inspection of the vagina will reveal a brownish foul fecal discharge even with a very small fistula. As this is wiped away the ostium may be visualized immediately as a pinkish dimple or pout of granulation tissue. Manipulation can express more material from the tract and from the bowel. The presence of a fistula may be assumed, also, when actually no fistula exists. As a case in point, the loss of the perineal body by previous delivery or surgery may allow fecal contamination of the vagina although no actual incontinence exists, simply the derangement of the rectal and vaginal relationship and faulty hygiene. An error can be made though in not making a complete search for a possible vaginal fistula which may coexist with the old third degree laceration.

The vaginal mucosa and the rectal mucosa must be minutely inspected by probing, transillumination, and adequate visualization by vaginal speculum and by rectosigmoidoscopy. There may be more than one fistulous opening on either the vaginal or rectal mucosa, particularly in those cases where previous surgery or abscess formation has occurred. The fistula tract may burrow and branch out in the rectovaginal septum giving an indurated maze of tracts and sinuses (Fig. 5.20). This may be particularly troublesome if these defects are in the lower vagina and burrow through the fibers of the sphincter. Extra care during dissection must be used to limit the destruction of this muscle tissue. If an error is made in overlooking any of these pockets and thus failing to excise all of the passages, the operation will likely fail. A valuable safeguard is injection of the fistulous openings with methylene blue from either side of the rectovaginal septum, then carefully dissecting out the various ramifications. In the great majority of instances, the tract will be found to be singular and direct. Instillation of a contrast solution such as methylene blue per rectum and above the anal sphincter may aid in the diagnosis of the presence of a small rectovaginal fistula. After care has been used not to spill any methylene blue into the vagina or on the perineum, a slightly moist tampon is placed to fill the vagina. The patient is instructed to walk or move about for a few minutes and the tampon withdrawn and inspected. Any blue color indicates not only the presence of the rectovaginal fistula but may also reveal its level.

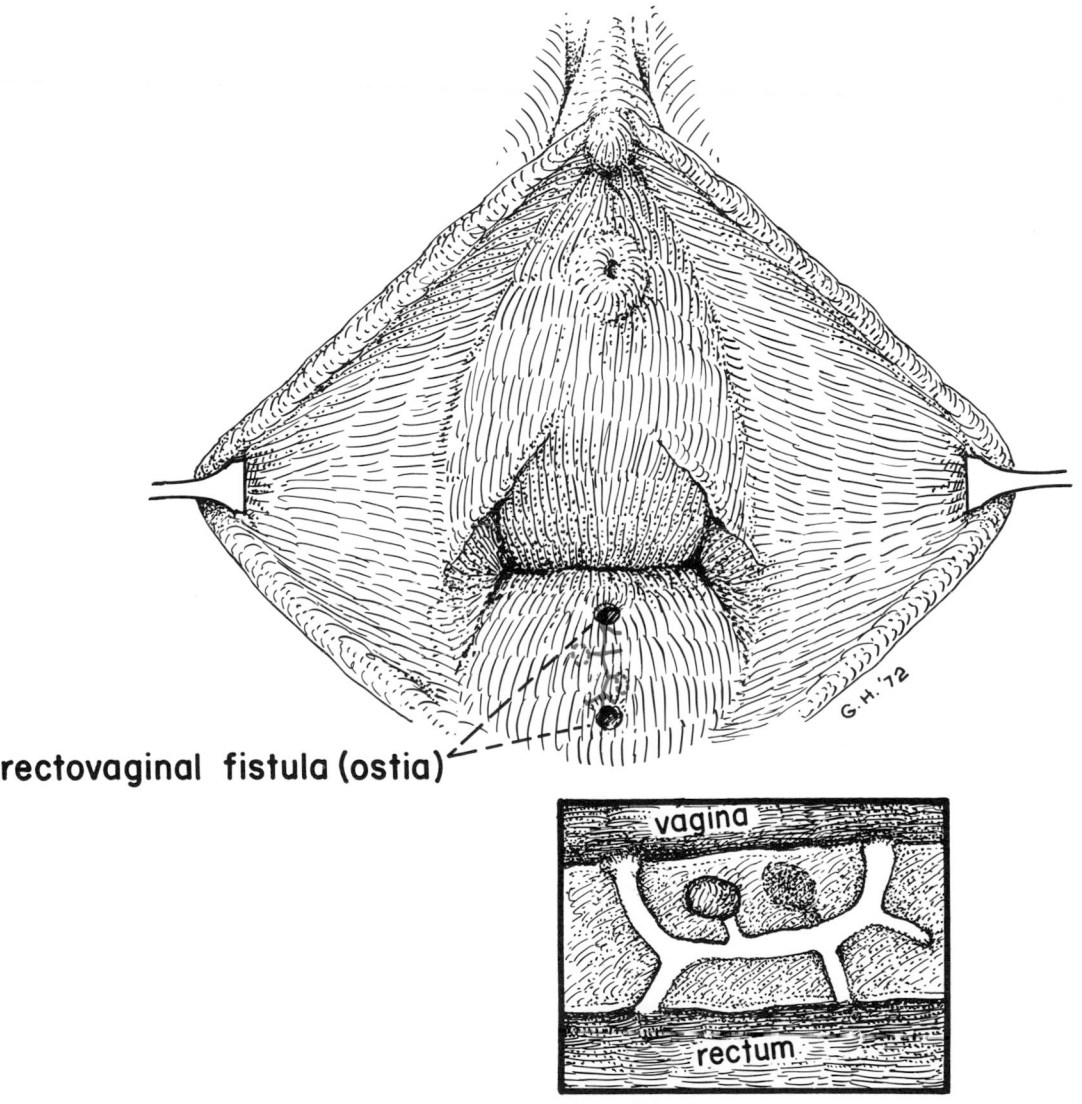

rectovaginal fistula (ostia)

Fig. 5.20. The complex rectovaginal fistula showing intraseptal ramifications of fistulous tract. What may be thought, at first, to be simply a double rectovaginal fistula can, in fact, have an indurated maze of pockets and tracts filled with pus and feces. This complex system must be dissected out, completely destroying the epithelialized passages, or removed *en bloc,* leaving a larger singular fistula to be repaired. A temporary diversionary colostomy must be considered when this condition is encountered.

The indication for the temporary sigmoid colostomy preoperatively or in conjunction with the fistula repair is dependent on the size and location of the fistula, and the amount of scarring or induration present from previous attempts of repair. The small rectovaginal fistula may be safely closed in three layers without undue tissue tension and circulatory embarrassment. To insure postoperative decompression of the bowel, a rectal tube of 1-cm diameter is anchored in place by skin sutures about the anal margin, being positive that there is no impingement on the repair area. The patient is given low residue diet and small rectal irrigations as needed to reduce any chance for distention of the rectal ampulla. Bowel antiseptics are given routinely in all cases of repair of rectovaginal fistula. We use the combination of sulfonamides and antibiotics given concurrently. Sulfasuxidine or Sulfathalidine with neomycin is currently used in the prescribed dosage for 2 or 3 days preoperatively and continued for 5 days postoperatively. This simple practice will very likely obviate the use of the sigmoid colostomy and incision of the anal sphincter.

However, where there has been obvious induration and circulatory impairment from previous surgery or irradiation, making it obvious that healing is jeopardized, temporary diversion of the fecal stream is advisable. This is also true in those cases of large rectovaginal fistula, or extensive involvement of the anal sphincter muscles. Here again, the gynecologist must explain it clearly to the patient that the repair of a vaginal fistula, whether it be of a rectovaginal or urinary type, is not just a "simple procedure," but may entail extraordinary effort such as fecal diversion to gain success. The patient must not be made unnecessarily apprehensive, but must be given a full understanding in layman's language of what the operation demands technically and what care preoperatively and postoperatively will be needed.

With proper bowel sterilization the temporary sigmoid colostomy is performed 10 to 14 days preoperatively to the anticipated repair of the rectovaginal fistula. Two days after the sigmoid loop is exteriorized it is completely transected with a cautery making sure that neither limb withdraws beneath the anchoring sutures. The distal loop is cleansed daily from

above and below to eliminate as well as possible any persisting harmful bacterial flora.

After the rectovaginal fistula has been repaired, the patient will be most anxious for the colostomy to be closed. However, 5 or 6 weeks must be allowed to elapse to guarantee complete healing of the fistula repair before the bowel is closed again. In the event of failure of this attempt at the fistula repair, the colostomy must remain open until a successful repair can be accomplished at a later date, allowing approximately 3 months to elapse between the rectovaginal operations.

Repair of Rectovaginal Fistula

The repair of any rectovaginal fistula whether large or small demands strict observance of the established surgical practices. The posterior vaginal wall is adequately exposed and the fistula injected with a small amount of methylene blue. A small amount of dilute Neo-Synephrine solution 1:1000 is injected into the tissues about the fistula. This is a helpful aid in dissection of the tissue layers and control of ooze bleeding which can obscure delicate dissection. This does not impair the circulation of the tissue permanently. The fistula margin is circumcised at least 5 mm from the opening and the vaginal mucosa mobilized from the underlying scar tissue and bowel wall (Fig. 5.21). The rectal ostium must be identified and the edges freshened using great care not to unnecessarily enlarge the opening. The rectal wall including the mucosa and muscularis are mobilized as well as possible to facilitate closure of the ostium without tension. Interrupted mattress sutures or a continuous locking suture is taken with 3-0 chromic catgut on a round atraumatic needle. An error of piercing into the bowel lumen must be avoided. The second layer of 3-0 catgut sutures is taken interruptedly in the muscularis in any axis of closure that gives least tension. The third layer, the vaginal mucosa, is closed with interrupted mattress suture of monofilament nylon #1 or silver wire (Fig. 5.21). These sutures of the vaginal layer are left in place for 21 days.

The closure of a smaller and uncomplicated rectovaginal fistula may be varied from the above described standard closure. After the fistula opening has been circumcised and the vaginal mucosa mobilized by undercutting, the

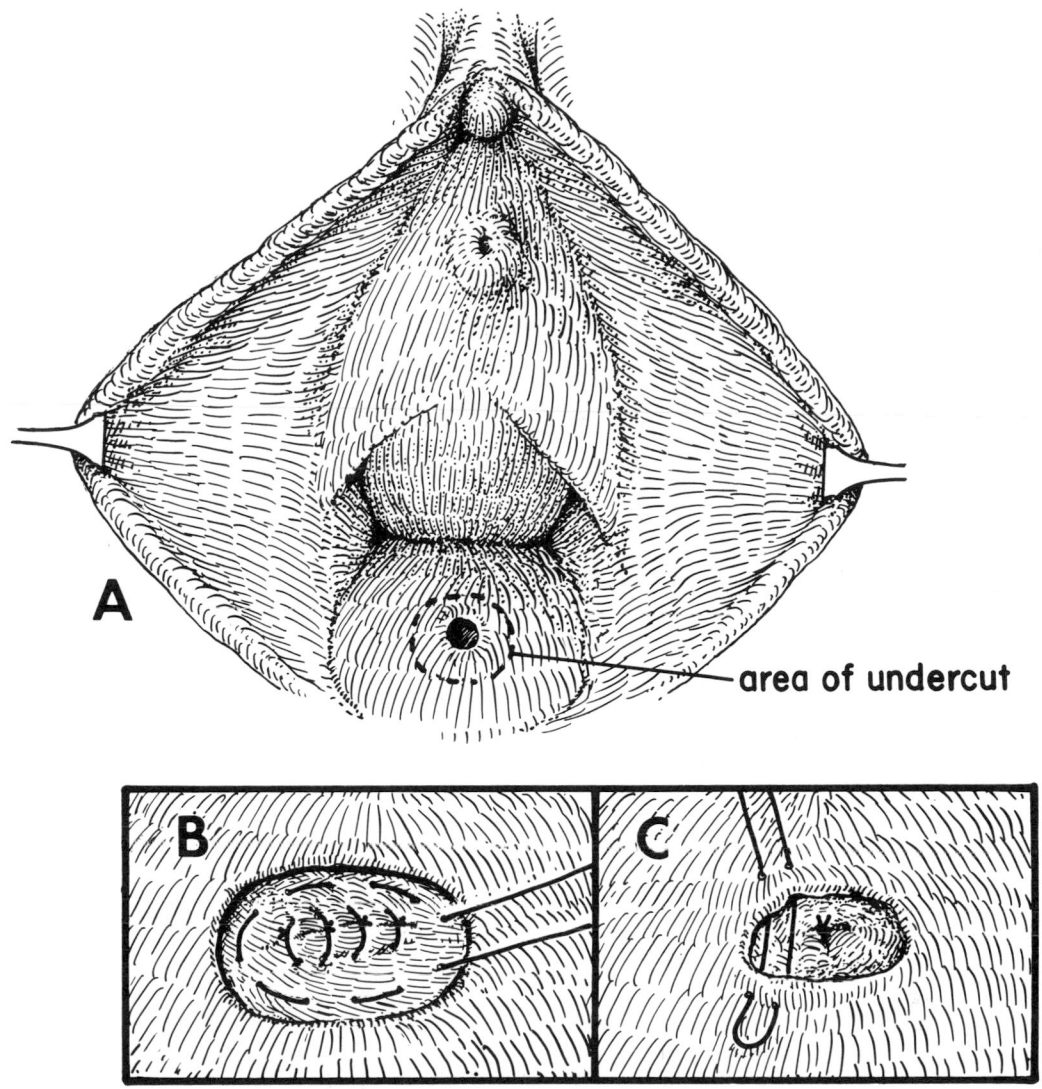

area of undercut

Fig. 5.21. The basic steps of closure of a small simple rectovaginal fistula. The area of undercut (A) about the fistula mobilizes the vaginal wall from the rectal wall. The amount of vaginal mucosa to be sufficiently trimmed away is arbitrary depending on the condition of this membrane. (B) The first line of sutures inverting the rectal mucosa has been taken, and a second layer in the submucosa and muscularis has been started as a pursestring closure in this case. (C) The final layer of closure of the vaginal mucosa by interrupted mattress sutures of monofilament nylon.

rectal ostium of the fistula may be closed by a pursestring suture of 3-0 chromic inverting the edges of the fistula into the rectal lumen (Fig. 5.21). The second or intermediate layer can be another pursestring suture using the same type 3-0 catgut on an atraumatic needle. The closure of the vaginal mucosa is best closed with the mattress suture of nonabsorbable material as described above.

A more serious problem of closure of the rectovaginal fistula arises if the rectovaginal septum is indurated and tunnelled by ramifications of the fistulous tract. Sigmoid colostomy is then indicated. An extra effort is needed at searching for additional ostia on either the rectal or vaginal aspect of the septum. The entire affected area must be resected *en bloc* to insure reapproximation of normal tissues for closure. Proper use of methylene blue and gentle probing can identify any diverging tracts and sinus cavities. The rectal opening of the fistula may have been necessarily or accidentally enlarged in this removal of the affected rectovaginal septum and must be closed as described previously with interrupted mattress sutures or continuous locking stitch in a line of least tension. The muscularis, if identifiable, is closed as the intermediate layer and the rather large defect of the vaginal mucosa closed with nonabsorbable nylon or silver wire suture. This might narrow the caliber of the vagina, and tension-relaxing incisions may be utilized. In any event, if the vaginal caliber has been narrowed enough to cause dyspareunia later, subsequent vaginal dilatations or vaginoplasty may be needed. This is not thought to be a prohibitive price to pay for the proper closure of a vaginal fistula.

The Latzko Operation for Closure of the Vault Rectovaginal Fistula

At times the bowel fistula may be high in the vagina and at the seam of the vault where previous hysterectomy or treatment of cancer has been performed. This may not be rectal involvement but could possibly be of a loop of sigmoid or ileum. If the vaginal vault is not inaccessible from below due to scarring, the Latzko vaginal operation is more desirable than using the transabdominal approach. In some rare instances it becomes necessary to use the abdominal approach as described, in principle, previously in Figure 5.18 discussing the vesicovaginal fistula.

Technique

For the Latzko procedure the patient is placed in the dorsolithotomy position and the fistula exposed. Traction sutures or clamps placed about the periphery of the fistula brings it into a more workable range. The fistula is circumcised about 1 cm from its edges and the vaginal membrane undercut and reflected outward (see Fig. 5.12). This bowel mucosa is identified and closed by inverting the membrane edges into the lumen of the bowel. A 3-0 chromic catgut on a small atraumatic needle is used. It may be necessary to employ some of the delicate traction instruments and needles

ordinarily used in closure of the vesicovaginal fistula because of the high location of this bowel fistula. A second layer of closure with the 3-0 chromic catgut is desirable if it is possible to mobilize the bowel wall well enough to permit it. The vaginal mucosa about the fistula is now removed for about 1 to 1.5 cm about the periphery of the fistula thus denuding the vaginal vault on the posterior and anterior aspects as needed. Interrupted sutures of 2-0 chromic catgut are taken to obliterate the dead space and further enfold the closed fistula area. The new edges of the vaginal mucosa are now closed with #1 monofilament nylon taken in a mattress fashion, thus creating a partial upper vaginal colpocleisis. Even with this necessary vaginal shortening, a functional vagina will usually be preserved.

Postoperative Care

The postoperative care of the repaired rectovaginal fistula is most important and demanding, but not so capricious as the postoperative care of the repaired vesicovaginal fistula. The lower intestinal tract is not so likely to become so acutely distended as the urinary tract. Adequate rectosigmoid decompression is usually easily accomplished by the proper use of an adequate sized rectal tube carefully held in place without trauma to the repaired area. If a sigmoid colostomy has been established preoperatively, the problem of decompression is completely controlled. In any event the newly approximated fistula margins must be protected from tension. The use of low residue diet, low pressure saline rectal irrigation when needed, and bowel antiseptics for 2 weeks postoperatively are recommended. The patient is kept on mineral oil and milk of magnesia regime to provide gentle laxative effect and lubrication. If this medication is intolerable to the patient, stool softeners given by mouth each night accomplishes practically the same thing. Low pressure, small warm saline enemas are given at any time the patient fails to have a bowel movement at least once per day. Coitus is prohibited for 2 months after the repair has been done. It is generally agreed that if the patient desires more children that cesarean section is indicated, as after any successful repair of a vaginal fistula.

In the event that the attempted repair of the

rectovaginal fistula is unsuccessful, subsequent attempts to repair the fistula will probably be more difficult. There must be at least 3 months elapsed time between the attempts in order that the tissues may return to their optimal condition. If a sigmoid colostomy has been used in the previous repair, it is best to allow this to remain functioning for the subsequent repair. The patient may first object to this thought, but she must be made to understand the importance of this temporary diversion of the bowel stream.

Complete Perineal Lacerations

The complete perineal laceration known also as the third or fourth degree tear is practically entirely caused by obstetrical injury. In rare instances the loss of the perineal body and sphincter control may be caused by trauma as falling astride a sharp object, or by slough from a perirectal abscess, or granulomatous lesion. As the baby's head is forced through the vaginal introitus, the complete tear may result from (a) uncontrolled precipitous labor, (b) unyielding scarred tissues of the perineal body, (c) inaccurate or erroneous use of forceps, (d) extension of the medial episiotomy, or (e) occasional extension of the mediolateral episiotomy. The incidence of this complete perineal laceration is less in those clinics where carefully controlled final expulsion of the head is accomplished by outlet forceps and liberal use of the episiotomy. However, in remote areas where less skillful deliveries are done by midwives or unskilled attendants, the use of the episiotomy and forceps is not used as a rule and the more extensive lacerations are common.

Immediate recognition and repair of the complete tear is paramount, because the chance of healing per primum is 97 per cent. This is done carefully in layer-for-layer manner a particular effort to reapproximate the torn levator ani muscles. Postpartum care must include a careful regime of stool control to avoid distention of the bowel and trauma. This is discussed further under postoperative control of the delayed repair of the complete perineal laceration.

The diagnosis of the complete perineal laceration is usually easy and made by the patient herself. There is a variable amount of loss of control of feces and gas. It may be so complete that the patient is made miserable by the leakage which can be as copious and constant as a large fistula. On the other hand, the patient may really complain of the leakage only with gas or loose stools when she has either taken too much of a laxative or developed diarrhea of other causes. Even though the true spincter ani muscles may be completely interrupted, the patient may have learned or at least been able to contain most bowel contents by constant, voluntary contraction of the weakened levators ani. In some instances, strangely enough, the patient may choose to forego an operation for correction of this tear, if she is tolerably comfortable and abhors surgery.

Continence is re-established by two basic techniques, each having its own indications. The most popular in our experience has been the "Warren flap" technique. The other has been the layer-for-layer technique used less frequently, but with good results when chosen in particular cases.

In 1882, Warren (25) described a new operation of turning outward from the posterior vaginal wall an apron flap which became the anterior margin of the divided rectal lumen and allowed reapproximation above the torn levator ani muscles. Then over the inferior portion of this mucosal flap as if it has been turned outward, the divided ends of the torn sphincter fibers are reapproximated. Several errors may be made, however, in this relatively simple procedure. Great care must be exercised to safeguard against the possible error of buttonholing the anterior rectal wall. On the other hand, the mucosal flap must not have been mobilized by cutting so thinly that the blood supply is endangered. It will be found that there is usually a plane to be developed between the vaginal and rectal mucosa. As the flap is completely turned downward as far as needed, care again is particularly taken to prevent perforation of this membrane in the region where the sphincter fibers are to be reapproximated.

The most useful landmark in delineating the mucosal flap and planning the procedure is the detection of the dimples that will most frequently be found indicating the contracted ends of the torn sphincter on either side. As the limbs of the inverted U-shaped incision are brought inferiorly, they are extended just lateral to and a few millimeters beyond these dimples of the sphincter muscle ends (Fig. 5.22). The flap is turned all the way outward (Fig.5.23) and the ends of the sphincter are probed with an Allis clamp. There will usually be some scarring here which will facilitate grasping these torn ends. The two ends are now brought to the midline completing again the circle of the sphincter and passing over the downward flap. These ends are now united with three interrupted sutures of 3-0 silk.

The levator muscles are reapproximated in the midline with interrupted sutures of #1 chromic catgut within the area denuded by the downturning of the mucosal flap. This rebuilds the perineal body. The rectovaginal fascia is reapproximated in the midline with the same caliber catgut, and the new edges of the vaginal mucosa are brought together with interrupted sutures of chromic 0 catgut to complete the operation (Fig. 5.24).

It will be noted that some of the flap will be

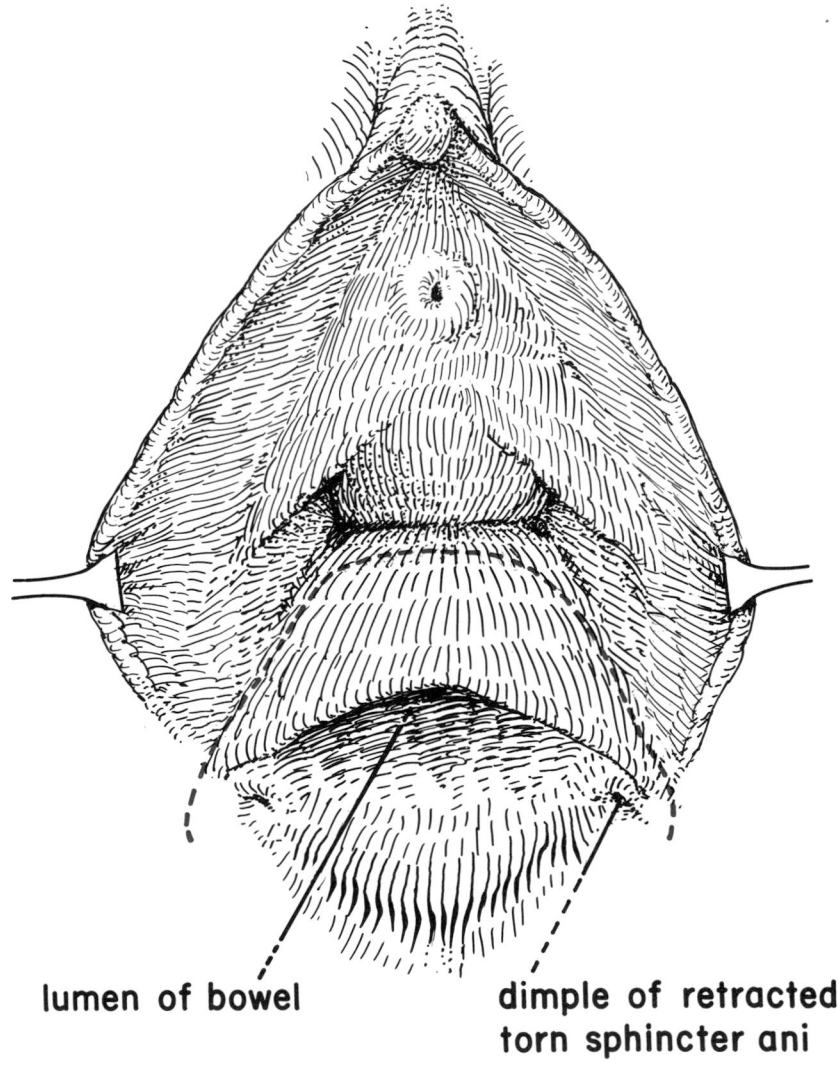

lumen of bowel   **dimple of retracted torn sphincter ani**

Fig. 5.22. Basic steps of the Warren flap procedure for the repair of complete perineal laceration. The perineal body is missing and the defect of the anterior rectal wall is no more than 2 cm. Particular notice is taken of the dimples laterally showing retracted ends of the torn sphincter ani. The inverted U-shaped incision (red) extends from at least 3 cm above the rectovaginal margin lateralward and downward just beyond and lateral to the important landmarks of the torn ends of the sphincter fibers.

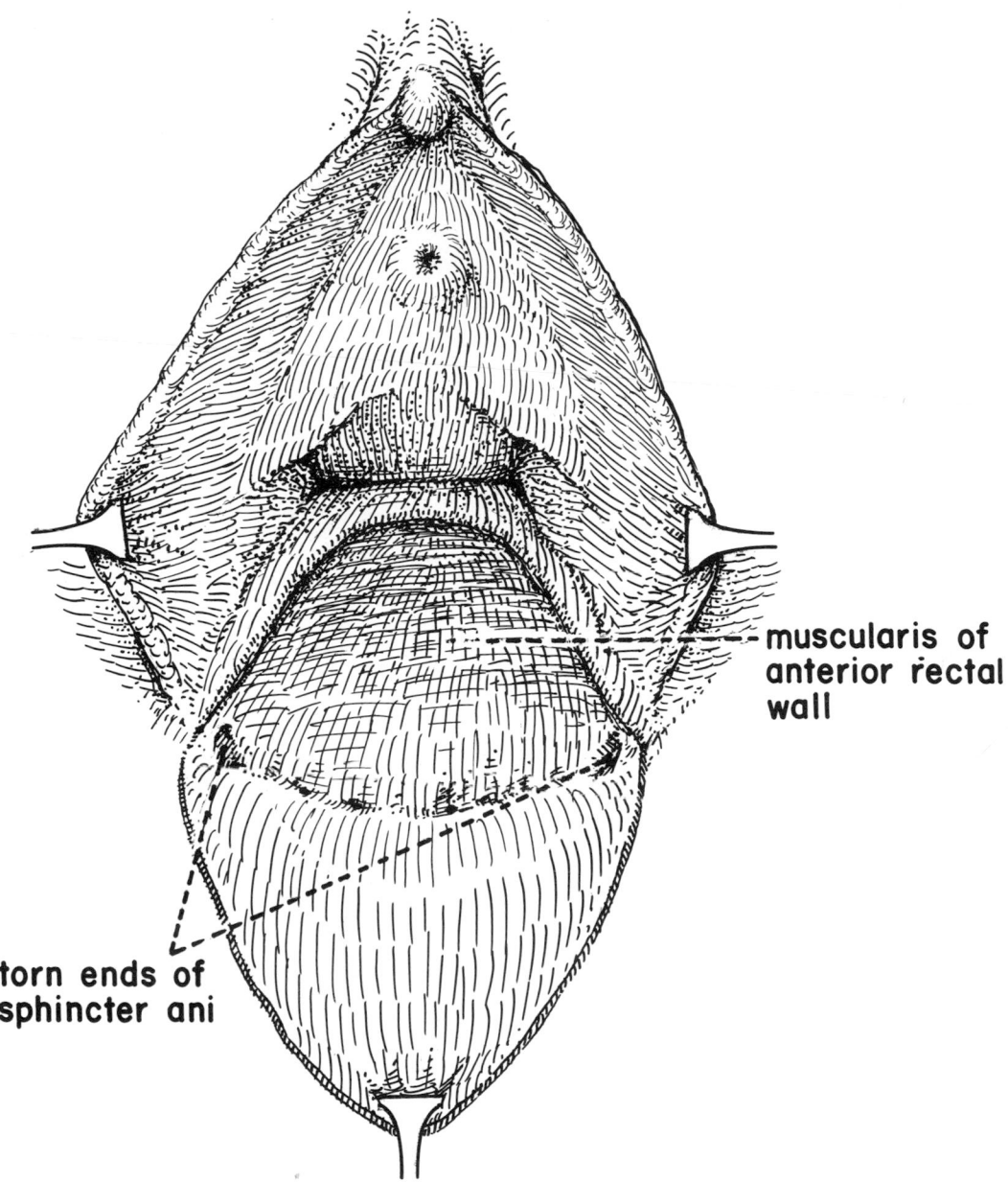

muscularis of anterior rectal wall

torn ends of sphincter ani

Fig. 5.23. The full thickness of the vaginal mucosal flap has been turned downward being particularly careful not to buttonhole this membrane nor the rectal wall. The area of the torn ends of the sphincter ani fibers is now exposed. These ends, although in scar tissue, may be probed for and grasped with an Allis clamp.

protruding from the anal opening. This is expected and most likely will undergo some partial necrosis and shrinkage in the following 10 days. Any redundancy can be trimmed away at a later date after healing is complete and if it is troublesome. At the end of the operation the sphincter is cut at right angles at 5 o'clock in

what is called Miller's "paradoxical incision." This relieves tension on the newly joined ends of the sphincter and thus aids in healing. We have had no instances of the paradoxical incision failing to heal within 10 days postoperatively. Statistically the use of this has been shown to increase the chance for complete

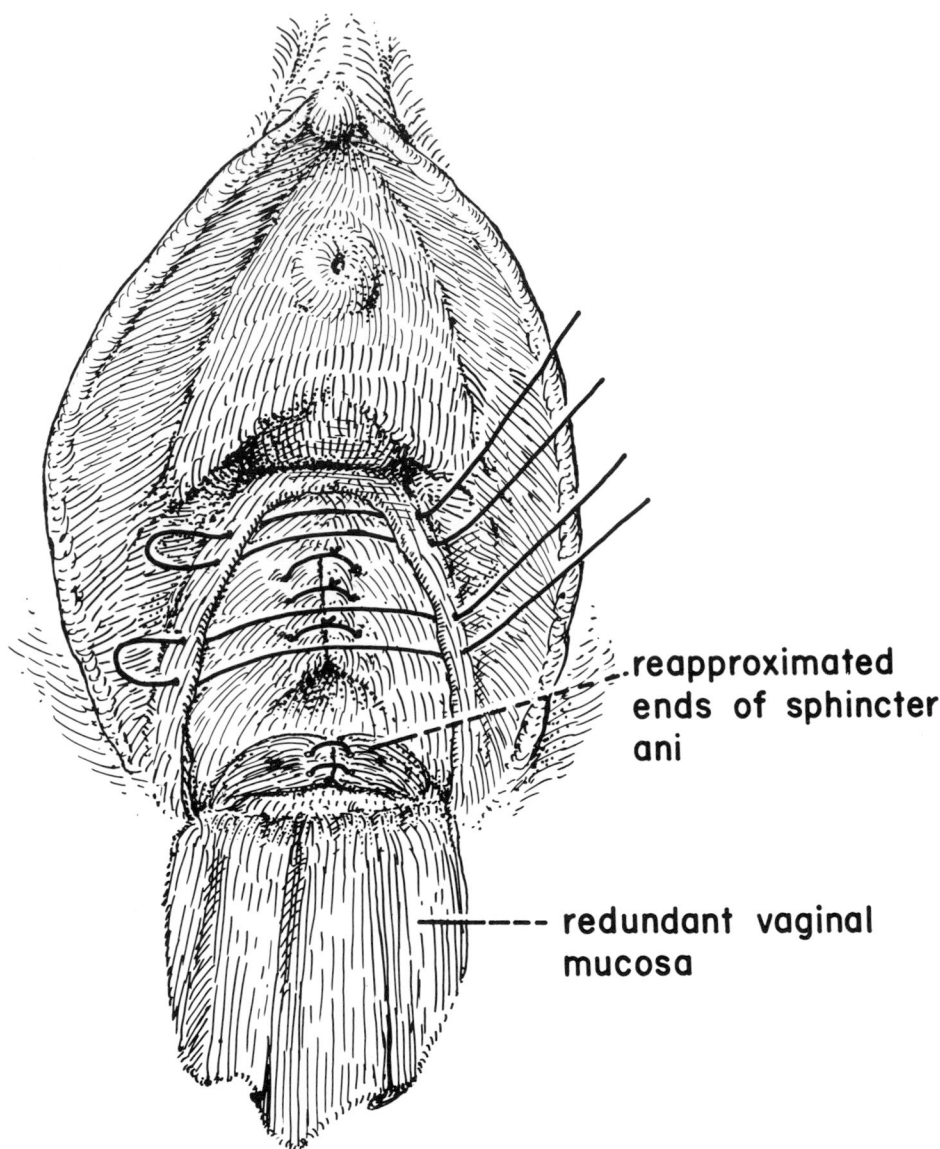

reapproximated ends of sphincter ani

redundant vaginal mucosa

Fig. 5.24. The vaginal mucosal flap has now been turned downward and outward to the junction of the rectal and vaginal membranes. The deep first layer of closure with chromic 1 catgut plicates the rectal wall to obliterate a rectocele, and reapproximates the torn and separated bellies of the levatores ani muscles, thus rebuilding the perineal body. Next and most importantly, the retrieved ends of the torn sphincter are reapproximated in the midline with interrupted sutures of 2-0 silk taken in mattress fashion. Finally, the vaginal mucosa is reapproximated with mattress sutures of #1 chromic catgut or monofilament nylon, depending on the operator's choice here. The redundant vaginal mucosa is allowed to remain and the excess can be trimmed away painlessly about 7 to 10 days later. A paradoxical incision through the sphincter ani at 5 o'clock is utilized by many operators (see text).

Technique of the Layer-by-Layer Operation

Although the Warren flap technique has established itself in our hands as the most popular and dependable procedure for the closure of the complete perineal tear, the layer method of repair is a valuable alternative. It is actually the procedure of choice, as has been mentioned in discussion of the immediate closure of the complete perineal laceration detected at the time of delivery. The other principal indication for its use is in those cases in which there has been extraordinary loss or wider separation of the anterior wall of the rectum. In this situation any attempt to turn down a long mucosal flap would jeopardize the blood supply of the flap, leading to possible necrosis and failure or formation of a recto-vaginal fistula.

The same bowel preparation regime is followed using the antiseptic of the operator's

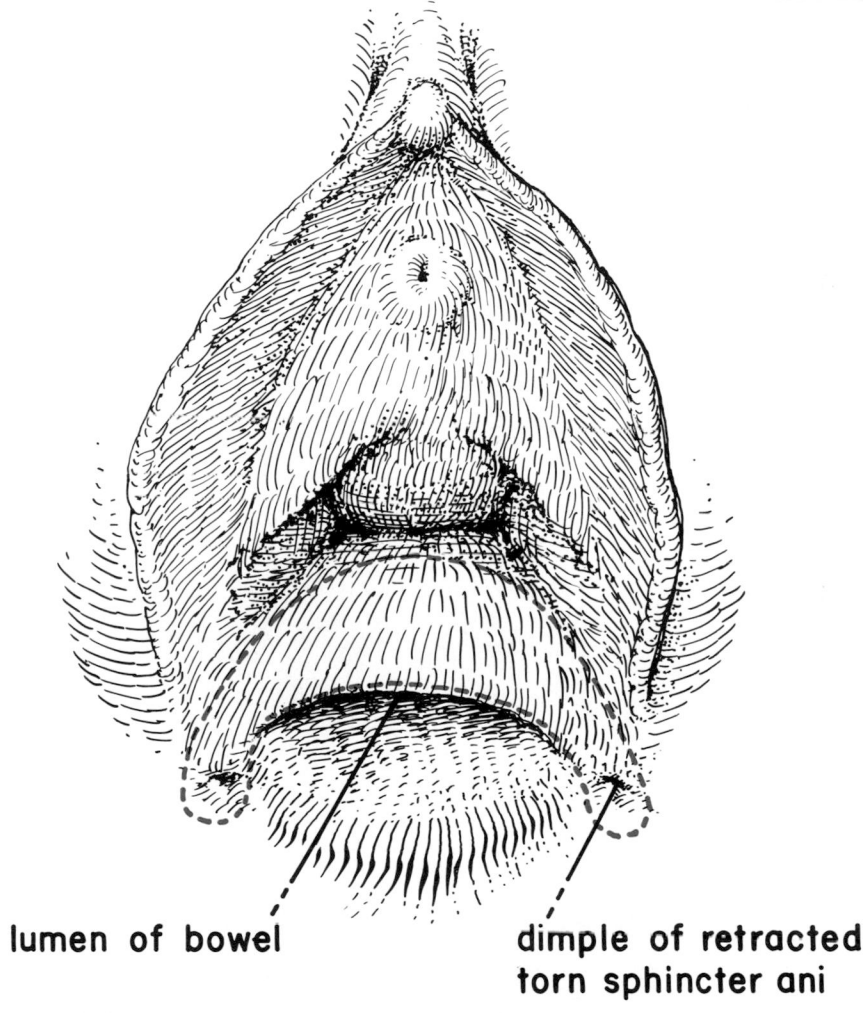

lumen of bowel   **dimple of retracted torn sphincter ani**

Fig. 5.25. The layer-by-layer technique of repair of the old complete perineal laceration. The proper incision (red) removes redundant vaginal mucosa, exposing the torn ends of the anal sphincter. The distal portion of the incision is accurately made at the margin of junction of the vaginal and rectal mucosas. Caution is used to prevent buttonholing the rectal wall.

current choice as would be used for repair by the flap technique or for the repair of the rectovaginal fistula.

The entire posterior wall of the vagina is exposed as well as possible. An incision is made just through the thickness of the vaginal mucosa about 2 to 3 mm from the margin of the rectovaginal defect, and the two structures are mobilized, being particularly cautious not to cut a bottonhole in the rectal mucosa, which might lead later to a rectovaginal fistula (Fig. 5.25). The rectal mucosa is now closed with a double layer of interrupted chromic 0 catgut inverting the edges into the bowel lumen tied snugly but without strangulating the tissues. This closure of rectal mucosa is carried down just beyond the part where the divided ends of the torn sphincter ani muscles can be reapproximated in the midline (Fig. 5.26).

As the vaginal membrane is dissected lateralward, particular attention is focused on exposure of the divided bellies of the levator ani muscles in the lower third of the defect being repaired. Two or three firm interrupted sutures of chromic 1 catgut are taken into these levator ani fibers which are brought together in the midline to reconstitute the perineal body (Fig. 5.27).

The torn ends of the sphincter ani muscles are probed for, grasped with an Allis clamp, and joined in the midline to complete the circle of the anal sphincter. Care is used here to be sure that the new junction is closed with three sutures of 3-0 silk and this area buried beneath the mucosa of the vagina as the repair is completed.

At the upper end of the repair above the newly joined levator muscles, the rectovaginal

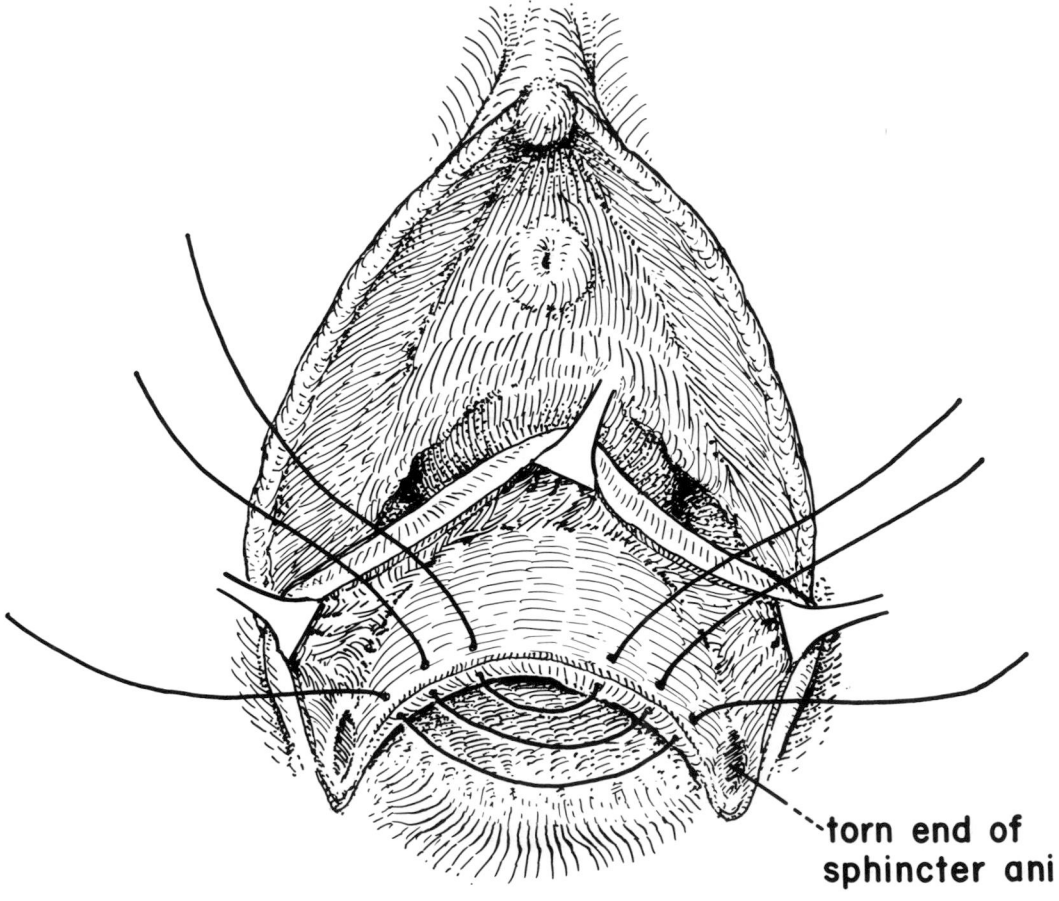

**torn end of
sphincter ani**

Fig. 5.26. The first layer of closure is the rectal wall. Sutures of 0 chromic catgut on an atraumatic round needle are passed through the bowel muscularis and submucosa but invert the edges into the bowel lumen.

fascia, if discernible, is reapproximated in the midline. A redundant vaginal mucosa is trimmed away and its new edges are reapproximated in the midline without tension with interrupted mattress sutures of chromic 0 catgut to complete the operation (Fig. 5.28). The sphincter fibers are now cut radially, at right angles to their course at 5 o'clock as a paradoxical incision.

A third type of procedure which was first described by Noble (27) in 1902 was rediscovered by Mengert (28) in 1952, who did not know of the original publication which had become buried and forgotten in old publications. This operation consisted of mobilization of the rectum sufficiently above the margin of the defect and sliding the structure inferiorly to re-establish a continuous rectal wall anteriorly. The vagina was then repaired with reapproximation of the sphincter fibers, the levator ani muscles, and the vaginal mucosa.

Postoperative Care of the Repair of the Complete Perineal Laceration

It is of paramount importance to avoid any trauma to or distention of the newly approximated tissues whether the flap or layer techniques have been used. The paradoxical incision of the sphincter ani muscle is well used but not always employed, if the operator is satisfied that there is not excessive tension on the newly joined fibers anteriorly. However, we have had no sequellae or lasting incontinence from its use. A small rectal tube fixed in place by interrupted silk suture to perianal skin is a good guarantee that distention of the rectum will not occur by gas and feces. The bowel antisepsis is continued for 10 days during which time a low residue diet is continued along with mild laxatives and lubricants such as milk of magnesia and mineral oil as needed. The patient is kept in bed for 10 to 14 days during which

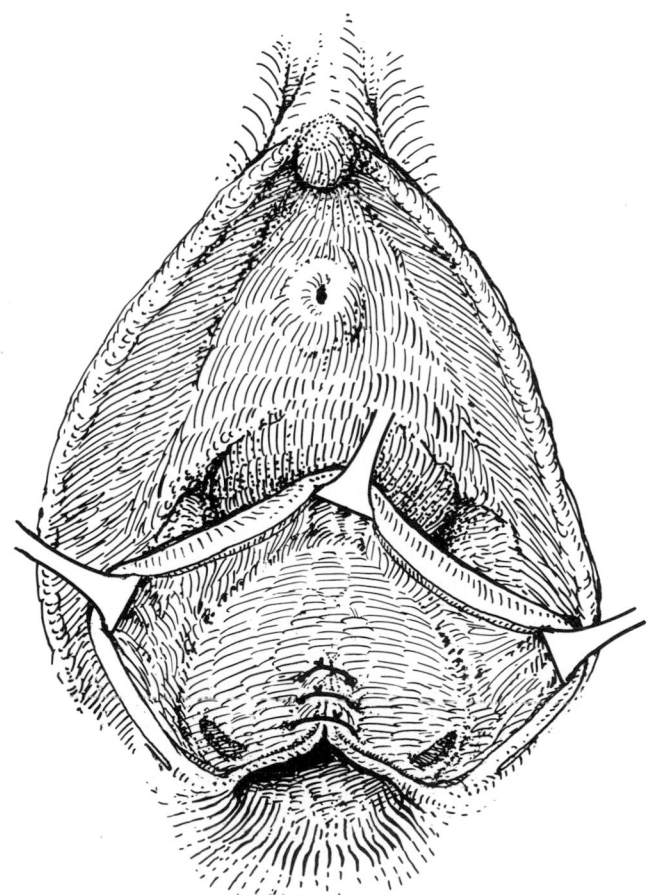

Fig. 5.27. As this first layer is closed, the torn edges of the sphincter ani muscle are identified and grasped with an Allis clamp preparatory to reapproximation in the midline.

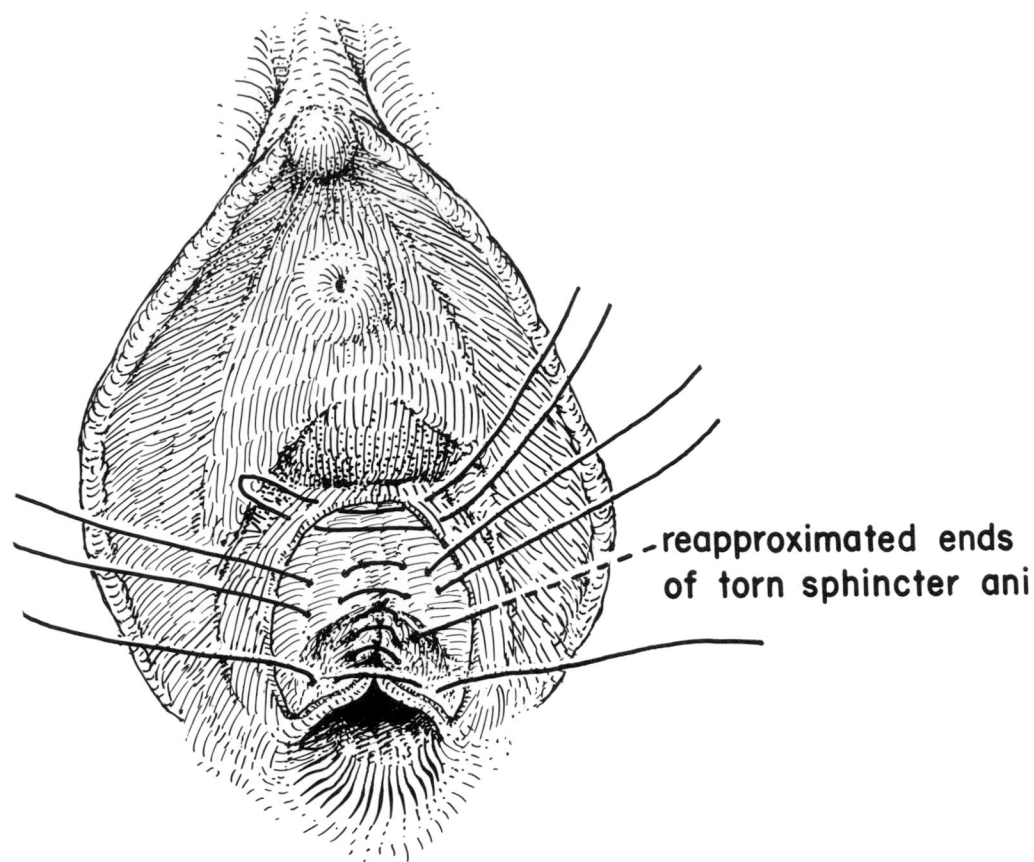

reapproximated ends
of torn sphincter ani

Fig. 5.28. Final steps of closure. The torn ends of the sphincter ani fibers are reapproximated in midline using 2-0 silk end-on mattress sutures. Above this, mattress sutures are used to reapproximate the separated bellies of the levator ani muscle, to rebuild the perineal body, and to reapproximate the layers of the rectum down to the new anal opening. Final layer of closure is by interrupted mattress sutures of #1 chromic catgut and a subcuticular stitch to close the anal skin anteriorly. The sphincter is now cut, paradoxically, at right angles at 5 o'clock.

time she may be allowed to turn from side to side, but not sit upright. A perineal heat lamp gives comfort and promotes healing. Sitz baths can be used after the 14th day. The patient is cautioned against coitus for 2 months postoperatively.

In the event of failure of these procedures either by complete reopening of the defect or the formation of a rectovaginal fistula through a partially healed suture line, the operator must wait at least 3 months before another attempt of salvage can be undertaken.

Recapitulation of Common Errors

1. Failure to give the patient an understanding of the problem, its cause, the magnitude of the attempt to repair, and the chances of success or failure.

2. Overlooking a concomitant fistula whether it be of bladder or bowel origin.

3. Improper preoperative preparation and investigation of patient to rule out malignancy or chronic infection.

4. Improper selection of the special instruments and suture materials.

5. Inadequate mobilization of the vaginal and bladder (or bowel) mucosa.

6. Failure to close antivaginal ostium by inversion of mucosa into lumen of bladder (or bowel).

7. Strangulation of tissue by sutures or tension.

8. Careless removal of nonabsorbable sutures.

9. Inadequate drainage of urinary or bowel tract.

10. Failure to anticipate or detect early postoperative infection.

11. Failure to properly emphasize to the patient the importance of her postoperative convalescence, *i.e.*, coital abstinence and avoidance of any vaginal trauma.

These more common errors are generalizations, but are enumerated to alert the operator to anticipate the possibility of occurrence so that proper safeguards may constantly be incorporated in the procedure.

References

1. Sims, J. M: On the treatment of vesicovaginal fistula. Am. J. Med. Sci. 23: 59, 1852.
2. Te Linde, R. W.: Textbook of Operative Gynecology, 4th ed., Chap. 28, p. 588. J. B. Lippincott, Philadelphia, 1970.
3. Gossett, T.: Fistula repair (Letter to Editor). Lancet, 1834.
4. Shaw, W.: Textbook of Operative Gynecology, 3rd ed. edited by J. Hawkins. E. & S. Livingstone, Edinburgh, 1968.
5. Ridley, J. H.: Indirect air cystoscopy. South. Med. J. 44: 114, 1951.
6. Moir, J. C.: The Vesicovaginal Fistula, 2nd ed., p. 55, Bailliere, Tindall, and Cassell, London, 1967.
7. Counseller, V. S.: Surgical and postoperative treatment of large vesicovaginal and rectovaginal fistula. Surg. Gynecol. Obstet. 74: 738, 1942.
8. Collins, C. G., Rent, D., and Jones, F. B.: Results of early repair of vesicovaginal fistula with preliminary cortisone treatment. Am. J. Obstet. Gynecol. 80: 1005, 1960.
9. Pearl, C. L., and Keizure, L. W.: Optimum time interval from occurrence to repair of vesicovaginal fistula. Am. J. Obstet. Gynecol. 104: 205, 1969.
10. Russell, C. S.: Vesicovaginal Fistulas and Related Matters. Charles C Thomas, Publisher, Springfield, Ill., 1962.
11. Clarke, B. G., and Joress, S.: Quantitative bacteriuria after indwelling catheter. JAMA 174: 1593, 1960.
12. Novak, F.: The prevention of ureterovaginal fistulas after Wertheim operation. Int. J. Gynaecol. Obstet. 7: 301, 1969.
13. Boronow, R. C., and Rutledge, F. N.: Vesicovaginal fistula, radiation and gynecologic cancer. Am. J. Obstet. Gynecol. 111: 85, 1971.
14. Martius, H.: Zur Auswahl der Harnsfestel- und Inkontinenz-Operationen. Zentralbl. Gynaekol. 66: 1250, 1942.
15. Betson, J. R.: Bulbocavernosus fat pad transplant. Obstet. Gynecol. 26: 135, 1965.
16. Latzko, W.: Postoperative vesicovaginal fistula, genesis and therapy. Am. J. Surg. 58: 211, 1942.
17. Falk, H. C., and Tancer M. L.: Urethrovesicovaginal fistula. Obstet. Gynecol. 33: 422, 1969.
18. Everett, H. S.: A condemnation of resectoscopic procedures upon the female vesical neck. Urol. Cutan. Review 52: 121, 1948.
19. Hamlin, R. H. J., and Nicholson, E. C.: Reconstruction of urethra totally destroyed in labour. Br. Med. J. 2: 147, 1969.
20. Symmonds, R. E.: The loss of the urethral floor with total urinary incontinence. Am. J. Obstet. Gynecol. 103: 665, 1969.
21. Roulston, J. M.: Repair of bladder neck fistula and reconstruction of urethra. Am. J. Obstet. Gynecol. 83: 453, 1962.
22. Ridley, J. H.: Appraisal of the Goebell-Frangenheim-Stoeckel sling procedure. Am. J. Obstet. Gynecol. 95: 714-721, July 1966.
23. Lee, R. A., and Symmonds, R. E.: Ureterovaginal fistula. Am. J. Obstet. Gynecol. 109: 1032, 1971.
24. Counseller, V. S.: Some urologic phases of vesicovaginal fistula. J. Urol. 47: 711, 1942.
25. Warren, J. C.: A new method of operation for the relief of rupture of the perineum through the sphincter of the rectum. Trans. Am. Gynecol. Soc. 7: 322, 1882.
26. Miller, N. F., and Brown, W.: The surgical treatment of complete perineal tears in the female. Am. J. Obstet. Gynecol. 34: 196, 1937.
27. Noble, G. H.: A new operation for complete laceration of the perineum designed for the infection from the rectum. Trans. Am. Gynecol. Soc. V. 27: 357, 1902.
28. Mengert, W. F.: Personal communication, 1972.

CHAPTER SIX

HOWARD W. JONES, JR., M.D., AND MASON C. ANDREWS, M.D.

SURGERY FOR CONGENITAL ANOMALIES OF THE UTERUS AND VAGINA AND FOR INFERTILITY

Congenital Absence of the Vagina and Uterus

Patients with congenital absence of the vagina most often lack the uterus as well. However, by common usage, the term *congenital absence of the vagina* is often used to describe the condition. Except for the genital defect, on physical examination most such patients appear to be entirely normal. However, on examination by intravenous pyelogram, approximately 10 per cent have anomalies of the urinary tract. These are usually not disabling, but may consist of such disorders as congenital absence of one kidney, pelvic kidney, etc. In addition, a much smaller percentage, perhaps 3 to 5 per cent, have anomalies involving the vertebral column, such as extra vertebra or congenital fusion of the vertebra. A rare patient will have serious defects in the bones of the extremities. Cytogenetically, such patients have a normal 46,XX chromosome complement. The differential diagnosis lies between this condition and male hermaphroditism with feminization (testicular feminization syndrome), and this differential may be easily made by an examination of a buccal smear. Failure to perform this necessary examination might result in a missed diagnosis resulting in the undesirable retention of testes which later in life could become malignant. A laparotomy for diagnostic purposes or visualization of the pelvic organs by laparoscopy or radiography is unnecessary. Such diagnostic meddling invites complications, may make an unnecessary scar, and is expensive. Ample studies have shown that the Fallopian tubes are usually normally developed. The ovaries themselves are normal in appearance and function. The uterus is represented by undeveloped muscular tissue resembling a very rudimentary bicornuate uterus. These nubbins are usually palpable on rectal examination (Fig. 6.1).

While suggested treatment has varied from the so-called Frank technique involving the prolonged use of dilators to make a vagina to the use of small and large intestine and other materials to line the surgically created vaginal space, our experience through the last 20 years with the use of a split thickness graft to line the neovaginal cavity has been so satisfactory that this operative procedure can be highly recommended.

Creation of an Artificial Vagina with a Split Thickness Graft (McIndoe)

The selection of the proper age to perform this operation is a very important consideration. There is a certain amount of discomfort associated with the postoperative care revolving around the self-manipulation of the vaginal form for a period of a few weeks after the operation. If the procedure is performed before the patient is sufficiently motivated to wish to have a vagina, the form is apt to be left out for prolonged periods of time with unfortunate results. In the only two unsatisfactory results that we have had with this operation over a period of years, the operation was carried out before the patients were 16 years of age. Even in this era of sexual revolution, it is our observation that young teenagers are not sufficiently motivated to wish to have a vagina prior to the age of about 17 or even later. Therefore, young patients who are discovered to have this defect may be told that a vagina can be created at any time, but that we believe it to be an advantage not to do it prior to about the age of 17. This fits in well with other practicalities, because often such patients have insurance coverage under a family policy until their 18th birthday, and it is obviously desirable to take advantage of this. Of course, the operation may be done at any later time.

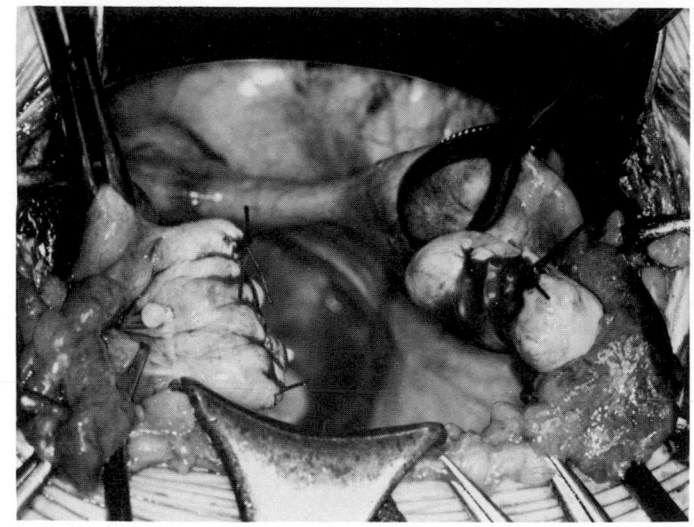

Fig. 6.1. Laparotomy of a patient with congenital absence of the uterus and vagina. There are normal Fallopian tubes bilaterally and deep in the pelvis may be seen the characteristic undeveloped Müllerian structures which do not contain functioning endometrium. These structures may often be palpated on rectal examination. The ovarian incisions are unrelated to the congenital defect.

While the McIndoe procedure is certainly easier to perform in a patient who has not previously been operated upon, it is certainly possible to use the procedure in patients with previously failed operations. In some instances, as in the two patients mentioned in the preceding paragraph, the failure resulted from an inability to maintain the vaginal cavity with the necessary postoperative stent. However, by far the most common indication for secondary operations has resulted from a missed diagnosis, when there has been an unwise exploration of the rectovaginal space by an operation undertaken in a patient who was mistakenly thought to have an imperforate hymen. There is really little excuse for making this error, but in the event that the rectovesical space is inadvertently opened (it usually happens about the age of puberty), there is no hope of maintaining the cavity by a simple cigarette drain, gauze pack, or some similar device. If this mistake is made, it is best to allow the dissected area to heal primarily. A secondary procedure at a later proper time is possible and much more preferred than attempting to create the neovagina in a patient who is 12 or 13 years of age. At the second operation, the scar tissue must be removed, but generally this is not too difficult, and the operation may be aided by a double gloved finger in the rectum. These secondary operations seem to be no less successful than the primary procedures.

To obtain a satisfactory split thickness graft is one of the most important steps of the operation. Such a graft can be cut freehand, with the Brown electric dermatome or with the Reese drum dermatome. We have used all techniques and find the Reese instrument using the adhesive tape on the drum to be most satisfactory. The Brown instrument even when open to its widest gives a strip of graft that is somewhat too narrow to cover conveniently and completely the usual size mold. The Reese dermatome gives a wide enough strip but requires a full drum of tissue for a strip of sufficient length. We have found a thickness of 14/1000 of an inch to be most satisfactory. A thinner graft will tend to fragment, and a thicker graft will sometimes remove so much dermis that healing of the donor site is delayed.

The assembly of the Reese dermatome requires special attention to two particular points which have from time to time given us trouble.

It seems to work best not to remove the covering from the dermatome tape until after the tape has been secured firmly to the drum. If it is removed earlier, the sticky part of the tape is very difficult to handle and fingerprints or other contact with the tape, prior to impressing it on the skin for the purpose of taking the skin graft, will make an area on the tape which will not have enough adhesive quality to function properly. However, the covering can be left on the tape and the tape inserted onto the dermatome with the greatest of ease. The winch used to tighten the tape needs to have very firm tension, but not enough to crack the fiber backing of the tape. Reasonably firm hand tension seems to be adequate. It works well to put the tape onto the drum prior to applying the cement to the patient's donor area and, when the cement is almost dry, to then remove the covering from the tape by incising the covering across the tape on the inside of the drum with a scalpel so that the tape on the external surface of the drum is unmarred. The covering will easily peel off. At this point, tension having been on the tape for a matter of 5 or 10 minutes, additional tightening is very desirable to take up the little stretching which will have occurred in the few moments of waiting.

A second point, which can give great trouble, arises from the loosening of the take-up knobs which hold the blade during the cutting of the graft. It is necessary that these knobs be very firmly secured. It is very difficult to do this by hand tightening, and a suitable instrument to grasp the knobs is very useful. The opened jaws of an Ochsner clamp with the teeth engaging the stria on the knob are very suitable, although probably not the best use of a surgical instrument.

In order to render the donor site invisible, it is convenient to remove the split thickness graft from the buttock. It is useful to determine from the patient ahead of time the upper and lower limits of her bathing trunks to try to stay within bounds. (This gets more difficult each year.) For mechanical reasons while cutting the graft, it seems easier to get it from the right buttock than the left, although either may be used (Fig. 6.2).

With the patient in the Sims' position, the uppermost thigh and knee must be secured on the table firmly by tape or other device. This is essential; otherwise when pressure is exerted with the dermatome, the uppermost knee may slip off the edge of the table making it necessary to start over, *i.e.*, resecure the patient, reclean, redrape, and restart.

The donor site must be carefully shaved. It is important that the skin not be nicked, as wet or semi-dried blood will cause failure of adherence of the dermatome cement and loss of capability to secure a graft in this area. The area is cleaned up only with ether or alcohol and ether, as detergents or antiseptics which leave a film on the skin interfere with adherence of the dermatome cement. The dermatome cement is applied in a thin, even layer over the entire area and allowed to dry for a full 5 minutes before the use of the dermatome. It is important to use cement only from a freshly opened tube. This extravagance is necessitated by the undesirable thick viscosity of the cement acquired in a half used tube. If the cement is too viscid, it cannot be applied evenly and a graft of irregular thickness will result. Such irregular grafts tear easily and are difficult to handle.

In taking the graft, firm pressure by the operator needs to be exerted to get good adherence. In somewhat obese patients this will

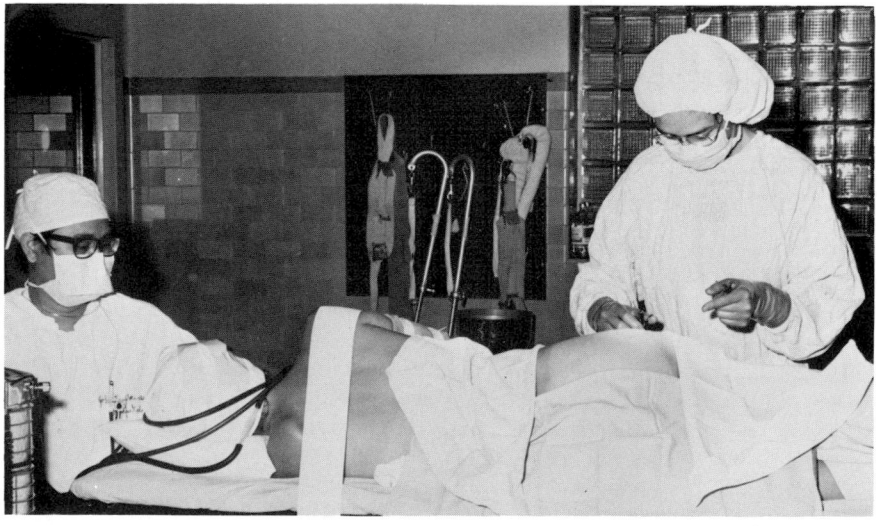

Fig. 6.2. A patient properly positioned on the operating table to obtain a graft from the right buttock.

cause the drum to sink below the surface into the buttock. This might cause gouging of the skin by the blade at the lateral limits of the drum unless an assistant with an instrument such as a tongue depressor holds down the overlapping skin edges. In the event that there is some gouging of the lateral limits of the donor site due to the strokes of the blade, it is very desirable to suture these gouged areas so that they will not curl and form an unsightly spot at the edge of the donor site. It is very important that pressure with a tongue depressor lateral to the excursion of the dermatome blade be just right for if the skin is depressed too vigorously, it will tend to pull the graft off the drum (Fig. 6.3). If the pressure is not sufficient enough, gouging of the skin lateral to the dermatome drum will prove to be a troublesome problem which will require the suturing of the edges to prevent an unsightly area (Fig. 6.4).

When the graft has been successfully cut, the tape may be removed from the dermatome with the graft still adherent. It may then be conveniently removed from the tape by rolling the graft on itself. Great care must be taken during this procedure to prevent tearing the graft. If the graft should be exceedingly thin in some areas due, for example, to the application of dermatome cement too thick or uneven, a

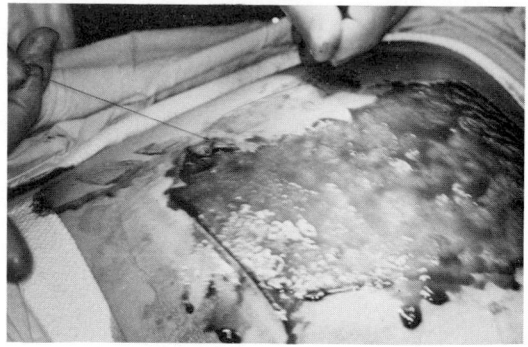

Fig. 6.4. A gouged area lateral to the graft site. Sutures are being applied to prevent curling of the skin.

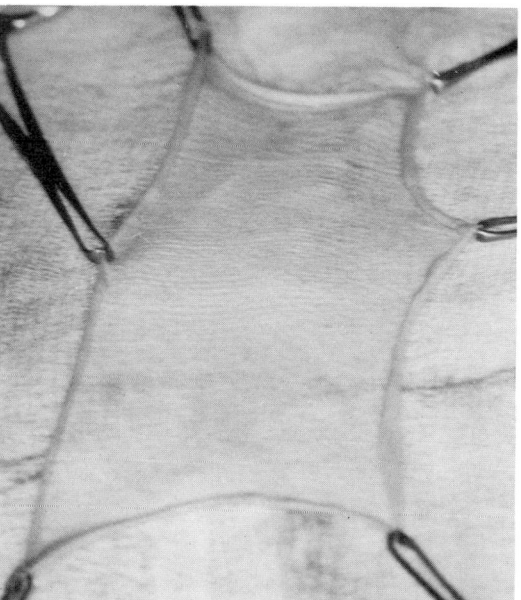

Fig. 6.5. A perfectly removed graft being unrolled and stored in gauze thoroughly moistened with salt solution.

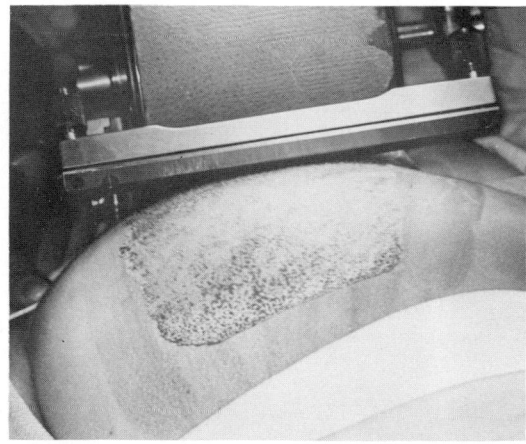

Fig. 6.3. The split thickness graft in the course of removal from the buttock. Note pressure being applied by tongue depressors laterally in an attempt to prevent gouging of the skin outside the path of the drum. Also note a defective area on the drum on the right where excess pressure by the tongue depressor pulled the graft off the drum.

sponge moistened in ether will greatly facilitate the removal of the graft, although this seems an undesirable thing to do for fear of fixing some of the cells of the graft. After the graft has been successfully removed from the dermatome tape, it can be opened out on a sponge which is moist with normal saline (Fig. 6.5). It is important to keep the graft thoroughly moist until it is ready to be applied into the neovaginal cavity.

The remainder of the operation is performed with the patient in the lithotomy position. A transverse incision at the site of the vaginal orifice is desirable, and this should tend to be

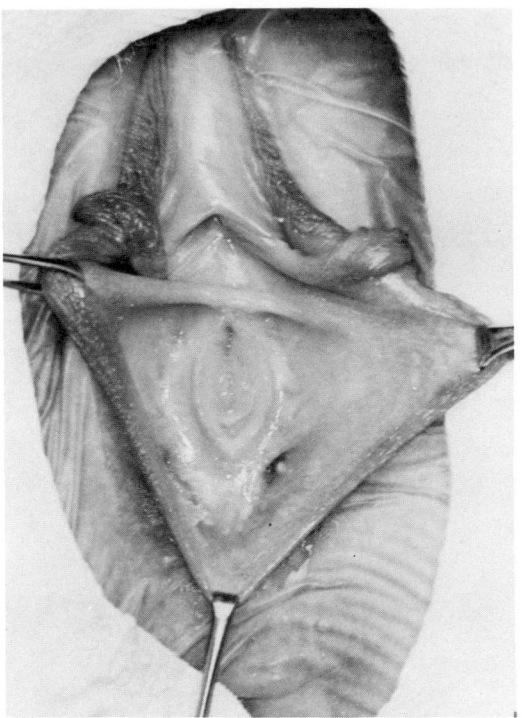

Fig. 6.6. The introitus prior to operation. The urethra seems rather patulous. There is no vaginal orifice.

incision. The most troublesome bleeding vessels are deep in the vagina laterally about two-thirds of the way to the apex. These can be caught with long Kelly clamp and tied with a small catgut free tie. If bleeding has not been adequately secured in the depths of the vagina, the accumulation of blood, after the insertion of the skin graft, can result not only in failure of the graft to take, but in the expulsion of the form with the graft in the early hours after operation. When this happened to us on one occasion, it was necessary to reinsert the mold with graft under anesthesia after securing the bleeding and washing the graft (Fig. 6.8).

Various materials for the prosthetic device over which the split thickness graft is attached have been suggested. These have varied from balsa wood to silastic or various other plastic materials and glass. The objective is to obtain a material that has a suitable resilience so that pressure is rather evenly distributed and hard areas which may result in necrosis of the skin graft are avoided. We have tried several substances but have found that ordinary foam rubber, such as may be obtained from an upholstery shop has about the desired consist-

more posterior than anterior in order to assure maximal protection to the urethra by any available vaginal flap (Fig. 6.6). The development of the vaginal cavity is usually not difficult in patients who have not previously been operated upon. However, the dissection is most easily developed on one or the other side of the median raphe where the tissue between the bladder and the rectum seems to be condensed almost enough to warrant the designation of a rectourethralis fascia. If, however, spaces are developed by blunt dissection with the two fingers on either side of this condensed tissue, the latter may be conveniently dispatched with a scissors. The dissection should be carried up to the peritoneum, but care must be exercised not to expose too large an area of peritoneum, for in one patient there developed what amounted to an enterocele several months subsequent to the skin graft, apparently as the result of too extensive an exposure of the peritoneum. The cavity must be reasonably dry (Fig. 6.7). The most frequent bleeding vessels are around the edge of the vaginal epithelium at the site of the initial

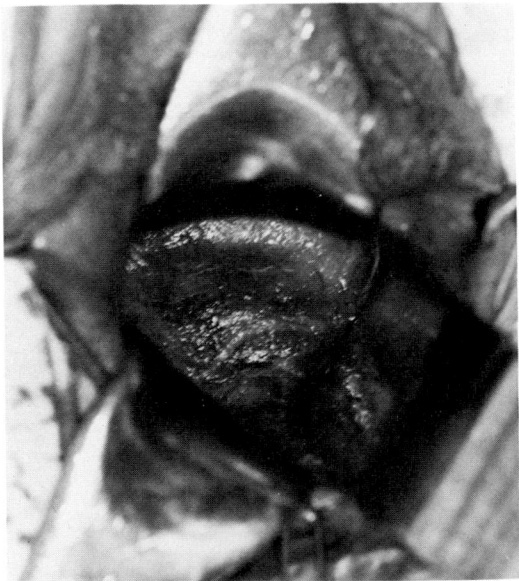

Fig. 6.7. The vaginal dissection has been completed. The cavity is approximately 10 cm deep. The peritoneum can be seen at the depth of the wound. The bladder is anterior. The rectum is not visible posteriorly, being covered by the retractors. The cavity is dry. No more peritoneum than is shown should be exposed.

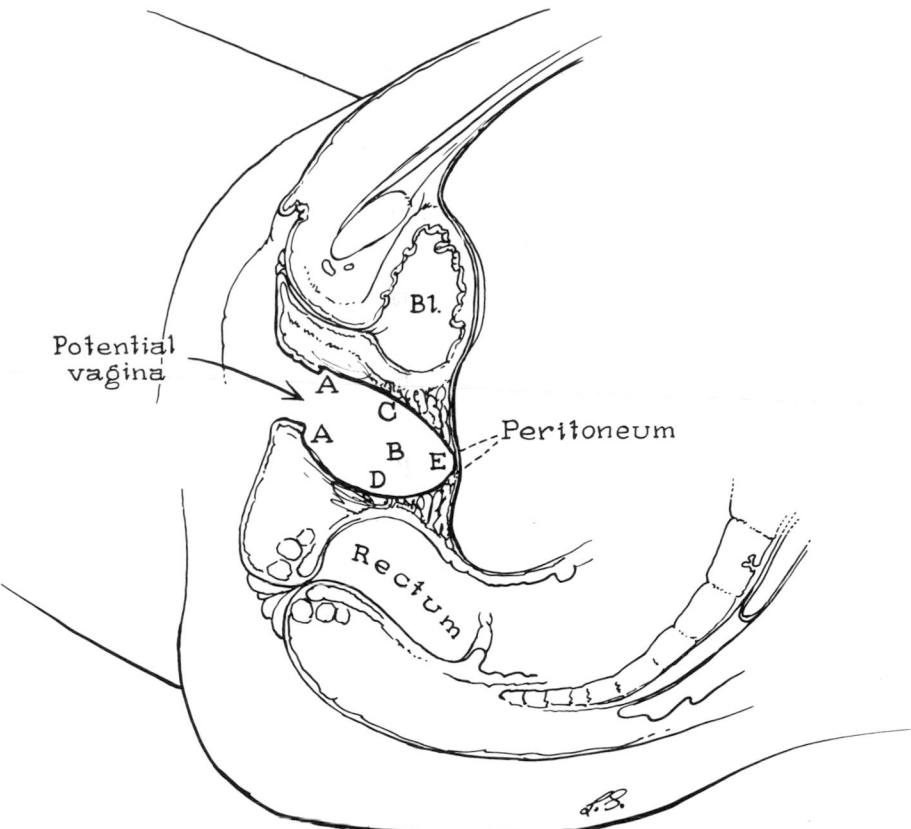

Fig. 6.8. A sagittal diagram showing trouble spots in the development of the neovagina. A. Troublesome bleeding often occurs at the edge of the original vaginal epithelium. B. A second area for troublesome bleeding occurs laterally on each side about two-thirds the distance up the vagina. It may be necessary to clamp relatively large vertical vessels with a long Kelly clamp and to ligate them with fine catgut. C. In the proper plane, the bladder is pale and feels firm in contrast to the peritoneum which will be encountered above it. D. The perirectal fasia is not as well defined as the bladder. Injury to the rectum has been reported much more frequently than injury to the bladder. It is difficult to be sure of the peritoneorectal fold; therefore, it is preferred to develop the peritoneum from an anterior dissection, *i.e.*, from the direction of the bladder. E. The peritoneum is thin. It is important not to expose more than 4 or 5 sq. cm for fear of entering the peritoneal cavity or of causing the subsequent development of an enterocele.

ency and can be readily sterilized. An initial block 10 x 10 x 20 cm is best. Such a large block has the advantage of furnishing sufficient material to cut the prosthetic device to a suitable size for the particular patient (Fig. 6.9). To accomplish this the form is cut about twice the desired volume and compressed by a covering of two rubber sheaths which are ordinary condoms. These are tied so that just the proper amount of air is trapped within the foam rubber to give the proper size form (Fig. 6.10). Prior to securing the graft onto the form, the form should be inserted into the neovaginal cavity as a test for size. If too much air has

been trapped within the condoms, they will bulge outside the vaginal outlet. Better this problem is adjusted at this point than after the graft is applied.

Dermatome cement can be used to secure the graft to the form. However, the application of the dermatome cement to the condom causes a considerable amount of wrinkling and buckling of the condom so that the graft is not smooth, and we much prefer to suture the graft over the form with interrupted stitches of #00000 chromic catgut on a reverse cutting needle. Interrupted vertical mattress sutures are used so that the exteriorized undersurface of the graft

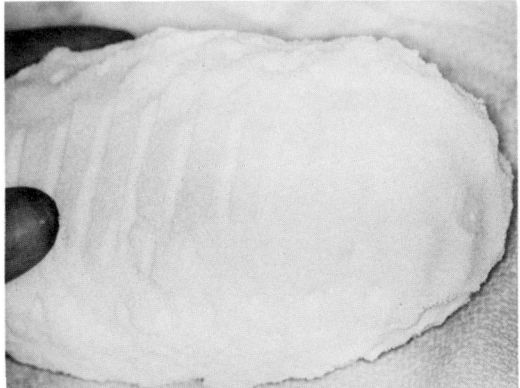

Fig. 6.9. Rough cut foam rubber ready to be compressed by the application of a covering rubber sheath.

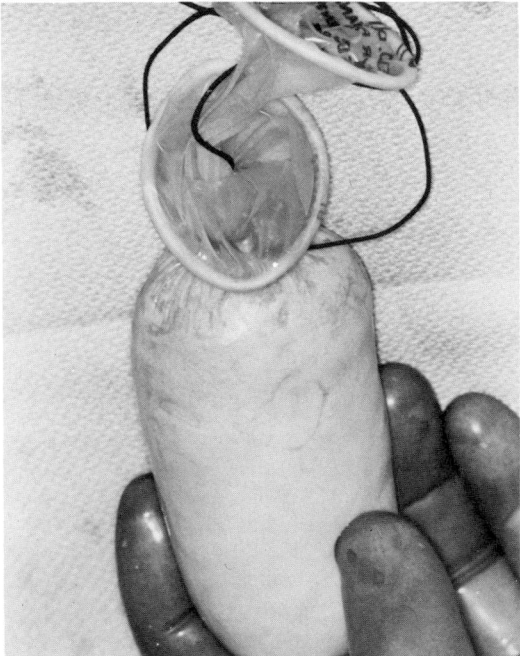

Fig. 6.10. The foam rubber with two rubber sheaths applied.

applied to the external surface of the graft on the mold is a very useful trick (Fig. 6.12).

After the graft has been inserted into the cavity, the edges of the graft may be sutured to the cut edges of the original vaginal mucus membrane (Fig. 6.13). However, if this is inconvenient to do, or inaccessible, these extra stitches may be dispensed with, as the graft will obviously take only on raw areas and, if there is any overlapping onto normal epithelium, that portion of the graft will, of course, not grow.

Although various types of straps and har-

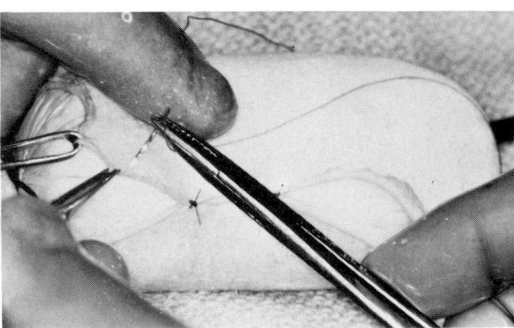

Fig. 6.11. Suturing the graft onto the vaginal mold.

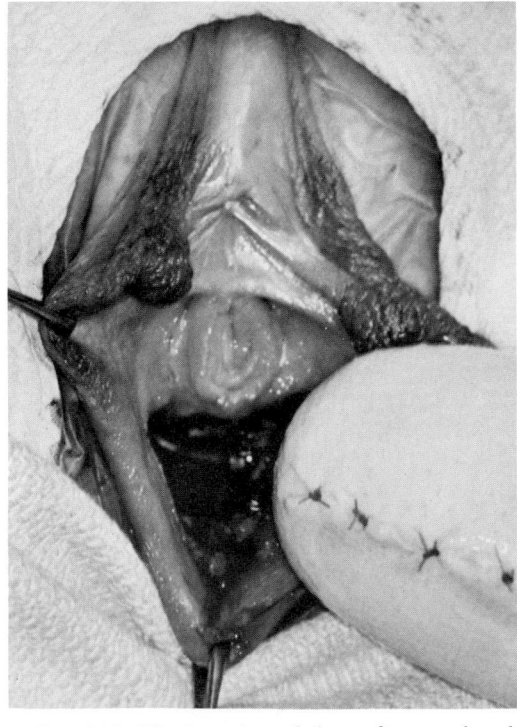

Fig. 6.12. The insertion of the graft-covered mold into the neovaginal cavity.

is approximated to exteriorized undersurface at the sutured edges (Fig. 6.11).

When all is ready, the mold covered by graft is inserted into the newly created space. In order to facilitate the insertion of the mold, it is very important that the cavity and the skin graft be well lubricated. To accomplish this, the cavity may be irrigated with salt solution and the same solution generously applied to the graft. It extra lubrication is desired, mineral oil nesses have been suggested for holding the form in place, in our experience none of these has been completely satisfactory. Indeed, if too much upward pressure is caused by such a contrivance, necrosis of the upper part of the graft may result. We, therefore, now use rather large braided silk sutures through the labia to prevent extrusion of the form (Fig. 6.14). These stitches are often uncomfortable, but they have been so satisfactory in holding the form in place that we have considered this an overriding consideration.

Formerly, an indwelling catheter through the urethra was used, but in a few cases, some slough at the distal end of the urethra, fortunately without incontinence, was caused by pressure of the form against the urethra. I am aware of instances where the whole urethra has sloughed. To avoid this, in more recent years we have uniformly used a suprapubic cystotomy device with great satisfaction.

Postoperatively, the patient is kept on a low residue diet, antibiotics, and a position in bed almost flat so that there will be exerted a minimal force which might cause expulsion of

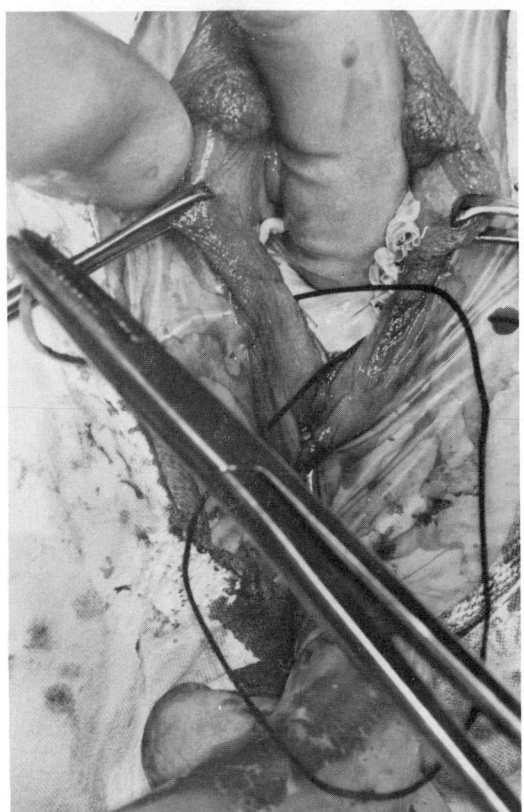

Fig. 6.14. Suturing the labia with heavy braided silk sutures.

the form. Formerly the graft was left undisturbed for 14 days, but during days 10 to 14 the patients became increasingly uncomfortable due to the labial stitches and malodorous discharge which often develops. Therefore, more recently, after 9 or 10 days the sutures are removed, the form removed, the graft inspected, and the vaginal cavity irrigated with copious amounts of salt solution (Fig. 6.15). This is conveniently done with light general anesthesia. At this time it is usually difficult from inspection to be sure whether the graft has taken satisfactorily. The foam rubber form, or a new one similar in size, is reinserted. A firmer form is not used until at least 6 weeks postoperatively, in order to prevent possible necrosis of some areas of the graft due to pressure. We think we have observed such a late loss of portions of the graft from harder forms.

Following the initial removal of the form and its reinsertion under anesthesia, it has been our practice to leave this *in situ* for about 24 hours

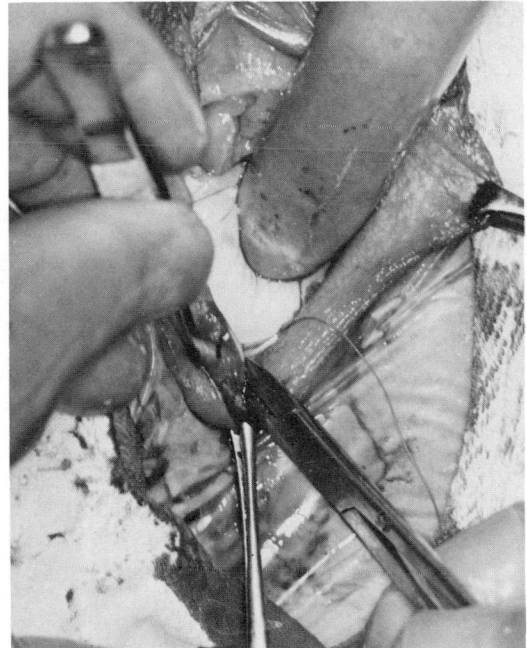

Fig. 6.13. Suturing the edges of the graft to the edges of the introitus, a desirable but not necessarily essential step. If these sutures can be applied, there is much less likelihood of granulations at the junction between the introital epithelium and the graft.

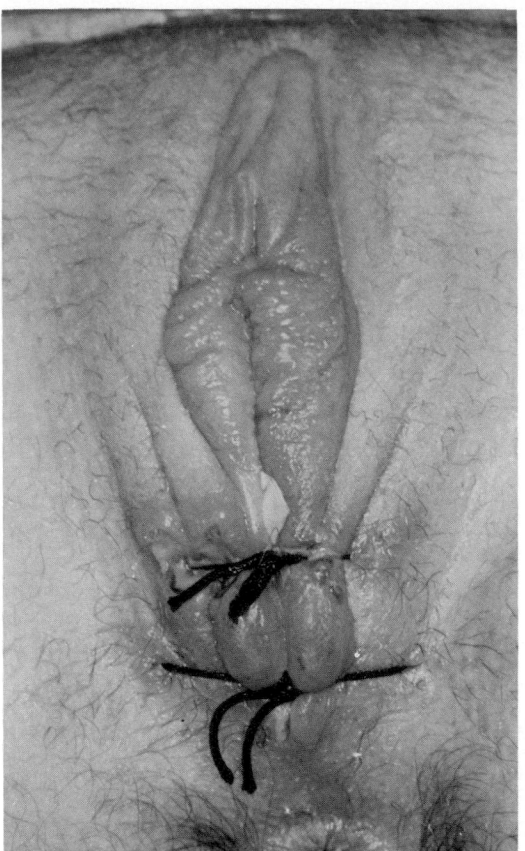

Fig. 6.15. The appearance of the labia 10 days after operation. The edema shown in the photograph disappears within 24 hours after the stitches have been removed.

in order to allow the discomfort and the edema in the local area to improve. This will also give an opportunity to see if the patient can void normally, as the suprapubic catheter is customarily removed under anesthesia at the time of the original dressing. The site of the graft on the buttock is dressed for the first time while the patient is under anesthesia for the first form removal.

About 24 or more hours after the original removal of the mold, the patient is instructed in the self-removal of the mold. The first time this is done, it is not undesirable to administer 50 mg of demerol or its equivalent a half hour prior to the first removal, although in many instances this is not really necessary. The patient is usually concerned that she can do herself some harm, but there is really very little damage that she can do, and she must be encouraged to grasp the form and to remove it

by traction. After the removal of the form, she takes a low pressure clear warm water douche. The mold is cleaned, covered with a new condom if necessary, and reinserted with a neutral vaginal lubricant. She is then instructed to do this daily; as soon as she has acquired the necessary skill in the self-removal of the form, the taking of the vaginal douche, and the reinsertion of the form, she is ready for discharge from the hospital.

After about 6 weeks, a silastic form, or one of similar material, is much easier for the patient to handle in that she can wash it off in tap water and does not have to replace the condoms (Fig. 6.16).

If there is 100 per cent take of the graft, most patients will have very little discomfort in the vaginal area 6 to 8 weeks or so after the operation. Many patients find the vagina comfortable and functional within this period of time.

In the event that there is some loss of the graft, granulation tissue will grow in the denuded area. It is necessary, therefore, in postoperative visits to keep the granulation

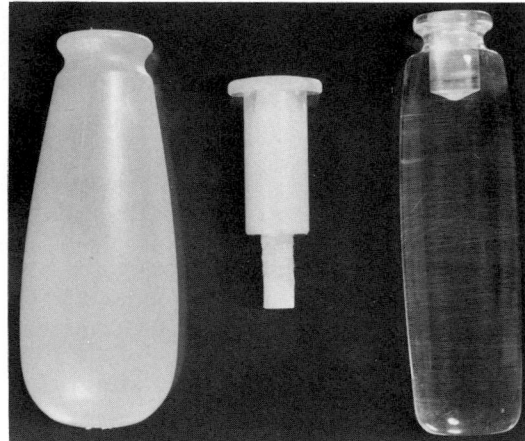

Fig. 6.16. Two types of more permanent vaginal molds which can be used beginning no sooner than about 6 weeks from operation. On the left is a silastic form which has proved to be very satisfactory. On the right is a lucite form. The latter is much firmer than the silastic form, and is useful only in special situations. In the center is a nylon tip which can be applied to either form for the purpose of attaching elastic bands to a girdle to secure upward thrust of the form. This is seldom if ever necessary for patients with a neovagina in a genetic female but is sometimes useful in genetic males whose perineal muscles do not allow self-retention of the mold as easily as in the genetic female.

tissue low so that epithelialization can take place from the edges of the graft. Generous use of silver nitrate for this purpose is probably undesirable due to its deleterious effect on the growing epithelium. It has, therefore, been our custom to keep a curet in the office so that the excess granulations can simply be curetted away, and the bleeding stopped by pressure.

In a few patients, a considerable portion of the graft is lost for one or another reason, although with experience with the operation, this complication seems to be less frequent. In the event this occurs, a decision must be made as to whether the area should be regrafted. In general, if the area of defect is as large as a 25¢ piece or larger, a secondary graft greatly shortens the period of convalescence, as the growing edge of epithelium from the new graft is sluggish at best. Secondary grafting may be carried out 3 months or more after the original operation. It is done exactly as in the original graft with no special preoperative preparation. At the time of secondary grafting, the base of the denuded area is thoroughly curetted with an ordinary serrated curet, so that a firm base with minimal granulations is obtained. Usually secondary grafts take very well.

The overall results of the McIndoe operation are quite satisfactory. Through 1973 approximately 150 patients have been operated on with generally satisfactory results. Major bleeding expelled the form and graft in one instance, but reinsertion under anesthesia ultimately gave satisfactory results. There were three small rectovaginal fistulae which healed spontaneously before the use of the hard wooden form was abandoned, and the distal 1 cm of the urethra sloughed in two instances without the loss of urinary continence when an indwelling catheter was used. The only cases that could be considered failures were two done in 15-year-old girls who were insufficiently motivated to endure the discomfort caused by postoperative self-manipulation of the form.

A secondary procedure at a later date was successful in one of these patients, but the other patient has been lost to follow-up.

Congenital Absence of the Vagina with a Normal Uterus

The condition with which we are here concerned is usually described in the literature under the rubric of "Congenital Absence of the Vagina with a Normal Uterus." This is indeed an accurate description of the condition, but it implies that the basic embryologic defect is somewhat akin to that which occurs with congenital absence of the vagina and uterus. However, it seems likely that the condition is developmentally more allied to a transverse vaginal septum, except that in those patients who might be considered to have congenital absence of the vagina with a uterus, the transverse vaginal septum is of very considerable length, so much so that the vagina seems not to have developed at all. The main point here is that in the condition we are discussing, not only is the uterus normally developed in most instances, but many times, although not always, there is a small normal upper segment of vagina. When present, this is a very fortunate circumstance for it is the key to its successful operative treatment (Fig. 6.17).

My personal experience with this disorder leads me to say that of all congenital anomalies of the female generative tract, serious mistakes are made more often with this disorder than with any other. This is probably due to its rarity, but it is doubly unfortunate because errors in handling can lead to loss of reproductive potential, whereas if the lesion is handled ideally, reproduction is not precluded.

As mentioned, this disorder is rare, and my own experience has been limited to only 10 patients, all of whom have been seen secondarily with some remaining unsolved problem. It has been extraordinarily instructive to realize that in each instance one or more deviations from an ideal method of treatment created problems which made the situation into a very difficult one. The basic problems are two: (1) a wrong preoperative diagnosis and (2) failure to provide egress for menstrual blood when creating a neovagina in a patient immediately after the menarche. The difficulties are compounded by the absolute necessity for perineal surgery in patients of this age (see section above on "Creation of an Artificial Vagina with a Split Thickness Graft" for the ideal age for vaginal construction). The surgical situation can rapidly deteriorate if the diagnosis is made for the first time at laparotomy especially if the operating surgeon is not prepared to handle the key problem of providing for menstrual egress from below.

Thus, in several instances in our series, the

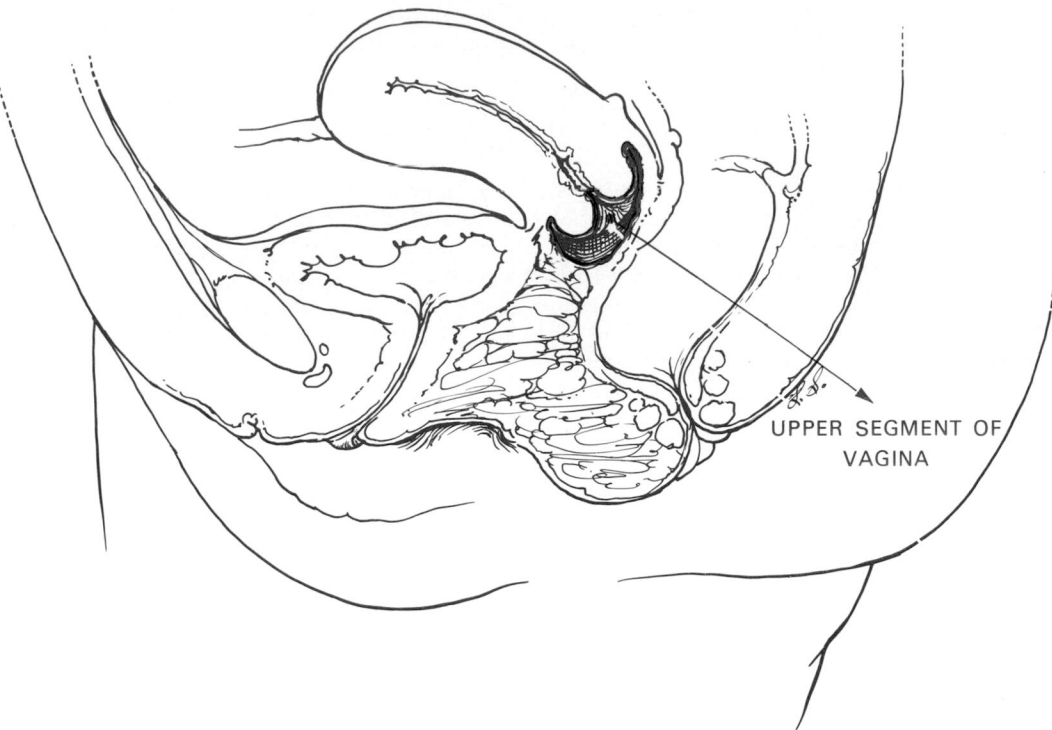

UPPER SEGMENT OF
VAGINA

Fig. 6.17. Diagram of sagittal view of pelvis showing the relationships when there is congenital absence of the vagina with a normal uterus. Note the segment of upper vagina which is most often, but not always, present in this condition.

patient was operated upon with a mistaken diagnosis. The abdominal pain in a young teenager led to an exploratorial laparotomy undertaken with the provisional diagnosis of acute appendicitis, ruptured ovarian cyst, or the like. With the abdomen open, the operating surgeon, who many times was a general surgeon, was confronted with an enlarged uterus or a uterus sitting on a mass that he did not recognize. At this point there are numerous opportunities for error. A major one, in my experience, is to aspirate or open the mass to evacuate the trapped menstrual blood. There are two reasons why this should not be done from above. First, the liberating of menstrual blood into the peritoneal cavity predisposes to endometriosis, and secondly, the collapse of the dilated upper vagina and uterus makes the approach through the perineum to the small upper vagina ever so much more hazardous. Dissection between the bladder and rectum to create a neovagina is relatively easy, but opening into structures at the apex of the dissection can be hazardous because it may be

difficult to distinguish between the rectum, the bladder and the upper vagina. However, if the upper vagina is distended and tense with menstrual blood, the operation is relatively easy, and the vagina can be opened in a way, which will be described, to provide for evacuation of the menstrual blood through the perineum. Therefore, in the event an error is made and the abdomen of a teenager with this difficulty is opened, it can be highly recommended that no further operative procedure be done from above, that the abdomen be closed, and that the remainder of the operation be performed from below.

Best of all, of course, is that a proper preoperative diagnosis be made, and that the abdomen not be opened. The diagnosis is to be highly suspected in a child of pubertal age who has had no external bleeding, who has had bouts of abdominal pain at about monthly intervals, and who has a midline pelvic mass. The mischief arises from failure to make a pelvic examination, for the mass can easily be felt by rectal examination, and no patent vaginal opening is present.

A second major difficulty in handling these cases is inadequate provision for the periodic escape of menstrual blood through the perineum in these pubertal children. It has been surprising that many times a perineal dissection has been performed, the upper vagina opened, and at this point the operation was abandoned, perhaps with no more than a cigarette drain or a gauze pack left through the perineum. In other patients, when the bladder was lacerated, the defect was closed, but no perineal path provided for menstruation. Such procedures are doomed to failure. The tract will scar down very promptly, and it is at this point that, if reproductive capacity is to be saved, prompt and definitive steps must be taken.

With a normal functioning uterus it is, of course, quite obvious that some provision must be made for the menstrual blood to repeatedly escape. Several methods to accomplish this have been attempted. Several years ago, we ourselves used a split thickness graft in a few patients, modifying the operation from the one for congenital absence of the vagina and uterus to the extent that a hollow tube was provided in the center of the vaginal mold to provide for menstruation. Perhaps this technique would work if it were applied to a patient who had not been previously operated upon. However, we did not succeed in getting the graft to take to any appreciable extent on the patients on whom it was tried, but in all instances this was a secondary procedure through a vaginal sinus tract which was scarred and infected.

The key to what seems to be the most satisfactory method yet devised for handling this condition was provided by an experience with a patient whose primary operation took place in Santiago, Chile. In this patient the proper diagnosis was made preoperatively. The pelvic mass was approached from below, the upper vagina entered, the menstrual blood evacuated, and the upper vagina and the neovaginal space was kept open by inserting a glass flask with the large bulbous end in the upper vagina (Fig. 6.18). The vaginal space was then allowed to contract down around this glass flask. This solved satisfactorily the motivational problem of the young teenage patient to maintain the form in the vaginal cavity involuntarily and without discomfort. The opportunity to see this patient was provided 6 months later

when an attempt was made to remove the glass flask, and it could not be retrieved. In actuality, the removal of the flask did not prove difficult and was accomplished by making a lateral incision down the side of the neovagina.

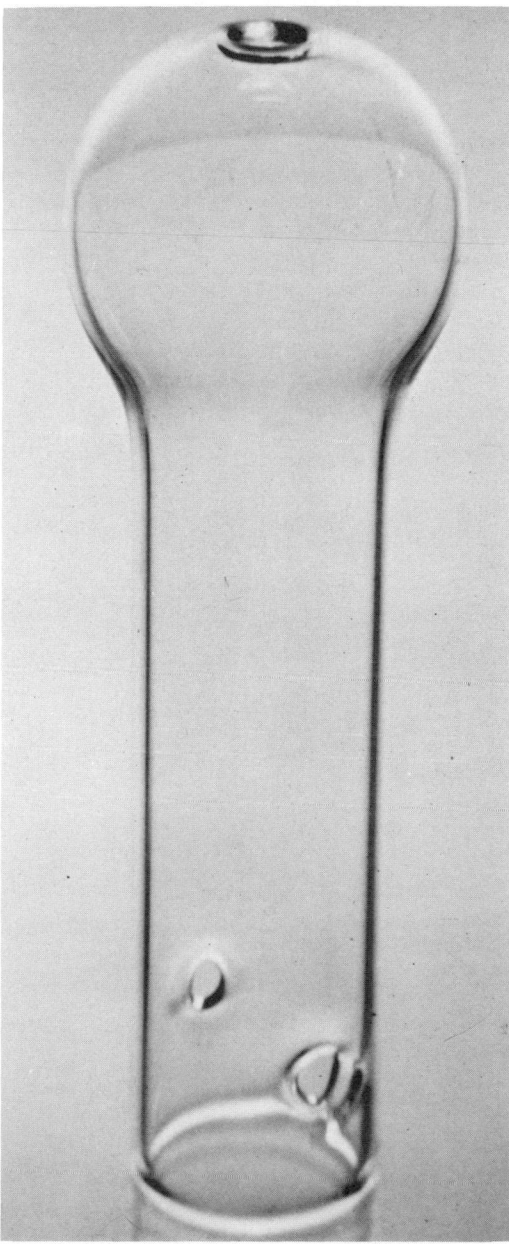

Fig. 6.18. Glass flask, the bulb of which provided self-retention in a patient with congenital absence of the vagina with a normal uterus. After being *in situ* for 6 months, the neovagina was satisfactorily epithelialized.

However, the amazing and indeed instructive point was that, in the 6 months in which the flask had remained *in situ,* the vaginal space had completely epithelialized along the glass flask presumably from the edges of the upper vagina growing downward to meet the epithelium growing up from the vaginal outlet. We have had the opportunity to apply this technique in secondary operations to four patients with results which are quite satisfactory. The only variation has been that a lucite form, instead of a glass flask, has been used (Fig. 6.19) to minimize the opportunity for breakage. With these lucite forms, which can be custom made to the appropriate size for each patient, no motivation is required on the part of these youngsters to maintain the form *in situ* or to remove and replace it. The form is allowed to remain *in situ* for a minimal period of 6 months, during which time epithelialization will hopefully take place, and indeed in all instances

it has done so. At a second operation, the lucite flask is removed and a silastic or other type of removable form is substituted, but at this point the original form has been in place so long that, even if the patient is not completely cooperative in maintaining the form within the vaginal space, there is little likelihood of losing the now completely epithelialized neovagina.

Myomata Uteri

The relation of multiple myomata to infertility has been difficult to establish with impeccable data. However, there seem to be instances where no cause except myomata can be found to account for the infertility. In the absence of an understanding of the mechanism of this infertility, the diagnosis is made by the exclusion of all other known factors. Under these circumstances, myomectomy may be indicated. Several authors have reported series of patients who seem to be infertile on the basis of myomata. Almost 50 per cent of those who have had a myomectomy, under this circumstance, subsequently become pregnant, but there is a troublesome miscarriage rate (Table 6.1).

Myomectomy for Infertility

Troublesome though the data are on the basic relation between infertility and myomata, they are virtually nonexistent on the details. Thus, there are no data on the relation of number, size, location, or mechanism of interference of myomata with fertility. Specifically, there are no data relating alterations in configu-

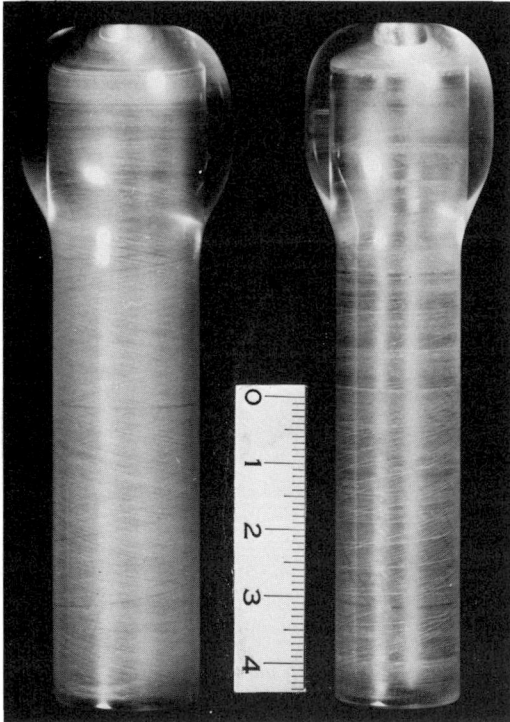

Fig. 6.19. Two lucite stents of different sizes. The bulb end is inserted into the small segment of upper vagina. A lumen provides egress for the menstrual blood. Such a stent requires no attention by the patient—an important consideration in a very young teenager.

Table 6.1. Pregnancy Results after Myomectomy

Reference	Patients	Pregnancies	Term Deliveries
Brown *et al.* (5)	21	11	9
Dearnley (6)	80	37	29
Ingersoll (7)	39	20	?
Stevenson (8)	35	18	?
Loeffler and Noble (9)	23	9	7
Total	198	95 (48%)	
Total term determinate	144	57 (46%)	45 (36%)

ration of the endometrial cavity with infertility. Therefore, it is necessary to assume that any reasonable enlargement of the uterus without regard to the configuration of the endometrial cavity may somehow interfere with fertility (Figs. 6.20, 6.21).

Myomectomy is not a difficult operation and errors are infrequent. It is almost unheard of not to be able to technically perform a myomectomy in lieu of a hysterectomy even when the myomata are symptomatic with respect to vaginal bleeding, but in an occasional, albeit unusual, circumstance, operative bleeding from the multiple myomectomy incisions may be so troublesome that hysterectomy is required. It is obviously necessary, therefore, before undertaking myomectomy to have some clear understanding with the patient that in the rarest circumstance it may not be possible to accomplish the operation which is planned.

Bleeding is essentially the only troublesome problem. While incisions to enucleate the individual tumors must be placed in the most convenient position in relation to the nodule, in general it is desirable to locate the incisions parallel to the major vessels (Fig. 6.22). Intramyometrial infiltration with an oxytoxic solution may be used to control bleeding and is not undesirable, but if this is used, it is nevertheless important to ligate visible major vessels, otherwise they may bleed after the effects of the oxytocin have worn off. Normally, only one set of major vessels seem to enter a myomatous nodule. Actually, even with relatively large intermural nodules, bleeding at the time of a nucleation is seldomly worrisome (Fig. 6.23).

However, as the incision is closed, bleeding is often annoying, so that sutures in excess of those required to approximate the edges of the

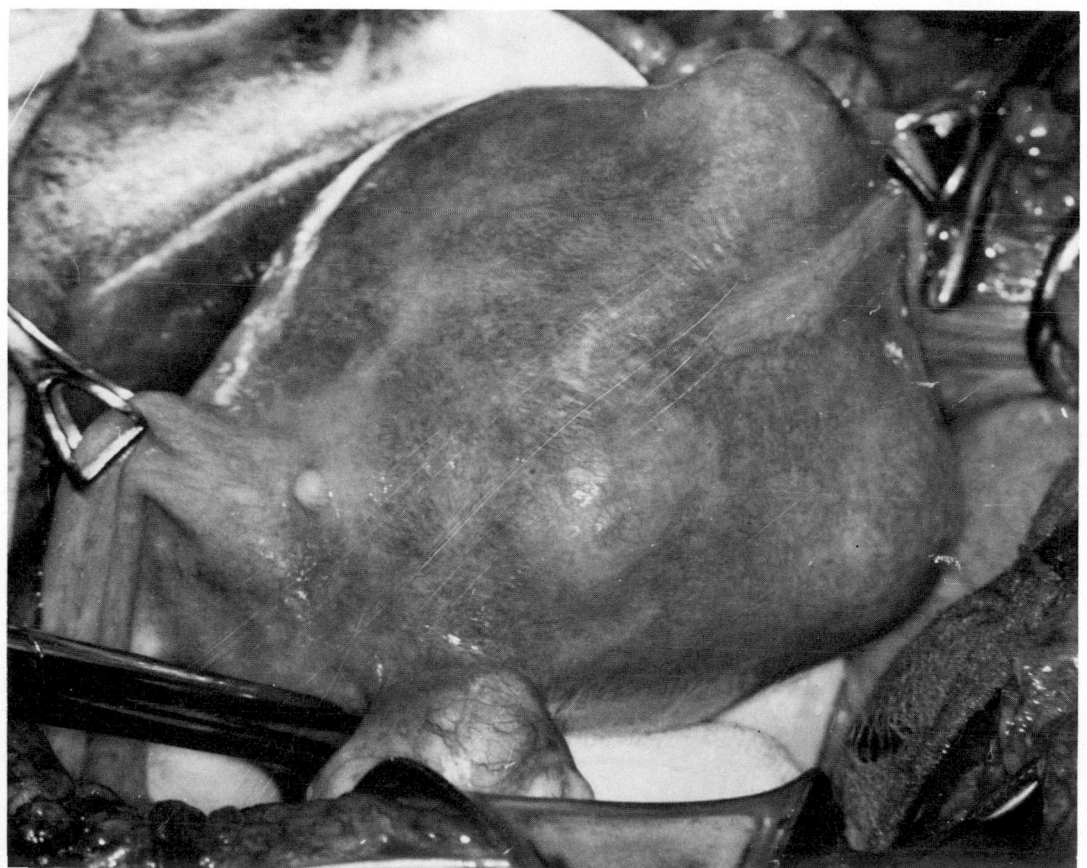

Fig. 6.20. Multiple myomas in the uterus of a patient who had been infertile after 6 years of marriage with no other identifiable cause for the infertility.

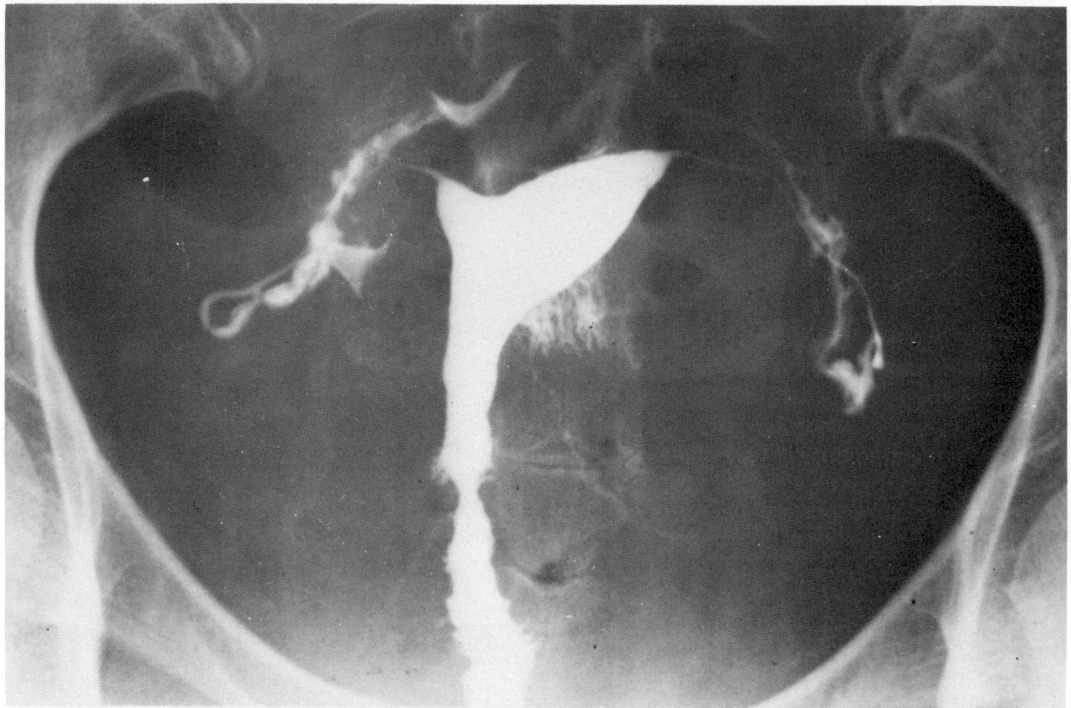

Fig. 6.21. Hysterogram of uterus shown in Figure 6.20. Note the deformity of the cavity due to the large intramural myoma being enucleated in Figure 6.23.

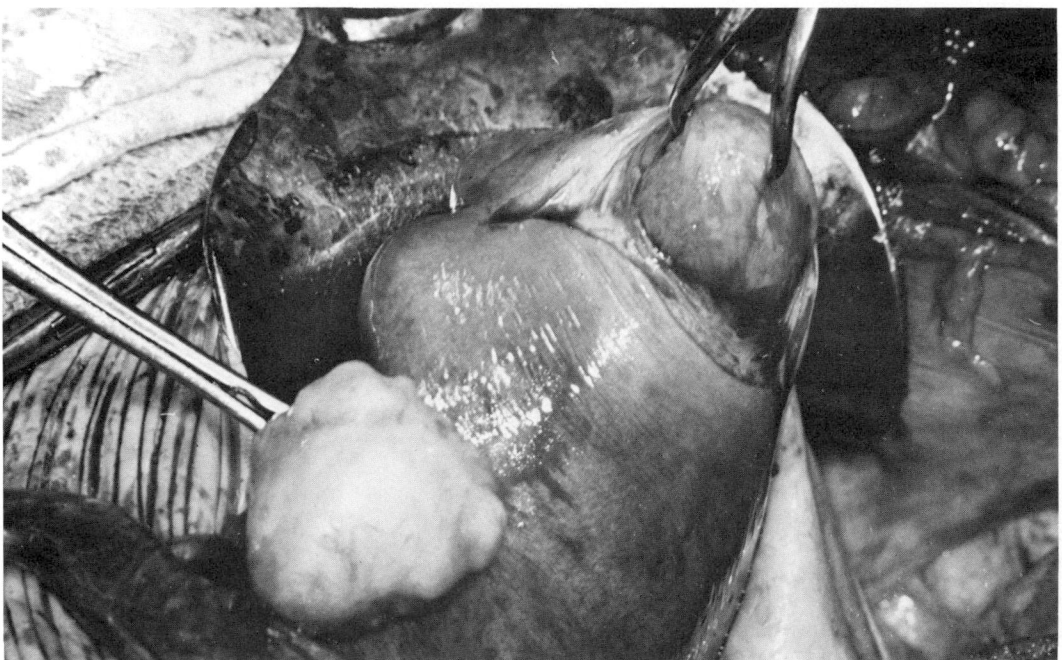

Fig. 6.22. Enucleation of a myoma through a crescentic vertical incision in an attempt to place the incision parallel to the vessels coursing into the myometrium from the lateral sides of the uterus.

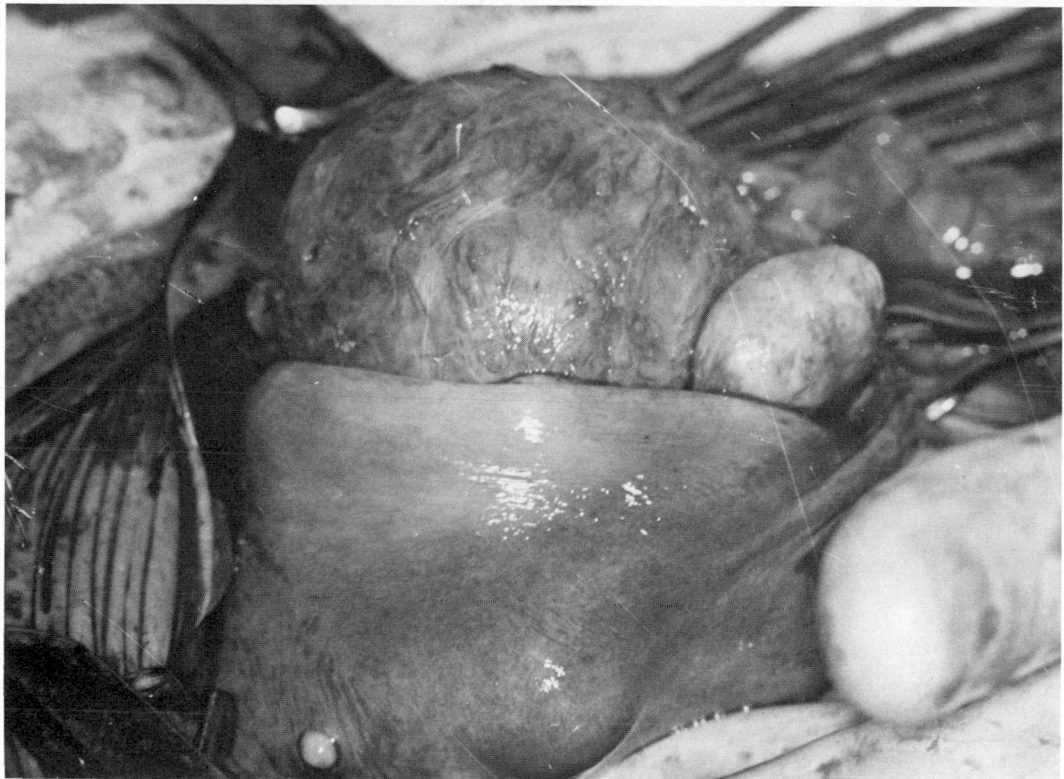

Fig. 6.23. Minimal bleeding from the enucleation of a relatively large intramural nodule. No oxytocin has been used in this patient.

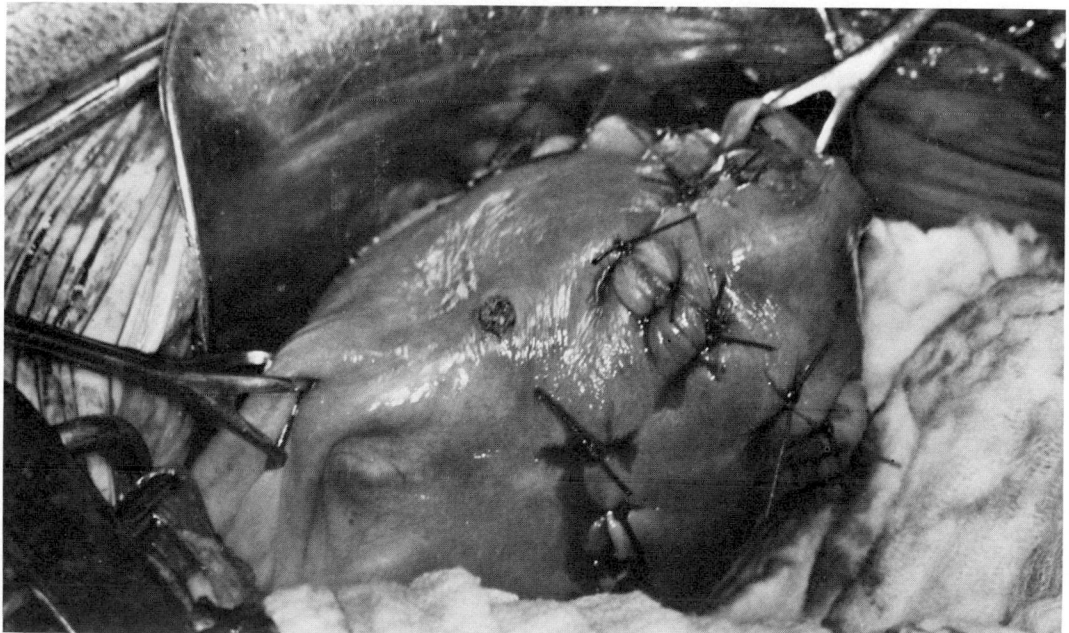

Fig. 6.24. Large numbers of sutures placed in the myomectomy incisions. The number of sutures required to control bleeding is in excess of those required to approximate the tissues.

incision are often necessary to control the bleeding (Fig. 6.24).

Because of the tendency of the incisions to delayed weeping and oozing, Dr. T. S. Cullen always insisted that his residents and assistants place one or more Penrose drains down to the uterus to remain in place for the first 24 hours after myomectomy. While this may not be required in every case, the principle just enunciated illustrates the problem of hemostasis, and it is often surprising to note the amount of oozing through an incision into which a Penrose drain has been placed after myomectomy.

Double Uterus

Reconstruction of a symmetrical double uterus, when there is no obstruction to either horn, is indicated when there is reproductive failure, most often if not always, consisting of repeated miscarriage. Naturally the best results are obtained when a proper diagnosis is made. It may be a mistake to operate for a double uterus upon a patient who has reproductive failure from a cause unrelated to the double uterus. For example, if the patient's problems are due to a metabolic difficulty and not to the double uterus, reconstruction of the double uterus will probably not be helpful. It has been clearly shown, and all obstetricians of experience are aware of the fact, that the patients with double uteri do not necessarily have problems of reproductive failure. Therefore, it is exceedingly important to be certain that in a particular case the reproductive difficulty is due to the double uterus. Before undertaking reconstruction of a double uterus, it is essential that the patient's reproductive problem be thoroughly investigated from all points of view and that the patient has demonstrated that either her problem cannot be solved by correction of the metabolic difficulty or that no metabolic difficulty can be found. This problem has been thoroughly discussed on previous occasions (11, 12).

If a thorough study of the individual problem indicates that surgical reconstruction is needed, several operative procedures have been suggested for this purpose. Strassmann (13) described the original techniques which did not remove any tissue. Tompkins (14) described a variation combining some of the features of the Strassmann procedure and the operation about to be described. However, through the years, we have preferred to excise surgically the septum and close the defect in the uterus. As the results from this operative procedure have been quite satisfactory, we can continue to recommend this method of operation.

Operation for Double Uterus

Most often, but not always, a patient who needs reconstruction of a double uterus will have a septate uterus as opposed to a bicornuate uterus. This is an important technical point, for when the septate uterus is exposed at operation, many times the abnormality is not appreciated from the external configuration of the uterus which tends to appear normal (Fig. 6.25). Often, the only abnormality which can be seen is a faint vertical depression in the midline. At other times a somewhat deeper medium raphe is apparent. It is important in excising the muscular septum to have a good concept of the location of the uterine cavity from a previously obtained hysterogram. We have previously advocated preoperative staining from below through the cervix of the endometrial cavity by some dye, such as methylene blue, in order to easily recognize the endometrium as one cuts into the cavity from above in removing the muscular septum. With experience, this is not entirely necessary, but for those who have not had great experience with the operation, it is probably desirable, as many times the endometrial cavity is somewhat difficult to recognize as one approaches it surgically from above, and it would be easy to completely transect one or the other of the horns before realizing it. This would obviously be undesirable as it would make considerably more difficult the final anastomosis of the unroofed cavities from each side. If staining of the endometrial cavity is undertaken, it is important not to inject into the cavity more dye than necessary, because excess dye will flow through the Fallopian tubes and stain the peritoneal cavity. About 3 to 5 ml of dye injected through a Rubin's cannula should suffice.

It is desirable to draw with brilliant green on the outside of the uterus the lines of incision for the excision of the uterine wedge. This is desirable because after the first incision is

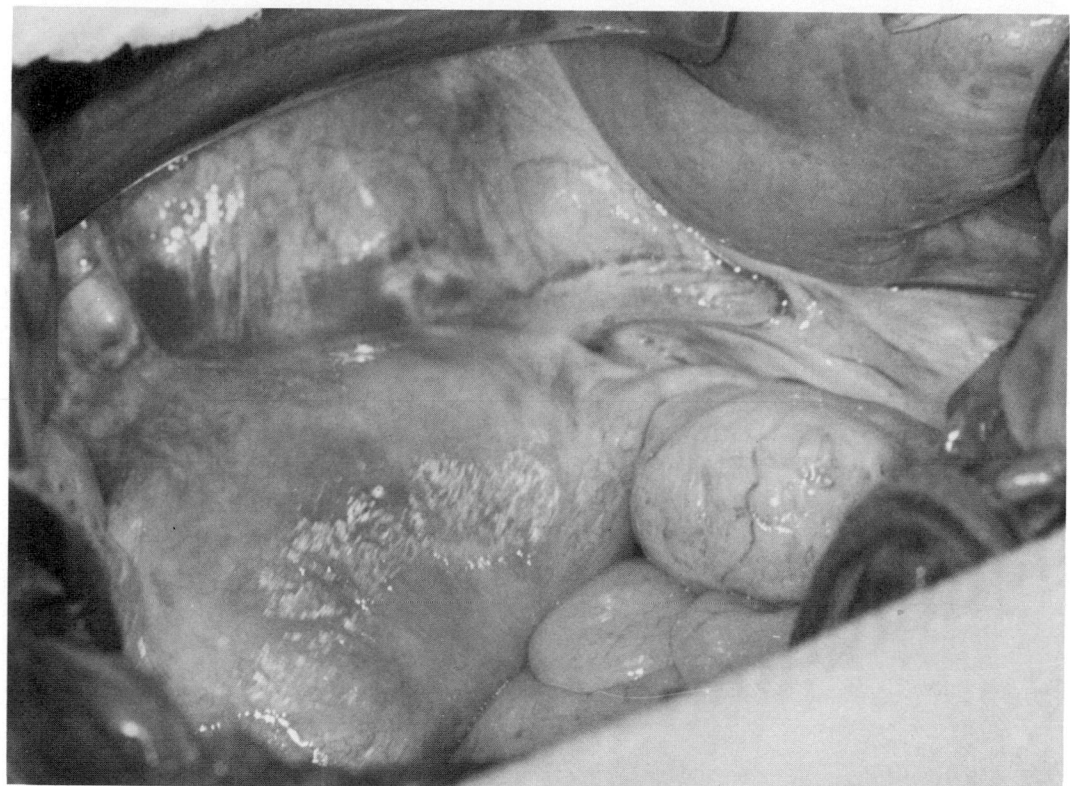

Fig. 6.25. External appearance of a septate uterus. Note the insignificant appearance of the median raphe. Many times a septate uterus is not recognized by its external appearance.

made, the uterus gets somewhat distorted, and unless one previously knows where one wishes to make the other incisions, it may be difficult to place them in the exact position. To stabilize the two horns after the initial incisions, a guy suture is suitably placed in each horn (Fig. 6.26).

While incision into the corpus of the uterus can be somewhat bloody, we have not found it necessary to employ mechanical devices such as a cervical tourniquet to reduce the amount of bleeding. In fact, this is not as effective as might be desired due to the rich vascular supply to the uterus from the utero-ovarian arteries. In some cases we have employed oxytocin, U.S.P. synthetic, for this purpose. This is supplied in 1-cc ampules which can be diluted to 10 cc with salt solution to thoroughly inject the myometrium. This makes for an almost completely bloodless operation. With this technique, visible vessels even though not bleeding should be tied. Obviously the anesthesiologist should be informed that such an injection is to be made (Fig. 6.27).

As the wedge is being removed (Fig. 6.28), it is desirable to identify the endometrial cavity to help prevent total transection of the cavity (Fig. 6.29). At times it is necessary to excise additional bits of myometrium if the two endometrial cavities have not been satisfactorily unroofed. In fact, in order to prevent removing too much of the endometrial cavity, it is desirable to err on the side of removing too small an amount of uterine septum than the contrary (Fig. 6.30).

Prior to excising the uterine wedge, all sutures for closing the defect should be in readiness so that there is no waiting while the nurse prepares the necessary stitches. The two sides of the uterus can be approximated by interrupted or continuous stitches, but we have found it somewhat easier using big bite interrupted stitches in the endometrium and including the inner one-third of the myometrium, being sure that the knots are tied inside the cavity (Fig. 6.31). The endometrium is friable, and it is important as the knots are tied down for the assistants to compress the two sides of

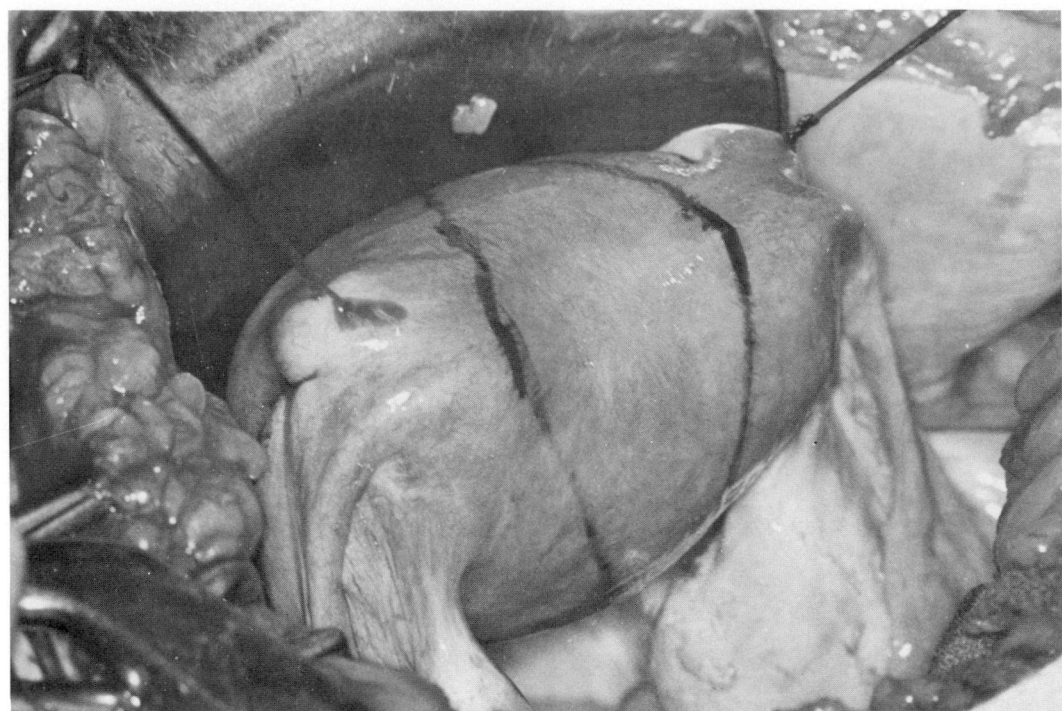

Fig. 6.26. The initial incisions have been outlined by brilliant green, and temporary guy sutures have been placed in each horn.

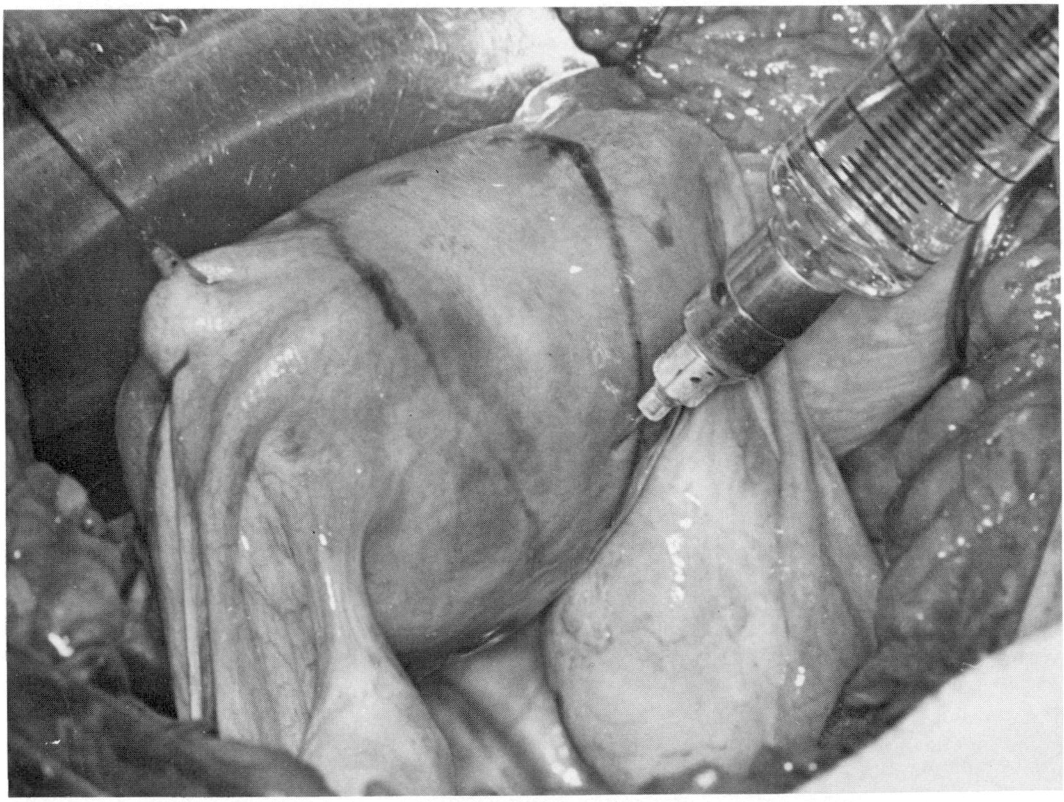

Fig. 6.27. The injection of oxytocin into the myometrium to reduce bleeding.

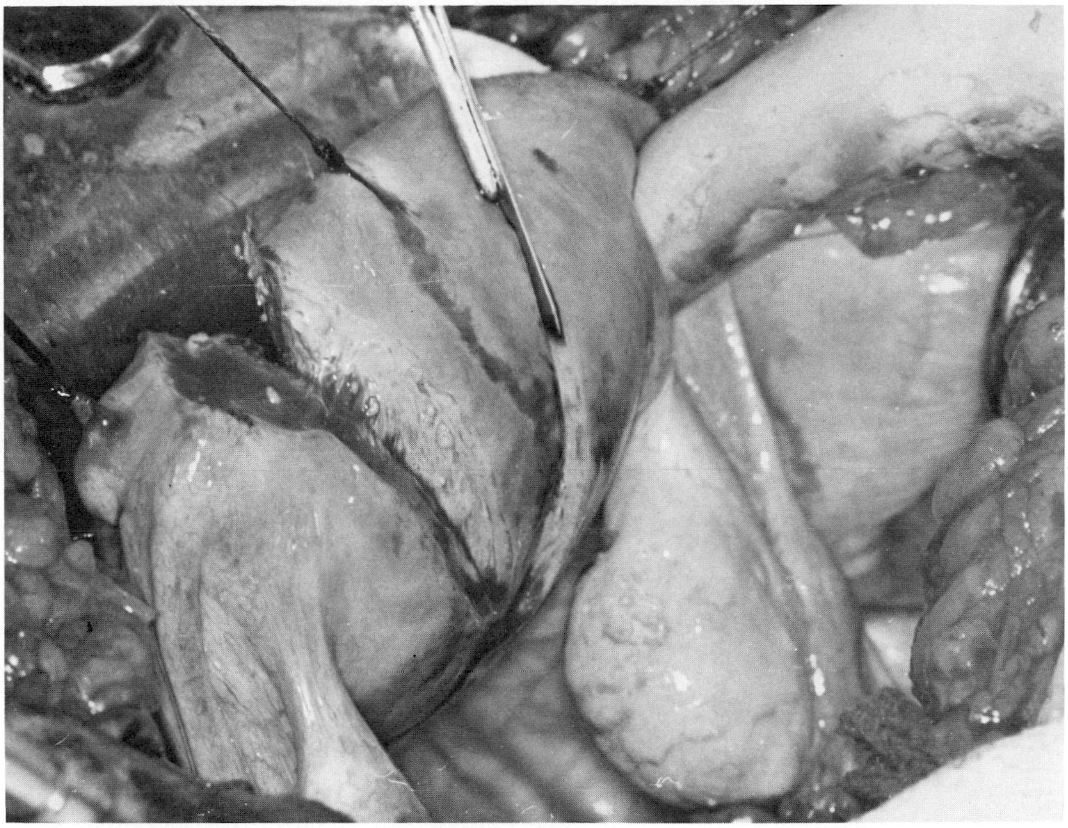

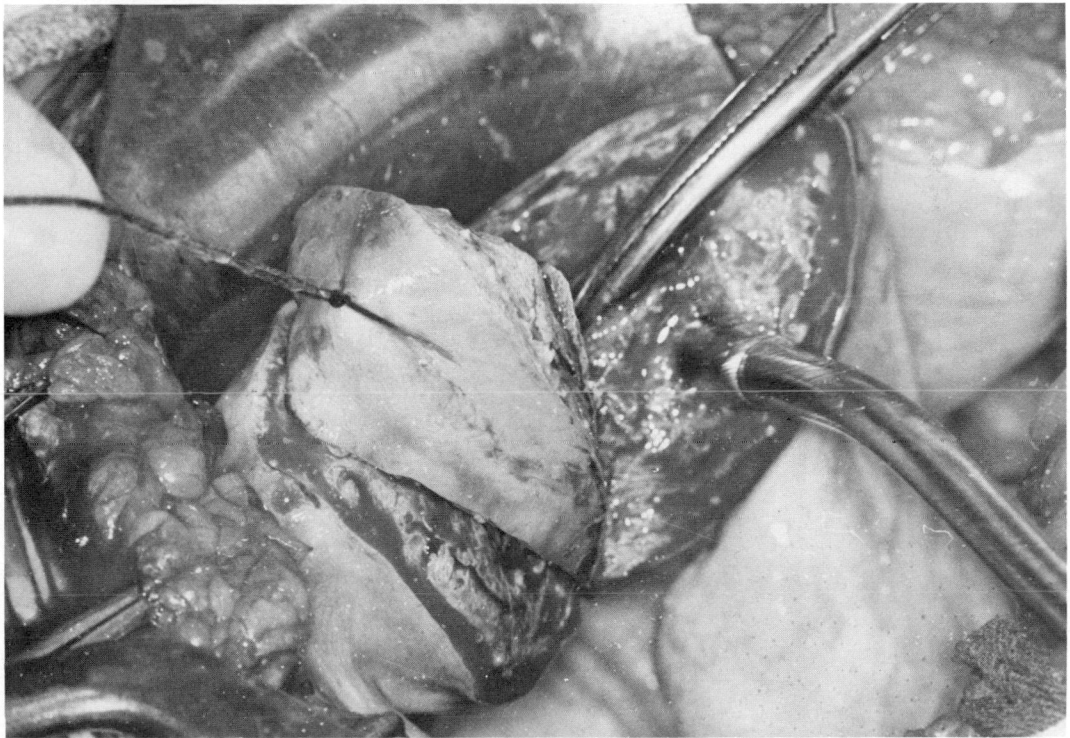

Fig. 6.28. Removal of the wedge containing most of the septum.

Fig. 6.29. Identification of the right endometrial cavity as the wedge is being removed. Such identification helps prevent the undesirable transection of the cavity. Similar identification of the left cavity is also important.

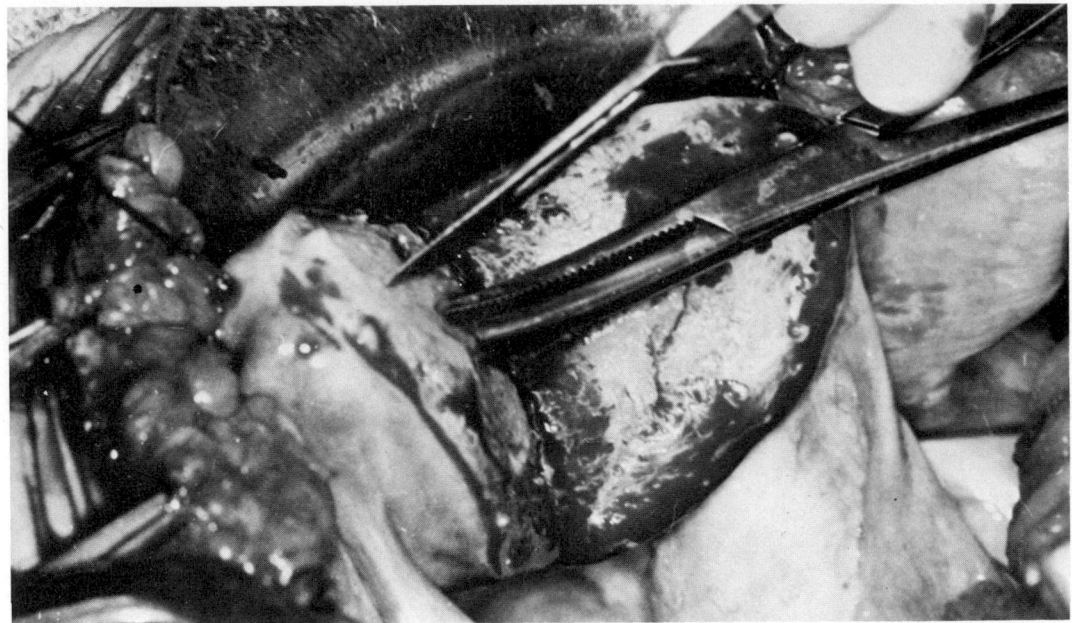

Fig. 6.30. Additional unroofing of the left cavity after excision of the main bulk of the septum.

Fig. 6.31. Drawing of the placing of sutures in the anterior endometrium. Note that the stitches are placed so that the knots are tied inside the endometrial cavity.

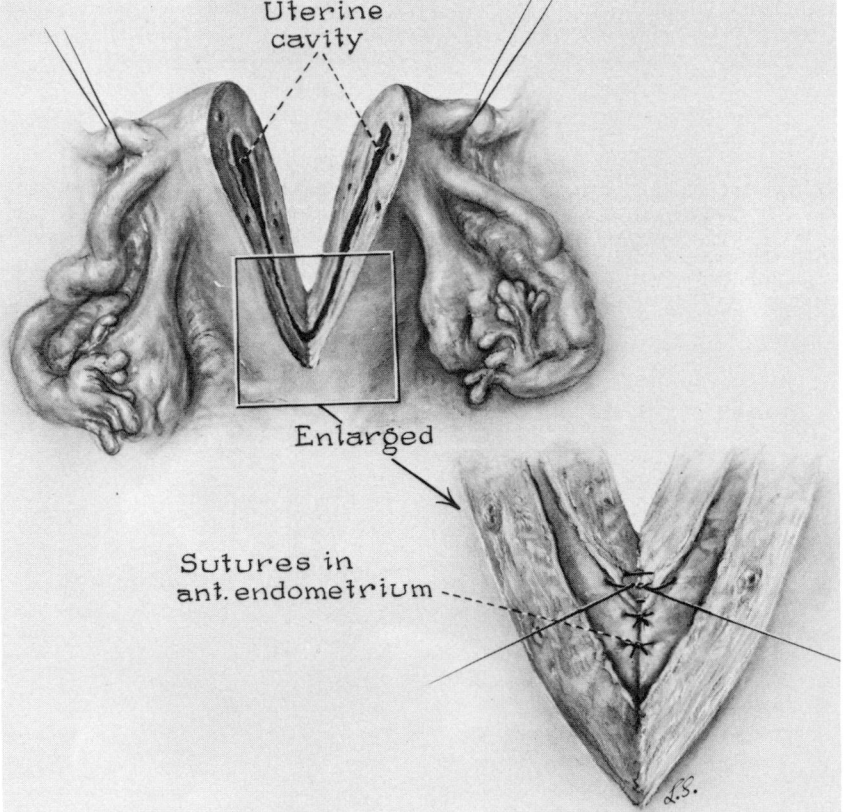

Uterine cavity

Enlarged

Sutures in ant. endometrium

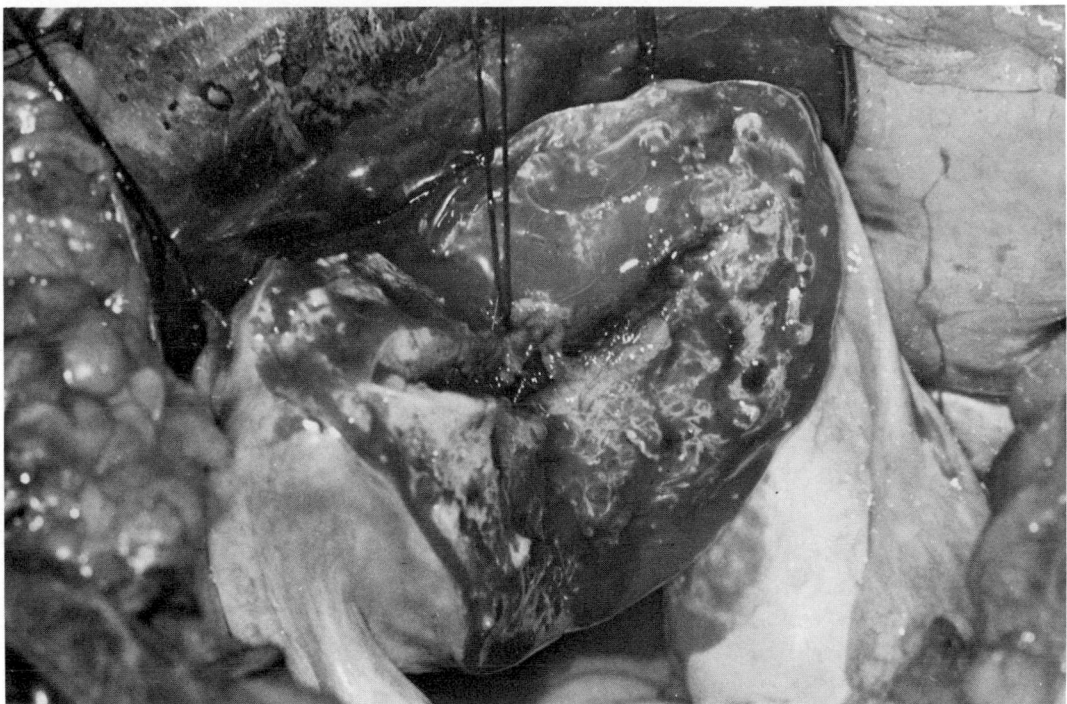

Fig. 6.32. The initial interrupted suture has been placed in the endometrium.

the uterus together, so that undue tension will not be placed on the tissue as the knots are tied (Fig. 6.32). Instead of continuing the stitches around the uterus to close entirely the endometrial cavity before introducing a second layer, it has proved desirable to place second layer myometrial stitches as the closure progresses in order to prevent the endometrial layer stitches cutting through under undue tension (Fig. 6.33). We have thought it important to limit the number of myometrial stitches in order to reduce the amount of buried catgut, although in no instance has lack of healing of the uterine incision seemed to be a problem (Fig. 6.34). The third layer of stitches through the serosal surface of the uterus can likewise be placed as the operation progresses (Fig. 6.35) before completing the endometrial closure (Fig. 6.36).

The operation is really not difficult, and there are relatively few opportunities for error, but on at least one occasion we have thought that we created an incompetent cervix by dividing the septum down through the cervix. We, therefore, now believe that with a complete double uterus, *i.e.,* one in which the septum penetrates the cervix, it is better to leave the septum intact in the lower uterine segment and the cervix. This will prevent the surgical creation of incompetence of the cervix and should not of itself cause reproductive failure. If the retained septum in the cervix should cause problems at delivery, it can be removed at that time, although delivery by cesarean section is usual.

There is no reason to believe that healing in the nonpregnant uterus is to be compared with healing in the uterus at the time of cesarean section. The importance of this statement is in the fact that there have been very few ruptures of scars in nonpregnant uteri. However, it has been our recommendation that these patients be delivered by cesarean section prior to going into labor. This stems from the fact that many times these are premium pregnancies, and it would seem unwise to accept any additional hazard of labor when the delivery of a normal term child is so near at hand. Indeed, I know of only one rupture of a scar of a uterus sutured in the nonpregnant state after an operation for duplication of the Müllerian ducts.

It is probably unwise to advise pregnancy before a suitable period of healing. There really are no good data on this point, but it has been

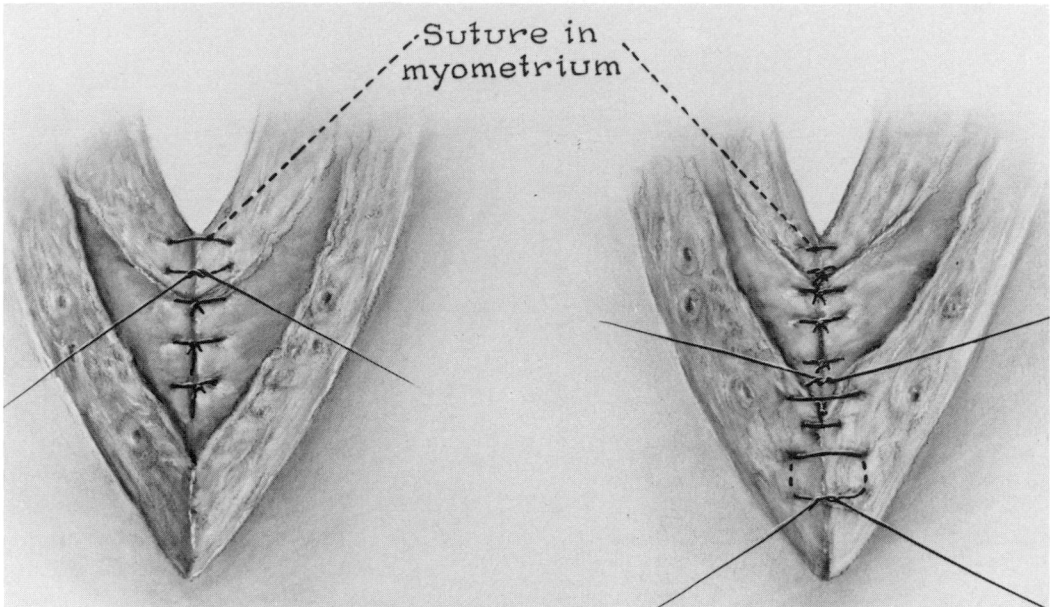

Fig. 6.33. The placement of the buried myometrial sutures. Note that sutures have also been placed in the anterior and posterior endometrium with the knots tied inside the cavity, but the knots for the buried stitches will obviously have to be within the myometrium.

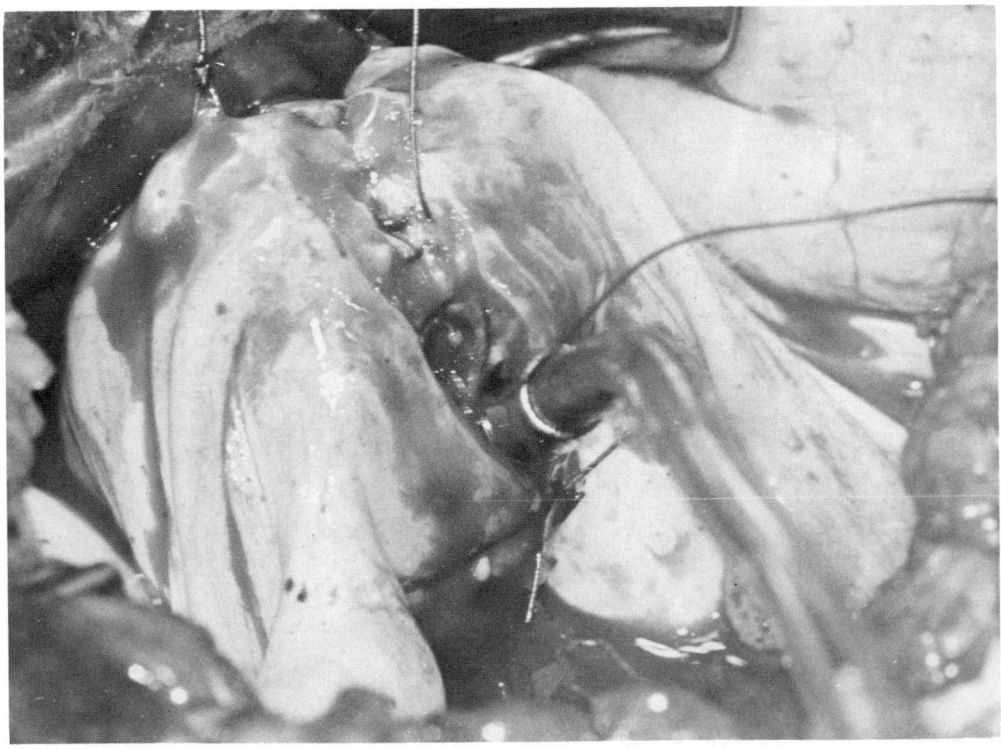

Fig. 6.34. A second layer, buried myometrial suture is placed.

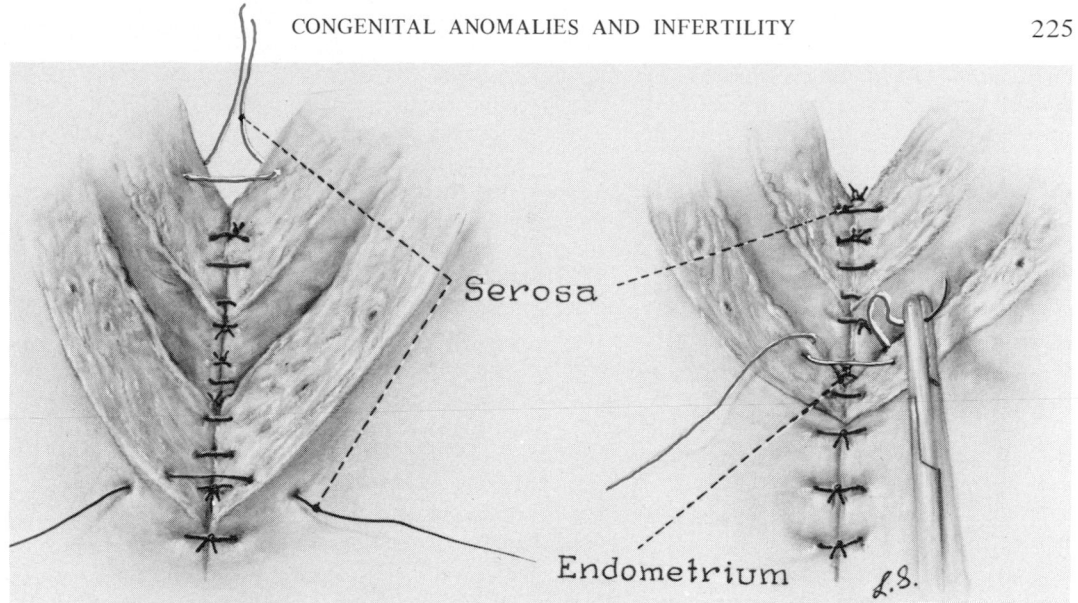

Fig. 6.35. The placement of sutures in the myometrium. Note that the sutures are placed in such a way that the knots are tied on the outside of the uterus.

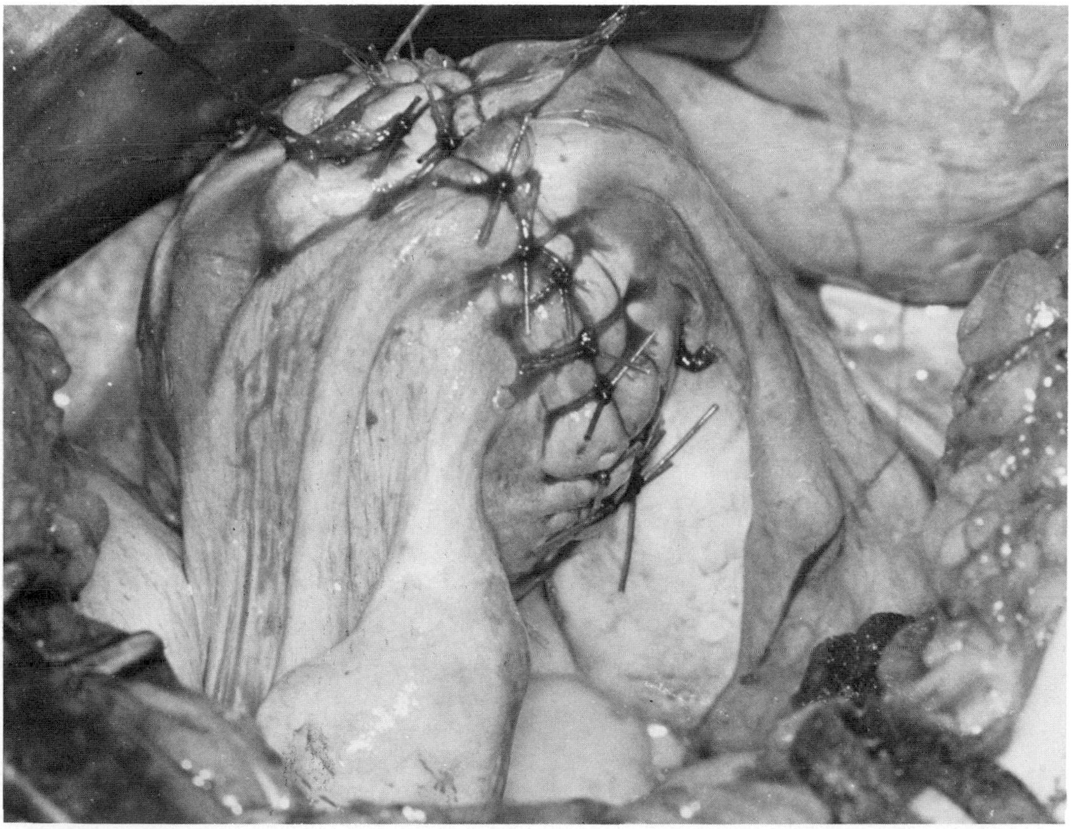

Fig. 6.36. The third layer of sutures is placed through the serosa. Note how close together the corneal portions of the tubes appear to be at the completion of the operation.

customary for us to recommend a minimal waiting period of 9 months. However, there have been some exceptions to this for we have had patients who became pregnant within 4 months of operation and had no undue difficulty.

With proper selection of patients, surgical reconstruction of the uterus is a very satisfactory operation. Approximately 85 per cent of patients with reproductive failure due to a double uterus will have a term delivery after operation.

Surgery for Impairment of Ovarian Function

Tumors, both benign and malignant, may interfere with normal cyclic function of the ovaries, even when unilateral. Removal when detected is beneficial. For patients whose families are incomplete, dissection of the benign cyst from the ovary should be attempted where salvageable tissue is present, including cysts of considerable size. Some adhesions, possibly incompatible with achieving pregnancy, may result from any incursion into the ovary. Corpora lutea and transient follicle cysts frequently distend to the ovary appreciably and the temptation to explore them when incidentally encountered should be resisted when future fertility is a consideration.

Stein-Leventhal Syndrome (Sclerocystic Ovarian Disease)

Although this is basically a medical disorder, it remains a rewarding target for surgery until more is learned about the medical treatment. This disturbance of the hypothalamic-pituitary-ovarian relationship which manifests itself in large smooth white ovaries, gross ovulation deficiency, infertility, and excess ovarian androgen production, responds remarkably well to wedge resection of the ovaries. The principal errors occur in improper selection of cases and inadequate resection of tissue.

Nature of the Disorder. The Stein-Leventhal syndrome, which is probably inherited as an autosomal dominant, involves fluctuating protracted elevation of luteinizing hormone (LH) levels (without ovulatory peak). Under this stimulus (accompanied by follicle-stimulating hormone (FSH) in smaller amounts) the ovaries develop multiple unruptured follicles sur-

rounded by excessive luteinized theca cells. Some similar cells appear in the hyperplastic stroma. The capsule, possibly as a result of the excess androgen, becomes thick and fibrous. Abnormal ovarian function accompanying these changes, and probably resulting from them, includes faulty synthesis of ovarian estradiol. Instead, the defective synthesis produces unusual amounts of androgen, especially androstenedione, dehydroepiandrostenedione, and testosterone. Some androstenedione thus produced is converted peripherally to estrogen which, when added to reduced amounts of ovarian estrogen and unopposed by progesterone in the anovulatory cycles, may stimulate endometrial hyperplasia, excessive bleeding, and even adenocarcinoma of the endometrium (15).

Clinical Indications. The ovarian failure results in skipped menstrual periods, irregular and excessive bleeding, and infertility. The distorted steroid synthesis, depending upon the amount and identity of androgens manufactured, produced recognizable hirsutism in 50 per cent of our cases.

Diagnosis. Recognition of the disease is based upon demonstrated persistent ovulation failure accompanied by bilaterally enlarged ovaries after elimination of other causes of anovulation and of excess androgen production (adrenal cortical hyperactivity, adrenal and ovarian steroid-producing tumors, or pituitary adenoma). Dexamethasone suppression test may be useful in separating adrenal cortical hyperactivity.

Endoscopy is very useful in confirming the diagnosis earlier than it might be otherwise and in reducing error.

Treatment. First, determination should be made as to whether any treatment is necessary to relieve symptoms. A period of observation may be useful. If fertility is not an issue, infrequent periods and the threat of hyperplasia and carcinoma may be satisfactorily and safely controlled by progesterone (75 mg I.M.) or Norlutin (5 mg × 5) every 2 months. Hirsutism is more troubling and is generally relieved very little by surgery. Plasma testosterone levels frequently fall some and remain less although usually do not return to normal. The net effect appears to be stopping the progression of the hirsutism.

Clomiphene has been used quite successfully

in inducing ovulation in patients exhibiting the Stein-Leventhal syndrome during the cycle of medication (77 per cent), but the pregnancy rates tend to be as low as 25 per cent (41 per cent of those induced to ovulate) (16, 18). Dosage should be approached cautiously (beginning at 50 mg daily for 5 days) because these ovaries appear particularly responsive. The patients who ovulate as a result of clomiphene medication but who fail to conceive have been shown to have an inadequate luteal phase in a high proportion of cases.

Except where ovarian masses remain large (5 to 6 cm), initial treatment should be with Clomid and, assuming satisfactory response, continued at least 6 months.

Wedge resection is highly successful in producing regular ovulation, and cases which respond usually continue indefinitely to ovulate regularly. A study of the long term results of 36 cases of wedge resection for Stein-Leventhal syndrome in a single practice at the Johns Hopkins Hospital showed 81 per cent ovulation induction (Table 6.2) and a pregnancy rate of 63 per cent of eligible patients (Table 6.3). Two more of these patients conceived after Clomid was added later when the operation failed to produce regular ovulation. These results are exactly comparable to others reported (17). Where a regular ovulatory cycle was restored following surgery, improvement usually persisted indefinitely. Contrary to Stein's original report, a quite consistent clinical feature of these patients was gross irregularity of the menstrual cycle from menarche (27 of 34 patients).

In a small but tragic number of cases the ovulation defect is corrected by wedge resection only to produce adhesive pelvic disease which prevents pregnancy. It would, therefore, seem preferable to attempt medical treatment first except where enlarged ovaries exist. Two of the 36 cases referred to above did have benign ovarian tumors accompanying Stein-Leventhal ovaries, and an additional one had a steroid-producing tumor of the adrenal cortex.

The principal surgical error is the excision of too little ovarian tissue. With enlarged ovaries, about one-half to two-thirds of the mass should be removed by wedge resection extending into the hilus, leaving ovaries approximately normal size. Results appear to be related to the adequacy of the wedge resection.

The Incompetent Cervix

The great variations in success of surgical correction of recurrent mid-trimester abortion due to cervical incompetence are due principally to differences in *accuracy of the diagnosis* and the *timeliness and adequacy of the surgery*. Reduction of these errors can substantially improve results.

Selection of Cases

A history of repeated painless effacement and dilatation of the cervix prior to bleeding or labor in the mid-trimester is highly suggestive of cervical incompetence. When first encountered during pregnancy, this has usually progressed too far for successful surgical repair. In the nonpregnant state, the incompetent cervix will admit easily the 8-mm Hegar dilator. Hysterosalpingogram can demonstrate the widening of the internal os. This technique was refined by Mann, McLarn, and Hayt (22) using a balloon. Since the cervix is most relaxed under the estrogenic influence of the proliferative phase, results may be misleading unless hysterograms exploring the possibility of incompetent cervix are done toward the end of a cycle. In the usual case the diagnosis is made on the basis of history of repeated mid-trimester abortion in

Table 6.2. Ovulation Induction after Wedge Resection for Stein-Leventhal Syndrome in 36 Patients

Follow-up	Patients	Regular Ovulation Postop.
<5 years	18	16 (89%)
5 to 14 years	14	10 (71%)
Total	32	26 (81%)

Table 6.3. Pregnancy Results after Wedge Resection for Stein-Leventhal Syndrome*

Term Pregnancy	Term Pregnancy after Clomid and Surgery	Total Pregnancies
12 (63%)	2 (11%)	14 (73%)

* A total of 19 patients were eligible for pregnancy and followed 1 year.

the absence of other identifiable cause.

It is important to exclude as far as possible other causes of reproductive deficiency through assessment of history, general health, hysterosalpingogram (double uterus or myoma), and endometrial biopsy (adequacy of premenstrual endometrium). Determination of pregnanediol excretion during the first and early second trimester will help to identify cases having a progesterone deficiency due to placental inadequacy and requiring only progesterone replacement.

Nonsurgical Treatment

The inability of the cervix to retain the growing pressure of a pregnancy may be due to (a) congenital deficiency of cervical fibrous tissue; (b) damage at delivery of prior pregnancy or dilatation of the cervix, especially that employed for therapeutic abortion; (c) deep cone biopsies or amputation of the cervix; or (d) premature initiation of whatever processes achieve softening and effacement of the cervix prior to labor. Except for the cases showing gross defects from trauma or surgery, it is usually difficult to know whether the valve (cervix) is giving way because of weakness of the valve or because of unusually increased pressure (hyperirritability of uterine muscle or multiple pregnancy). Mid-trimester aborters usually do demonstrate adequate progesterone production, but may benefit from supplementation with *large doses of Delalutin* to reduce uterine irritability. Sherman (23) obtained remarkably good results without surgery by treating habitual mid-trimester abortion patients with doses approximating 1000 mg of Delalutin initially and 500 to 1000 mg twice weekly. The use of such a regime is appealing (at the 500-mg, twice weekly dose), when uterine irritability is detectable, as an adjunct to surgery and may be useful alone when the diagnosis is uncertain.

The *Smith-Hodge pessary* alone appears to benefit some patients by changing the location of the cervix so as to bear the weight of the uterine contents through the lower uterine segment rather than through the weakened os. *Increased rest* will similarly reduce pressure and may be a useful adjunct in certain cases, but this is neither practical nor sufficient as the sole treatment. *Smoking and intercourse* should be restricted. The Baylor balloon (24) is an experimental silicone device which has been applied to the presumably incompetent cervix in a limited number of patients who have reached viability in gratifying proportions, but they have usually delivered prematurely. This nonoperative method must be used more before it can be evaluated.

Timing of Surgery

The common errors in timing of cerclage for a repeated aborter are (1) waiting for effacement and even dilatation to occur to reassure the operator that it really needs to be done, and (2) attempting surgical correction after dilatation in excessive (< 2 to 3 cm) or painless labor is in progress. The former is avoided by making the diagnosis on the basis indicated above and operating before effacement when possible or between pregnancies. The latter is avoided by using conservative measures in lieu of surgery and looking to a future pregnancy if untimely expulsion proceeds. When there is any question of labor, an observation period of 24 hours is indicated. Rest and Delalutin may be used during this interval.

Results are clearly better if cerclage is performed before effacement and dilatation have occurred. If the procedure is to be performed during pregnancy as is the general preference, it is best to wait until the pregnancy has grown successfully through the 12th week and therefore past the time for most genetically and environmentally predetermined abortions. Surgery after the 12th week and before the 15th week therefore seems preferable.

Repair prior to pregnancy is desirable for severe specific lacerations of the cervix and may be preferred when previous cerclage has failed. Such prepregnancy procedures involve permanently buried band or suture and must avoid fistula formation to the suture because of the troubling infection so generated over the time required for conception and an entire pregnancy. Keetle (25) obtained 19 living children from 20 operations on patients with two prior mid-trimester abortions using such an interval Shirodkar procedure. Mann *et al.* (22) using two buried polyethylene-enclosed dacron sutures had 32 of 36 such patients deliver successfully at term.

Type of Surgical Procedure

Installing a durable, nonabsorbable band around the incompetent cervix during pregnancy appears to be almost equally successful whether a buried permanent synthetic band is used (Shirodkar-Barter) (Fig. 6.37) or a removable suture is placed around the cervix (McDonald). Results, which were reported range from 60 to 80 per cent, but it is impossible to compare the severity of the cases and one suspects that the most difficult tend to be treated with the Shirodkar procedure. Failures most often involve the cerclage slipping off (usually the posterior lip), and selection and execution of the procedure should respect this fact.

Shirodkar-Barter Procedure (26). This technique employing a 5-mm wide mersilene band buried beneath the mucosa involves upward dissection of the bladder through a transverse incision in the anterior vaginal mucus membrane near the junction with the cervix (Fig. 6.38). This permits the band to be placed as high as possible toward the level of the internal cervical os. Shirodkar emphasized the importance of high posterior dissection to place the supporting band nearer the internal os there and reduce the tendency to slip off. The dissection with an aneurysm needle around both sides of the cervix has served well, but the use of a swedged-on needle appears to be simpler and to facilitate fixation of the encircling band into the cardinal and uterosacral ligaments and into the cervical muscle anteriorally and posteriorally (Fig. 6.39). If the dissection button-holes the mucus membrane, a fistula may be created and the band must be removed at delivery to reduce the risk of troubling infection. The successfully buried

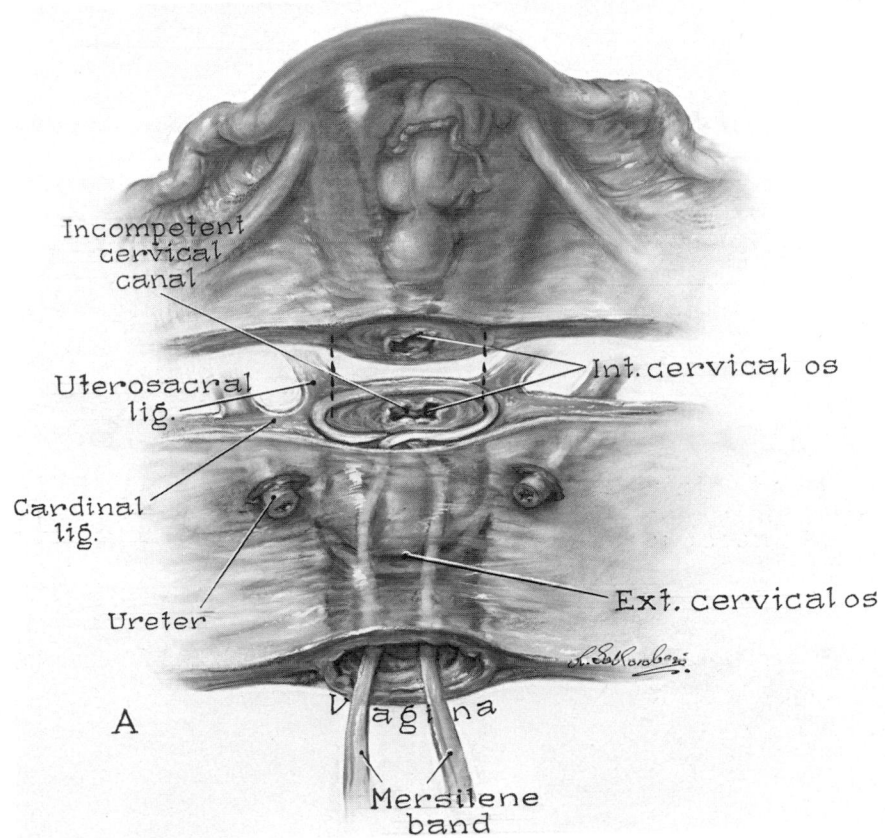

Fig. 6.37. Buried cerclage band in Shirodkar-Barter procedure, penetrating cardinal and uterosacral ligaments for more durable fixation. Installation as high as possible toward the internal os reduces slipping off, a common cause of failure.

band should usually be left in place and delivery accomplished by cesarean section.

Fistulae are more likely to occur if the mucus membrane has been penetrated during the procedure at other than the incision sites. However, the incision over the knot may fail to heal if the knot is too bulky. A remedy is to set only one layer of the knot with an extra loop and secure the knot arms with transfixing sutures of 00 silk (Fig. 6.40).

Jennings (28) has used successfully a temporary Shirodkar buried cerclage leaving the ends deliberately exposed for later removal prior to delivery. The installation of the sewed-in mersilene band is simplified by bringing the needle out at 9 and 3 o'clock and sewing back through the same hole. The possible fistula formation from this procedure is not of consequence since the band will be removed and the knot is already forming a fistula. The theoretical disadvantage of such a procedure is the tendency toward infection along the buried band, but none was encountered in the 48 cases reported.

The McDonald Encircling Suture (29). This method has the advantages of somewhat simpler installation and removal prior to delivery thereby permitting vaginal delivery. McDonald uses #4 braided mersilene sewed into the cervical mucus membrane and tissue in four quadrants, encircling the cervix as high as

possible. Hofmeister *et al.* (30) have used two mersilene bands on a swedged-on needle placed 1-cm apart for such a cerclage. A suitable compromise may be two #4 mersilene sutures similarly placed.

A transabdominal cerclage described by Benson and Durfee (31) offers a method of placing the band really high enough in selected patients where the cervix has been diminished by surgery, there is deep uncorrectable laceration, or previous cerclage has failed.

Although his experience has been principally during pregnancy, and there was troubling bleeding from distended veins in several cases with possibly interference with fetal oxygenation in one, overall results were good. The procedure can be accomplished probably more simply between pregnancies.

Problems Associated with Cerclage

1. Rupture of the uterus has been reported when unrecognized labor proceeded without removal of the band or the fetus. The procedure should not be performed in labor.

2. Infection is a lurking danger if the buried band is exposed to the vagina through a fistula over the months of exposure and resistant and virulent organisms tend to accumulate. Given the opportunity to invade, such as occurs with ruptured membranes without prompt evacua-

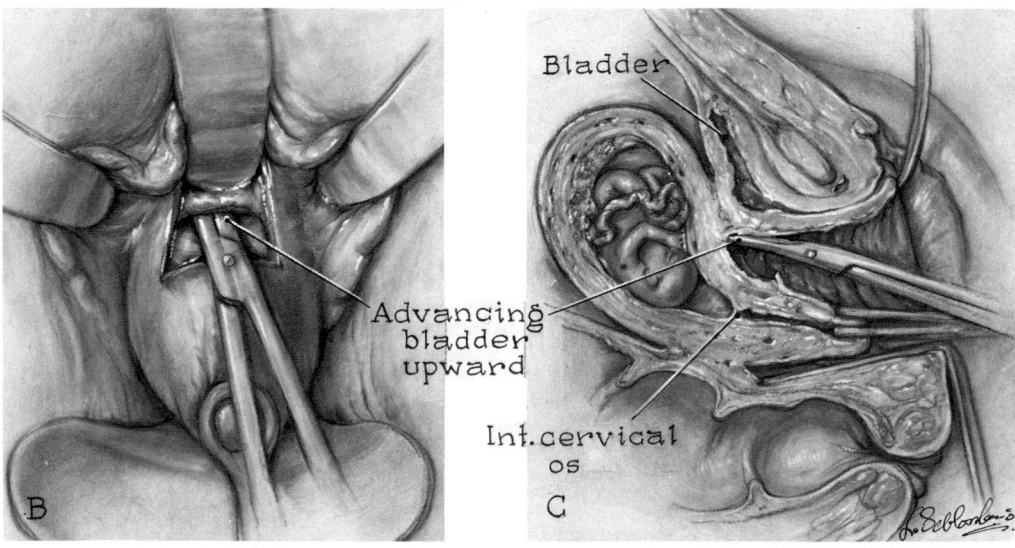

Fig. 6.38. B. Transverse incision into the anterior vaginal wall just above attachment to cervix. Bladder dissected up exposing bladder pillars and anterior cervix (C).

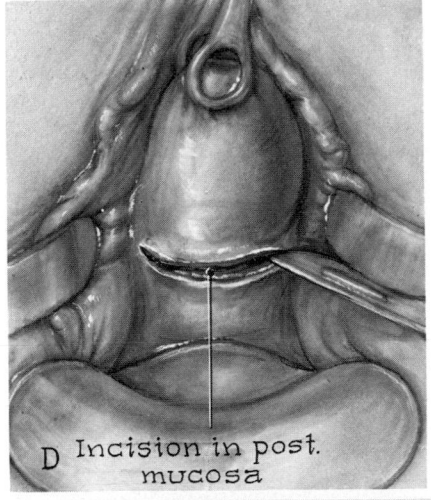

D Incision in post. mucosa

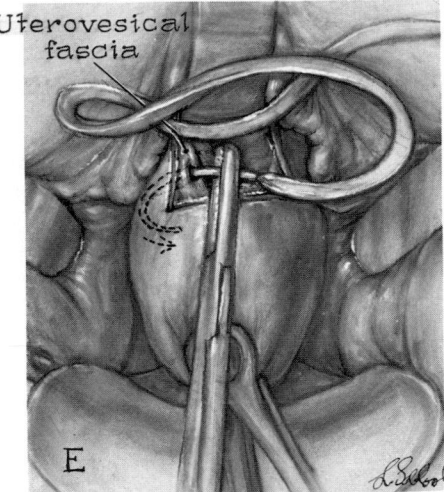

Uterovesical fascia

E

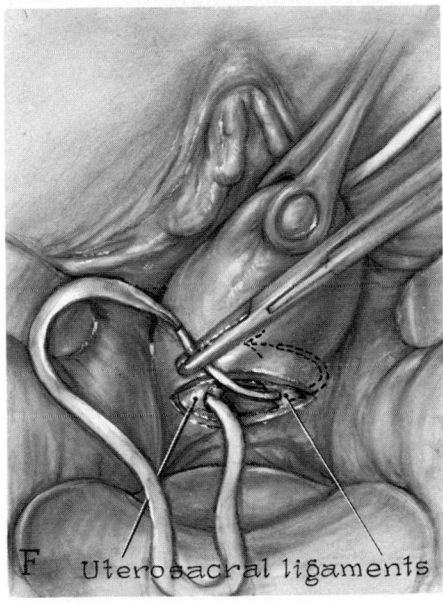

F Uterosacral ligaments

Fig. 6.39. D. Wide incision in posterior vagina just below cervix permits dissection posteriorly for high placement of suture. E. and F. Mersilene band sewed through cardinal ligaments and uterosacral ligaments for fixation to reduce slippage under subsequent stress.

tion of the uterus, serious consequences can be expected. If infection occurs, vigorous treatment is necessary.

3. Fistulae can be prevented as indicated above. The presence of a fistula should be investigated during pregnancy and suspected if unusual discharge occurs. If found, the band must be removed at delivery to reduce the danger of infection.

4. Cerclage slipping off can be reduced by placing it as high as possible, operating before effacement, and sewing it into the ligaments and the cervix.

5. Cerclage cutting through one or both lips of the cervix may be reduced by tying the band only as tight as will admit the tip of the index finger.

Tubal Surgery for Infertility

Surgery for the relief of infertility due to the incompetence of the Fallopian tubes is among the most unsuccessful in gynecology. This is due principally to (1) the extent of irreversible damage to the tube frequently present prior to operation, (2) the need for the repaired tube not only to be patent but to be functionally competent, and (3) the frequent failure to make best use of existing knowledge concerning selection of patients, techniques, and post-operative care.

The success rate of 9 per cent living children reported by Hellman based from questionnaire response may actually be better than overall experience, but the all inclusive 35 per cent success rate of Arronet, Eduljee, and O'Brien (36) reflects the consequences of concentrated attention to these patients. Surgery for the correction of lesions where the fimbriae have not been damaged should yield better results. A review of the overall experience in 43 cases operated upon by various surgeons, including residents, at the Johns Hopkins Hospital in the 3 years preceding 1971 shows a yield of 21 per cent living children (Table 6.4). Improved selection of cases and concentration of attention should improve results.

Prevention of Damage

Since surgical repair leaves so much to be desired, attention to the apparent genesis of tubal damage and its prevention is important. The apparent cause of tubal obstruction in various locations in these cases is indicated in Table 6.5. The importance of special vigilance in the diagnosis and treatment of pelvic infection in patients whose family is not complete is apparent. Attention to the following in nullipara will reduce sterility. (1) There should be greatly increased *suspicion of gonorrhea* and the use of cultures, with persistent treatment of patient and consort to negative cultures. (2) *The early diagnosis* and treatment of *endometriosis* are needed before the symptoms and physical findings are sufficient to

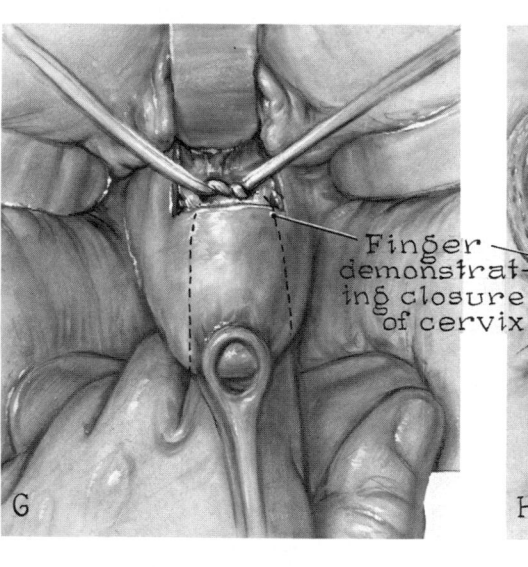

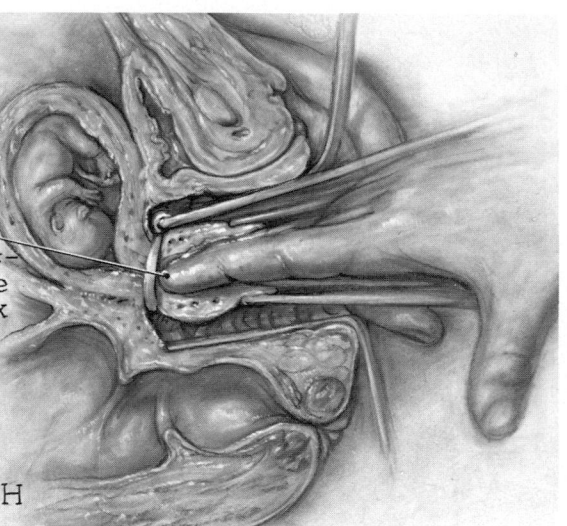

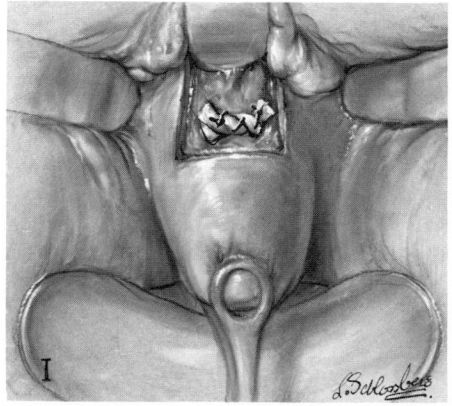

Fig. 6.40. G and H. Band secured by silk suture after double loop set snug for fingertip but not tight. I. A full square knot is bulky and tends to erode through the vaginal mucous membrane.

Table 6.4. Results of Tubal Surgery
(43 Cases, 1967-1970)

	Cases	Patient	Pregnant	Term Delivery
Peritubal adhesions	10	7	4	3 (30%)
Cornual implantation	10	8	4	4 (40%)
Cuff Fimbriolysis	16	11	4	2 (13%)
Hood	6	3	1	0
Mid-portion	1	1	1	0

Table 6.5. Probable Causes of Obstructive Tubal
Disease in 43 Cases

	Cornu	Fim-bria	Mid-por-tion	Peri-tubal Adhe-sions
Salpingitis		6		2
Salpingitis isthmica nodosa	3			
Prior acute appendicitis		1		3
Prior abortion	3			
Parovarian cysts		2		
Prior ectopic pregnancy	1	1		
Postpartum infection	1	1		1
Prior abdominal surgery	2	2		1
Endometriosis	2	2	1	1
Tubal ligation			1	
Unknown	1	2		3
	—	—	—	—
	13	17	2	11

make the diagnosis clear. More prompt endoscopy will conduce this. (3) *Every abortion* should be suspected of having retained tissue as a focus of infection until ruled out through exploratory gentle curettement with or without anesthesia. Antibacterial coverage is useful when any suspicion of contamination exists. (4) Surgery for *ectopic pregnancy* in nullipara is best not accompanied by appendectomy, and prophylactic antibiotics are helpful to reduce the frequency of infection and adhesive pelvic disease after the hematoperitoneum. (5) *All laparotomies* in such patients deserve special effort to prevent inflammatory adhesions, including elimination of glove powder. Maximal diagnostic effort to prevent unnecessary laparotomies, particularly in the young patient, will reduce tubal impairment.

Selection of Patients for Surgery

Desiderata. Successful pregnancy depends not only on achieving patency of the tubes but also on sufficient functional efficiency to transport and capacitate the sperm, capture the ovum after it bursts out of the ovary, provide a suitable milieu, and conduct the fertilized egg into the uterus at just the proper rate. This requires delicate, freely movable fimbria to move over the surface of the ovary and the cul-de-sac and considerable mobility of the entire tubes. It requires that the muscular wall be unencumbered by fibrosis and adhesions so that its peristalsis can conduct the ovum on its precise schedule. Healthy ciliated epithelium along the entire length including the cornu is also important to this journey.

Infertility Probably Due to Tubal Impairment. It is important to avoid surgery on patients where there is little hope of achieving pregnancy. It is also important to identify for surgery patients whose fertility is due to correctable tubal impairment of such a minor nature that no palpable or X-ray changes are found. *Thorough fertility investigation* should first exclude all other causes through general evaluation of the patient, including endometrial biopsy, husband's semen analysis, X-ray of the uterine cavity, and postcoital test of cervical mucus. Suitable cases may or may not involve total obstruction.

Three types of evidence are usually necessary to evaluate surgical potential, and at least two patency tests should be negative before obstruction is presumed. (1) *Hysterosalpingogram* should usually show whether the tubes are patent and, if not, the location of the obstruction. Any hydrosalpinx suggests probable damage of irretrievable proportion and low salvage possibility. Certainly one 3 cm or more in diameter should rarely be operated upon. Water-soluble dyes are preferable since oil-based material introduces small but definite risk of damaging foreign body inflammatory reaction before and after surgery (up to 6 months from installation). If obstruction at the cornu is found, the condition of the tube beyond must be assessed by endoscopy. It is quite possible to be mislead by one or more hysterosalpingo-grams showing no spill or no filling on one side when both tubes are normal. (2) *Rubin's tests,* recording the pressure at which carbon dioxide passes into the peritoneal cavity through the tube, give usually reliable evidence concerning patency and the adequacy of the opening. It is a useful initial test and supplements information from the salpingogram. (3) *Endoscopy* by laparoscope or culdoscope is important in estimating whether the extent of damage is essentially irreparable (large hydrosalpinx), the condition of the fibria, and if otherwise undetectable peritubal adhesions or endometriosis may, unsuspectingly, be impairing tubal function. Correctable cases so identified may demonstrate little or no impairment of tubal function as determined by hysterosalpingogram or Rubin's test.

Failure to obtain maximal preoperative information about the nature of the tubal factor in infertility is a common error. Also, nullipara requiring pelvic surgery for other reasons occasionally require a second operation because the tubal status was not considered prior to tubal surgery.

Corrective Surgery

When obstruction due to *peritubal adhesions* only is corrected surgically in patients shown to have no other impediment and to have significant interference with tubal freedom, results tend to be the best and have been reported as 53 per cent (38) and 59 per cent (36). Distinguishing between adhesions which are causative and those which are incidental is not precisely possible.

Obstruction at the mid-portion (Fig. 6.41) is most commonly encountered secondary to tubal ligation and may occasionally result from local infection. Success rate should exceed 65 per cent where the proximal portion is patent as shown by the hysterosalpingogram (Fig. 6.42). Resection and anastomosis over a splint are quite successful provided that 2 cm or more of the proximal portion are patent. Implantation into the cornu is required if the proximal portion of the tube is occluded. The largest splint which can be threaded into the anastomosis side is desirable, but since the tube narrows as it approaches the cornu, anastomosis near it requires a rather small splint (outside diameter .05 inches to .062 inches, PE 90 to 160). The anastomosis using 5-0 chromic catgut in four quadrants should seek to approximate the endosalpinx and the tubal wall without entering the lumen. To secure the splint in place, a suture (5-0 chromic) to the fimbriated end or, preferably, inside the tube .5 cm proximal to the anastomosis is quite satisfactory. Although the results with this procedure have been gratifying, the fixation suture in either location is an undesirable feature. The alternative of forcing a probe through the cornu into the uterus or opening the uterus and forcing a probe outward through the cornual portion seems even more traumatic. Where the tube stump is too short and small to accept the splint, a fine probe can lead small polyethylene (PE 90) through the cornual tube into the fundus. Through a small incision in the fundus, this can be threaded on a similar probe inserted through the opposite cornu and fixed to an IUD as described in the implantation procedure.

Usually, the distal end of the splint is brought through the lower abdomen on each side with a cutting needle and fixed to an occluding lead shot or button and sewed to the skin. It is essential that the lumen of the splint be unequivocally closed to prevent serious infection descending to the lumen. The securing suture in the splint will be dissolved in 14 to 20 days, and the splint should then be removed (see "Splints" below). Transuterine insufflation of the tube at this time and every 2 days thereafter until normal pressure readings occur appears to improve results.

When *obstruction at the cornu* is encountered in the presence of normal fimbriated ends and otherwise normal tubes, results of implantation are surprisingly good in experienced hands, although reports vary greatly (Table 6.6). The greater the length of the tube which can be preserved, the better the results. Determination of the extent of patency from the fimbria to the cornu is notoriously misleading. Probing with a normal size probe will certainly indicate obstruction sooner than it actually exists because of the naturally small diameter in that region. Probing with a fine flexible probe with or without a small bulb tip may be necessary. Retrograde insufflation through a large splint threaded into the tube is helpful in estimating the extent of patency. The pressure of this insufflation should not exceed 250 mm Hg to prevent blowouts and damaging of the tube. Passage of the gas into the uterus is palpable and audible.

The occluded cornual portion is excised (Fig. 6.43) and the endometrial cavity entered. Accurate identification of the site of the cornu is desirable because the uterus is thinner at that point and entry is more physiologic. A probe plunged through this area may be useful as a guide. A large cork borer may be used for this purpose. However, excision of the occluded portion and opening the cornu sufficiently to approximate the endosalpinx and the endometrium precisely are desirable. Shirodkar opened the entire fundus transversely from one cornu to the other for this purpose. A splint of the largest diameter which can be drawn easily through the patent portion of the distal tube is then selected. A silastic splint with an outside diameter of .065 inches is usually suitable. When the distal tube accepts it, sizes up to .095 inches diameter may be used. Equivalent polyethylene sizes are PE 160 and 240. The mid-portion of the splint may be retained in the uterine cavity for later removal by forming a Shirodkar loop with a small wire in the lumen or by securing this splint to an IUD. Bringing the ends of the splint through the cervix predisposes to ascending infection, and the

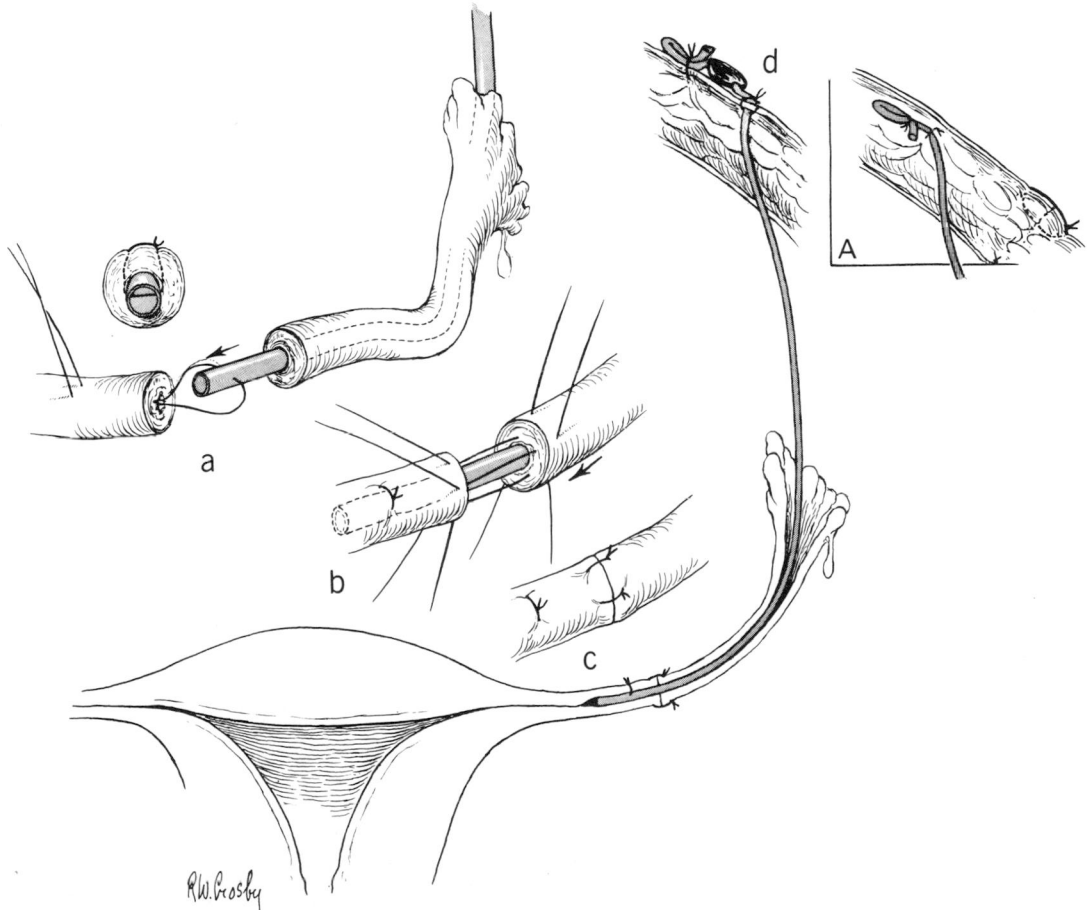

Fig. 6.41. Repair of occlusion at mid-portion (including tubal ligation). Obstructed portion has been resected using sharp knife to obtain fresh edges. Catheter threaded through distal tube following fine wire probe (a). Suture (5.0 chromic catgut) transfixing catheter sewed through its lumen 1 cm into proximal tube. Catheter fed into proximal tube (b) and four fine sutures set for anastomosis (c). All layers of the tube wall are included in the suture, including the endosalpinx, attempting to avoid the lumen. d, Tube drawn through lower quadrant of abdomen with stay suture needle (or through incision if transverse), tied, closed carefully, fixed with lead bead, and fixed to skin. Inset A, alternative fixation under skin. Pre- and postoperative medication is important to success (see text).

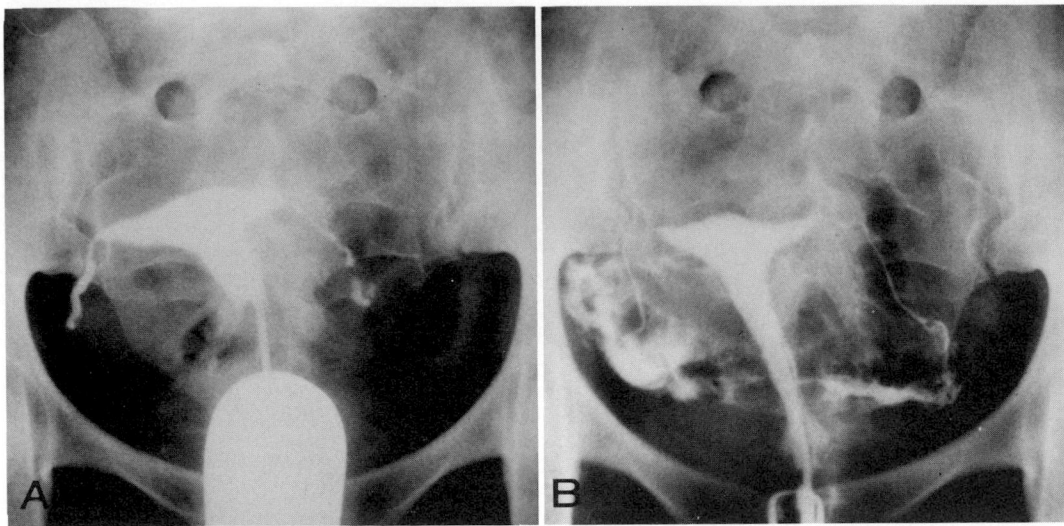

Fig. 6.42. Hysterosalpingogram (A) after tubal ligation and (B) after reanastomosis. Slight dilatation of the proximal portion of the ligated tube is not uncommon, occasionally due to endometriosis in this portion. Also, the pressure of the instilled liquid may contribute to this appearance. Six weeks after reanastomosis, both tubes appear delicate and patent with peritoneal spill (B).

Table 6.6. Results of Implantation Operation for Obstruction at Interstitial Portion of Tube

Author	Cases	Patient	Pregnancies
Green-Armitage (1957) (43)	38		14 (37%)
Mulligan (1953) (44)	48	24	5 (10%)
Shirodkar (1960) (45)	140	90	49 (35%)
Garcia (1968) (39)	14	8	2 (14%)
O'Brien et al. (1969) (46)	36		15 (41%)

fixation to the cervix tends to slip after days or weeks. A 000 chromic suture is placed on both sides of the proximal portion of the remaining patent tube. Individually the two arms of each suture are sewed through the open cornu from the endometrial cavity out through the uterine wall on the side of origin, the tube drawn into the junction with the endometrial cavity, and these sutures tied to each other to secure it. The cornu is then approximated and the last suture includes the wall of the tube to further secure it in place. Certain failures occur when the tube becomes displaced from its cornual implantation to the endometrium. The protruding ends of the splint are trimmed to project

about 1 cm from the fimbria. The splint is left in place for 3 months (Shirodkar used 6 months), and the intrauterine loop or IUD is easily retrieved without anesthesia with any suitable IUD removal hook or with a closely bent probe. When patients bear children following this procedure, cesarean section should be elected because of the danger of rupture of the cornu even where the opening is no greater than that formed by the borer.

Occlusion at the fimbriated end (Fig. 6.44) is the most unlikely site to be successfully repaired because of the difficulty of restoring free functioning fimbria. Table 6.7 shows some results. The repair of significant hydrosalpinx should usually be avoided. Amputation of the clubbed end and turning back the remaining end of the tube (Sovak cuff) has produced predictably dismal results in terms of pregnancies, and alternative methods should be used if surgery is attempted.

Careful dissection of adhesions which close the fimbria may result in restoration of rather natural and functioning fimbria. Insufflation through the uterus during surgery may identify thin areas where such separation of adhesions may best be approached. Penetration with a fine hemostat and blunt dissection may be necessary. A dimple or fine groove may suggest the optimal point of entry, but this must be quite thin if results are to be successful. When the best practical opening and fimbria exposure have been achieved and hemostasis is carefully obtained, preferably with electrocautery, a decision as to measures to conduce maintenance of patency during healing is necessary. Sutures to hold open the fimbria have a disadvantage of compromising the future freedom to function in seeking and capturing the egg, and they tend to generate more adhesions around the site of their location. When used, they should be of 5-0 plain catgut and placed very close to the natural position of the fimbria.

The results with silastic hoods in the hands of Garcia and Mulligan command respect. This requires a second operation, and our results have been discouraging probably because of selection of the worst patients. The second operation frequently permits release of fine postoperative adhesions which do not reform. When silastic is used in any form, its tendency

to attract lint because of static electricity should be appreciated, and the contact with cloth avoided both in sterilization and at surgery. The spiral stent of Roland (37), which can be removed through traction on its transabdominally exposed end, offers some promise of a simpler procedure. Since soluble sutures are used to hold it in the tube, it cannot be expected to remain in that location much beyond 3 weeks. The use of no stent after dissection is another acceptable course for appropriate cases provided that careful pre- and postoperative programs indicated below are used to minimize adhesive consequences.

Medical Measures to Improve Surgical Results

During the days following surgery, and especially the first 48 hours, a competition of some importance occurs between tubal epithelium attempting to line the operative area and

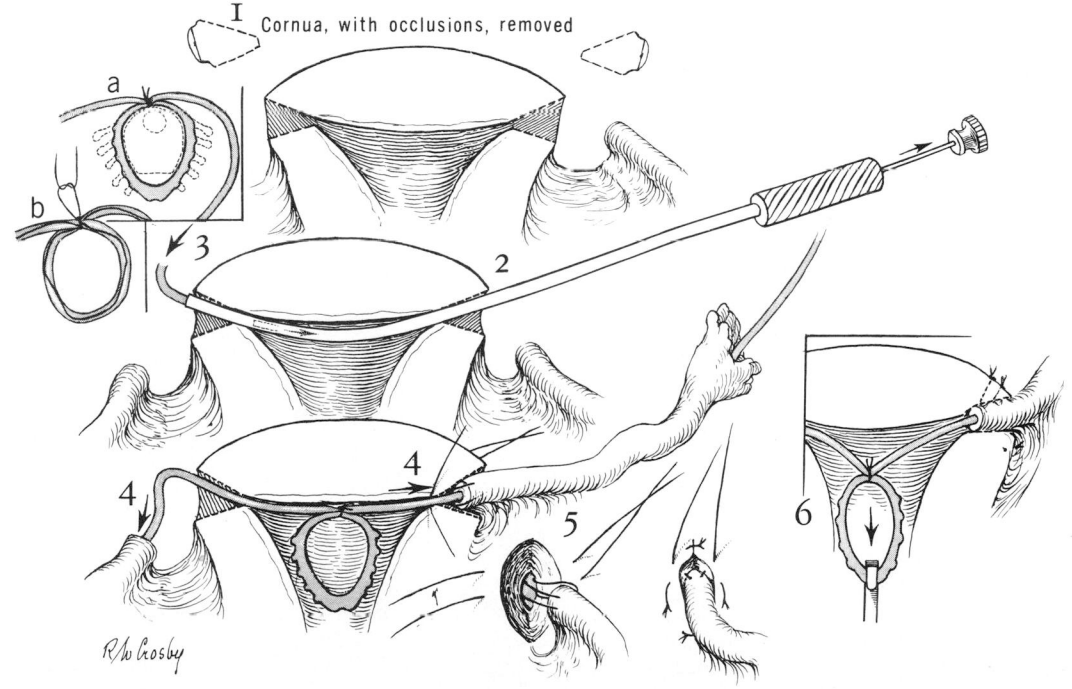

Fig. 6.43. Repair of cornual occlusion. (1) Occluded cornua excised (knife or cork borer), (2) curved cannula or long Kelly clamp introduced from one cornu through the other, (3) prosthesis introduced in the uterus and protruding ends threaded through tubes (4). Prosthesis made at operating table (a) of silastic tubing (autoclaved) tied to trimmed Dalkon shield (presterilized new or gas-sterilized) with dacron or nylon suture (four tight knots). Silastic protected from touching cloth. Silastic with wire obturator (b) (Shirodkar loop) (¾ inches in diameter). (5) Tubes sewed to cornua approximating endosalpinx to endometrium. Cornua closed, one suture catching serosal surface of tube. (6) Removal of prosthesis by hook passed through cervix.

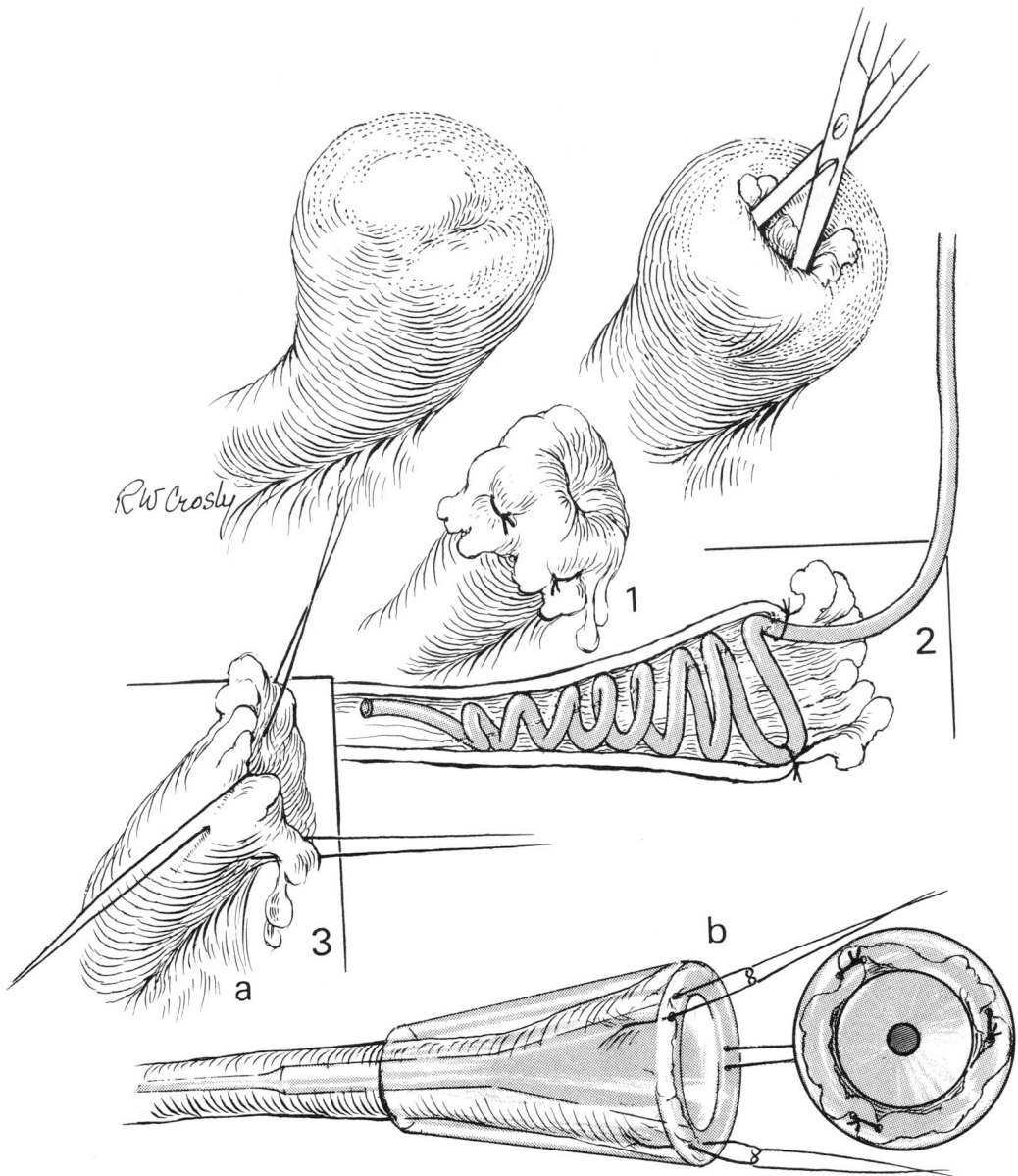

Fig. 6.44. Repair of occlusion at fimbriated end. Dissection of adhesions, especially those of tube to ovary, may release delicate functional fimbria. Where occlusion persists and the tube is not extensively damaged by hydrosalpinx, fimbria may be released by penetrating the thinnest spot in the occlusive adhesions—usually a slight dimple—and delicately dissecting adhesions. In ideal cases, where no raw surfaces result from dissection, no further surgical procedure may be needed to conduce persisting functional freedom of the fimbria. Usually some further protection against readhesion is prudent by one of the following: (1) holding fimbria open by two or three sutures of 5-0 plain catgut as close to the natural position as possible (a "cuff" looks appealing but is unphysiologic); (2) the Roland splint sewed into the opened fimbria with two or three sutures of 5-0 chromic catgut, combining simplicity, removal without future abdominal surgery, and a physiologic status of the tube; or (3) the fimbria drawn into the Mulligan silastic hood by 3-0 dacron sutures and anchored at the base of the hood by the same material. These knots untie easily unless tightly tied four times. The reoperation for removal of the hoods often confers the additional benefit of separating filmy adhesions which may not recur.

Table 6.7. Results Following Surgical Correction of Obstruction at Fimbriated End

Author	Technique	Cases	Patient	Pregnancies
Ingersoll (1949) (47)	Cuff salpingostomy	18	6 (33%)	0
Pratt (1956) (48)	Salpingostomy	15		0
Mulligan (1953) (44)	Polyethylene hood	21	13 (64%)	2 (9%)
Mulligan (1966) (49)	Silastic hood	45	39 (87%)	9 (21%)*
Garcia (1968) (39)	Silastic hood	25	19 (76%)	7 (28%)†
O'Brien *et al.* (1969) (46)		80	20	24%

* Plus three miscarriages and four ectopic pregnancies.
† Plus one miscarriage and two ectopic pregnancies.

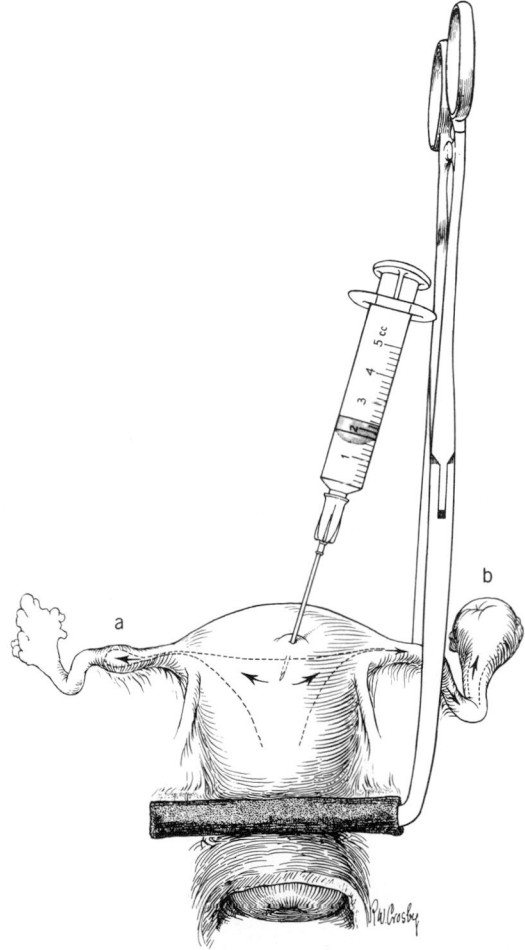

Fig. 6.45. Retrograde determination of patency at surgery. Cervix occluded with Siegler-Hellman clamp and dye (diluted indigo carmine) injected to determine site of obstruction shown here as mid-portion (a) and fimbria (b). Carbon dioxide insufflation connected to Rubin's pressure gauge through same needle is also useful to determine the degree of obstruction before

combat inflammation and fibrous tissue seeking to close the tube and form adhesions. *Unopposed estrogen* produces proliferation and heightening of the tubal epithelium and appears to reduce tubal susceptibility to inflammation (38). Therefore, in anticipating the postoperative period, it is necessary to block ovulation in the cycle of operation with estrogen (stilbestrol 2 mg daily from day 5 of cycle), operate at about mid-cycle, and continue this beneficial influence for 2 weeks postoperatively. *Cortisone* in adequate doses inhibits fibrous tissue growth and may reduce occlusive tendency and adhesion formation. The continuous presence afforded by the systemic route of administration is beneficial on a schedule approximating 125 mg the first day in divided doses, 100 mg on days 2 and 3, and 75 mg on days 4 and 5. No difficulty with incision healing has been encountered by us, although animal experiments suggest some retardation therein. It may be prudent to close the abdomen with nonabsorbable sutures if this medication is anticipated.

Broad spectrum antibiotics to reduce the incidence and extent of bacterial infection and consequent adhesions appear indicated prophylactically in this type of surgery.

Hydrotubation with antibiotics and cortisone has been used to facilitate the above objectives and as a dilator of tubal patency. The intermittent and superficial presence of these medications would not appear to make it a suitable substitute for systemic medication. As an adjunct it may or may not be beneficial, since some degree of bacterial invasion may be generated. One suitable solution includes neo-

and after repair. Excessive pressure on syringe can create false passages and misleading results.

mycin ½ per cent and 25 mg cortisone in 30 cc of normal saline or 0.5 per cent neomycin.

General Principles of Tubal Surgery

Too frequently, because life is not threatened, tubal surgery does not receive sufficient attention to confer upon the trusting and deserving patients the maximal opportunity of success. Adequate preoperative investigation, preoperative preparation of patient and apparatus, and adequate time, incision, instruments, and devices are all needed.

Gentle handling of tissues requires small instruments and adequate exposure. Fine flex-ible probes with and without small bulb ends are important in exploring the extent of patency and in leading splints through. A choice of sizes of tubing is helpful, both for use as a vehicle for retrograde insufflation to determine the extent of patency, as well as for use as splints. The pressure applied to gas so introduced should be limited to 250 mm Hg to avoid damage to the tubes. Preoperative work-up should reduce the need for trans-uterine insufflation during operation, but this can be helpful. It can be accomplished during abdominal surgery by occlusion of the cervix with the Siegler-Hellman clamp and injecting saline or indigo carmine solution (Fig. 6.45).

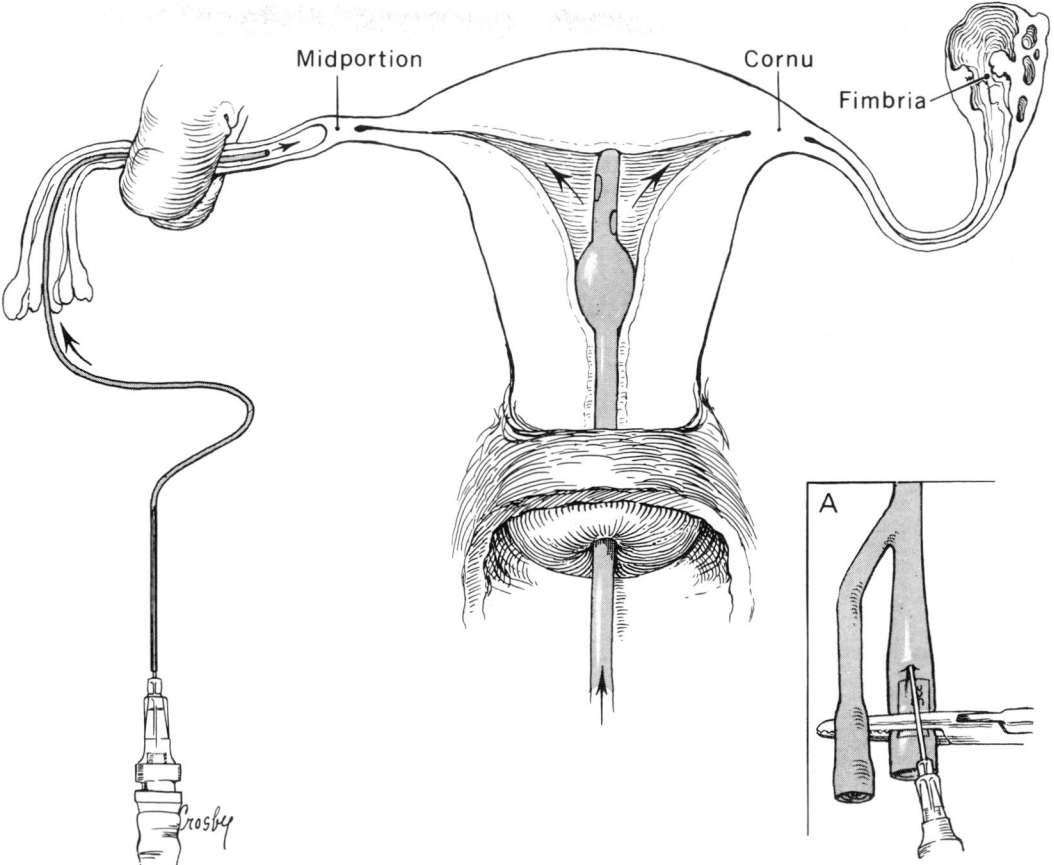

Fig. 6.46. Locating obstruction and determining extent of patency. Foley catheter (#14) inserted, inflated with 1½ cc saline, occluded, and needle inserted and connected by sterile plastic extension to syringe for dye injection or to Rubin's apparatus for CO_2 insufflation and determination of pressure required for patency, pre- and postoperatively. Extent of tubal patency determined at left by retrograde threading polyethylene catheter into tube and gently insufflating. Patency is frequently found to be greater than the probe has detected. This arrangement is most useful for instillation of dye during culdoscopy. Needle shown in inset A is connected to a plastic extension tubing or rubber tubing from Rubin's manometer in order to be clear of drapes.

Pressure should be controlled to prevent damage. A #14 Foley catheter inserted into the fundus preoperatively and held in place with 1½ cc of saline in its balloon is usually satisfactory for connection to a Rubin's tubal insufflation apparatus (Fig. 6.46).

Splints. The importance of intraluminal inert splints during the regenerative postoperative period is amply demonstrated in reported results. *Polyethylene tubing* has been used the longest and is still useful because it is pliable and soft and can be sewed with less tearing and breaking than silastic.

Silastic stimulates less reaction from tissue in contact with it, but is so soft as to tear easily, especially if sewed in sizes smaller than .065 inches diameter. Care to avoid acquisition of lint through contact with cloth is necessary.

Teflon is also especially nonreactive but is stiffer than either of the above and may cause concern (and pain) as the end protruding from the tubes impinges upon intestines.

For tubal anastamosis such small diameters are required (PE 90 or 160; .050 to .062 inches) that polyethylene or Teflon are necessary.

For cornual implantation the larger silastic tubing can be handled satisfactorily, and since the prosthesis will remain in place for 3 months, its lower tissue reactivity is an advantage. The Shirodkar loop must retain some diameter or it will deliver through the cervix. A steel wire in the loop portion serves this purpose but, if forced through a small opening at the cornu, will be compressed and not regain the loop configuration. The IUD avoids this problem.

Fixation of splint through the abdominal wall is useful for retrieval where the uterine cavity cannot be entered without damaging the tube or uterus. It is conveniently fixed by passage through a lead shot which grips it when compressed. Serious infection descending into the repaired tube has precluded success when the splint has been incompletely occluded or traumatized and opened accidentally. Antibacterial ointment is useful when this is sewed to the skin where short duration of placement is expected (2 to 3 weeks). Where the splint will be left in place for longer periods and recovered through the abdominal wall, the splint may best be buried just under the skin and removed under local anesthesia, eliminating the risk of accidental descending infection.

Bibliography

Congenital Absence of the Vagina and Uterus

1. Cali, R. W., and Pratt, J. H.: Congenital absence of the vagina. Long-term results of vaginal reconstruction in 175 cases. Am. J. Obstet. Gynecol. 100: 752, 1968.
2. Ulfelder, H.: Agenesis of the vagina. A discussion of surgical management and functional and morphologic comparison of end results, with and without skin grafting. Am. J. Obstet. Gynecol. 100: 745, 1968.
3. Counseller, V. S., and Davis, C. E.: Atresia of the vagina. Obstet. Gynecol. 32: 528, 1968.
4. Page, E. W., and Owsley, J. Q., Jr.: Surgical correction of vaginal agenesis. Am. J. Obstet. Gynecol. 105: 774, 1969.

Myomata Uteri

5. Brown, A., Chamberlain, R., and Te Linde, R. W.: Myomectomy. Am. J. Obstet. Gynecol. 71: 759, 1956.
6. Dearnley, G.: The place of myomectomy in the treatment of primary infertility. Proc. R. Soc. Med. 49: 252, 1956.
7. Ingersoll, F. M.: Fertility following myomectomy. Fertil. Steril. 14: 596, 1963.
8. Stevenson, C. S.: Myomectomy for improvement of fertility. Fertil. Steril. 15: 367, 1964.
9. Loeffler, F. E., and Noble, A. D.: Myomectomy at the Chelsea Hospital for Women. J. Obstet. Gynaecol. Br. Commonw. 77: 167, 1970.
10. Jones, H. W., Jr., Davis, H. J., and Frost, J. K.: Opportunities and procedures for the early diagnosis of carcinoma of the cervix. Md. State Med. J. 21: 54, 1972.

Double Uterus

11. Jones, H. W., Jr., Delfs, E., and Jones, G. E. S.: Reproductive difficulties in double uterus. The place of plastic reconstruction. Am. J. Obstet. Gynecol. 72: 865, 1956.
12. Jones, H. W., Jr., and Wheeless, C. R.: The salvage of the reproductive potential of women with anomalous development of the Mullerian ducts: 1868-1968-2068. Am. J. Obstet. Gynecol. 104: 348, 1969.
13. Strassmann, P.: Die Operative Vereinigung eines Doppelten Uterus. Zentralbl. Gynaekol. 31: 1322, 1907.
14. Tompkins, P.: Comments on the bicornuate uterus and twinning. Surg. Clin. North Am. 42: 1049, 1962.

Surgery for Impairment of Ovarian Function

15. Jackson, R. L., and Dockerty, M. B.: Stein-Leventhal syndrome: Analysis of 43 cases with

special reference to association with endometrial carcinoma. **Am. J.** Obstet. Gynecol. 73: 161, **1957.**

16. Greenblatt, R. B., Zarate, A. T., and Mahesh, V. B.: Gynecological Endocrinology, edited by J. J. Gold, p. 406. Hoeber Division, Harper and Row, New York, 1968.

17. Goldzieher, J. W.: Progress in Infertility, edited by S. J. Behrman and R. W. Kistner, p. 371. Little, Brown and Co., Boston, 1968.

18. Kistner, R. W.: Progress in Infertility, edited by S. J. Behrman, and R. W. Kistner, p. 419. Little, Brown and Co., Boston, 1968.

19. Kistner, R. W.: Principles and Practice of Gynecology, 2nd. ed. Year Book Publishers, Inc., Chicago, 1970.

20. Leventhal, M. L.: Gynecological Endocrinology, edited by J. J. Gold, p. 478. Hoeber Division, Harper and Row, New York, 1968.

21. Goldzieher, J. W., and Axelrod, L. A.: Clinical and biochemical features of polycystic disease. Fertil. Steril. 14: 631, 1963.

The Incompetent Cervix

22. Mann, E. C., McLarn, W. D., and Hayt, O. B.: The physiology and clinical significance of the uterine isthmus. Am. J. Obstet. Gynecol. 81: 209, 1961.

23. Sherman, A. I.: Hormonal therapy for control of the incompetent os of pregnancy. Obstet. Gynecol. 28: 198, 1966.

24. Yosovitz, E. E., Haufrect, F., Kaufman, R. H., and Goyette, R. E.: Silicone-plastic cuff for the treatment of the incompetent cervix. Am. J. Obstet. Gynecol. 113: 233, 1972.

25. Keetle, W. C.: Discussions of paper by R. H. Barter *et al.*, 1963 (ref. 27).

26. Barter, R. H., Dusabeck, J. A., Aiva, H. L., and Parks, J.: Closure of incompetent cervix during pregnancy. Am. J. Obstet. Gynecol. 75: 511, 1958.

27. Barter, R. H.: Further experience with the Shirodkar operation. Am. J. Obstet. Gynecol. 85: 792, 1963.

28. Jennings, S. L.: Temporary submucosal cerclage for cervical incompetence. Am. J. Obstet. Gynecol. 113: 1097, 1963.

29. McDonald, I. A.: Incompetent cervix as a cause of recurrent abortion. J. Obstet. Gynaecol. Br. Commonw. 70: 105, 1963.

30. Hofmeister, F. J., Schwartz, W. R., Vondrak, B. F., and Martens, W.: Suture reinforcement of incompetent cervix. Am. J. Obstet. Gynecol. 101: 58, 1968.

31. Benson, R. C., and Durfee, R. B.: Cervicouterine cerclage. Obstet. Gynecol. 25: 145, 1965.

32. Hefner, J. D., Paton, W. E., and Ludwig, J. M.: A new procedure for the correction of the incompetent cervical os during pregnancy. Obstet. Gynecol. 18: 616, 1961.

33. Lash, A.: Habitual abortion: The incompetent internal os of the cervix. Am. J. Obstet. Gynecol. 59: 68, 1950.

34. Nishijima, S.: Antepartum cervical cerclage operations. Am. J. Obstet. Gynecol. 104: 173, 1969.

35. Shaalan, M. K.: A simple midcervical cerclage for cervical incompetence during pregnancy. Am. J. Obstet. Gynecol. 107: 969, 1970.

Tubal Surgery for Infertility

36. Arronet, G. H., Eduljee, S. Y., and O'Brien, J. R.: A nine year survey of fallopian tube dysfunction in human infertility. Fertil. Steril. 20: 903, 1969.

37. Roland, M.: Spiral Teflon stent for tuboplasty involving fimbria. Obstet. Gynecol. 36: 359, 1970.

38. Andrews, M. C., and Andrews, W. C.: Plastic reconstruction of the Fallopian tubes using polyethylene catheters. Am. J. Obstet. Gynecol. 70: 1232, 1955.

39. Garcia, C. R.: Surgical reconstruction of the oviduct in the infertile patient. In Progress in Infertility, edited by S. J. Behrman and R. W. Kistner, Little, Brown and Co., Boston, 1968.

40. Murray, E.: Peritoneal factor in sterility. Clin. Obstet. Gynecol. 5: 836, 1962.

41. Siegler, A. M.: Salpingoplasty: Classification and report of 115 operations. Obstet. Gynecol. 34: 339, 1969.

42. Shirodkar, V. N.: Plastic surgery of Fallopian tubes. West J. Surg. Obstet. Gynecol. 69: 253, 1961.

43. Green-Armitage, V. B. Tubo-uterine implantation. Brit. Med. J. 1: 1222, 1952 and J. Obstet. Gynaec. Brit. Emp. 64: 47, 1957.

44. Mulligan, W. J. et al.: Use of polyethylene in tuboplasty. Fertil. Steril. 4: 428, 1953.

45. Shirodkar, V. N. Contributions to Obstetrics and Gynecology. Livingstone, Edinburgh, 1960. p. 65.

46. O'Brien, J. R. et al.: Operative treatment of Fallopian tube pathology in human fertility. Am. J. Obstet. Gynec. 103: 520, 1969.

47. Ingersoll, F. M.: Plastic operation on fallopian tube. N. Eng. J. Med. 241: 686, 1949.

48. Pratt, J. H. et al.: Reconstruction operations for obstruction of fallopian tubes. Am. J. Obstet. Gynec. 71: 1097, 1956.

49. Mulligan, W. J.: Results of salpingostomy. Int. J. Fertil. 11: 424, 1966.

50. Umezaki, C., Katayama, K. P., and Jones, H. W., Jr.: Pregnancy rates after reconstructive surgery on the Fallopian tubes. Obstet. Gynecol. 43: 418, 1974.

CHAPTER SEVEN

J. DONALD WOODRUFF, M.D., AND CONRAD J. JULIAN, M.D.

SURGERY OF THE VULVA; VULVECTOMY

A wide variety of surgical procedures have been employed in the treatment of vulvar disease ranging from the minor coagulative approaches to the simple, but often recurrent vulvar wart, to the extensive radical vulvectomy and node dissection currently accepted as the therapy of choice for vulvar cancer. In general, complications may be avoided by the correct evaluation of the pathologic process, knowledge of the anatomy of the area, utilization of the proper procedure for the patient and her disease, and meticulous attention to technique and postoperative care.

Trauma

Minor trauma to the vulva is not uncommon, affords little if any discomfort to the patient, and thus is seldom brought to the attention of the physician. Major trauma is rare but occurs particularly during the first and second decades of life. Hematomas usually develop as the result of "a fall astraddle" a rigid object and, as a rule, are self-limiting (Fig. 7.1). However, it is important to recognize that the tissues of the external genitalia are extremely loose and as a result, extravasated blood may dissect cephalad over the mons and caudally into the perineum to be limited only by the restricting fascial planes. If the patient is seen immediately after the accident and the spread of the hematoma cannot be controlled by pressure, an attempt to evacuate the accumulating clot and to ligate the bleeding vessel should be undertaken.

The recovery period may be reduced strikingly if ligation can be accomplished promptly. Accurate knowledge of the vascular supply to the vulva is critical if the procedure is to be performed efficiently (Fig. 7.2). The most common major vessels suffering traumatization are one or more branches of the pudendal artery or vein; however, the congeries of veins comprising the pampiniform plexus, or branches of the hemorrhoidal and clitoral vessels may be involved. Nevertheless, a majority of hematomas are seen after the major bleeding has subsided, and in these instances bed rest with the application of an agent such as Burrow's solution to reduce the edema is usually sufficient.

As in the male, the pampiniform plexus, closely associated with the round ligament in the female, contains the venous channels often involved in the formation of a varicocele. Nevertheless, the association of varices in the buttock indicates the participation of the pudendal vessels in certain cases. As noted previously, ligation can be performed more easily with a thorough knowledge of the vascular tree and its associated structures. Excision of the mass of dilated veins should accompany ligation in order to avoid distortion of the labium.

Perineal Scars

Lacerations of childbirth are well known and are usually repaired at the time of delivery. The occasional painful perineal scar may result in stricture of the outlet with disturbing dyspareunia, particularly in later years with postmenopausal changes, and may be a cause of concern for the patient and her husband since postcoital bleeding results from a tear in the tight band of skin at the fourchette. Revision of such scars at the fourchette with amplification of the introitus is simple but is among the most satisfying of all local surgical procedures. A triangular flap of skin with its apex at the anal orifice is excised from the fourchette (Fig. 7.3 A-D). The underlying fibromuscular tissue is incised in the midline almost to the anal sphincter. The posterior vaginal mucosa is dissected from the underlying tissue thus freeing sufficient mucosa to cover the defect produced by the initial excision (Fig. 7.3 E,F).

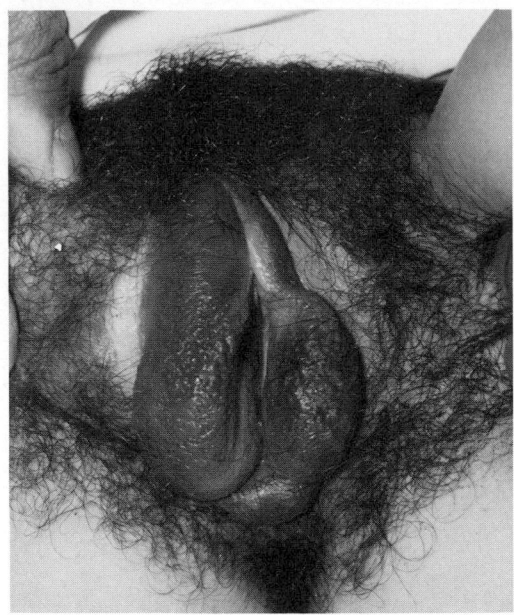

Fig. 7.1. Post-traumatic vulvar hematoma.

A small 1- to 2-cm incision in the midline of the freed mucosa may be necessary to establish an outlet adequate to admit three fingers. Skin edges are approximated to the mucosa with interrupted sutures of Dexon (Fig. 7.3 G). Pressure bandage for 24 hours will help eliminate hematoma formation. The latter is rare, however, if hemostasis is meticulously observed. Postoperative sitz baths or ice packs usually assist in reducing the local discomfort. Breakdown of the incision is reduced if Dexon rather than catgut is used to close the incision. It is important, of course, to avoid the development of stenosis, and care at the time of either episiotomy or rectocele repair may eliminate the necessity for revision. Vaginal mucosa should be used to cover the posterior midline rather than approximating the skin tightly in this area.

Condylomas (Knobs)

A variety of benign neoplasms arise in the vulva. Excisional surgery, however, is usually simple and uncomplicated. The condyloma acuminatum, of viral origin, is to be distinguished from the secondary syphilitic lesion and is generally treated with cauterizing solutions such as podophyllin (the resin of podophyllum). Since the infecting agent is a parasite and thus usually associated with local infections and their resultant irritating discharges, careful attention to the toilet of the area must be pursued vigorously if long term results are to be obtained. Sulfonamide therapy may prove to be a worthwhile adjunctive treatment, and systemic vitamin A has been successful according to certain clinicians. In the authors' experience, however, neither have been useful. When recurrent on large, extensive lesions, surgical removal may become necessary. The merits of knife excision vs. electrocoagulation have been debated. In the essayist's opinion, the latter is more easily accomplished and does not result in a major degree of local discomfort to the patient. Heat to the perineal area decreases the local postoperative reaction. The successful use of cryosurgery in the treatment of condyloma acuminatum has been reported, although opinions vary as to the efficacy of this methodology. Looking into the future, it is quite possible that recurrent warts may well be treated by topical chemotherapeutic agents.

Bartholin Gland

The Bartholin duct and gland are commonly involved in both inflammatory and traumatic processes. Although a variety of medical therapies have been proposed for the abscessed gland, none is as therapeutically successful as "incision and drainage" performed under local anesthesia. Initial drainage may be accomplished by insertion of a small "wick" deep into the sac; however, this drain is usually extruded spontaneously in a few hours and is of questionable value. The "bulb" drain is more effective but unnecessary at this stage of the disease. Sitz baths and systemic analgesics are important adjunctive measures.

In the chronic stage with cyst formation, therapy is unnecessary since in a majority of cases the lesion is asymptomatic. Occasionally, the cyst may be uncomfortable or become recurrently infected. In most such cases marsupialization is a simple and eminently satisfactory approach. During the quiescent stage a 1- to 2-cm incision should be made at the mucocutaneous border. The position of the incision allows the secretions, if still present, to assist in lubrication of the outlet (Fig. 7.4). Several fine catgut sutures approximate the mucosa of the duct to the skin, and the use of a

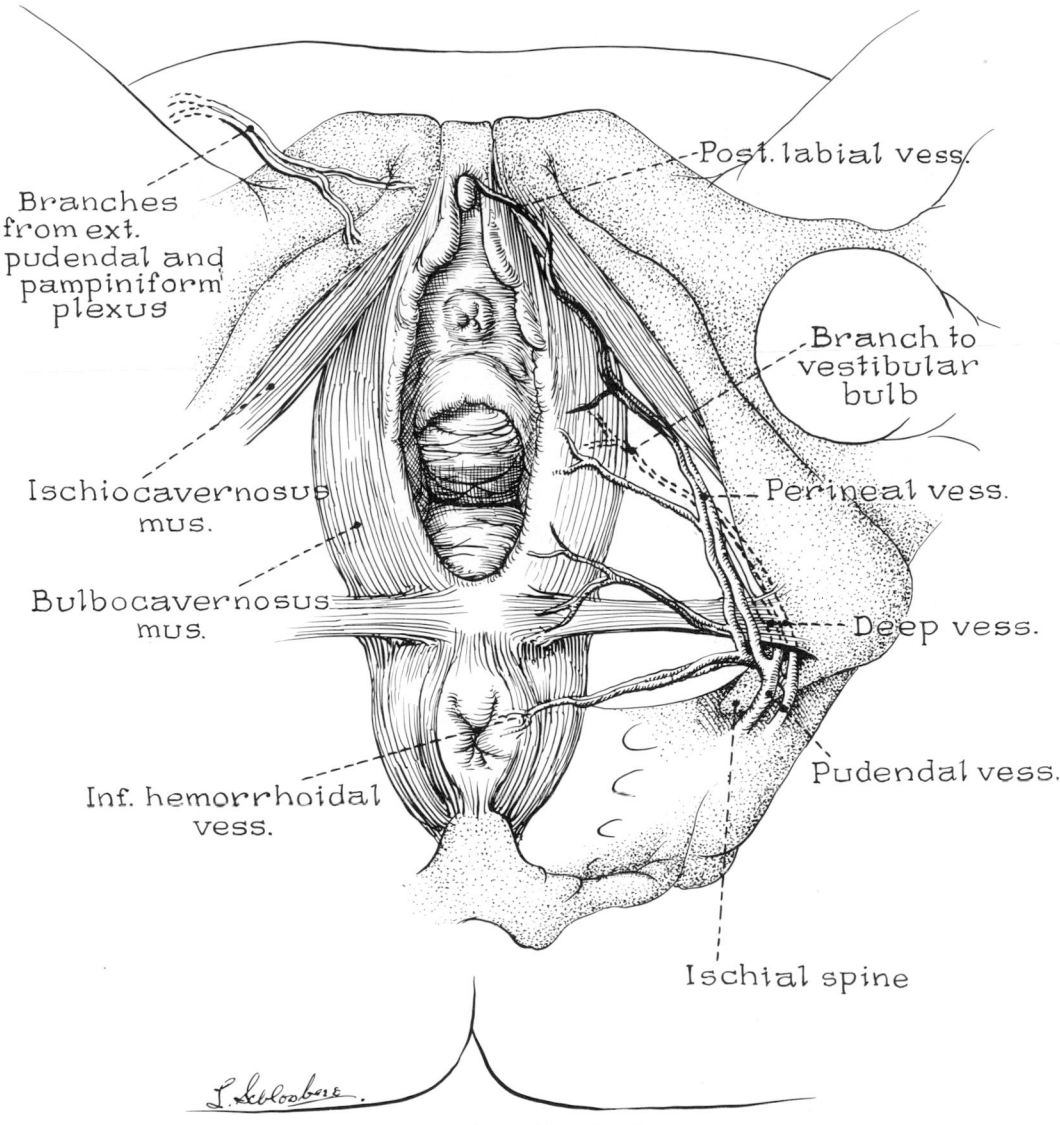

Branches
from ext.
pudendal and
pampiniform
plexus

Post. labial vess.

Branch to
vestibular
bulb

Ischiocavernosus
mus.

Perineal vess.

Bulbocavernosus
mus.

Deep vess.

Inf. hemorrhoidal
vess.

Pudendal vess.

Ischial spine

Fig. 7.2. Anatomic relationships of perineal vasculature.

small drain, preferably the "bulb" type, is usually successful in preventing postoperative stricture (Fig. 7.5). Goldberg (1) has applied this diversionary approach satisfactorily in 20 patients. In spite of all precautions, these neo-orifices may become reoccluded even though the patient has been symptomatically and psychologically relieved, and thus further excisional surgery is unnecessary.

Excision of the duct and its associated glandular elements should be pursued only if recurrent infections or uncomfortable enlargements are not prevented by marsupialization or

if neoplasm is suspected. Removal of the gland has been known as the "biggest little operation" in gynecology. Troublesome bleeding from branches of the pudendal and hemorrhoidal vessels is often difficult to control, and drainage should be instituted to prevent the deeply dissecting hematomas which prolong healing and add to the postoperative discomfort. Rare complications are the formation of rectoperineal fistulae and fenestration of the labium minus as the result of interruption of the blood supply by deep "blindly placed hemostatic" sutures. Removal of the thinned,

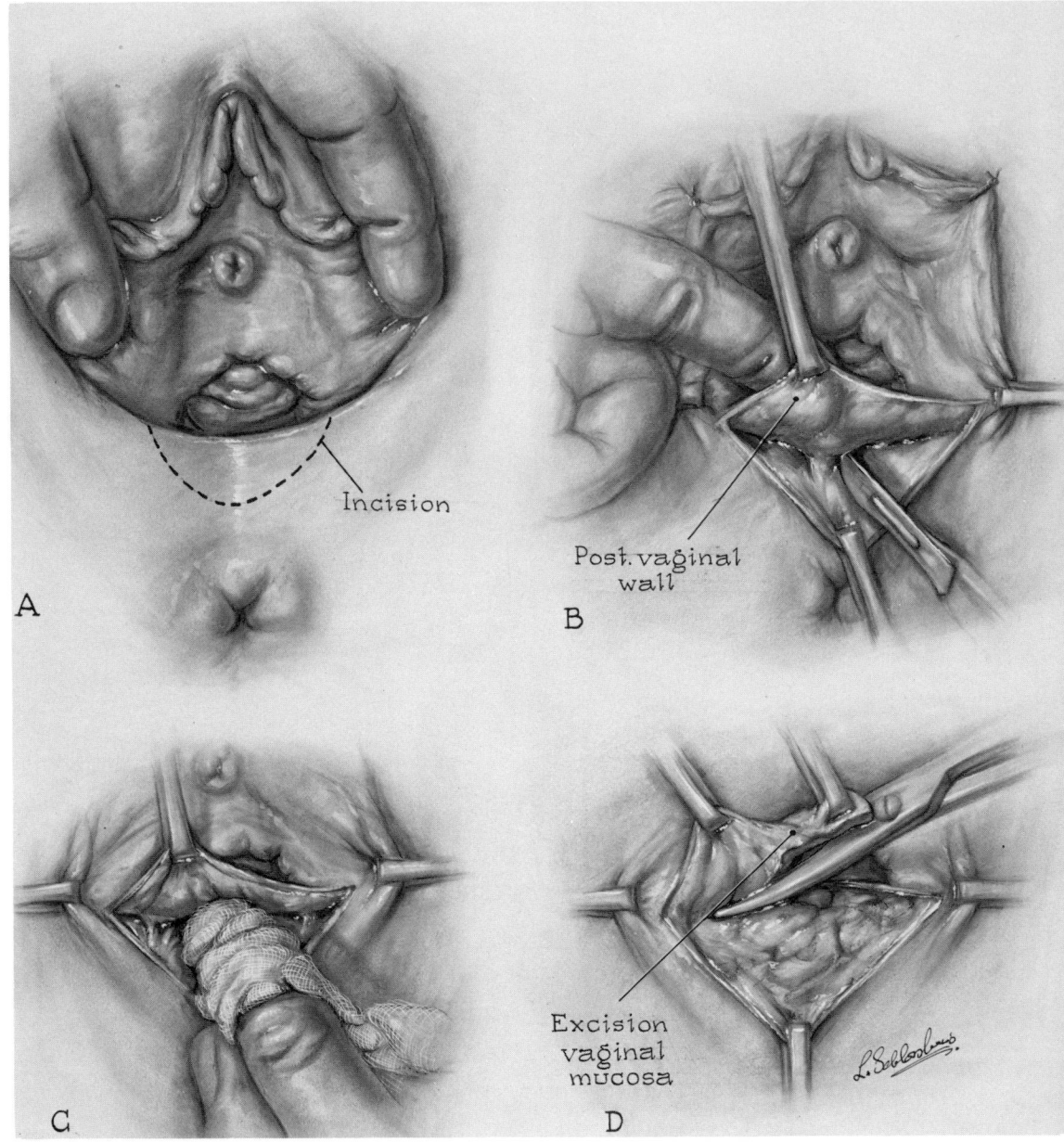

Fig. 7.3. Surgical correction of perineal scars. See continuation on next figure.

devitalized superficial skin over the cyst will assist in the prevention of a distorted vulva and will provide the surgeon with a skin section for traction in performing the dissection. Incising the cyst and inflating a Foley bag within the cavity can perform the same function. To prevent fistula formation, a finger in the rectum will guide the placement of sutures; and if the rectal wall is in jeopardy, packing is preferable to the risk of the development of a fistula. An alternative approach to hemostasis may be accomplished by placing deep mattress sutures from the vagina through the excisional defect to a parallel area on the perineal skin.

During pregnancy, it is important to avoid any surgical therapy to the Bartholin gland or to the external genitalia. The increased vascularity and edema often lead to excessive bleeding, and on rare occasions transfusion has been necessary to replace blood loss from

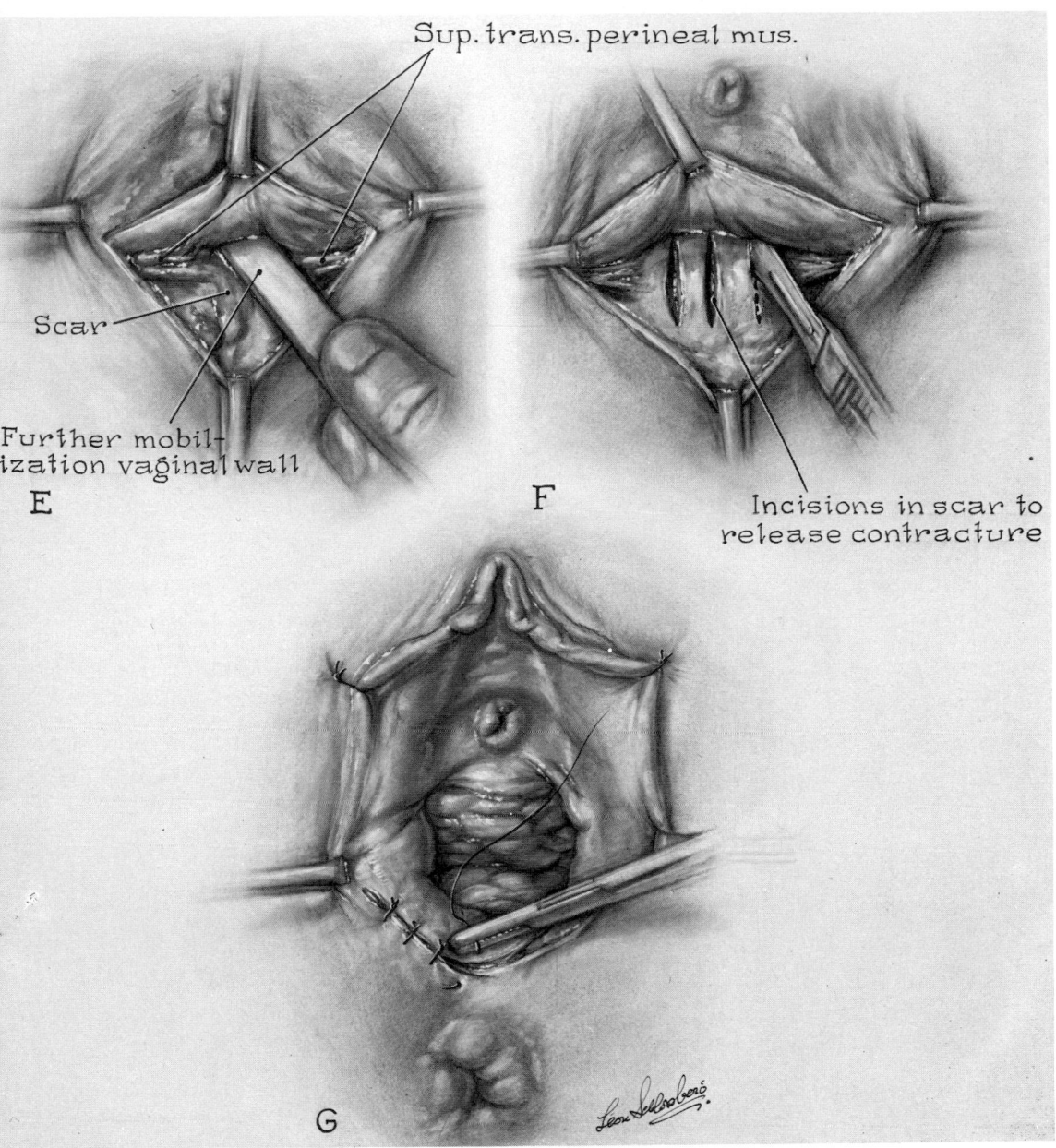

Fig. 7.3. Continued.

simple incision and drainage of a Bartholin abscess. Such procedures are to be avoided unless imperative.

Phimosis

Phimosis or paraphimosis rarely is a problem in the female. Nevertheless, the condition may result from or be associated with other conditions, particularly "lichen sclerosus." Occlusion of the paraclitoral space by agglutination of the folds of the prepuce may lead to recurrent infections and pseudocyst formation. In such cases, circumcision is indicated. If the accumulation of smegma and irritating debris between the remaining skin folds is to be prevented, excision of the prepuce to the base of the clitoris is necessary. Gentle massage of the incisional area with mineral oil assists in the healing process.

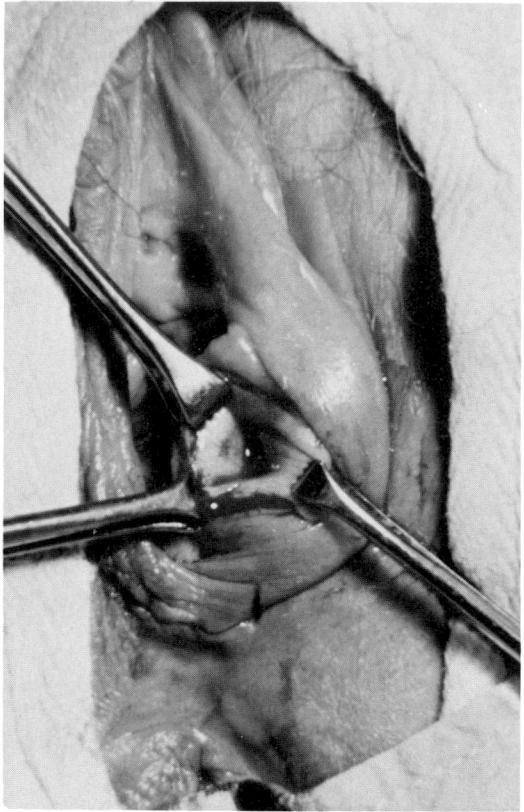

Fig. 7.4. Marsupialization of a Bartholin duct cyst.

Labial Agglutinations

Such complications occur most commonly in infancy and are undoubtedly related to the thin, watery, vaginal discharge and the resultant irritation to the labial folds so frequently noted in the prepubertal girl. Simple massage with Vaseline followed by the use of intravaginal estrogen and the avoidance of tight-fitting, nonabsorbent underclothing will usually produce satisfactory long term results. The counterpart of this condition, infibulation, was a well documented ritual among certain societies, and surgery was occasionally necessary at the time of marriage in order for coitus to take place. Such procedures are rarely necessary today; but if the agglutination is of long standing, a separation under anesthesia may seem wise. Again, meticulous care in the form of gentle massage with oil or Vaseline to the incisional lines is important if recurrence is to be prevented. Finally, estrogenic creams do not alter the texture of the skin and do not create a more resistant tissue.

White Lesions

Historically, the persistently irritating vulvar lesion, particularly that which appears grossly as a "white patch," has created controversy as to differential diagnosis and therapy. Much of the confusion has stemmed from use of the term "leukoplakia," a poor definition of its histologic features, and the relationship of the vulvar lesion to the buccal lesion, described by Schwimmer (2) in 1877 and well established in the latter area as a precursor of malignancy. A great variety of white lesions on the vulva, varying from simple depigmentation to invasive cancer, have been designated as "leukoplakia." Undoubtedly a specific "true leukoplakia" does exist and is characterized grossly by elevated, white, hyperkeratotic patches often associated with linear excoriations, superficial ulcerations, and distortion of the vulvar architecture. However, since such a variety of lesions may appear white, it is imperative that a better correlation between the gross and microscopic features must be made in each case prior to therapy, and that the characteristics of the true precancerous lesion of the vulva be defined more specifically. Thus to avoid incorrect diagnosis and therapy, it is wise to describe

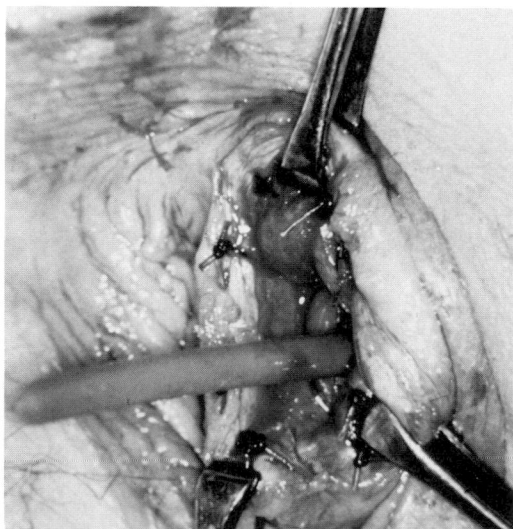

Fig. 7.5. Approximation of Bartholin duct epithelial lining to the skin with drain *in situ.*

accurately and give examples of the various pathologic entities which may appear as "white or grayish-white" patches.

Chronic Dermatitis

Because of the great number of local and systemic irritants to which the external genitalia are exposed, pruritis is a common and recurrent complaint. Acute problems are caused by local vaginal infections with "reactive" vulvar irritation, the use of local agents to which skin may be sensitive, the moisture which accumulates and is maintained in the area by tight-fitting clothing, and systemic medications, particularly the antibiotics and the often resulting mycotic vaginitis. These are usually treated successfully by local application of antipruritic agents, such as the hydrocortisones; the elimination of local irritants and the "nonbreathing, tight-fitting" synthetic underclothing; the systemic use of antihistamines; and specific agents for the vaginitis.

Conversely, chronic disease produces a more complicated situation. Since the skin commonly has been irreversibly changed, although the symptoms may be controlled temporarily by local agents, recurrences are common and alterations in the gross and microscopic appearance of the vulvar tissues are unmodifiable. In the therapy of such chronic conditions (Fig. 7.6), it is imperative that suspicious areas be biopsied in order to establish the correct diagnosis.

As noted previously, criteria for the acceptance of the designation "leukoplakia" must be rigidly defined. Too often the histologic alterations associated with chronic dermatitis, namely, hyperkeratosis, acanthosis, and chronic inflammatory infiltrate, have been designated as "leukoplakia" (Fig. 7.7), and therapy for a presumed premalignant lesion has been instituted. Vulvar biopsy is a simple and eminently satisfactory technique. Under local anesthesia, the Keyes punch produces little trauma, delineates the localized lesion readily, and results in a specimen that can be easily fixed in the paraffin block for better tissue orientation.

In a patient with diffuse disease, if the histologic alterations are not suspicious of malignancy, symptomatic relief may be accomplished by local alcohol injection. On the other hand, if the lesion is well localized in an area

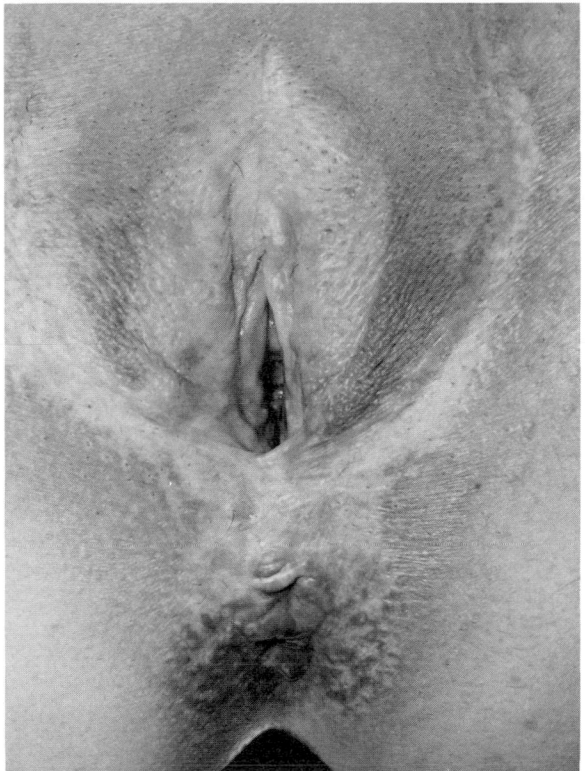

Fig. 7.6. Gross appearance of the vulva in a case of chronic dermatitis.

other than the clitoris, regional excision may be performed with ease and an assurance of symptomatic relief. Such a procedure obviously has the effect of nerve section as well as the elimination of the affected tissue. Furthermore, the distortion which may be produced by vulvectomy is avoided. Alcohol injection produces a local block that is effective from 4 to 6 months (Fig. 7.8). Usually by this time the patient has been relieved of the local irritation, the "scratch reflex" has been interrupted, and the minimal residual symptoms can be controlled adequately by topical medication.

This procedure is not without hazard. If the injection is too deep or too superficial, slough of the tissue may occur; if the sphincter ani is injected, temporary paralysis may result. Similar unpleasant complications may ensue if the tissues are acutely infected at the time of injection. In approximately 2 per cent of our cases, there have been varying degrees of tissue loss (Fig. 7.9). Fortunately, although the local tissue destruction is disturbing, the eventual

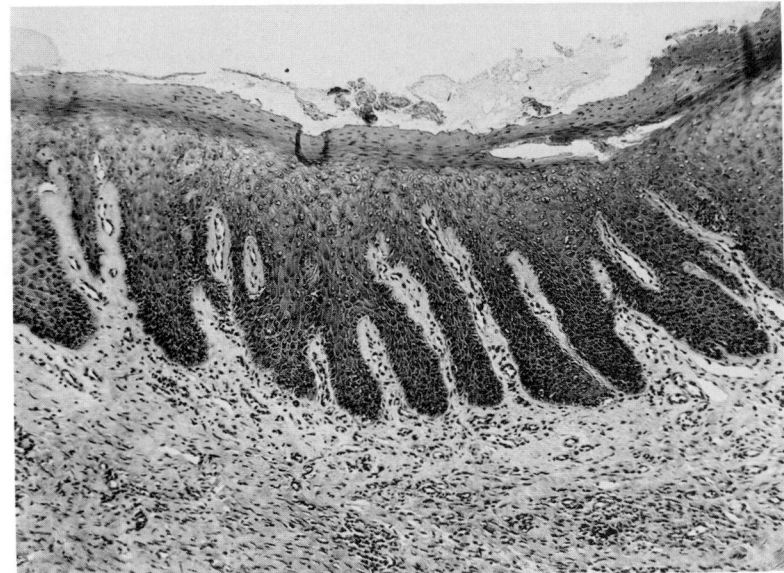

Fig. 7.7. Chronic dermatitis characterized by hyperkeratosis, acanthosis, and chronic inflammatory infiltrate. Hematoxylin and eosin; ×75.

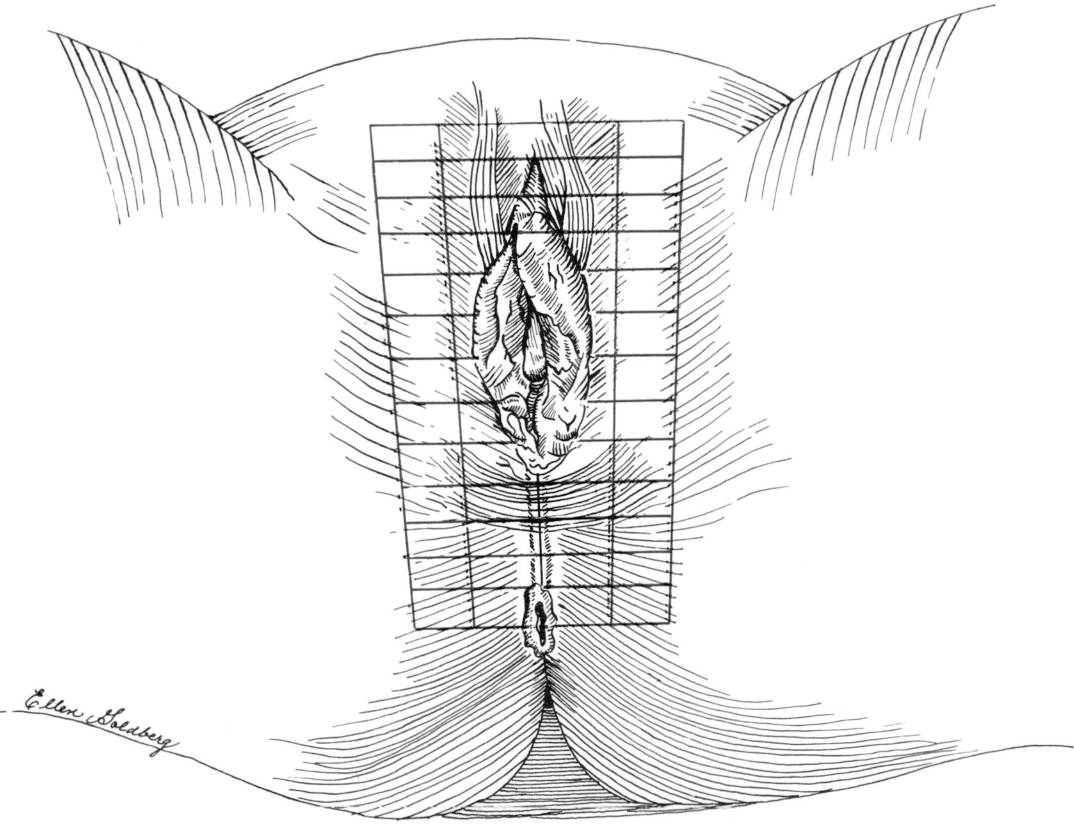

Fig. 7.8. Plan for systematic alcohol injection for relief of vulvar pruritis. Injection is made at the point where the lines intersect.

healing is satisfactory, and symptoms are relieved since nerve block is effected by such "excavations." In approximately 5 to 10 per cent of the cases, the minute needle holes will become thickened and focally indurated. In these situations, however, breakdown does not

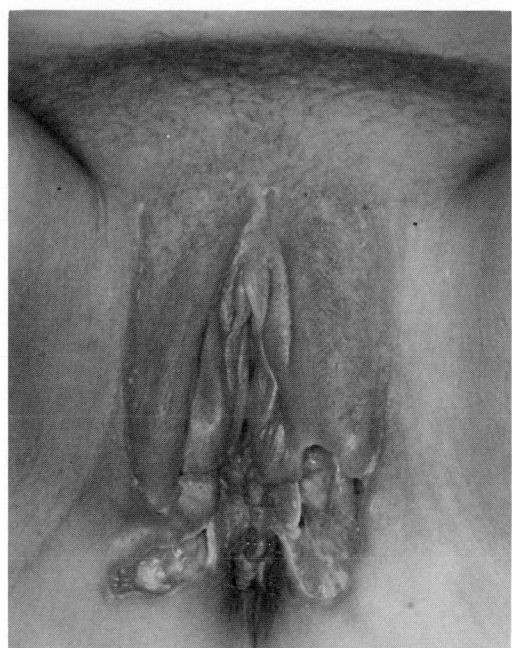

Fig. 7.9. Perineal slough following alcohol injection.

occur and local supportive therapy is sufficient to prevent more serious local complications.

In the recurrent case, not relieved by topical agents or alcohol injection, more extensive nerve block may be entertained. Again, it should go without saying that accurate diagnosis must be established prior to therapy. It is also of major importance that persistent vaginal infection, *e.g.*, trichomonas and moniliasis, must be ruled out since vaginal itching will not be relieved by a vulvar nerve block. Definitive neurectomy has been described by Mering (3). The rationale for this procedure is based on the anatomic arrangement of the nerve supply to the vulva (Fig. 7.10). Linear incisions parallel to the long axis of the outlet on the most lateral aspect of the labia majora extend from a point directly lateral to and on a line with the clitoris, a similar point lateral to the upper level of the anal orifice (Fig. 7.11). Incision is carried down to the fascia and the tissues are undermined widely by finger dissection (Fig. 7.12). The fingers extend above the clitoris on either side to meet in the upper midline so that all sensory nerve fibers in the entire area including those directly beneath the skin are disrupted. Similar blunt dissection is performed with the fingers meeting behind the anal orifice. Hemostasis must be accurate. Incisions are closed using catgut for the underlying tissues and Dexon for

the skin. Dependent drainage, as suggested in the section on "Simple Vulvectomy" below, may be instituted in selected cases. The area is packed tightly for a period of 72 to 96 hours. Suprapubic catheter drainage for the bladder is preferred by the authors. The patient experiences little discomfort from the procedure and healing is eminently satisfactory.

The results of this procedure have been excellent; and although the approach may seem radical for benign disease, the patient with severe, intractable pruritis will consider it a godsend.

Professor Bela Horn, of Budapest, has described a similar procedure which has a simpler technique. A small incision is made lateral to and just above the fourchette at right angle to the outlet. Scissors are inserted through these incisions, simply dissecting the underlying tissue by opening and closing the blades as they are directed upward toward the level of the clitoris and then downward to the level of the anal orifice. Professor Horn closes the incision with three or four silk sutures, using no packing, and suggests that the routine vulvar hematoma which develops is an important feature of the procedure and increases its effectiveness. We have had no experience with this technique. It must be emphasized that with proper diagnosis and therapy, there is rarely a need for such surgery. Only six cases have been performed in the Johns Hopkins Hospital in 16 years.

Simple Vulvectomy

In the past simple vulvectomy has been the procedure of choice for many of the "white lesions," and was performed on the false assumption that these alterations were premalignant. The satisfactory results in a majority of such cases were produced by the "modified" neurectomy accomplished by the vulvectomy incisions. Unfortunately, in some patients on whom simple vulvectomy was performed, postoperative constriction of the outlet occurred with resultant increase in local discomfort produced by any attempt at entry into the vagina. In a series of 80 cases reviewed by the author and Baens (4), 15 patients complained of dyspareunia preoperatively and 15 had a similar problem postoperatively. Unfortunately, because these two groups did not include the same patients, a certain number had been made

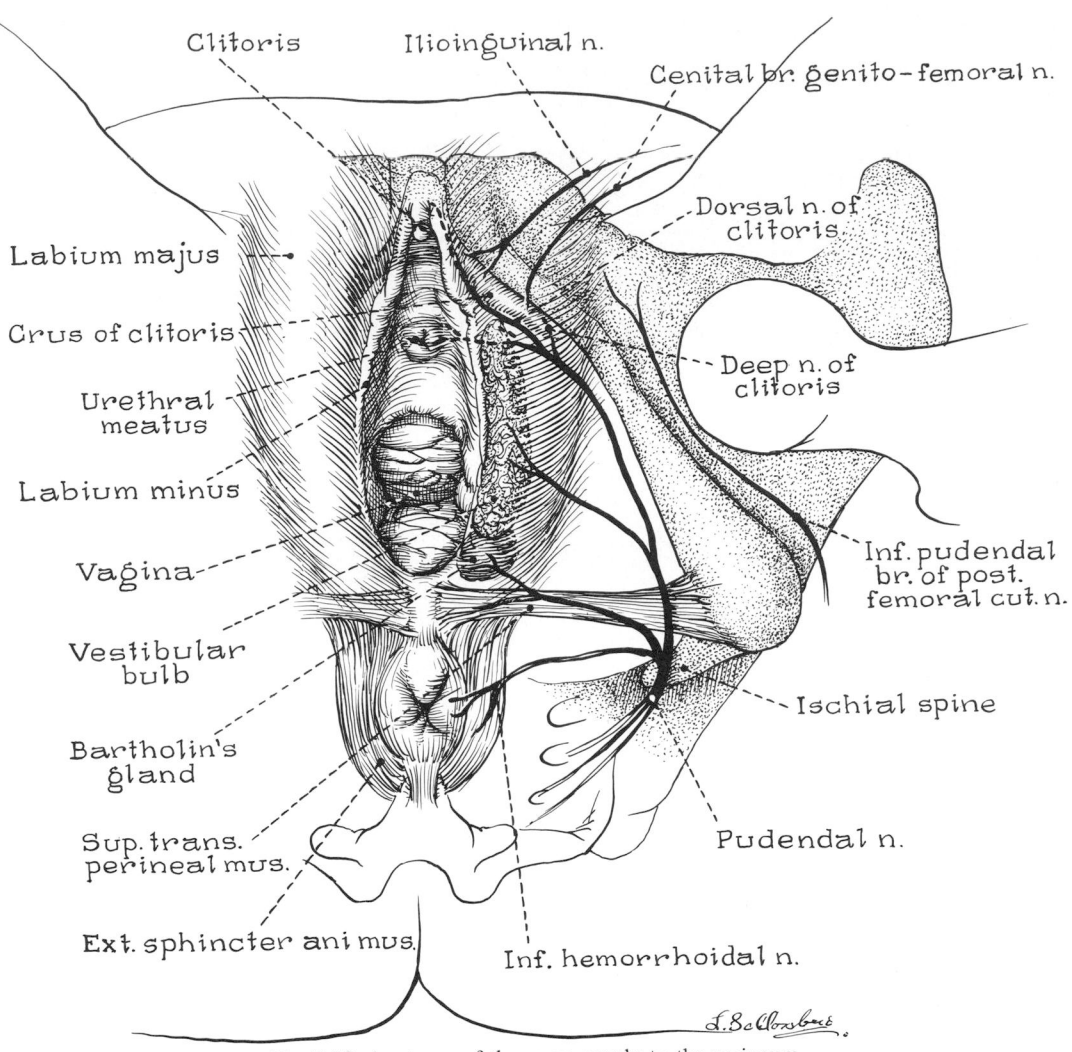

Fig. 7.10. Anatomy of the nerve supply to the perineum.

worse by the procedure.

In the authors' opinion simple vulvectomy should be limited to therapy for carcinoma *in situ* and "histologically well defined" pre-malignant disease of the vulva. It should be noted that isolated and well circumscribed lesions in both of the above categories may be widely excised with satisfactory results. Nevertheless, it also must be recognized that both of these conditions are frequently characterized by multicentric foci and particularly in cases of carcinoma *in situ*, gross delineation of the diseased areas may be impossible. Therefore, it is imperative that every effort be made to discover the grossly normal but histologically atypical epithelium. The use of toluidine blue as described by Collins (5) has been of value in demonstrating the metabolically active skin if the abnormal nuclei are exposed. Unfortunately, many of the preinvasive lesions are hyperkeratotic, and in such situations the dye penetrates poorly into the underlying, well protected anaplastic cells. Although multiple biopsies may be helpful, often these are purely "blind" punches since no gross lesion is visible.

Cytologic study has not been helpful in most of the vulvar lesions unless again the abnormal nuclei are exposed and available to the instrument. Furthermore, because the surface is dry and hard, and the cells are often keratinized, obtaining such specimens is difficult. The surface moistened with saline and a firm, but gentle scraping will add to the accuracy of the cytologic study.

More complicated techniques such as colposcopy and tissue incubation for the determination of differential metabolic activity are either
not available or impractical on a routine basis.
Some degree of success has been obtained in the
treatment of these multiple areas of neoplasia,
particularly in the young individual, by the use
of topical chemotherapeutic agents. In the
future such agents may be widely employed in
selected cases.

The difficulty in determining early anaplastic
changes may account for the frequency of local
"recurrence" in cases of both invasive and
preinvasive disease. Furthermore, the inability
to eliminate the carcinogenic agents undoubtedly results in the production of new lesions.
Such a sequence of events may be appreciated
in the case of vaginal carcinoma *in situ* which
developed in the new vagina after vaginectomy
for intraepithelial disease. An additional demonstration of the validity of this thesis is the
high incidence of local "recurrence" of vulvar
cancer. Many late appearances of malignant
disease, either invasive or *in situ*, after removal

of the primary focus suggest the persistence of
an area carcinogen. Finally, the recognition of
the many unusual gross pictures which may
suggest neoplasia may prevent the development
of invasive cancer. The characteristic erythro-
plastic alteration with its white epithelial
islands is typical of Bowen's disease. The
unusually pigmented lesion, however, is less
well known but equally important.

In the surgical approach to simple vulvectomy, it is important to note that the major
postoperative complication, particularly for the
younger individual engaged in active sexual life,
is stricture of the outlet. A majority of these
strictures may be avoided by excising the skin
at the fourchette as described earlier in this
chapter. It is important to recognize that the
exposed vaginal mucosa covering the incisional
area is quite pliable, and in the postmenopausal
patient it will respond readily to local estrogen.
Conversely, skin is relatively rigid and has a
tendency to tear at the incisional line, producing a chronic "fissure." Furthermore, particularly in the postmenopausal patient, the skin

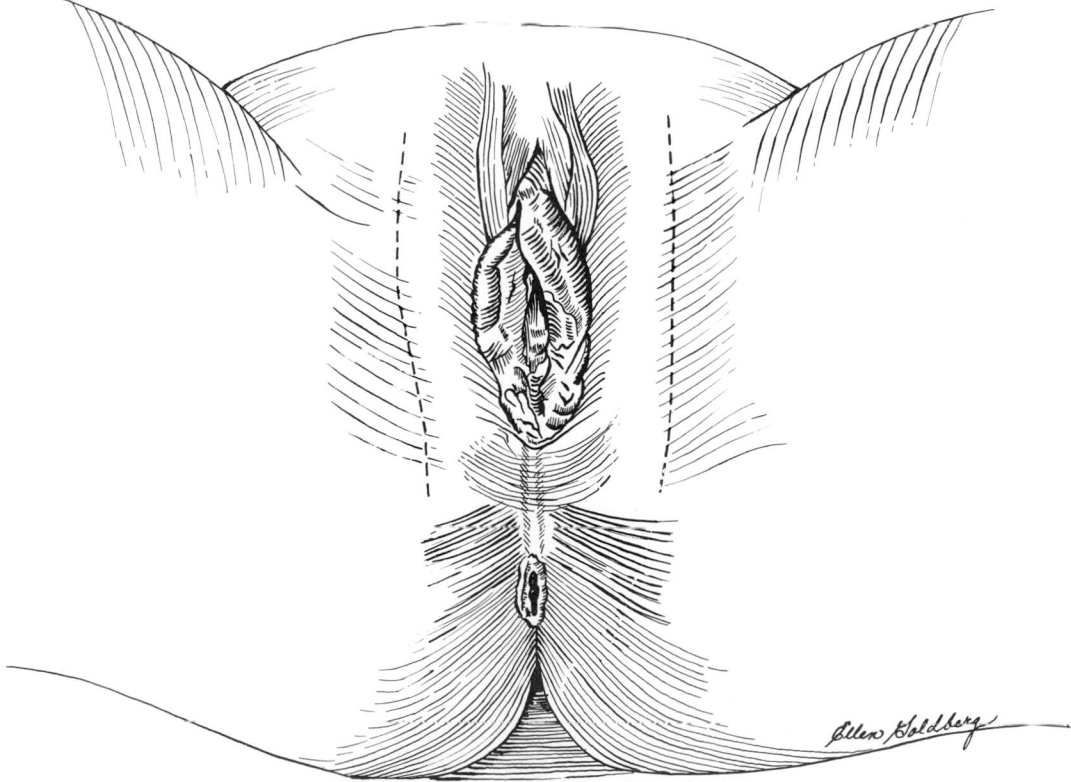

Fig. 7.11. Placement of incisions for the "Mering procedure."

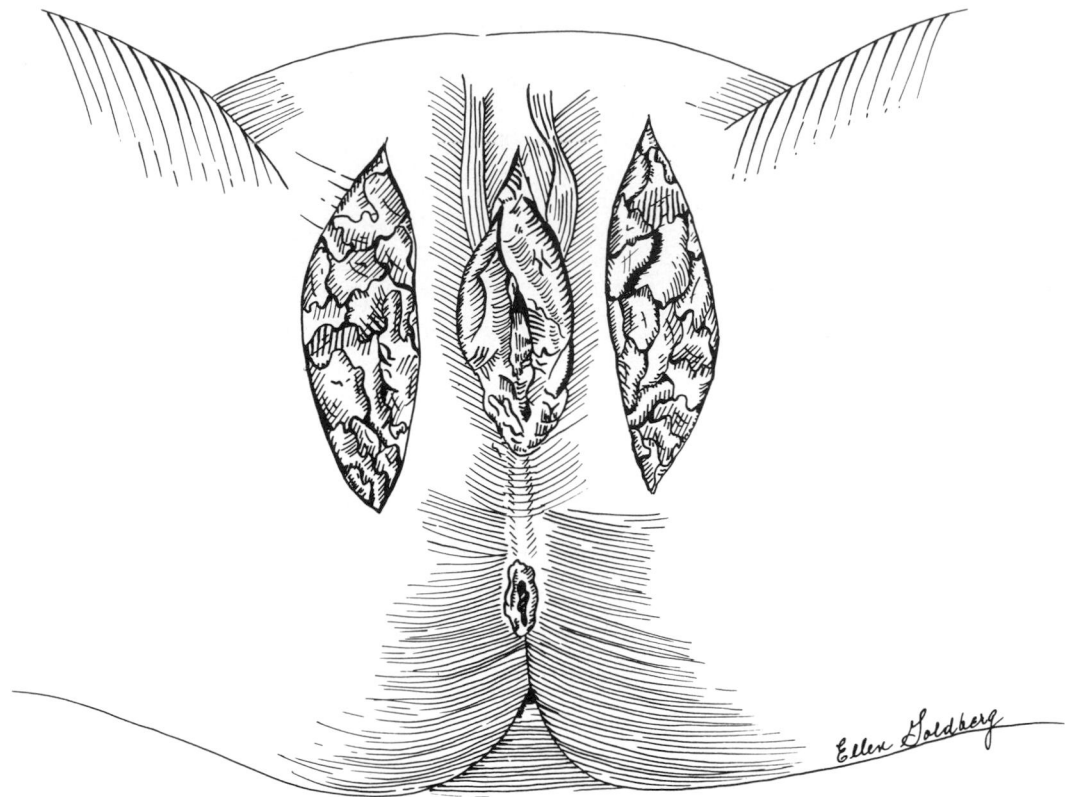

Ellen Goldberg

Fig. 7.12. Appearance of the vulva following wide blunt dissection to achieve neurectomy.

does not respond to topical therapy as does the vaginal mucosa. A preoperative outline of the incisional lines prevents the trauma of defining the extent of dissection and the possibility of an irregular, distorted scar. An initial incision to delineate the margins at the introitus facilitates the final union of the vulvar and vaginal lines of dissection. Incision above the external urethral meatus early in the dissection allows the surgeon to boldly remove the tissue from the mons through the clitoris without fear of urethral injury. Mattress or figure-eight sutures are necessary at the clitoris. Except for the skin edges, the generous use of the electrosurgical unit reduces the time and minor traumas imposed by ligation of the myriad of small vessels. Nevertheless, sutures are necessary for the pudendal vessels. Closure with Dexon rather than catgut reduces the breakdown often coincident to the dissolution of the absorbable material (Fig. 7.13). Standard precautions to avoid hematoma and excessive edema include meticulous hemostasis, pressure dressings for 48 hours, and adequate dependent drainage if hemostasis seems inadequate.

Finally, surgical interruption of the local blood and nerve supply to the vulvovaginal area occasionally results in vaginal relaxation, particularly if minor degrees of the latter have been present preoperatively. Such complications are difficult to predict. However, if the patient's condition warrants, repair may be in order at the time of primary surgery. The surgeon should resist the temptation to further impair the blood supply with tightly constricting sutures in the restoration of the pelvic floor. Close approximation of tissues without constriction is the main thrust in such procedures.

Radical Vulvectomy

Since the introduction of the Bassett operation by Taussig (6) more than 40 years ago, carcinoma of the vulva has been treated by radical vulvectomy with inguinal and femoral lymph node dissection. The importance of extraperitoneal lymphadenectomy is being seriously challenged today. With involvement of

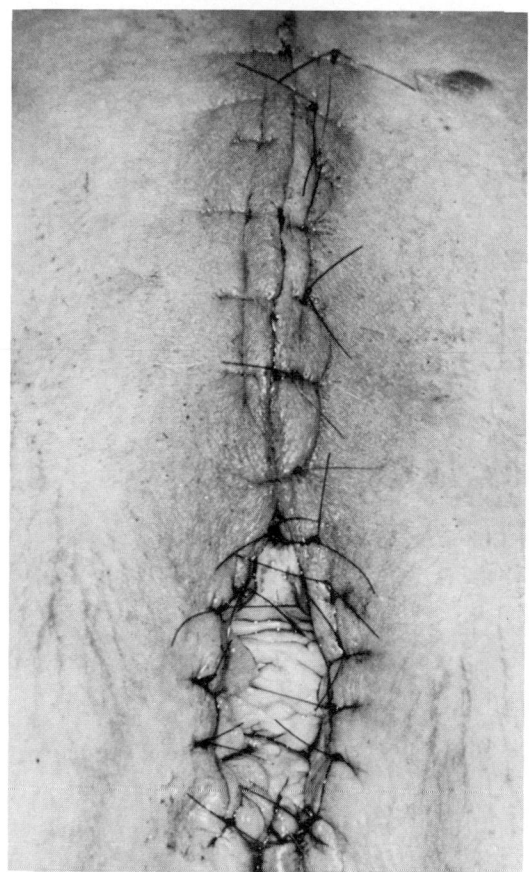

Fig. 7.13. Closure with nylon suture material following simple vulvectomy.

the hypogastric, illiac, and/or obturator nodes, the salvage rate is improved so slightly that the addition of this procedure at the end of the primary surgery must be questioned. It is important not to be too impressed with 5-year salvage rates, for many patients with widespread local disease have survived many years and others appear with local recurrences 10 or more years after initial therapy. A study of the autopsy findings in 168 cases (7) revealed widespread extrapelvic disease in less than 10 per cent of the patients.

The one exception to this rule is basal cell carcinoma, and although the suggestion has been made that such lesions differ from basal cell carcinoma elsewhere on the skin and should be treated radically, a majority opinion opposes this approach. It must be understood that there is a vulvar lesion which superficially resembles basal cell carcinoma but actually should be categorized as a "cloacal" or "transitional cell"

cancer. The latter is in every respect as malignant as the squamous cell carcinoma. Conversely, basal cell neoplasia behaves biologically like histologically similar lesions elsewhere on the skin, and wide local excision is adequate if multiple foci have been excluded.

In the therapy of invasive squamous cell, cloacal carcinoma, Bartholin gland cancer, malignant melanoma, and the rare sarcomas, the Bassett two-stage procedure of vulvectomy followed by regional lymph node dissection has been superseded by the one-stage approach. A single crescent-shaped incision from iliac crest to iliac crest with the midpoint over the mons has been most frequently used. In the latter procedure the skin is undermined for several centimeters on either side of the incision in an effort to remove all of the adipose tissue which might contain superficial lymphatics. This undermined, devitalized skin was a frequent site of extensive local necrosis. More recently a crescent-shaped area of skin has been excised so that undermining is reduced to a minimum and the incidence of incisional breakdown has been greatly decreased (Figs. 7.14 and 7.15). In spite of this modification, the area directly over the mons where the edges of the vulvar incision are approximated to the abdominal skin remains a vulnerable point. In an effort to eliminate this focal point at which the blood supply is in jeopardy, a tongue-shaped flap skin has been left at the midline border of the incision over the mons and eventually brought down to the urethral meatus. In order to avoid tension on this flap, the skin and underlying adipose tissue in the lower midline must be freed from the fascia, and, if necessary, a "wedge" of skin removed from the cephalic portion of the flap at the iliac crests.

Initial results with this incision have been satisfactory, but too few cases have been performed to give an accurate evaluation of the efficacy of the procedure. Of major importance in attempting to prevent wound separation and to promote better approximation of the skin to the underlying tissue is the employment of methods to reduce the accumulation of fluid and to avoid dead space. To accomplish this, drainage tubes are inserted lateral to the lower ends of the vulvar incision and carried up into the inguinal regions. Constant low pressure suction to these tubes results in better primary healing. Injudicious use of pressure dressings

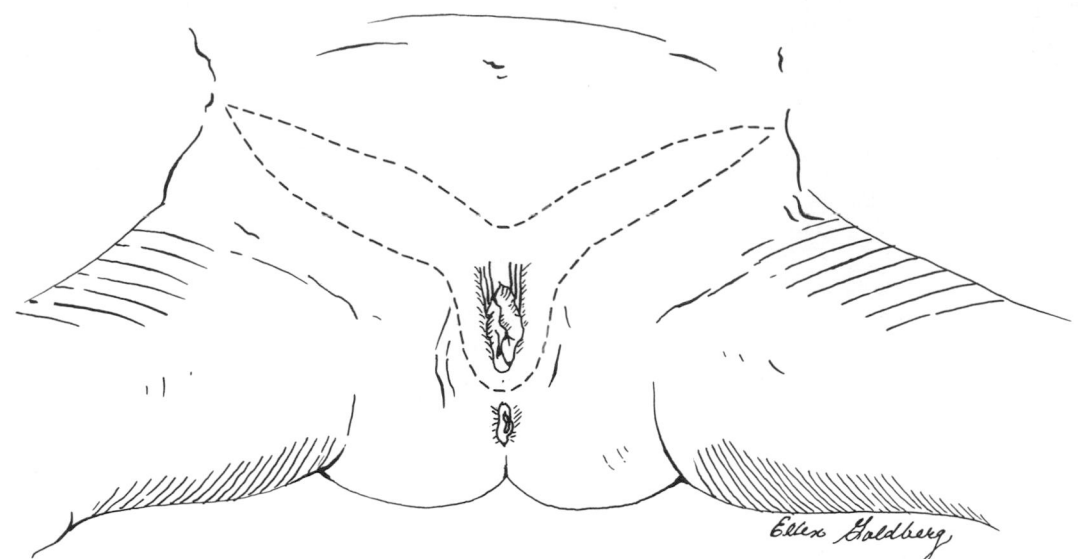

Fig. 7.14. Outline of the incision used for the one-step radical vulvectomy and groin dissection.

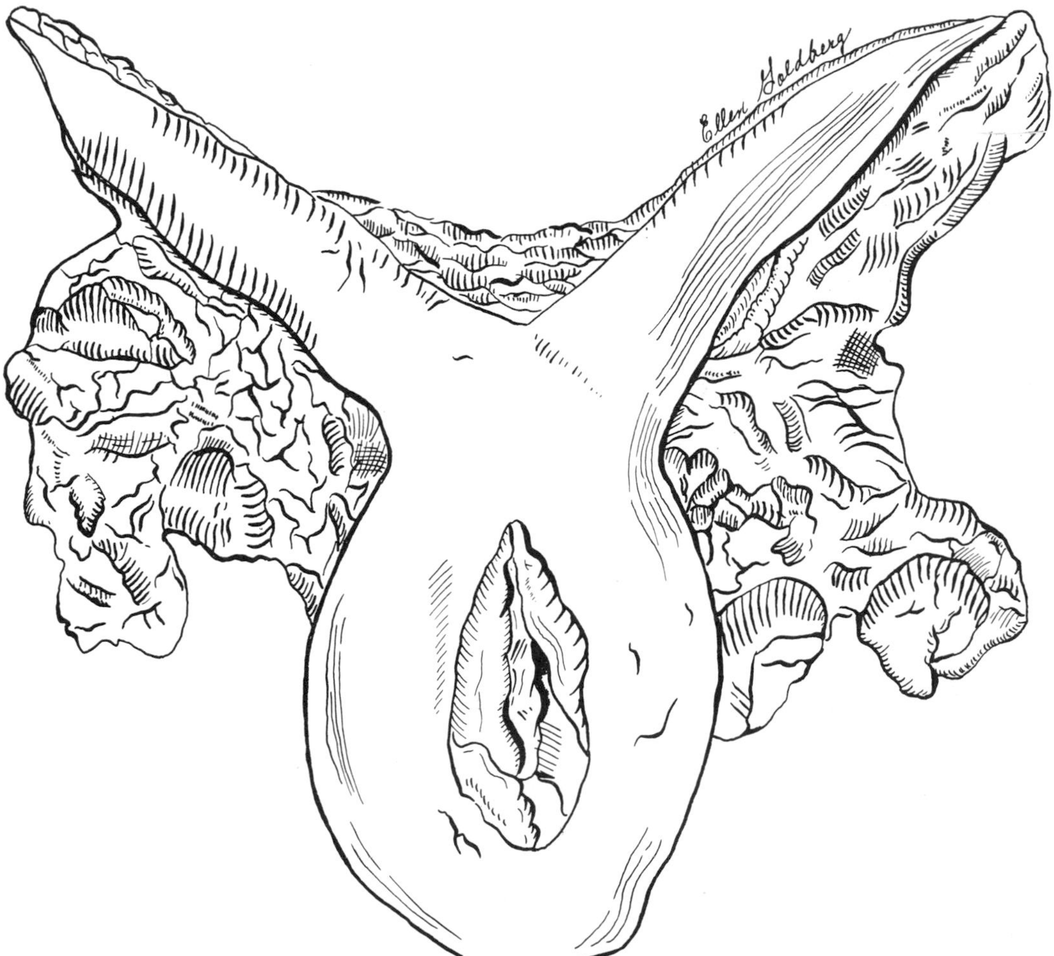

Fig. 7.15. The appearance of the excised specimen.

can lead to impairment of the blood supply to healing wound edges.

The basic prime factors which tend to reduce the operating time and the morbidity are a thorough knowledge of the anatomy of the area, the use of sufficient personnel to reduce operating time, and obvious proper pre- and postoperative care. Details of the operative procedure are documented in several operative texts.

Features of importance in avoiding complications in radical vulvectomy:

1. *Incision*: outline incisional lines with dye.

a. Two-team approach has been time-saving and effective for the authors. Primary surgeon makes the initial incision; the groin and femoral dissections are carried out by teams. One team closes while the second performs the vulvectomy.

b. Excision of skin with underlying tissue to prevent slough resulting from "skinning the skin."

c. Development of a "tongue-shaped" mid-incisional flap to prevent breakdown at the "3-point skin union" over the symphysis. Prior to final incisional closure, adequate blood supply to the tip of the flap must be established by cutting back on skin edge until brisk bleeding results.

d. Avoidance of extra incisions, *e.g.*, over the femoral triangle and through the inguinal ligament unless absolutely necessary for exposure.

e. Electrosurgery may be used but *not for skin incision*.

f. Dissection of Cloquet's node may result in entrance into the peritoneal cavity. Careful closure and repair are important if a hernia is to be prevented.

2. *The Vascular System*

a. Knowledge of the vessels causing common problems, *e.g.*, circumflex and epigastric arteries, avoids troublesome bleeding.

b. Care in the femoral triangle. Dissection from the lateral aspect uncovering the nerve through the fascia investing the ileopsoas muscle.

c. Double ligation of the saphenous vein first at its entrance into the femoral and later at the deepest point of origin approximately mid-thigh.

d. The major clitoral and pudendal vessels should be sutured and ligated.

e. Ligation of the bundle of lymphatics at the apex of the femoral triangle inferiorly and at the femoral canal superiorly will prevent lymphocyst formation in most instances.

3. *Drainage and Closure*

a. Suction drainage in the thigh adjacent to the lower point of the vulvar incision is necessary. The femoral area should be included or drained separately.

b. Approximation of subcutaneous tissue and skin to the deep fascia.

c. Covering of the femoral vessels with the transplanted sartorius muscle (Fig. 7.16).

d. Careful cleansing of operative area. Antibiotic spray, as recommended by Way, or similar agent.

e. Skin edge approximation with Dexon or similar nonabsorbable material.

f. Pressure dressing for 48 to 72 hours *only* if hemostasis has been questionable. Careful observance of exposed incision is preferable.

g. Catheter or suprapubic drainage for bladder.

4. *Postoperative Care*

a. Binding of legs individually and together. The former for 2 weeks at least, the latter for 4 to 5 days.

b. Care of suction to assure adequate drainage, usually 1500 to 2000 cc per 24 hours.

c. Use of anticoagulants or dextran. Obviously careful follow-up of prothrombin time is necessary to avoid massive bleeding from the multitude of large and small vessels in the extensive operative site.

d. Suture line care with careful massage using mineral oil or a similar agent frequently.

e. Emphasis on fluid and electrolyte balance particularly in view of the fluid loss through drainage.

f. Adequate antibiotic coverage—cellulitis is not uncommon.

It is important to recall that the vessels which cause a majority of problems are the circumflex, the epigastric, and the saphenous

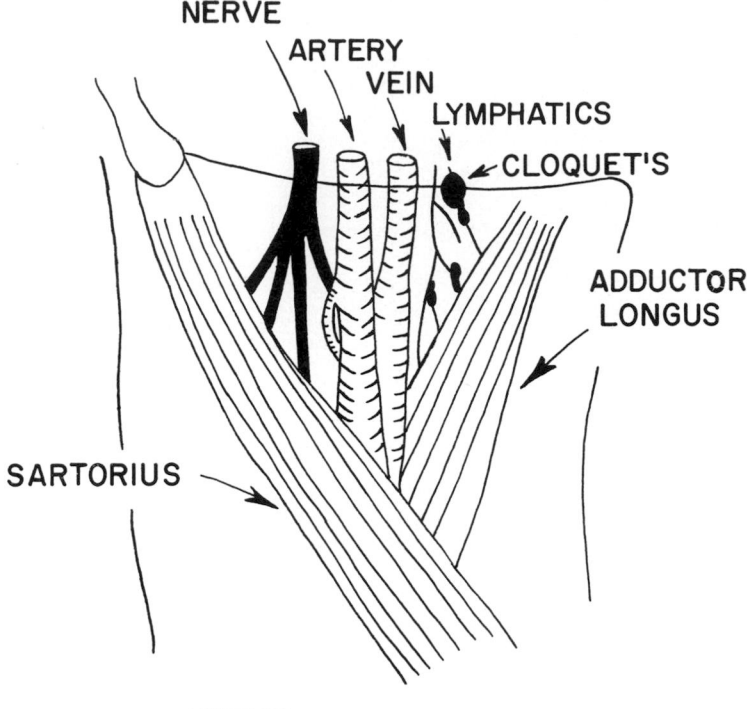

NERVE
ARTERY
VEIN
LYMPHATICS
CLOQUET'S
ADDUCTOR
LONGUS
SARTORIUS

Fig. 7.16. Transplantation of the sartorius muscle over the femoral vessels.

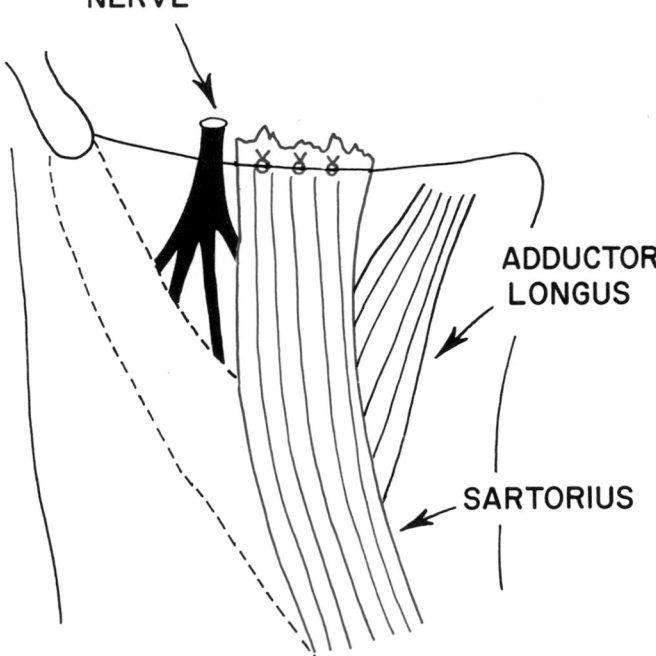

NERVE
ADDUCTOR
LONGUS
SARTORIUS

vein. The greater saphenous vein must be ligated near its junction with the femoral to eliminate bleeding from many minor branches. Obviously great care should be taken with the femoral vessels. In a majority of cases there is no need to sever the inguinal ligament since the node of Cloquet can be generally dissected from the area with little difficulty. Furthermore, reapproximation of the ligament often results in weakness with a tendency to pseudohernia formation. Transplantation of the sartorius muscle from its tendonous attachment at the anterior superior iliac spine to the inguinal ligament will cover the major vessels. This is accomplished easily and affords a sense of security should incisional breakdown develop in this area.

In the authors' experience the two-team approach to the groin dissection reduces the operative time, and in general the entire

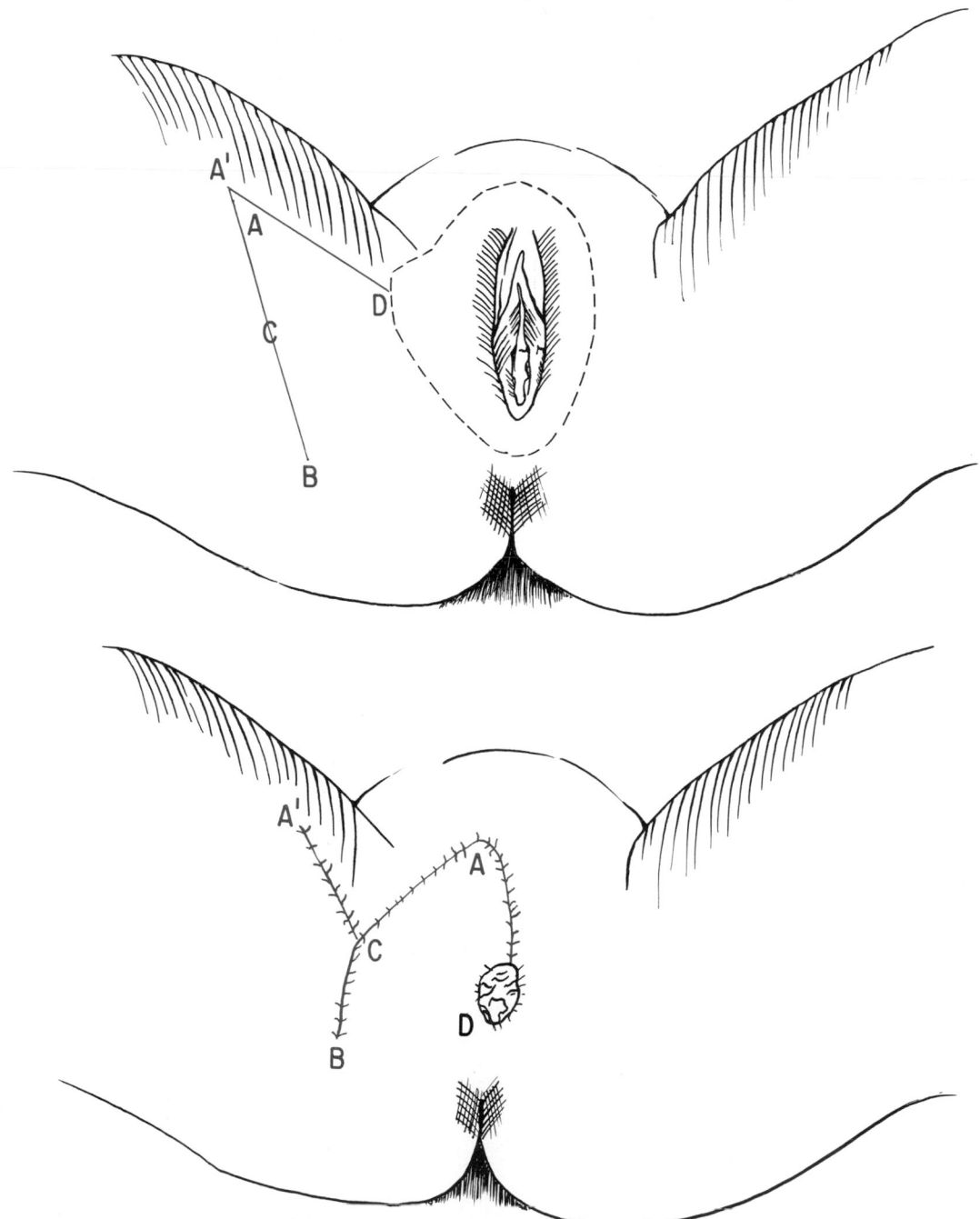

Fig. 7.17. Development of a full thickness flap from the medial aspect of the thigh to cover extensive defects in the perineum.

procedure with vulvectomy can be accomplished in approximately 2½ to 3 hours. In the absence of apparent involvement of the superficial glands, the iliac and hypogastric nodes will be invaded in approximately 2 to 3 per cent of the cases, and with this extensive involvement cure is unlikely. Thus, if adequate study of the superficial nodes reveals no metastases, in the authors' opinion extraperitoneal pelvic node dissection is not necessary. Lymphocyst resulting from such procedures is discussed in another chapter.

Carcinoma in Situ

In the study and treatment of carcinoma *in situ*, it must be repeatedly emphasized that the entire lower genital canal is subject to the effects of carcinogenic agents. Therefore, the patient with such alterations on the vulva must have a thorough evaluation of the vagina, cervix, and perianal skin, not only by inspection and cytologic study but also by use of various adjunctive techniques, *e.g.*, the Schiller reagent on the cervix and toluidine blue. Finally, careful follow-up of the patient with such lesions is imperative; surgical removal of an isolated lesion does not eliminate the carcinogenic agent.

Plastic Procedures

Occasional extensive defects are created in the external genitalia when disease has progressed beyond the confines of the area or recurrent disease in old scars of previous surgery or irradiation make primary closure impossible. Grafts for foreign donor sites are suggested by Rutledge and Sinclair (8) or simple packing of the area with healing by secondary intent are possible approaches to this problem. The former necessitates an additional procedure and a second scar at the donor site while the latter creates a long term healing process by granulation. The authors have had success using full thickness "flap grafts" from the adjacent thigh and recommend this procedure, since it avoids the problems created by the other proposals (9) (Fig. 7.17).

In conclusion, the vulva offers a great variety of operative experiences for the surgeon, and results are in general excellent if the following are observed: (1) accurate diagnosis is established prior to the institution of therapy; (2) care is taken with hemostasis; and (3) care is taken in repair of the fourchette.

References

1. Goldberg, J. E.: Simplified treatment for disease of Bartholin's gland. Obstet. Gynecol. 35: 109, 1970.
2. Schwimmer, E.: Die idiopathische Schleimhautplaques der Mundhohle: Leukoplakia Buccalis. Vierteljahrschr. Dermat. Syph. 4: 511, 1877.
3. Mering, J. H.: A surgical approach to intractable pruritis vulvae. Am. J. Obstet. Gynecol. 64: 619, 1952.
4. Woodruff, J. D., and Baens, J. S.: Interpretation of atrophic and hypertrophic alterations in the vulvar epithelium. Am. J. Obstet. Gynecol. 86: 713, 1963.
5. Collins, C. G.: Discussion of paper by J. D. Woodruff *et al.*: Metabolic activity in normal and abnormal vulvar epithelia. Am. J. Obstet. Gynecol. 91: 809, 1965.
6. Taussig, F. J.: Diseases of the Vulva. D. Appleton & Co., New York, 1923.
7. Lundwall, F.: Cancer of the vulva. Acta Radiol. (Stockh.) (Suppl.) 208, 1961.
8. Rutledge, F., and Sinclair, M.: Treatment of intraepithelial carcinoma of the vulva by skin excision and graft. Am. J. Obstet. Gynecol. 102: 806, 1968.
9. Julian, C. G., Callison, J., and Woodruff, J. D.: Plastic management of extensive vulvar defects. Obstet. Gynecol. 38: 193, 1971.

CHAPTER EIGHT

FELIX RUTLEDGE, M.D.

RADICAL HYSTERECTOMY

Radical hysterectomy is an effective treatment for carcinoma of the cervix. Its success has been defined and its limitations exposed by comparison with radiation therapy, an able competitor for this role. That radical hysterectomy has survived as a complete treatment for this disease, however, affirms some advantages over irradiation therapy. Nevertheless, these advantages are only evident when the operation is used properly.

Selection of Patient

The most frequent mistake in primary surgical treatment of carcinoma of the cervix is the misapplication of the hysterectomy. The able surgeon can attempt to excise advanced lesions, and by doing so, diminish the margins about the specimen. The resection is insufficient and fails to cure because recurrences appear. The uncertain surgeon resects too near even the earlier and smaller lesions and also fails because the cancer recurs at the margins. In either situation, nothing is accomplished and much is lost, because the patient's disease is now more disseminated, and the opportunity for intracavitary radium is unretrievable. Unless the surgeon can encompass the cancer and provide a margin of normal tissue which is clinically negative at the periphery, the outcome will be poor. Misapplication of the operation is an error that should be credited against the surgeon.

The type of cervical cancer which is suitable for treatment by radical hysterectomy must be either confined to the cervix or with only minimal spread to the vagina, in the immediate vicinity of the cervix. Lesions which extend a distance into the parametrium involve the ureter and the base of the bladder with cancer that cannot be resected by means of this operation. The physician who chooses operation for cancer of the cervix in stages more advanced than Stage I or IIA must have a special reason. Proper selection of the stage of cancer greatly determines the percentage of cures by radical hysterectomy; therefore, thorough preoperative study of the disease must not be neglected.

Pelvic Examination

The inaccuracies of the clinical examination are well known; nevertheless, this estimation is singularly most useful. The exactness of the bimanuel pelvic examination and the accuracy of staging depends on the physician's experience, the cooperation of the patient during the examination, the thickness of the abdominal wall, the normality of the other pelvic organs, and the spread pattern of the cancer. With so many influencing variables, the physician must be deliberate and thorough, because omitting these essential steps leads to unfortunate discoveries at laparotomy.

A pitfall exists in our common practice of referral of patients. In the transfer of patients from physician to physician, such as for the physician who establishes diagnosis to the physician to be responsible for treatment, the surgeon must make his own assessment of the disease by pelvic examination. Often, for the convenience of the patient and to hasten the definitive treatment of her disease, the surgeon may rely upon the examination performed by others and upon their findings base the treatment plan. A misunderstanding and a difference in the estimation of the amount of cancer can lead the surgeon into an awkward position at laparotomy.

Bimanual examination of the anesthetized patient allows the best assessment obtainable by pelvic examination. Therefore, each patient should be rechecked before the abdominal incision is made. Because of the distinct advantage of an examination with the patient under anesthesia, this extra effort is justified when the conditions for examination are unusually difficult or when there is some doubt about the significance of the palpable findings.

The decision as to whether to treat the patient by radical hysterectomy should remain open even after the abdominal cavity is incised. There is still an opportunity to change treatment plan, although such changes are best made before the operation is begun. Errors tend to be compounded when the operation proceeds upon a patient who has been selected poorly.

Intravenous Pyelogram

Selection of a patient with cancer which lends itself to resection may be facilitated by several tests which have become a standard practice during the preoperative study to delineate the cancer. The abnormal intravenous pyelogram often reflects extension of disease that would be better treated by irradiation. More advanced degrees of ureteral obstruction indicate more advanced cancer; however, any amount of hydroureter, not otherwise explained, should deter the pelvic surgeon. The cause of abnormality in the intravenous pyelogram may be checked by cystoscopy. However, cancer which is suitable for operation should not have extension into the bladder. Such abnormalities are more likely due to encroachment into the lower portion of the ureter invisible to cystoscopy. Caution should limit forced catheterization of the obstructed ureter, since pyelonephritis may be introduced. The threat of dangerous sepsis from an infected obstructed renal unit should discourage probing when it is not essential.

There are other special methods for gaining information about the renal reserve and the obstruction sites, but the routine intravenous pyelogram usually answers the surgeon's needs. In summary, ureteral obstruction in any patient not otherwise explained must be the result of cancer which is unsuitable for resection by radical hysterectomy.

Lymphangiogram

The value of the lymphangiogram remains controversial. Certainly, the usefulness of this test for lymph node metastasis will depend upon the local facilities for performing and interpreting the examination. At our institution, we have confidence in the study when positive nodes are seen, yet we realize that there are important nodes which are not opacified and therefore not assessed. The lymphangiogram may miss positive nodes not filled with dye, or metastases too small to cast a recognizable shadow. At present we would say that the omission of such a study before operation was not an error. Although this study is not an essential preoperative requirement, some patients with Stage I and Stage IIA disease will show metastasis by lymphangiography. Whether the surgeon agrees with the interpretation, this advanced information will guide the exploratory laparotomy to earlier and more certain localization of lymph node metastasis.

Other Tests

When the battery of routine roentgenograms (chest X-ray, intravenous pyelogram, and lymphangiography) are reported, additional clarification studies of these reports may be needed; therefore, it is wise to allow an extra day or more before the operation to conduct these added studies. For example, should a suspicious chest lesion require tomography studies, or a renal shadow necessitate renal arteriography, or a large para-aortic node require a venogram, the surgeon would like these questions resolved before the operation. A routine test, such as the chest or intravenous pyelogram, supplies the basic information of unsuspected metastasis to the bones for this selected group of patients. Such tests give an adequate routine bone survey, since most of the common sites of skeletal metastasis are included in these studies.

Technical Considerations

The Incision

In order to obtain a specimen from this area, the incision must be long enough to expose the lower aortic nodes. The incision may be too long, however, and then will not retain the abdominal gauze packs used to support the intestines which then fall into the pelvis or out of the abdomen during the operation. The usual incision for pelvic lymphadenectomy is longer than that for the conservative hysterectomy because additional exposure is needed. The transverse incision of the lower abdomen increases access to the pelvic walls but severely restricts exposure for dissection above the pelvic brim. Generally, the vertical midline incision provides the best exposure.

Search at Laparotomy

The laparotomy provides an opportunity to search the abdominal cavity for signs of metastasis. Failure to inspect the abdominal viscera, to palpate the para-aortic nodes, and to lavage the peritoneal cavity for cytologic study of the free cells may result in inaccurate treatment. At the least, failure to perform these functions leaves the prognosis more uncertain.

Examination, by palpation alone, of the pelvic ligaments supporting the uterus may disclose new evidence of metastasis; however, palpation may be insufficient. Therefore, to avoid both premature disruption of the blood supply to the uterus and commitment of the surgeon to the operation, entry of avascular spaces will improve palpation (Fig. 8.1). These spaces are anatomic avenues which facilitate the search for metastasis without committing the surgeon to radical hysterectomy. The para-vesicle and pararectal spaces may be entered quite simply; since they are on opposite sides of the parametrium, this structure, which is so important as the pathway for metastasis, may be checked with accuracy. (This dissection does not add unnecessary time to the duration of the radical hysterectomy for early entry of these spaces also facilitates subsequent lymphadenectomy.) The operation seems feasible when the paravesicle and pararectal spaces are open on each side and the tactual conditions are favorable. In this case, the cancer has not extended to the pelvic wall, and there is a tumor-free space about the specimen. However, there are still other sites to be checked.

For radical hysterectomy the attachment of the base of the bladder and the rectum to the cervix and vagina must not have been infiltrated by carcinoma. Palpation first, and then dissecting this attachment will indicate the amount of spread fore and aft of the cervix. The size of the primary growth and any contiguous extensions can now be judged suitable or not for radical hysterectomy. Having cleared the condition of the primary growth as operable, the regional nodes may be attacked for excision.

Whether the surgeon performs the lymph-

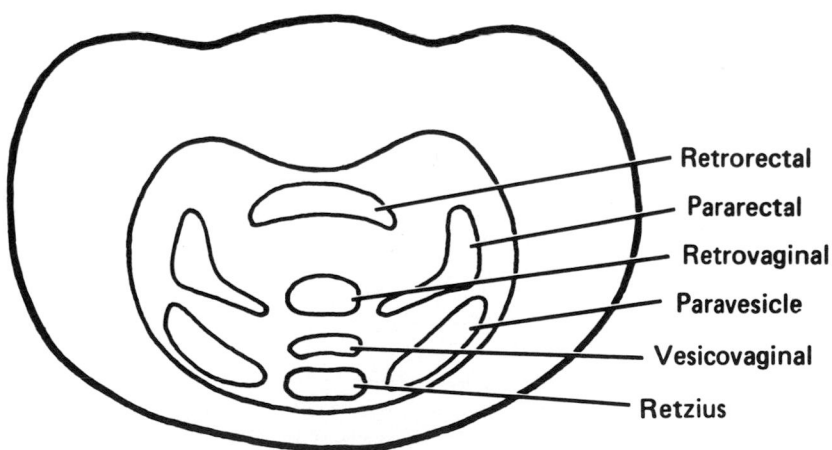

Fig. 8.1. Pelvic avascular spaces

These potential spaces within the pelvic cavity which separate the pelvic viscera from each other and from the pelvic side walls provide the surgeon access for discovering metastases and facilitate controlled excision of all or selected pelvic organs.

These spaces are created anatomically with loosely related boundries which permit a viscus, like the bladder or colon, to distend or to change its position in relation to other structures. Opening these spaces for investigation creates no permanent injury. Through these passages the surgeon may palpate and biopsy without committing the organ to excision.

When excision is decided hemorrhage control may be improved by utilizing the avascular spaces of the pelvis to prepare vessels for ligation with maximal security.

adenectomy before or after the hysterectomy is a matter of personal preference. There are advantages to starting the operation with the lymphadenectomy because information about the size of the node, how many sites of metastases, and height of cephalad spread alters the decision to remove the uterus. The planned radical hysterectomy may be cancelled if adverse conditions are found, for lymphadenectomy will not impair irradiation treatment. Should an unfavorable cancer become evident by discovery of disseminated nodal metastases, external therapy will be needed.

Sometimes large retroperitoneal nodes indicating unforeseen spread are discovered in the exposure created by the lymphadenectomy dissection. Although lymphadenectomy alone controls about half of the patients with positive nodes, when a large group of matted nodes are found, postoperative irradiation therapy to the area becomes essential. Such findings should arouse suspicion that the primary tumor also is larger than estimated, and the surgeon should suspect the cervix and its surrounding tissues of harboring subclinical metastasis. If this concern is sufficient, termination of the operation after the lymphadenectomy may be wise. Irradiation therapy employing both intracavitary and external techniques can then proceed quite satisfactorily. Certainly, unless there is the expectation of a definitive cure by operation, the risk of complications from both radical hysterectomy and subsequent irradiation is not justified.

Lymphadenectomy

Para-aortic Nodes. A specimen of node containing fibrofatty tissue may be safely removed near and immediately above the bifurcation of the aorta, providing the surgeon has an abdominal wall incision which exposes this region and enough assistance to retract (Fig. 8.2). Effective retractors, a functioning aspiration suction, and a supply of hemostatic metallic clips are basic tools. A confident knowledge of the regional anatomy will protect the right ureter and the inferior mesentery artery while the specimen is being approached (Fig. 8.3). An incision in the dorsal peritoneum below and parallel to the route of the terminal ileum mesentery will open the retroperitoneal

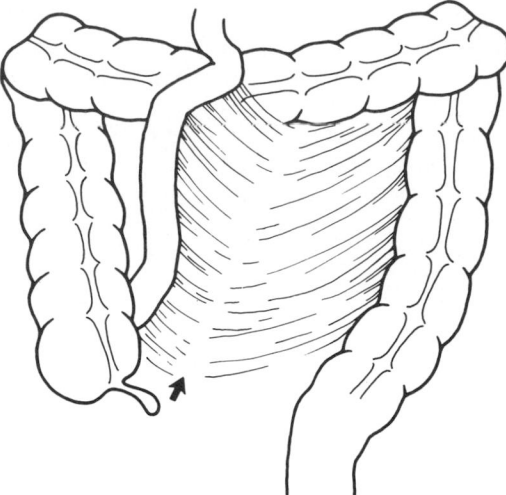

Fig. 8.2. Precaval and para-aortic exploration

The precaval and para-aortic nodes may be approached by reflecting either the right or left colon mesially after incising the restraining peritoneum of the respective lateral gutter. The direct approach may be simplier.

For sampling the nodes and biopsy needs, the direct approach through the parietal peritoneum by incision along the base of the small bowel mesentery serves most occasions. Upward traction upon the terminal ileum will create a groove in the parietal peritoneum parallel to the right ureter. This will guide the surgeon to the underlying fibrofatty tissue which contains lymph nodes that lie within the pathway for metastasizing carcinoma of the cervix.

(The beginning site and direction of the incision are noted by the arrow.)

space. The group of nodes of interest is approached from all sides and dissected free (Fig. 8.4), and the small peripheral blood vessels are secured with ligature or metallic clips. When the specimen seems ready for removal, a critical phase is near because the remaining attachment is to the vena cava. Short veins join the nodes and the vena cava, and these require special care to avoid causing a rent in the vena cava. These are also occluded with metal hemostatic clips and severed.

Pelvic Wall Nodes. The retroperitoneal space is entered by dividing the round ligament about an inch from its exit through the internal inguinal ring. The peritoneum is incised along the route of the iliac vessels upward to the level where the ureter crosses the common iliac vessel. The peritoneal incision is directed downward to the pubis. The ovarian vessels are

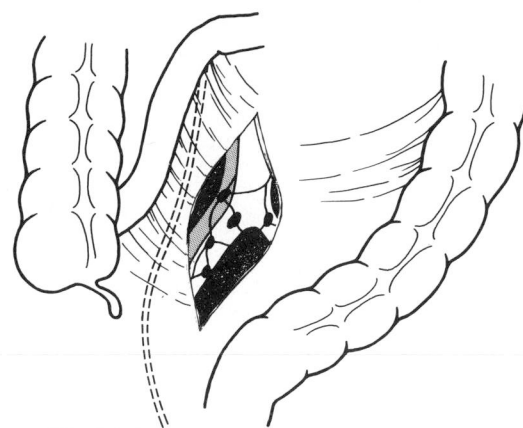

Fig. 8.3. Para-aortic lymph node investigation

The superior level of the common iliac nodes and the lower para-aortic nodes compose part of the secondary nodes which become positive by metastasis from carcinoma of the cervix. Since these nodes are difficult to excise completely by lymphadenectomy and are badly positioned for irradiation therapy, the patient's prognosis is strongly influenced when they are positive. The answer for patients suspected to have positive nodes may be essential for the radiotherapist to design the treatment and fundamental for the pelvic surgeon who may be planning extended resection.

The incision of the peritoneum described in Figure 8.2 may be extended conveniently to higher level aortic nodes until dissection becomes restrained by the renal vessels and the transverse portion of the duodenum or the incision may be lengthened caudad to the level of the right ureter as it crosses the pelvic brim. Thus the right side precaval, para-aortic, and common iliac nodes are exposed.

stripped back from the overlying peritoneum, cleaned of loose fibrofatty tissue, and ligated as close as possible to the cecum on the right and the sigmoid on the left, without detaching the vessels from these structures. Isolation and ligation of the ovarian vessels high on the pelvic brim facilitates exposure of the common iliac nodes and reduces the chance of tearing the ovarian vein by retraction. A lateral flap of peritoneum is lifted by bluntly pushing off the attached fibrofatty tissue to become part of the specimen. The medial peritoneal flap, with the attached ureters, likewise is retracted medially by bluntly dissecting it from the pelvic wall structure. The node containing specimen is now exposed but still attached to vessels.

There is a cleavage plane vertical to the course of the internal iliac artery which can be extended downward along the lateral side of

the superior vesicle artery and the side of the bladder to the pubic ramus. Care should be taken to remain lateral to the superior vesicle artery with the dissection because on this side, no significant bleeding will be encountered before the bottom of the obturator fossa is reached. The specimen is now isolated for removal.

Mishaps with Vessels

The nodes can be removed in three main specimen blocks. The largest block contains the external iliac, hypogastric, and obturator nodes. About the common iliac vessels, removal of the specimen in a common block becomes more difficult. A dissection in this region becomes more risky also because the vessels are less mobile and the vein wall thinner. Some of the

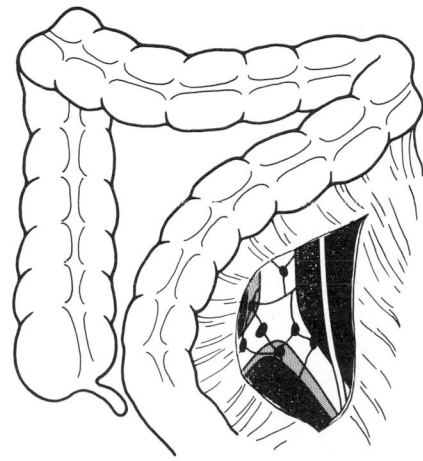

Fig. 8.4. Left side approach to the para-aortic region

Utilizing the precaval incision subperitoneal tissues may be dissected across to the left side of the aorta; however, exposure becomes more limited because the inferior mesenteric artery and vein limit mobility of the mesentery to the left colon. Without sacrificing the inferior mesenteric vessels, an improved exposure for dissecting the left para-aortic lymph nodes may be had through another incision in the left peritoneal gutter along the base of the mesentery to the descending colon and sigmoid colon.

Again on this left side the ureter must be protected while dissecting. Usually the left ureter will remain attached on the mesentery of the descending colon; however, para-aortic fibrosis created by irradiation treatment or by cancer in the area may cause the ureter to remain within the pathway for dissection as pictured here. With either condition the left ureter must be considered in jeopardy.

deeper nodes lie below the internal iliac vein between its divisions, thus less accessible. Dissection first on one side and then on the other may be necessary in order to extract the nodes from between the perforating branches of the internal iliac vein. The sacral nodes are quite variable in size and are the least likely to be removed *en bloc.* Except for the region of the bifurcation of the vena cava, they are the least important locations for metastases.

The caudal end of the lymphadenectomy operation is the easiest and safest part, and this part of the operation should be done first. The troublesome venous bleeding happens most often in the areas of the common iliac artery and aortic bifurcation. This phase of the operation should be reserved for the last because blood staining of the operative field is best delayed as long as possible. Also venous bleeding can usually be controlled best by direct pressure from a gauze pack if the dissection has been completed. The common technical errors are hemorrhage and incising or severing an essential structure.

Retraction in dissection about the perforating division of the internal iliac vein should be done very cautiously for bleeding from these venous branches may be quite profuse. The threat of hemorrhage during pelvic lymphadenectomy remains with the veins for they are more fragile. Injury by penetration during dissection and laceration during retraction has occurred but control is regained by suture or ligature. The more resistant, thicker walled arteries tolerate the dissection best. Except for variability in the origin of the obturator artery, their course is consistent and they can tolerate retraction and stripping more vigorously than the pelvic wall veins which are more fragile and have a less dependable course.

Variation in the take-off site may cause the surgeon to sever large veins inadvertently because its course is unexpected. The obturator, the circumflex iliac, and the inferior epigastric veins are unpredictable because they frequently branch out of the internal iliac at a higher-than-usual site and may be severed without sufficient stump for easy ligation. Although the initial venous hemorrhage can be frightening, it can be temporarily stopped by direct pressure while preparing to repair the defect in the vein by suture with fine material. Repair should be attempted, for although the external iliac vein may be ligated, this is not desirable since lower extremity edema may result. The surgeon who hastily places a hemostat in the general direction of hemorrhage often aggravates the problem.

Lymphocysts

Following completion of the lymphadenectomy, the best possible hemostasis and lymph stasis do not assure that the defect will remain empty of serous drainage material. The many severed lymph vessels continue to deposit fluid into the dissection site. Absorption of the fluid and recanalization of these lymphatics is usually adequate, but for some patients the area accumulates sufficient fluid to be encapsulated into a lymphocyst. These fluid-filled tumors compress neighboring veins and often produce hydronephrosis by ureteral obstruction. The lymphocyst may block urinary drainage by compression or angulation of the ureter. Resulting impairment of the renal function forces the surgeon to drain the lymphocyst, whereas the preferred treatment would be to allow it to resolve without interference. Evacuation by needle aspiration provides transient relief of a lymphocyst but carries with it the hazard of introducing infection. Also, a single aspiration is ineffective because of prompt refilling which shortens the relief. Total excision of the lymphocyst wall is definitive but formidable, requiring laparotomy. Although spontaneous resolution of a lymphocyst is desirable, incision sometimes is necessary. Chronic drainage, infection, and slow recovery may be the outcome. There is no reliable technique to prevent lymphocysts; therefore, their appearance is not an indictment against the surgeon.

The surgeon must be aware of the threat of lymphocysts and should ligate all identifiable lymphatic trunks leading to the dissection site. Suction evacuation of the pelvic wall spaces has been a most successful preventative. Catheter tubes are effective if placed at the termination of the operation into the retroperitoneal space and aspirated with a strong negative pressure so long as the drainage collects. Lymphocysts are often a development after lymphadenectomy. They cause the patient considerable extra discomfort for a prolonged postoperative period. There is no simple and effective way of erradicating the lymphocysts, thus prevention is the best method of control.

(The surgeon should check the strength of the catheter if additional holes are made in the wall. These additional holes are often desirable; however, if they are cut too large or too near each other, the wall of the tube may be weakened sufficiently that it will break when traction is exerted to remove it. Also avoid placing a hole in the tube in direct contact with large, thin walled veins. Prompt application of suction to these catheters will prevent coagulation of accumulated material within the tube. Regular irrigation of the tubes is not suggested since infection may be introduced. The tubes are removed when they cease to function.)

The Hysterectomy

Basic Technical Steps

Of all the abdominal operations, the radical hysterectomy should be considered as demanding the most technical skill. The steps of the operation are sequentially dependent, and each phase is performed best when the previous one is uneventful. If mishaps do occur, the surgeon should be in control sufficiently to correct accidents and re-establish the orderly dissection. Individuality in operative techniques among pelvic surgeons indicates the superior understanding of the anatomy and the mechanical elements of the procedure. The surgeon who has a preference for a technique probably has a skill in depth to deal with contingencies. A stereotype technique is not admirable for it suggests a lack of imagination in performing the procedure most efficiently. The complexity of the dissection and the chance of adversity require a repertoire of alternate surgical approaches. These may be needed when the usual planes of dissection are obliterated by fibrosis, when previous operations have altered the normal anatomy, when tumor growth obstructs a standard approach, or when hemorrhage occurs which necessitates control by packing and approaching the specimen from an alternate direction. The hysterectomy involves five basic steps:

1. Separation of the bladder and the rectum from the specimen.
2. Liberation and retraction of the lower ureter.

3. Isolation and division of the ligaments that are attached to the uterus and vagina.
4. Amputation of the vagina.
5. Reconstruction.

Detachment of the Bladder

A critical point in the radical hysterectomy dissection is separation of the bladder from the vagina. Ways of eliminating common technical errors which cause injury to the bladder are:

1. Avoid establishing a false plane in the muscular wall of the bladder which weakens this structure. The correct space is superior to the pubocervical fascia and this space may be missed or lost as the bladder and vagina are separated. The surgeon should suspect that part of the bladder musculature has been left on the vagina if the texture and color of the tissue change. The pubocervical fascia should continue to be smooth and gray at the vaginal level and on the cervix.

2. Maintain traction while dissecting, thus stretching the surface of the bladder wall and the anterior vaginal wall laterally. This flattens creases and folds of the bladder wall which are more likely to be cut with injury to a full thickness of the wall.

3. In the separation of the bladder from the vagina, use a broad frontal approach. If the dissection proceeds far in advance on one side, the opposite side is more susceptible to injury.

4. Perform this critical dissection early in the operation because safe separation depends upon the distinctive color and texture of the organs that are to be detached. These differences are blurred by blood staining.

5. Avoid blunt dissection. The muscular wall of bladder will separate by this technique, thus leaving part of the bladder musculature on the vagina. Blunt dissection produces interstitial hemorrhages in the bladder wall which are traumatizing, and this aggravates the postoperative problem on bladder atony.

Separation of the Rectum from the Vagina

Injury of the rectum should be avoidable since carcinoma of the cervix rarely spreads in this direction; nevertheless, entry of the bowel occurs unless care is practiced. The sites for caution have a basis in the anatomy.

1. The posterior vaginal wall is quite long so the rectum must be detached for a considerable distance. If visualization becomes difficult, it will improve if, while dissecting, upward and posterior traction is maintained on the bowel.

2. Blood vessels are avoided by separating the bowel from the vagina in the midline. There are two firm attachments of the bowel to the vagina in this zone which will require separation. One forms the bottom of the cul-de-sac and the other is at the level of the middle third of the posterior vaginal wall. The latter attachment is less obvious; however, this second attachment of the bowel is especially susceptible to injury at this level. Although attached firmly, it creates a knuckle of intestine which is vulnerable to entry as the posterior vaginal wall is freed by sharp resection.

3. If large hemostatic clamps are applied while dividing the uterosacral ligaments and their continuation downward as the pillars of the rectum, injury to the bowel may be caused and this in turn is conducive to fistulization. The uterosacrals are usually divided very close to the bowel wall; thus when large hemostatic clamps are applied, they can accidentally include some of the wall.

Liberation and Retraction of the Lower Ureter

The ureter commands the respect of the surgeon since the life of the kidney depends upon its function. Not only must it contain the urine, but the passage must also be free. It must be an active participant in urine excretion by peristalsis because stasis of urine flow or reflux invites pyelitis. Things to be avoided are devascularization and trauma and injury caused first by the surgeon and secondarily by pelvic infection. A ureteral fistula may be caused by a single one of these mechanisms; more often, however, several etiologic forces contribute.

Within boundaries resected by radical hysterectomy, some vessels to the ureter will be sacrificed. The manner in which the surgeon treats the ureter and the ease with which the operation proceeds affect the degree of devascularization of the ureter. The ureter is in the midst of the operation and, consequently, some trauma is unavoidable. Postoperative infections are not totally preventable; however, the incidence and severity will be influenced by the surgeon's management of the pelvic cavity at the completion of the operation and during the postoperative care. Adjustments of the pelvic tissues displaced by the dissection may ultimately distort the course of the ureter and lead to kinking and obstruction. A technical error may cause obstruction or subsequent fibrosis which produces compression and distortion of the ureter at its junction with the bladder.

There is much about the etiology of the ureteral fistulae which remains unknown. There is an abundance of recorded clinical observations, suppositions, and theory. Such material has been recorded regularly in the literature, yet scientific evidence based upon the laboratory investigation to prove the mechanism of ureteral fistulae is lacking. Available knowledge based upon observation of clinicians is loaded with personal bias and prejudice and may not qualify as scientific evidence. Yet this recording of clinical events appears to be accurate and useful and may serve as a basis for a plan to lessen the incidence of ureteral fistulae.

Conserving Vascularity to the Ureter

Probably as a result of the embryology and migration of the renal system during early development, the ureter has a specially contained vasculature which courses along its surface interconnecting the supply branches into a vascular network throughout the entire length. This network of blood vessels ensheaths the ureter at various intervals along its course, and arterial supplies connect to the regional vascular trunks. This system compensates remarkably well for the loss of the ureteral supply at any segment, and makes the ureter especially tolerant of the devascularization necessary to perform the radical hysterectomy.

Survival of the devascularized ureter has limits. Exceeding these limits is one of the more frequent causes of slough and ureteral fistulae. The vascular anatomy has never been portrayed better than by the drawings of Max Brödel (27) in 1900. In his artistic portrayal, Brödel supplied the pelvic surgeon a picture of the ureter with emphasis upon the blood supply, so that one can easily see the limitations imposed upon the pelvic dissection by the anatomy of the vascular supply to the ureter. The branches of the superior vesicle artery, the internal iliac artery, and the common iliac arteries are of special concern. Certain of the ureteral branches must be sacrificed for radical hysterectomy; the uterine branch is lost regularly, and sometimes the branch from the superior vesicle, and even the common iliac, must be severed. The more supply of these vessels to be disrupted, the greater the chance of ureteral fistula formation; therefore, the vascular supply is of prime importance. Whether one, two, or three of these vessels can be lost depends upon other contributing etiologic factors.

Although the surgeon is constrained by the effort to protect the ureteral blood supply, reluctance to disrupt the ureteral blood supply near the bladder may incur the risk of not resecting sufficient tissue to cure the cancer. In the radical hysterectomy, there is always the calculated risk involving ureteral survival *vs.* the effort to widely encompass tissue which may harbor metastasis. The key to the number of vessels that can be sacrificed with safety is the preservation of the periureteral network of blood vessels, for their collateral circulation will replace the loss of at least two of the contributing ureteral arteries. Excessive stripping of the adventitia by too close dissection about the ureter, or injury by careless retraction will destroy the periureteral vascular network. Obviously, technical accidents such as clamping of the ureter not only injure the blood supply but also destroy the vitality of the ureteral wall. Certainly, transection of the ureter during the operation disrupts this interconnection of vascular network. Although reanastomosis is performed, the efficiency of the network is impaired. Such unplanned injury certainly charges the surgeon with an error which may be costly to the patient.

Special Techniques for Avoiding Ureteral Fistulae

Surgeons have devised procedures as guides for lessening the risk of postoperative ureteral vaginal fistula from devascularization. Stallworthy (28) has validated his theoretical observations for avoiding ureteral vaginal fistulae by successful clinical application. He has a very low incidence of ureteral vaginal fistula, resulting no doubt, from his great technical skill, his acute clinical judgment, and the application of some surgical principles which he advises others to adopt. For surgeons, he recommends preservation of the mesentery to the ureter by careful dissection of the ureter from the pelvic wall location while preserving its attachment mesially to the peritoneum. This thin mesentery of fibrofatty tissue and small blood vessels contributes to the ureteral blood supply by branches from the internal iliac artery.

Green *et al.* (9) advised splinting and supporting the ureter to conserve its vasculature. Although the ureter is dissected from its pelvic wall position and mobilized, the terminal portion is reattached by delicately suturing the wall of the ureter to the superior vesicle artery. Green believes that the normal course of the ureter is thus restored by the splinting action of the attached artery. By this maneuver, a new blood supply develops faster from the superior vesicle artery to the ureter, thus improving nutrition of the ureter. In addition, the ureter is held at a high position in the pelvic cavity; thus if infections develop postoperatively, the ureter is less involved.

Symmonds and Pratt (25) have suggested that more effective drainage of the dissection site will reduce the incidence of pelvic infection by preventing serous fluid collection since such material nourishes bacterial contamination which is inevitable from an open vagina. Symmonds has suggested that the common practice of providing dependent drainage through the vagina can instead be improved by continuous aspiration of the pelvic cavity with suction catheters. This evacuates the media for bacterial growth and reduces the amount and severity of pelvic infection, since aspiration both evacuates and collapses the space in which the fluid accumulates. The suction catheters are more efficient for clearing the area, and there is also less risk of feeding the area with new bacteria from the vagina, as is likely with vaginal drains. The other function of the continuous suction catheter, as mentioned above, is to prevent the formation of lymphocysts which may indirectly contribute to ureteral fistula formation by blockage of the ureter through direct compression or by distortion of its course.

Frank Novak (16) has transplanted the ureter within the peritoneal cavity to protect the ureter from the injurious environment of the postoperative retroperitoneal space. Within the peritoneal cavity, the ureter is not attacked by infection so frequently. The ureter may gain nourishment from the peritoneal and omental vessels. Except for a few technical cautions to avoid angulation of the ureter at entry and exit through the peritoneum, this approach appears sound. The suggestion of Novak has been modified by O'Kawa of Tokyo; he suggests transfer of the ureter into the peritoneal cavity plus creating a tunnel of peritoneum for the pelvic portion of the ureter. Instead of approximating the sheaths of pelvic side wall peritoneum edge to edge, they overlap sufficiently to house the ureter in the space or tunnel created.

The many methods proposed to avoid ureteral fistulae are an indication of the universal concern for this complication of radical hysterectomy. The attention given to protecting this structure during and following operation has minimized the incidence of ureterovaginal fistulae. No longer should this complication blemish the records of surgical treatment after an effective operation without postoperative complications. There can be assurance that later a serious complication will not develop. The surgeon has better control over complications than the radiotherapist; thus the source of trouble can be traced when radical hysterectomy is the treatment.

Isolation and Division of Pelvic Ligaments

The cardinal, uterosacral, superficial, and deep pubocervical ligaments must be dealt with separately. Any attempt to apply clamps to any of these ligaments prematurely before they are isolated results in uncertain control and hindrance of the operation. A bundling of two ligaments by common ligature contracts avenues of exposure. This gross handling progressively narrows the range of the dissection. Since individual ligaments diverge outward from the specimen, they must be dissected free to be isolated for clamping if they are to be divided wide laterally—a requirement for radicality. The approach to isolation of these structures involves avascular planes of tissue.

Certain potential spaces within the pelvis have evolved embryologically and are maintained for physiologic reason. Expansile organs such as the bladder and rectum cannot be fixed to a rigid structure if they are to function; therefore, tissues in the zone neighboring the viscera are loosely structured. Where free movement of organs is necessary, a potential plane is maintained which the surgeon may dissect easily and safely. The paravesicle and pararectal spaces are utilized most for the radical hysterectomy. Surgeons who do not develop these avenues miss an advantage to enter the deeper zones of the pelvis.

Reconstruction

Closure of the Vagina. The management of the open top of the vagina after the specimen has been excised has long been discussed. Some points for consideration are:

1. The open vagina may efficiently drain the foci of hemorrhage and the serous exudate which continues after the operation; yet this open vagina is objectionable for it may feed bacterial contamination and be responsible for pelvic cellulitis or abscess.

2. Closure of the vagina covers the denuded portion of the bladder and rectum reinforcing this weakened area of the visceral wall. This technique helps reduce risk of fistulae.

3. The open top of the vagina preserves the maximal length of the vagina. This is a factor for coitus when a long part of the vagina must be excised. Procedures have been suggested to annex the cul-de-sac space as part of the vaginal depth. The sigmoid and pelvic peritoneum serves to cover the space when the vagina is not closed.

I would favor routinely closing the vagina to avoid fistulae; however, there will be situations when the reverse would be preferable to gain length to the vagina. At this time, no error can be imposed by using either the open or closed procedure.

Postoperative Care

Infection

Postoperative infections are a constant threat to the radical hysterectomy. Serous fluid collections that leak from the surface of the incised tissue of the severed lymph vessels, plus variable quantities of hemorrhaging to the dissection site, continue after the operation is completed. All efforts should be directed toward avoiding the development of bacteria into a full infection. Efforts such as an injection of a bolus of antibiotics at the termination of the pelvic dissection may deposit antibacterial agents into the accumulated serum and blood. Such antibiotics, when deposited directly into the media for bacterial growth, make it less suitable for infection to progress.

The additional efforts to reduce the number of bacteria caused by contamination from the vagina are profitable. Thorough lavage of the pelvic cavity after the removal of the specimen and before closure of the vagina reduces the population of bacteria and thereby the severity of the infection.

Atonic Bladder

Micturition disturbances are well known, but little understood consequences of radical hysterectomy. Because corrective operations are not required and no effective preventative is known, the topic receives little attention in discussion. However, much disability is caused by the atonic dysfunctional bladder. The patient is susceptible to recurrent cystitis; therefore, unless attention is paid to the prevention and treatment of cystitis and pyelitis, some of the years of life due a patient having undergone a successful operation for carcinoma of the cervix will be lost because of earlier death from renal failure. Repeated or chronic pyelonephritis may destroy kidney function; thus shortening the life span of the patient. To ignore or to be unaware of this hazard is an error in the follow-up care of patients who have had a radical hysterectomy.

The follow-up care should begin promptly while the indwelling catheter is still in place. Meigs (14) was one of the first to advocate prolonged drainage of the bladder after a radical hysterectomy. Although his stated purpose for retaining the indwelling catheter was to lessen the risk of ureteral fistula formation, he must have been treating the atonic bladder as well. His logic was founded in preventing the sequence of overdistension by retained urine followed by urinary tract infection. Deflating the bladder with an indwelling catheter for many weeks after the operation prevents the undesirable effects of a large amount of residual urine which destroys the bladder wall and causes recurring chronic cystitis.

The literature about the problem supplies practical advice for postoperative deflation of the bladder both by urethral and suprapubic drainage. Points of concern are (1) the duration

of the drainage, (2) the drainage system and its attachment which will allow maximal mobilization of the patient and protection from contamination, and (3) prevention of infection. Presently, these postoperative care practices are based mainly upon clinical observations because our knowledge of the physiology of the bladder altered by radical hysterectomy is incomplete. Some recent studies have contributed new information that promises to clarify the subject.

Cystometric studies of the postoperative bladder demonstrate pressure curves that are hypotonic as a result of denervation alterations in about half of the patients who had a true radical hysterectomy. Signs of a neurogenic bladder may be found in the symptoms of frequency of micturition, straining, urgency, and stress incontinence. Diminution of bladder sensation develops abnormally high bladder capacity. Incomplete micturition creates a high amount of residual urine which is responsible for the symptoms and also for the repeated episodes of acute or chronic infection. Postoperative management should precede the appearance of these symptoms because the incidence of the problem is sufficient to institute prophylactic management on a routine basis. Volumetric and urine flow studies may help the physician decide when to discontinue the bladder drainage after operation. Rehabilitation measures such as informing the patients of their problems and teaching them to use accessory forces to evacuate the bladder all are helpful. The informed patient certainly can cooperate better and do much to correct micturition problems.

Finally, the physician who is well aware of the effects of the radical hysterectomy knows the location of the nerves and can design the radicality of his operation to match the needs of the patient's disease. By avoiding an excessively radical resection for those patients with minimal cancer, he can spare the patient the inevitable consequences of radical hysterectomy.

*Management of Patients with Recent
Ureterovaginal Fistula*

Localization of the site of defect may not be simple. The intravenous pyelogram is most helpful, particularly if it shows unilateral obstructive uropathy or if there is extravasation of the dye from one side. Such findings are workable evidence of ureteral fistula, but they must be checked by further cytoscopic observation of the dye as it is excreted from the ureteral orifice. Retrograde sounding and even retrograde pyelography may confirm that one ureter is injured but the other is not. Uncertainty may remain after these tests because bilateral hydroureters are a common event following a radical hysterectomy even when there is no fistula. Thus a unilateral fistula may not present a distinctive picture in the intravenous pyelogram test. Instillation of methylene blue into the bladder and a check for staining of the vagina, followed later by the injection of indigo carmine for staining of the vaginal lining or a dry gauze placed into the vagina, may distinguish the simple vesicovaginal fistula from the ureterovaginal fistula. The difficult-to-diagnosis patients are those who have a combination ureterovaginal and vesicovaginal fistula. In these complicated cases, identification of the involved side may be delayed until near the time when corrective surgical treatment is contemplated. Thus, the conditions of the pelvis are returned to a more normal state. During this observation time, interval checks on the status of the urinary tract are essential since obstructive uropathy may lead to loss of renal unit.

The insistence of the uncomfortable, apprehensive patient, plus the surgeon's drive to resolve the problem may induce premature operation for correcting the fistula. Generally, this operation should be delayed until the inflammatory reaction of the pelvis has subsided. Spontaneous closure of the fistula during the waiting time has been recorded, but there is a hazard that the renal unit may be lost and that the cessation of drainage may also be a cessation of urinary production. The operation to correct a ureterovaginal fistula will be easier if it is not done until several months following the diagnosis. An earlier repair, however, may be necessary if the renal unit is threatened by blockage of the lower ureter.

Radical Hysterectomy and Irradiation

Preoperative Irradiation

The surgeon who ignores the current radiotherapy opportunities or does not stay informed of radiotherapy capabilities is likely to err in his practice by omission. The surgeon who ignores the opportunity to use radiotherapy for the difficult problem is forced to operate upon patients not ideally suited for surgery. Irradiation may offer much help to the surgeon who is planning to manage the disease primarily by operation. For example, the literature records experience and establishes the benefit of preoperative irradiation of the primary lesion before radical hysterectomy. Preoperative irradiation is a recognized, established concept, employed successfully for many years to accomplish several things.

1. By first irradiating the cervix, a foul lesion may be cleansed lessening the risk of postoperative pelvic infection.

2. The bulky cancerous lesions may be regressed by preoperative irradiation, creating more space within the pelvis for the surgeon to maneuver.

3. Perhaps most importantly a conservative dose of irradiation administered before operation reduces the ability of neoplastic cells which may contaminate the dissection site to produce a regrowth. This preoperative irradiation may make benign tissue less favorable for cells to implant and impair the growth ability of the cancer cells such that implantation does not occur. The threat of implantation during operation is real and is not infrequently a source of recurrence.

Combination Management Surgery and Irradiation

The distinction between preoperative irradiation followed by radical hysterectomy and combination therapy must be made. The purpose of preoperative irradiation is to prepare the cancer for a cure by excision alone. The dose would never be enough for a cure, while a larger dose or irradiation within cancerocidal range followed by operation is combination therapy. While preoperative irradiation may add little to the complication incidence of radical hysterectomy, the more cancerocidal dose used for combination therapy seriously restrains the radicality of subsequent operation.

Serious error can be made by the surgeon who chooses to perform a radical hysterectomy after high dose of irradiation. This applies to both dose irradiation from radium and/or from

X-ray therapy. High dose of external therapy is especially threatening because the bladder and rectum must receive the full effects when directed toward the cervix, whereas intracavitary irradiation is more confined about the uterus and upper vagina. The latter is, however, still dangerous for a radical hysterectomy since much of this irradiated tissue is included in the specimen. For both situations the incidence of vaginal slough, vesicovaginal fistula, and pelvis cellulitis rises sharply when a high dose of irradiation is combined with a radical hysterectomy. This has been observed sufficiently that the surgeon who insists on performing a radical hysterectomy after a high dose of irradiation therapy almost invariably commits a mistake that proves catastrophic.

Radicality of the Hysterectomy

A variety of operations may be termed radical hysterectomy or Wertheim's operation. Variation in radicality of hysterectomy for cancer of the cervix is useful because the treatment by operation should be an individualized plan—based upon the size of the cancer and whether this is primary treatment or treatment or recurrence. Also to be considered is whether an allowance should be made in the radicality for the effects of prior irradiation. Radicality suggests the distance the surgeon extends the resection away from the cervix; and it involves such factors as the nearness to the pelvic wall which the parametrium divided, the length of upper vagina removed, the amount of mobilization of the ureter from its bed, and the sacrifice of vasculature. The surgeon needs several extended hysterectomy operations to suit the patient's needs. Early lesions may be cured with the safer radical resection, but this same operation would be inadequate for more advanced and more complex problems.

The classic radical hysterectomy as practiced by Meigs (14) is the operation employed more frequently for invasive cancer of the cervix. Other patients may be considered for less extensive and safer operations, for example, (1) extensive cancer *in situ* involving the deeper parts of glands; (2) microinvasive cancer where there is uncertainty about deeper extension or concern about the involvement of lymphatics; and (3) the patient who has received rather large doses of irradiation, and there is doubt about the completeness of the total destruction

of this carcinoma by irradiation.

For these patients a procedure more extended than the conventional hysterectomy but less than the Meigs procedure could be adequate and free of postoperative complications. A bolder approach than the Meigs procedure may be warranted if a portion of the urinary tract is involved with cancer. The radical hysterectomy may be extended to resect and reconstruct this portion of the urinary tract, an ultraradical hysterectomy.

As mentioned earlier, the surgeon's responsibility ranges well beyond the operating room; he is the physician who should know what patients are better treated by operation; having decided on treatment by radical hysterectomy, he is responsible for proficiency in a variety of procedures depending on what his individual patient may require.

This individualized surgical treatment of carcinoma of the cervix is emphasized at the University of Texas M. D. Anderson Hospital by a classification for radicality in hysterectomy. There is nothing unique about the classification or the procedures described, and revisions are likely for the future. However, its use has simplified communications and recording among our staff. In this regard a classification of some type is recommended. The following definitions have proved useful for the precision and ease of documenting the radicality of hysterectomy.

Type I (Fig. 8.5)

This extrafacial hysterectomy, which is essentially the modified radical hysterectomy described by Telinde, separates the cervix and upper vagina in a plane outside the pubocervical fascia. The technique assures complete removal of the cervix and 1 to 2 cm of vaginal cuff. The inclusion of some paracervical tissue reduces a risk of dissecting into the cervix as the cardinal ligaments are detached. The additional vaginal cuff may be included when the vagina in this area is involved or suspected. The extrafacial hysterectomy needs additional preliminary dissection of the paracervical tissue to "skeletonize" the vessels for more lateral division; thus the ureter is deflected outward without removal from the ureteral tunnel. This is made possible by more complete exposure of the uterine artery and vein. The uterosacral ligaments are detached separately. The vagina becomes more

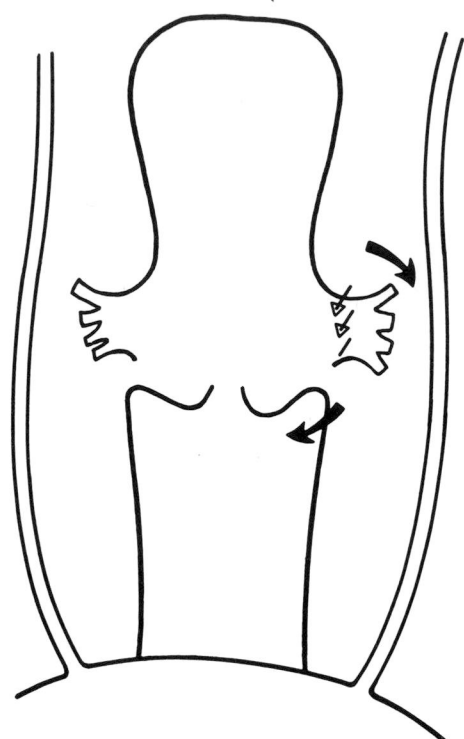

Fig. 8.5. Type I radical hysterectomy
(modified radical)

The endeavor is to excise totally the cervix with a margin of vagina while not mobilizing the ureter, *i.e.,* to carry the excision of the parametrium lateral without approaching near enough to the ureter as to incur risk of injury or ligation. This may be accomplished by dissecting the uterine and cervical vessel clean of surrounding tissues such that hemostats may be applied outward from the lateral limits of the cervix.

The initial dissection separates the anterior and posterior sheaths of the broad ligament. Fibers of the cardinal, uterosacral, and pubocervical ligaments are severed before hemostats are applied to the uterine vessels; thus precise application with a minimal size pedicle of tissue is ligated. When small purchases of tissue are clamped, a gathering of tissues is avoided. Successively the parametrium with the ureter falls away from the uterus and cervix. A wider sweep around the cervix results.

The purpose for this special treatment is to avoid dissecting into the sides of the lower uterine segment and cervix and to assure that all of the cervix is excised.

mobile prior to amputation, making it possible for the surgeon to select the amount of cuff to be included.

Type II (Fig. 8.6)

This moderately radical operation preserves the blood supply to the lower ureter and vagina while removing medially two-thirds of the parametrium and upper third of the vagina. The ureters are mobilized, but the uterine artery stays attached for they are ligated on the medial side of the ureter. The arterial branches from the superior vesicle artery to the ureter remain intact.

Type III (Fig. 8.7)

This truly radical hysterectomy may be used as primary treatment for Stages I and II cancer of the cervix. The resection follows the pelvic wall for the parametrium, the uterosacral ligament, and also removes about half the vaginal length. The extensive resection of the pubocervical ligament sacrifices vasculature to lower ureter and bladder not lost by the less extended procedures noted above; thus there is a greater risk of fistulae than is incurred in the Type III. Bladder atony becomes evident with this complete dissection of the uterosacral ligaments and the rectal pillars.

Types IV and V

These procedures are more extensive than usually implied by radical hysterectomy. When the internal iliac system must be resected, the superior vesicle supply is completely sacrificed. Therefore, this greater resection and greater expectation of postoperative complications are designated Type IV, while actual removal and reconstruction of a portion of the involved urinary tract are designated as Type V procedure.

Summary

This discussion has indicated the many difficulties which confront the surgeon who assumes responsibility for curing a patient with carcinoma of the cervix by radical hysterectomy. The number of possible errors introduced may seem exaggerated, interest in the operation may appear discouraging, and even trust for the procedure may seem fainthearted, but such is not intended because the radical

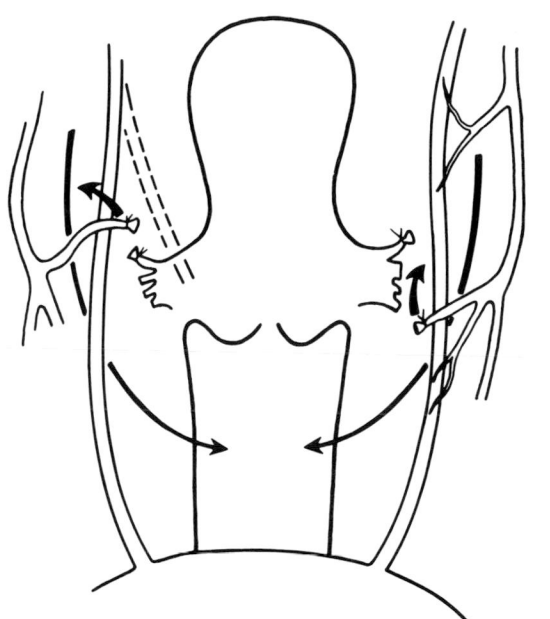

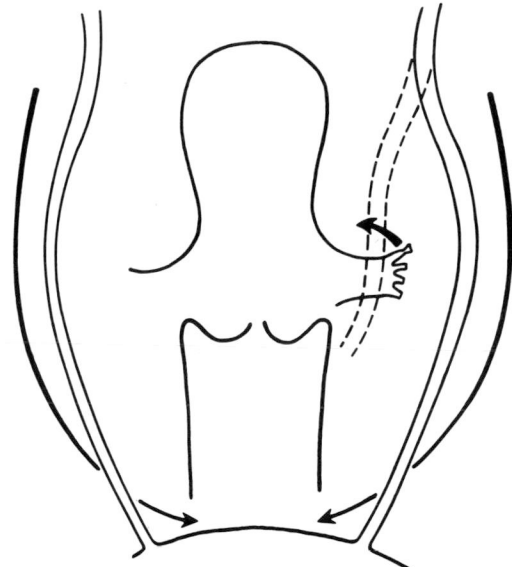

Fig. 8.6. Type II radical hysterectomy

The plan for this operation is complete excision of the uterosacral ligament, mesial half of the parametrium, and the upper one-third of the vagina. The ureter is lifted from its bed, but the blood vessels from the uterine artery and the supervesicle artery are not disrupted. Thus the risks of ureteral necrosis and fistulation are minimal.

This is accomplished by maintaining the ureter attached to the pubovesicle ligament. The ureter is lifted upward and swung outward from the uterus in a hinge manner (noted by short arrows). This allows the parametrium and paravaginal tissues to be amputated laterally such that 50 per cent or more of these structures may be included with the specimen (noted by long arrows).

My personal preference for proceeding with the hysterectomy follows this sequence: Divide the cul-de-sac and posterior peritoneum in preparation for dividing the uterosacral ligaments and upper pillar of the rectum at their base. This releases the uterus and vagina posteriorly and mobilizes the ureteral structures involved with dissection such that they can be retracted upward out of the deeper pelvis. Improved access and exposure usually result. Now the ureters can be freed.

After the bladder is freed down from the upper half of the vagina, the dissection directs toward the area of the ureterovesicle junction until the lowermost ureter is identified. All the overlying tissue retaining the ureter along side the cervix and upper vagina are now divided along the medial side of the ureter. As the ureter is freed, it can be swung upward and outward exposing the parametrium for applying clamps at a

Fig. 8.7. Type III radical hysterectomy

This operation involves extensive resection since the parametrium and uterosacrals are severed at the pelvic wall with about half of the length of the vagina removed.

The technical approach differs from the Type II where the uterine vessels are severed mesial to the ureter and the proximal pedicles are swung up and outward. The Type III operation severs the uterine vessels at their origin from the internal iliacs, and the distal stumps of the uterine vessels are swung upward and mesial (short arrows). Thus the ureters are liberated from beneath the uterine vessels and are then reflected laterally out of the way for applying hemostats across the parametrium along side the pelvic wall.

The long arrows indicate the wider range and direction of the resection. The original position of the ureters is indicated by the broken line. The position for displacement of the ureters possible after mobilization is portrayed by the solid line.

Type IV radical hysterectomy (not portrayed schematically) excises the internal iliac vascular system on one or both sides (in addition to the Type III range) to encircle carcinoma metastases in the lateral parametrium.

Type V radical hysterectomy (not portrayed schematically) excises a portion of the lower urinary tract. This may be a segment of ureter and/or bladder. The defect may be managed by closure, reimplantation, or ileoneocystotomy.

---

position more than half way from the cervix to the pelvic wall. Successively the paravaginal tissues and the vagina are severed. (The extent of resection is noted by the long curving arrows).

hysterectomy is a very valuable and effective treatment in gynecologic oncology. The operation may become more useful in the future as the current detection methods bring younger patients with smaller cancers of the cervix for treatment. The intention of the presentation is to advocate radical hysterectomy when its use gains the maximal benefit to the patient and preserves the reputation of the procedure. Technically, the operation appeals to the pelvic surgeon as an exciting challenge. There is a need to fit skills against the obstacles—an opportunity to maneuver and apply different attacks. There is acute responsibility. Technically the operation is the pinnacle and can be the enticement for a young physician to adopt gynecologic oncology for a career. Certainly in gynecologic oncology there are other procedures which are equally complex and longer in duration, but the radical hysterectomy is the pride of this surgical specialty. Naturally the pelvic surgeon seeks first to perfect his technical skill. This is soon followed by experience which shows that the treatment of cancer of the cervix involves problems of both surgical technique and clinical judgment.

Bibliography

1. Averette, H. E., LaPlatney, D. R., and Little, W. A.: Current role of radical hysterectomy as primary therapy for invasive carcinoma of the cervix. Am. J. Obstet. Gynecol. 105: 79, 1969.
2. Brunschwig, A., and Barber, H. R. K.: Surgical treatment of carcinoma of the cervix. Obstet. Gynecol. 27: 21, 1966.
3. Calame, R. J., and Nelson, J. H.: Ureterovaginal fistula as a complication of radical pelvic surgery. Arch. Surg. 94: 826, 1967.
4. Currie, D. W.: Operative treatment of carcinoma of the cervix. J. Obstet. Gynaecol. Br. Commonw. 78: 385, 1971.
5. Decker, D. G., and Smith, R. A.: Sequential radiation therapy and surgery for stage I and stage II cancer of the cervix. Am. J. Roentgenol. Radium Ther. Nucl. Med. 102: 152, 1968.
6. Fletcher, G. H.: Textbook of Radiotherapy. Lea & Febiger, Philadelphia, 1966.
7. Fletcher, G. H., and Rutledge, F. N.: Overall results in radiotherapy for carcinoma of cervix. Clin. Obstet. Gynecol. 5: 958, 1968.
8. Funnell, J. W., Kelso, J. W., and Funnell, J. D.: Combined surgical and irradiation treatment of invasive carcinoma of the cervix. J. Oklahoma State Med. Assoc. 64: 123, 1971.
9. Green, T. H., Meigs, J. V., Ulfelder, H., and Curtin, R. R.: Urologic complications of radical Wertheim hysterectomy: Incidence, etiology, management, and prevention. Am. J. Obstet. Gynecol. 20: 293, 1962.
10. Greiss, F. C., Blake, D. D., and Lock, F. R.: Treatment of cancer of the cervix by radiation and elective radical hysterectomy. Am. J. Obstet. Gynecol. 82: 1042, 1961.
11. Hsu, C-T., and Cheng, Y-S.: Clinical significance of preservation of the superior and inferior vesical arteries in the recovery of bladder function after radical hysterectomy for uterine cervical cancer. Am. J. Obstet. Gynecol. 111: 391, 1971.
12. Masterson, J. G.: Radical surgery in early carcinoma of the cervix. Am. J. Obstet. Gynecol. 87: 601, 1963.
13. Masubuchi, K., Tenjin, Y., Kubo, H., and Kimura, M.: Five year cure rate for carcinoma of cervix uterii with special reference to comparison of surgical and radiation therapy. Am. J. Obstet. Gynecol. 103: 566, 1969.
14. Meigs, J. V.: The Wertheim operation for carcinoma of the cervix. Am. J. Obstet. Gynecol. 49: 542, 1945.
15. Navratil, E.: Radical vaginal hysterectomy. Clin. Obstet. Gynecol. 8: 676, 1965.
16. Novak, F.: Procedure for the reduction of the number of uterovaginal fistulas after Wertheim's operation. Am. J. Obstet. Gynecol. 72: 506, 1956.
17. Parson, L., Cesare, F., and Freidall, G. N.: Primary surgical treatment of invasive carcinoma of the cervix. Surg. Gynecol. Obstet. 109: 279, 1959.
18. Roman-Lopez, J. J., and Barclay, D. L.: Bladder dysfunction following Schauta hysterectomy. Am. J. Obstet. Gynecol. 115: 81, 1973.
19. Rutledge, F. N.: Progr. Gynecol. 4: 619, 1963.
20. Rutledge, F. N.: Combination Irradiation and Surgical Therapy for Carcinoma of the Cervix: Cancer of the Uterus and Ovary, p. 216. Year Book Medical Publishers, Chicago, 1969.
21. Rutledge, F. N.: Surgery versus x-ray for treatment in cancer of the cervix. In Controversy in Obstetrics and Gynecology, edited by Reid and Barton, p. 397. W. B. Saunders Co., Philadelphia, 1969.
22. Rutledge, F. N., and Fletcher, G. H.: Transperitoneal pelvic lymphadenectomy following supervoltage irradiation for squamous cell carcinoma of the cervix. Am. J. Obstet. Gynecol. 76: 321, 1958.
23. Rutledge, F. N., Fletcher, G. H., and MacDonald, E. J.: Lymphadenectomy as an adjunct to radiation therapy in treatment for cancer of cervix. Am. J. Roentgenol. Radium Ther. Nucl. Med. 93: 607, 1965.
24. Schlink, H. H.: Cancer of the uterus: The Wertheim operation. Med. J. Aust. 1: 503, 1953.
25. Symmonds, R. E., and Pratt, J. H.: Prevention of fistulas and lymphocysts in radical hysterectomy: Preliminary report of a new technique. Obstet. Gynecol. 17: 57, 1961.
26. Symmonds, R. E., Pratt, J. H., and Welch, J. S.: Extended Wertheim operation for primary, recur-

rent, or suspected recurrent carcinoma of the cervix. Am. J. Obstet. Gynecol. 24: 15, 1964.

27. Brödel, M.: Fig. 107, p. 173, in Diseases of the Kidney Ureters and Bladder, by K. Burnam, Vol.

1. D. Appletons and Co., New York, 1914.

28. Stallworthy, J.: Radical surgery following radiation treatment for cervical carcinoma. Ann. R. Coll. Surg. Engl. 34: 161, 1964.

CHAPTER NINE

FELIX RUTLEDGE, M.D.

PELVIC EXENTERATION

Clinical experience has established pelvic exenteration as an acceptable treatment for patients with cancer which is either too advanced for conventional treatment or recurrent within the pelvis after previous irradiation. Exenteration, however, carries a great risk because the margins for safety and recovery are limited; thus, a single error in management may result in a fruitless operation. Since the complexities of pelvic exenteration are well appreciated, the suggestion that errors may occur will be readily accepted. But the first thought is likely to be of technical errors during the operation itself. In an operation of this magnitude, there are obviously many chances for technical errors. Yet, there are many other facets of management in which the reason for failure may be found. An error of omission in the preparation of the patient, for example, may be responsible for a lost opportunity for cure, even when the disease is amenable to resection. Postoperative mistakes can reverse progress when success is near, and inattention to follow-up care may shorten the patient's time for enjoying the benefits of the arduous treatment which she has survived.

Successful exenteration depends upon (1) wisely selected patients, (2) thorough preoperative study, (3) a perfect design for resection and reconstruction, (4) an uneventfully executed operation, and (5) diligent attention to postoperative care and support of the patient. These criteria are, of course, applicable to less radical procedures, but for exenteration, they are critical. Success is obtained by very narrow margins and there is no leeway for error or mishap.

Selection of Patients

At present, the risk of exenteration can only be justified when there is a good chance for long term cancer control. Two basic criteria of operability are that the tumor must be totally resectable and the patient must have an adequate physical reserve to recover. Unless these criteria are fulfilled, the decision must not be use of exenteration but instead institution of palliative treatment.

Clinical Examination

The first step in evaluation of the patient is a thorough clinical examination, including close attention to her history. At this time, some patients can be eliminated as candidates for this operation and thus be spared an array of laboratory and X-ray studies, as well as laparotomy; obviously, however, every patient deserves sufficient attention to avoid a premature decision against treatment.

The initial physical examination must be comprehensive and preferably should be done by the surgeon. The gynecologic oncologist knows the growth behavior and spread pattern of the various pelvic cancers, and this knowledge is helpful in the search for metastases. The responsibility for selecting patients for exenteration should not be delegated to physicians any less skilled in this speciality.

Particular attention should be given to such cancer-related factors as inadequate renal reserve, advanced cancer, or disseminated cancer. Other important factors unrelated to cancer include age, obesity, systemic disease, previous irradiation, and emotional adequacy.

Factors Related to Cancer

Obviously, an extensive pelvic operation such as exenteration would be a serious mistake if sufficient renal function was not in reserve to mitigate the added injury present in the postoperative stage. Uremia occurring in the first 3 or 4 weeks after surgical therapy could be fatal. Therefore, preoperative determination of the renal status is essential. This problem will be discussed further under "Special Tests."

Also, when disseminated disease is present, exenteration should not be performed. Such symptoms as cachexia, cough, severe anemia, low serum globulin, and leg edema are well recognized symptoms of disseminated cancer. The implications of pain patterns as reported by the patient are less generally appreciated, however. Distortion and pressure on large nerves, veins, the urinary tract, and the lower part of the large bowel may indirectly point to the amount and position of cancer. Severe pain which courses posteriorly down the leg from the sacrum along the sciatic nerve distribution indicates deep-seated cancer which is causing pressure upon the sacral nerve plexus. Cancer located more anteriorly in the pelvis affects the obturator nerve and causes discomfort in the region of the anterior and medial upper thigh. Severe leg pain associated with edema points to both venus and lymphatic obstruction caused by massive metastases along the pelvic wall or about the sacral promontory and is inevitably inoperable.

Cancer which does not cause pain is more often resectable than that which does although the type and location identify the more significant symptoms. When cancer is centrally located within the pelvis, pain is not usually severe until the ureters are blocked. Then both lumbar backache and pain radiating down the thigh to the knees develop. At first, the pain is severe but transient; ultimately, the obstruction produces a marked hydroureter and hydronephrosis which no longer hurts.

The bimanual rectovaginal examination is a valuable means of determining local cancer resectability although such an assessment is by no means infallible. The boundaries and fixation of the pelvic component of the cancer are often overestimated because firm tissues may be benign; likewise, metastases above the pelvis are usually not palpable. Conclusions based on pelvic findings may be erroneous; still, this examination provides our best information for judging operability and it must be performed thoroughly.

A search for the nodal groups most often affected by metastases can be made by palpation. The supraclavicular area, especially the left side nodes, may be felt as hard and enlarged when they contain cancer and such findings indicate the need for biopsy. Clinically abnormal inguinal nodes must be biopsied, for they,

too, often contain metastasis when the lower vagina is involved. Enlarged aortic nodes are rarely detected by palpation of the abdomen.

Other masses, the result of metastases to the omentum or to the liver such as abdominal ascites, may be palpated. Such findings, although not necessarily decisive in determining operability, are valuable. They may require special studies such as liver scintiscan to search for metastasis, a peritoneal tap for cytologic examination, or gastrointestinal roentenographic series.

Factors Not Related to Cancer

Certain physical disabilities unrelated to cancer are equally important in the selection of patients for pelvic exenteration. Failure to recognize these factors before surgical treatment is a serious error in clinical judgment and can only lead to numerous complications and high operative mortality.

Age. Generally, patients who are more than 70 years of age have some serious physical impediment that will eliminate them as candidates for exenteration. Individual variability exists, of course, and an occasional patient in this age group may have sufficient physical stamina to justify the operation. For most of these patients, however, the risk is too great.

Obesity. Obesity, especially when the abdomen is large, will pose some frustrating problems to even the most skilled technician. Tumor excision will be less complete, hemorrhage will be poorly controlled, and the anastomosis will be jeopardized. Guidelines in the case of excess obesity are elusive. The actual difficulty encountered may only become evident after laparotomy, since the proportion of exogenous fat varies. In the obese patient, both the ileostoma and the colostomy are exposed to greater tension and mobilization is poor. In addition, the obese patient is subject to cardiovascular strain which will be aggravated by the operation. During recovery, the presence of excess fat conceals the development of intra-abdominal complications.

Systemic Disease. The importance of the vascular system in determining eligibility for a prolonged operation is well known. Nevertheless, when the complications of pelvic exenteration are tabulated, deaths from myocardial infarction and cerebrovascular accidents are usually present. Therefore, particular attention should be given to the status of the vascular system. It should be remembered also that middle-aged patients may be "old" from the standpoint of vascular age, especially if the blood sugar and serum cholesterol levels are elevated. Some conditions can be improved with preoperative treatment; others are permanent impairments.

Varying degrees of vascular impairment may be detected. Some of these may be severe enough to be absolute contraindications; multiple unfavorable factors may also accumulate to become absolute contraindications to operation.

Prior Irradiation. Ranking high as a factor in the selectivity of patients for exenteration is the dose and distribution of any previous irradiation. Patients who have received a dose of external X-ray therapy of 5000 rads or more, at rates of 1000 rads per week, to the pelvic region must be evaluated with caution because their postoperative recovery is risky. High dose external irradiation applied through large portals involves the abdominal wall, the pelvic organs and vasculature, and especially large segments of intestine. Irradiation obliterates tissue planes, and a loss of these landmarks may result in prolonged, bloody operation. This effect is less important, however, than is the poor health of heavily irradiated tissues. Megavoltage X-ray equipment has the power to alter tissues so severely that they remain viable only by a tenuous reserve. Previous treatment with high dose irradiation to the pelvis and abdominal viscera induces profound permanent injury, and these organs will not survive the additional strain of operation. There is danger of disruption of the anastomosis and reconstruction; hemorrhage and infection with necrosis then ensue and the patient deteriorates rapidly. At this point, everyone involved knows that the extended operation was a mistake and that a limited survival with untreated cancer would have been preferable to an earlier painful death caused by the severe postoperative complications.

Irradiation from intracavitary radium, while it also contributes to the unfavorable condition of the pelvic tissues, is a less weighty factor because the tissues most affected are removed with the operative specimen and because of the rapid lateral diminishing dose. Also, unless the type of applicator and the distribution of radium sources are known, the dose levels cannot be estimated with any degree of precision.

Emotional Factors

Candidates for exenteration need emotional maturity and stability to endure the course following operation. Although this factor may not be as decisive in selecting a patient as are those factors related to the growth of cancer, it is an important consideration. There must be adequate emotional stamina to withstand the discomfort, isolation, and strain of this operation. Individuals with fragile emotional stability may collapse under the stress of a prolonged postoperative course. The emotional strain continues after discharge from the hospital because of the added need for personal care which is created by pelvic exenteration. Unstable persons may withdraw from society, lose interest in life, and neglect the care of the stomas; this in turn leads to illness as the diverted urinary and fecal streams fail to function. Adaption to the crippled sexual state will also test the patience of both the patient and her husband. Unless the patient has adequate emotional maturity to re-establish social relationships after she recovers, the operation can be considered only partially successful.

Special Tests

Excretory Urography

Among the most important preoperative tests is the excretory urogram. Distortion and obstruction observed on the roentgenogram tell the surgeon how much cancer is present; how much of the urinary tract must be resected; and, most important, the amount of dependable renal reserve. The urinary system must be studied thoroughly even if the operation must be delayed. If the excretory urogram does not serve decisively, then other tests will be necessary. The urinary tract status is so important that the search and evaluation should continue until the surgeon is satisfied with the results. The dye may have to be given as an intravenous drip when a greater filling of the renal pelvis and ureters is needed because of hydronephrosis or the fact that the patient cannot be properly dehydrated. The problems of iodine-reactive patients may be solved by retrograde pyelography. A good preoperative study of the renal units is important enough to justify these added efforts when routine techniques fail. Preoperatively the surgeon should study carefully these films and, preferably, have them in the operating room for review. A case study will relate an experience that illustrates this point.

In January, 1965, a 68-year-old woman had a total pelvic exenteration for an adenocarcinoma involving the bladder, cervix, and rectum. The urinary tract was diverted by an ileal conduit. The exenteration was technically uncomplicated and well tolerated by the patient. The first 5 days after the operation were uneventful, and during postoperative days 3, 4, and 5 the pack was progressively removed. After complete removal of the pack in the pelvic cavity, an outpouring of fluid from the perineal defect was noted and proven by injection of indigo carmine dye to be urine. The initial assumption was that a disruption of the ureteral ileoconduit anastomosis had developed or that a fistula through the conduit wall was responsible. Prior to laparotomy, however, the true situation was discovered by review of the excretory urograms. A double collecting system was proven on the right side, and only one of the two right ureters had been implanted at the time of the exenteration. At laparotomy, the third ureter was implanted into the conduit and the patient remained continent.

Lymphangiography

Obviously, every effort should be made to keep to a minimum the number of patients with inoperable cancer who undergo laparotomy. We have found the lymphangiogram particularly valuable in this respect because signs of positive nodes are interpreted very accurately. Even after extensive prior radiotherapy, the lymphatic channels remain patent and the lymphoid tissue usually persists, although there may be fewer and smaller nodes after irradiation. Previous operations on the lymphatic channels do cause distortion of the usual patterns; nevertheless, lymphangiography should be used for these patients because the lumbar and aortic nodes may still be visible and accurately interpreted. Despite the occasional false negative interpretation, we consider lymphangiography an essential part of the preoperative work-up for these patients.

Chest Examination

Pulmonary metastasis from carcinoma of the genital organs is so common that the chest X-ray is standard practice for both preoperative and follow-up examinations. Since metastasis to the lung may be noted at any time, all patients should have a chest X-ray within 1 week of exenteration. In addition, the information obtained may well reveal some recently developed inflammatory infectious processes.

Barium Enema

The barium enema is not routinely necessary before pelvic exenteration for recurrent cervical cancer. The need for this type of examination, as well as for proctoscopy, can be determined by review of the organ systems, symptoms, and physical findings. If there is a possibility that the pelvic tumor may be a primary carcinoma of the colon rather than recurrent genital cancer, then, of course, both proctoscopic and barium enema X-ray studies are essential. Cystoscopy to determine if invasion has occurred is routine.

The physician or service who performs exenteration regularly will benefit by a printed list of standard tests. To prevent omissions each test may be noted on the list as it is completed. The list may be used as a check, for instance, in ordering tests, or as a check for certainty that they are performed, or serve as a summary of preoperative results.

Preoperative Screening to Determine:
　　Amount of cancer
　　Location of metastasis
　　Status of vital systems
　　Range and radicality of resection required
I.　Routine test
　　A.　Regional biopsies to prove cancer and establish extent of spread
　　B.　Conference with pathologist to review extent and viability of neoplasia

C. Excretory urogram (I.V. pyelogram)
D. Lymphangiography
E. Chest X-ray (within 1 week of operation)
F. EKG
G. Laboratory test—liver function, coagulation profile, blood sugar, urine examination

II. Common elective test
  A. Cystoscopy search for signs of metastases to bladder by inspection and biopsy
  B. Proctoscopy as for above
  C. Barium enema search for evidence of metastases and associated bowel disease
  D. GI series as above
  E. Venography signs of metastasis noted roentenographically by deformity and narrowing lumen of pelvic veins and aorta
  F. Sociopsychiatric evaluation seeking additional appraisal by an especially skilled consultant

III. Uncommon elective test
  A. Intravenous drip pyelogram (for hydronephrotic kidneys)
  B. Renal scintiscan (Hippurate) for patients sensitive to iodine or those who show no kidney opacity by I.V. pyelogram
  C. Biopsy (palpable supraclavicular node or inguinal node)—clinically suspicious examination
  D. Liver scan to determine if liver contains metastatic cancer
  E. Peritoneal cytology (paracentesis): applicable if physician suspects cancer has surfaced into the peritoneal cavity
  F. Bromsulphalein: more complete liver function test
  G. Pelvic arteriography: The merit of this test remains to be established. If the study can be done conveniently it may show cancer by the regional vascularity.

Preparation of the Patient

Psychologic Preparation

When the results of the various examinations and tests show that the cancer can be removed, the physician is then faced with the task of discussing the situation with the patient and her family. The approach he uses must vary with the degree of intelligence and emotional stability of the patient.

The goal of these talks—for usually more than one conference is indicated—is to have the patient accept the proposed treatment, to allow her to acquire an impression of the risk, and to help her understand the physical conditions that will exist after the operation. The first conference brings frightening news to most patients, and their response may be irrational. How well the physician manages these talks may determine whether the operation is accepted. Although the magnitude of the procedure should not be concealed, some details, such as the chance of hemorrhage and the prolonged recovery period, might well be omitted at the first conference because some patients may be so horrified that they will block out further communication. If the patient gets the impression that she may die during the operation or that she will be bedridden, she will probably refuse the operation. The surgeon should not minimize the risk, but he should be reassuring; he should assure her that facilities will be available to cope with all events and that safety measures have been provided.

The surgeon's manner, dignity, composure, and actions portray dependability to the patient, and her confidence is developed by unhurried personal discussions. Delegating the necessary interviews to junior members of the staff is often a mistake because the patient recognizes the hierarchy of the surgical team and expects facts to be presented by the surgeon who is the most capable, best informed, and most authoritative source.

The following suggestions are made for conducting conferences with patients.

1. More than one conference may be necessary. A common mistake during the first conference is assuming that the patient comprehends. The patient may be learning for the first time of the diagnosis of recurrent cancer. This knowledge alone may make her so distraught that a detailed discussion of treatment should be delayed until she can adjust to this information and regain her composure. However, the conference should not end without encouragement and a promise of successful treatment.

2. The results of the many studies done as

part of the preoperative evaluation should not be reported to the patient in incomprehensible technical terms. The multiple tests that have been made of the various organ systems provide the opportunity to present encouraging results. Results related in uninterpreted technical terms leave the patient uneasy for fear that she is not physically suited for the major operation. One thing in particular—a patient is always concerned about the status of her heart. Her spirits are buoyed if she is told that her heart is normal and functions well.

3. The amount and distribution of cancer should be discussed in nonspecific terms such as "favorable early disease," "seems not to have spread," "appears still confined," "judged moderate or advanced," "the growth is not as early as we would like," or "because of tissue changes caused by prior irradiation, one cannot be certain about the amount of the disease." Some hedging is needed in this presentation in case metastases are found at laparotomy; however, there is no need to be grim. Certainly, the international staging terminology will not be meaningful to the patient, and it may be misinterpreted. An approximation of the degree of seriousness of the disease, expressed in customary language, will be appreciated by most patients and their families.

4. The chances of success should not be expressed in percentages because these are frightening to the patient and they commit the surgeon unnecessarily. Discussions of prognosis should be encouraging but not specific. The patient should be reassured that treatment is possible and that a chance for cure exists.

5. The details of treatment and the management of the ileostomy and colostomy should not be outlined until necessary, although the general functioning may be described. Presentation of too many details at this time is both inefficient and excessively alarming. To the patient, the prospect of having urine and feces flow out openings on the abdomen is repugnant. She should be assured that it is possible to continue much of her normal activity. It is usually helpful to have her meet a patient who has recovered from pelvic exenteration and who can show her that it is not necessary to live an isolated life. Institutions which have a stoma therapist have an outstanding advantage because this phase can be skillfully presented. A member of the staff must reassure the patient

that special support will be given her in mastering the system of stoma care.

Physical Preparation

Lungs. Patients with chronic bronchial reactions resulting from allergies, smoking, etc., should be prepared by several days of separation from the respiratory irritant and by cleansing of the respiratory tract with intermittent positive pressure treatment. A look at the list of postoperative problems will show that some of the first to occur are related to the respiratory tract. Failure to identify and correct pulmonary problems before prolonged anesthesia permits unnecessary complications to develop. When the patient is sedated, she is less able to evacuate the bronchi and to clear out the obstructing mucous secretions; the essential respiratory exchange is hampered. Also, poor mobilization of the lungs, with excess secretion and poor expansion in the immediate postoperative period, causes early temperature elevation. These problems must be overcome because if they are uncorrected, pneumonia may ensue.

Infections. Patients who have cancer extending into the vaginal canal will have a slough of the pelvic tissues from growth of the cancer and prior treatment; they will also have associated local infection. Although this infection cannot be completely eradicated, it should be dealt with as effectively as possible before surgical treatment. The use of antibacterial medicated douches, such as Betadine, significantly diminishes the risk of secondary infection from this source. Infections of the urinary tract are a common problem and will be discussed with other postoperative complications. Existing skin infections should be treated because postoperative infections of the incision are prevalent. Surface skin bacteria can be reduced by preoperative pHisoHex baths.

Bowel Preparation. No uniform plan exists for the preparation of the colon before surgery, although it is generally accepted that cleansing of the colon reduces local bacterial contamination. Some objections have been made to antibiotic bowel "preps," especially to their prolonged administration. Although these are still commonly used, the present trend is to omit the antibiotic bowel prep and depend on a thorough mechanical cleansing, since cleasing of the colon does reduce the chance of contamination during open bowel anastomosis. The collapsed and empty bowel interferes less with the displacement for exposure. The presence of stool in the colon is a needless hazard and one which complicates the working of the colostomy. A preoperative low residue diet, associated catharsis, and a cleansing enema accomplish significant cleansing of the lower colon. A low residue or liquid diet also lessens refilling so that the large intestine should be quite collapsed at operation.

It must be remembered, however, that evacuation of bowel with catharsis and enema causes fluid loss on the day before operation because all intake is stopped about the same time that the "prep" is completed. Intravenous fluids, with Ringer's lactate solution, must be given the evening before the operation so that the patient has normal fluid and electrolyte balance at the time of operation.

Blood Volume. The need for assuring adequate blood volume, good hydration, chemical and electrolyte balance, regulation of diabetes, and control of hypertension all are commonly accepted principles. It is well known that disability caused by chronic infection or malignant disease creates a relative intolerance to operation, probably because of diminished blood volume. Because extensive blood loss can be anticipated with subsequent dissipation of proteins, it is wise to make an effort to re-expand contracted blood volume and place the patient in maximal protein balance. Rules for preparation of the patient for operation are an evolution of experience and changes by observation and new developments in medication and knowledge of human physiology. The life value of documentation of a routine is short, rapidly outdated, and unretractable yet there is transient use.

Preoperative Preparation and Medication

1. The patient should be admitted at least 3 days and possibly 4 or 5 days prior to the operation, depending upon her physical status.
2. Intensive pulmonary care, including intermittent positive pressure breathing or bronchodilators, may be started at this time.
3. The minimal acceptable hematocrit should be 36, and preferably 39 to 40. Blood transfusions should be given at the earliest possible time to allow for adjustment of blood volume.
4. The following laboratory studies should be obtained: urine culture, colony count, complete blood count with platelets, blood-urea-nitrogen, creatinine, electrolyte, total protein and agglutinin ratio, liver function test, and coagulation profile.
5. The patient should be started on a low residue diet with only clear liquids for 48 hours preoperatively, and a low pressure suction of intestinal tract tube for 8 to 10 hours immediately preoperatively.
6. The following medications should be given.
   a. $MgSO_4$, 50 cc of 50 per cent solution t.i.d. for 48 hours preoperatively; this should be decreased if patient has had severe diarrhea.
   b. Multivitamins—one daily.
   c. Synkayvite, 25 mg I.M. 24 hours postoperatively.
7. At 6 p.m. the day before operation, 2000 cc of 5 per cent D/Ringer's lactate with 20 meq KCl are started and at least 1500 cc given by 8:30 a.m.
8. Adequate sedation is given the night before surgery to insure sleep.
9. Enema 36 hours preoperatively. Enema until clear 12 hours preoperatively.
10. Betadine douche preoperatively for several days for an infected lesion.
11. Skin care for the obese patient should start on admission.
12. The site of the proposed ileal and colostomy stoma are best marked, with the patient standing, the day prior to surgery. A dot of methylene blue dye is placed subcutaneously.
13. Should the patient have poor veins, either a subclavian or forearm intracatheter should be inserted prior to surgery.
14. The patient should be weighed preoperatively on a metabolic scale.
15. I.V. pyelogram should be reviewed carefully preoperatively especially if a double ureter is suspected.
16. Repeat chest X-ray, including oblique views, should be obtained in the week prior to surgery.
17. Daily pHisoHex bath should be given for several days prior to surgery.

Evaluation of Resectability

Decision to perform pelvic exenteration depends upon the upper abdomen being free from metastases and the resectability of the pelvic component. In some instances, the final decision cannot be made until laparotomy; after the abdominal organs are exposed, a significant amount of time may be necessary to ascertain that there are no metastases. Extensive adhesions may discourage a careful search, but short cuts at this stage may be regretted. The surgeon must not neglect this last chance to gather data and to consider again the chances of success before he passes the "point of no return" in the dissection.

Generally, the search starts in the upper abdomen. Metastases in this region may be obvious, but if the initial search is casual, positive sites may be missed. The preaortic node, especially, may feel deceptively benign upon casual palpation. The investigation for metastatic disease should include regular sampling of the more conspicuous preaortic nodes.

After the upper abdomen has been explored, an estimate of the amount of spread within the pelvic cavity should be made. The omentum and loops of intestine are commonly adherent within the pelvis. When they are grossly infiltrated with cancer or firmly adherent to the cancer mass, segmental resection of the intestine must be added to the exenteration. These findings mean an unfavorable prognosis and may be a contraindication to proceeding with the exenteration. Adherence of the small intestine or omentum to the pelvic tumor provides an opportunity for cancer to spread upward along additional lymphatic routes. Little success has been achieved for patients who have had this problem. Likewise, cancer that spreads to the peritoneal surface of the uterus, penetrates into the cul-de-sac, or otherwise extends into the peritoneal cavity may deposit free cancer cells which have the potential to metastasize throughout the peritoneal cavity. Peritoneal cytology has proven valuable in assessing the prognosis under such circumstances; however, with present techniques, reports of findings are delayed. Newer methods of peritoneal cytology assessment which can provide an immediate answer may eventually become part of the standard search technique at exploratory laparotomy, but at present the surgeon has no infallible method by which to make his decision.

Abdominal Findings

Contraindication for exenteration:
1. Metastasis to aortic nodes
2. Metastasis to abdominal viscera (omentum, small intestine, liver, etc.)
3. Metastatic implant upon peritoneum (above the pelvis)
4. Bilateral common iliac node metastases
5. Metastasis and tumor fixation over broad area of pelvic wall
6. Tumor densely adherent to iliac vessels
7. Tumor not totally removable

Debatable contraindication for exenteration:
1. Exposure of tumor surface in pelvic cavity
2. Positive peritoneal cytology
3. Positive pelvic wall nodes (especially if bilateral where very few cures have resulted)
4. Extensive parametrial cancer necessitating excision of internal iliac vessels for removal

Choice of Procedure

Anterior, Posterior, or Total Exenteration

Some surgeons believe that the bladder, the vagina, the uterus, and the rectosigmoid are so intimately related that cancer which has spread to either the bladder or the rectum must be presumed to have extended to the other structures, even if such involvement is not apparent. Consequently, they believe, that if exenteration is to be done, it is an error in judgment not to perform a total operation.

We, however, have practiced selected use of the anterior exenteration when the cancer is clearly spreading anteriorly and the rectum appears to be normal. One factor in the decision may be the total dose of irradiation which the patient has received. If, for example, the intestine has been injured by irradiation, its usefulness is diminished, and there is less reason to risk the chance that it might harbor cancer if not removed.

It is less common for cervical cancer to spread posteriorly than to extend along the anterior course. Few of these patients have rectal involvement but most have bladder metastases. In cancer of the vulva or primary vaginal cancer, posterior exenteration has proved more useful than it has for cervical cancer patients.

Technical Problems

Blood Loss

The possibility of hemorrhage has placed a stigma on pelvic exenteration from the inception of this procedure. Although intraoperative death resulting from hemorrhage rarely occurs, blood loss is still excessive and, consequently, there is a greater risk of early postoperative death. Despite routine replacement of blood and prompt correction of shock, considerable blood loss is hazardous and must be guarded against. Proper positioning of the patient is of utmost importance in aiding visibility and conserving blood (Fig. 9.1). In case of hemorrhage, an unusual tumor growth or the presence of tissue fibrosis may exonerate the surgeon, but the majority of causes for hemorrhage are avoidable and are the result of technical error. To improve this situation, we must study the problem objectively.

The sites most likely to develop uncontrolled bleeding have been well documented from experience. The single greatest threat is acute hemorrhage from the veins, especially the large veins. The reasons for this may be the greater frequency of veins encountered during the procedure, their less constant distribution, or their greater fragility.

Bleeding from the internal venous system is perhaps the most hazardous single source of serious hemorrhage. Here the veins are multiple, large, and difficult to expose. They are in the pathway for excising the pelvic specimen and are often injured before the dissection.

The cephalad end of the internal iliac veins to be excised should be ligated last. Failure to do so increases pressure in the occluded internal iliac venous system so that an accidental rent in the vein may develop. This then becomes the route which will force all the blood that usually flows through this route out through the opening. Also, by the same mechanism should hemorrhage from the internal iliac vein occur, ligation of the main trunk will make the condition worse. The leak must be corrected first.

Control of bleeding from the pelvic wall veins is especially difficult when the defect develops near the exit of these veins from the pelvis. Without adequate stump for ligation, vessels exiting the pelvis may be evulsed, and tamponade is the only method which can be used to control bleeding.

Veins which present similar hazards are also present in the hollow of the sacrum. These may be evulsed with removal of the specimen if the dissection plane is too deep. Usually such hemorrhage can be avoided if a plane outside the fascia which lines the sacral hollow is chosen. The correct zone can be found by forcefully retracting the sigmoid colon forward to indicate the avascular plane anterior to the pelvic fascia.

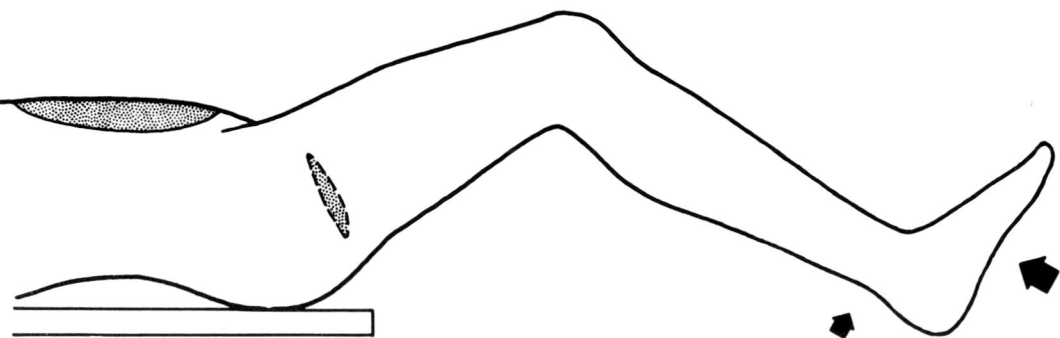

Fig. 9.1. Positioning a patient for pelvic exenteration. A dual approach to the pelvic cavity may be provided via an abdominal and perineal incision. Each direction may be approached simultaneously by separate teams of surgeons. The advantages in lessening the duration of the operation and conservation of blood are well known. Essential to accessibility to the patient for the surgeons and protection of the patient's back and lower extremities during the operation is proper support of the legs while the patient is on the operating table. Properly designed stirrups which exert the major force for support through the bottom of the feet are commercially available.

Other sites where excessive bleeding commonly occurs are the vena cava and the common iliac veins, since part of the routine search for subclinical metastasis is the excision, early in the operation, of a sample of fibrofatty node-containing tissue near the lower aorta and vena cava. The branches of the vena cava and the common iliac veins are easily torn away from the larger structures evulsing a defect in the vein wall without adequate stalk for ligation.

The surgeon's immediate response to hemorrhage is fear for the patient's life, but haste often compounds the problem. The too hasty application of an instrument without adequate exposure of the bleeding site may result in added damage to this vital structure and may make suture repair or ligature more difficult. Each additional clamp inserted into restricted space further limits visibility and the working area. The thin wall vena cava tears easily when hemostats are applied or the rent may be enlarged.

If hemorrhage does occur during the operation, the first step should be to try to control the bleeding by tamponade, either hand pressure or pressure with a pack. A hemostatic clamp may be used later when the bleeding site has been exposed and the clamp can be placed more precisely. In this situation, a well functioning suction is invaluable. If a fall in the patient's blood pressure has followed the initial hemorrhage, the tamponade should not be released in an attempt to repair damage until the anesthesiologist has improved blood volume and has stabilized the anesthetic. When the hemorrhage has been temporarily controlled, the field should be cleared of extraneous instruments, and the incision enlarged if necessary. Pressure on each side of the defect may keep the area clear of blood until it is repaired by sutures.

Although injury to the arteries is more avoidable than that to the veins, it sometimes occurs during removal of a lymph node from the lumbar area. Persistent dissection in an obscure region with sharp instrument accounts for arterial hemorrhage. Division of the inferior mesenteric or lumbar branches of the aorta may occur if the tissues are excessively fibrotic. In these situations, if the conditions for dissection cannot be improved, the effort must be discontinued.

Blood Replacement

A sufficient amount of matched blood and provisions with which to replace blood and fluid rapidly are mandatory during pelvic exenteration. Neglecting this precaution can be disasterous.

In our institution, we prefer subclavian or jugular vein catheterization for fluid replacement as well as for the monitoring of central venous pressure. The subclavian catheterization has been described and its advantages enumerated. The technique can be hazardous if attempted by the inept. Even after considerable experience, one must be alert for certain complications.

Urinary Diversion

The long term success of the ileal and sigmoid conduits justifies the additional technical complexities in creating them. The ureteral sigmoid implantation into the intact colon, the isolated rectal pouch, the wet colostomy, and the cutaneous ureterostomy should only be employed when a simpler method is needed to terminate the operation. Generally, it is simpler to use the sigmoid segment because intestinal reanastomosis is avoided, but obviously this advantage does not apply with an anterior exenteration. Also, a sigmoid conduit is not desirable if there is considerable cancer spread to the colon or if these segments of sigmoid colon are altered by diseases or prior irradiation treatment. Therefore, the ileal conduit is more generally applicable.

Few alterations have been necessary in Bricker's original description of the operation. The procedure can be adapted well to the usual situations; however, when a patient has received high doses of X-ray therapy to the lower abdomen, the terminal ileum which supplies the segment for the conduit often will have been injured by irradiation. This effect may not be visible; therefore, all patients who receive dosages beyond a critical level need special attention. First, a healthy segment should be used for the conduit. Any portion of the lower small intestine will adapt readily to the Bricker technique. Second, the anastomosis should be protected by splinting the juncture. Intubation of the ureters with a short segment of silastic tubing, serving as a catheter while the remainder of the tube extends through the conduit and out through the stoma, functions well for this purpose (Fig. 9.2). This arrangement temporarily conducts the urine flow from the respective kidney during the healing process. The splints function in several ways to improve healing: (1) facilitate the accurate approximation of the ureter and bowel by clearly showing the tissue margins, (2) prevent stenotic constrictions resulting from poorly placed sutures, and

(3) assure a competent suture line without excessive tension. Although most pelvic surgeons do not practice such splinting, for us the benefits have been evident in improved anastomosis and a reduced incidence of leak and fistulae.

The Stoma

Within the area, each person has an optimal location for the stoma—one which allows an adequate margin of skin on all sides for adherence of the appliance (Fig. 9.3). Prominences produced by bones or ligaments, or defects created by scars or skin irregularities should be avoided. The hang of the abdominal wall while the patient is standing, and the bulges of the visceral organs must be studied when the site of the stoma is selected. The selection may be tested before the operation by having the patient move about with the appliance held in place by the belt.

Before the incision in the abdomen is made, the crest of the ileum, the umbilicus, the symphysis, and the flank are concomitantly visible. This is the best time to mark the site of the stoma, since it must be related to these anatomic structures. A secure and continuous grip of the bag receptacle to the skin about the stoma depends upon a flat surface, and only a limited region of the abdominal skin offers a flat contact for the appliance. An appliance placed too low and too near the bony prominences will be pried loose on one side and a leak will develop. A stoma site that is too high interferes with wearing apparel about the belt line. In this case, even if the apparatus is not uncomfortable, it is unduly conspicuous. Even though urine may be successfully diverted by a poorly located stoma, the patient's adaptation depends upon the ease with which she can manage the appliance.

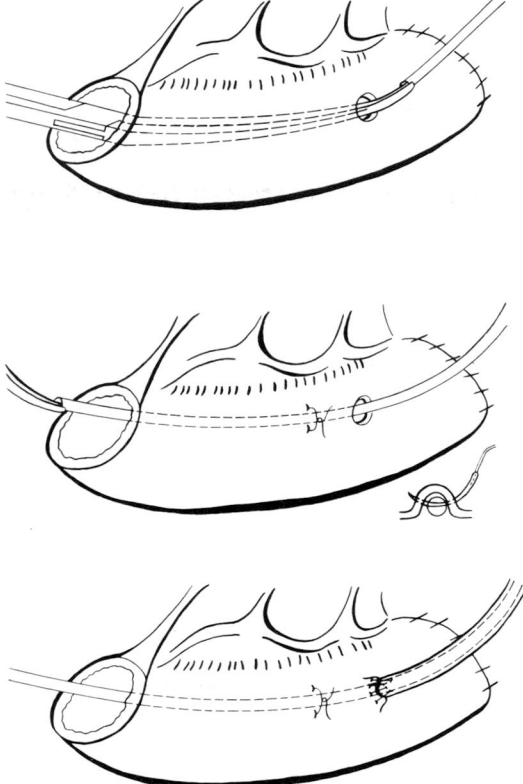

Fig. 9.2. Placement and securing silastic tube stents into ureters and urinary conduit.

Top: Long forcep-type instrument protrudes the bowel wall at the site selected for implantation of ureter. The bulge is amputated and through the opening the silastic tube is threaded into the lumen of the conduit and out the stoma. A length of tubing sufficient to catheterize the ureter half way to the kidney is scoured and sutured into the bowel wall with 4-0 catgut.

Middle: The securing suture passes through the tubing as well as the bowel wall.

Bottom: The ureter has been threaded onto the tubing and the anastomosis to the conduit made with 4-0 chromic material which attaches the full wall of the ureter to the entire thickness of the conduit wall.

Another important consideration in creating a satisfactory stoma is the construction. The tract through the abdominal wall should be created by excising a core of the layers. A simple stab wound has proven a technical error because stenosis frequently develops. The core method is superior when it is accurately directed and care is exercised so that openings in all layers will be superimposed after the abdominal incision is approximated. The movement of skin fascia and muscle layers may produce a "shearing action" upon the abdominal portion of the ileal conduit. An example of this complication led to our routine practice of simulating the closed incision by mesial traction upon the skin and fascia while making the stoma opening. Failure to do so in one patient caused blockage of the conduit at the abdominal wall level with urinary retention.

The opening within the abdominal wall should be about the size to permit two fingers to fit snugly in it. The passageway is created so that it does not become too tight by later contracture nor so excessive that herniation can occur.

Another common error in the construction of the stoma is neglecting to "mature" the exteriorized end of the intestine. A spout or nipple covered by bowel mucosa empties the urine more directly into the appliance and reduces the incidence of stricture. A full thickness eversion of about 5 to 8 mm may be created with specially placed sutures. The catgut suture attaches the bowel wall directly to skin margins while the end is turned inside out. The number of sutures needed to evert the bowel end and fix the circumference to the skin margin varies but should not be excessive. Too rigid fixation must be avoided because early postoperative edema will take place; this edema will subside without any detachment occurring if an allowance is made for swelling.

Other common sources of error in construction of the ileal conduit are listed.

1. Improper length of the conduit. Some clinical judgment is required to divide the intestine at the proper place. Making the segment too short or too long is a mistake. A too short conduit creates tension and causes the stoma to retract. If the conduit is too short to anchor the butt end, a strain develops upon the ureteral implantation site and causes disruption of the anastomosis. A short bowel segment must also have a reduced mesentery with less adequate reserve in blood supply.

The disadvantages of a too long conduit appear much later in the recovery. Ultimately, its inadequate function becomes evident in retained urine and recurrent urinary tract infections resulting from incomplete emptying.

The usual length of the intestinal segment is about 12 cm. The location supplying the intestinal segment should be selected taking into consideration the blood vessel patterns of

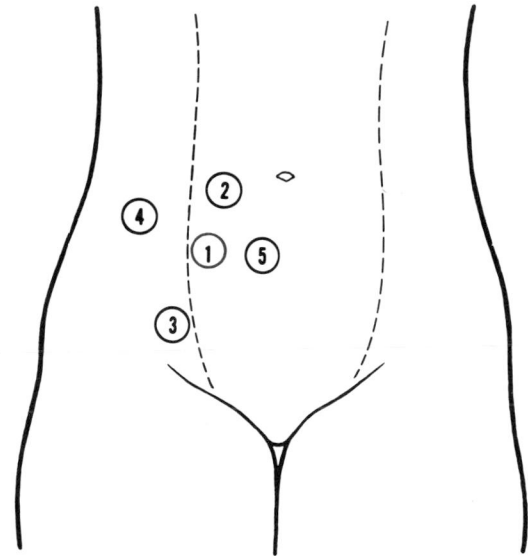

Fig. 9.3. Evaluation of selection of the site for the ileal conduit stoma.

1. Favorable because (a) it allows bag to hang in concave portion of abdomen for minimal distention of clothing thus being less conspicuous; (b) the site is visible to the patient as she attaches the bag; and (c) small intestinal mesentery to conduit is usually long enough to reach this site.

2. Unfavorable because it lies along belt line of many styles of garments which distorts clothing and compresses the appliance.

3. Unfavorable because the rigid bony and ligamentous structures within the area prevent a flat surface contact and will not adhere properly.

4. Unfavorable because the conduit bag is more apparent in this region in the fully dressed condition. This more prominent position upon the abdomen is thus undesirable.

5. Unfavorable because this site is too near the incision. This location is undesirable because the unhealed incision may delay application of the most secure-type bag, or after the incision is healed the scar may not tolerate the appliance as other areas of abdominal wall skin.

the mesentery. The arched pattern of anastomosing blood vessels in the mesentery supplying branches to the bowel wall is such that the surgeon may take advantage of a complete arch of blood vessels supplied by two or more trunks.

The segment of the mesentery should be selected to retain the maximal blood supply.

2. Reanastomosis of the intestine with the conduit below or ventral to the ileum forces bringing the ureters through the small bowel

mesentery. Although the surgeon usually recognizes and corrects the error, fruitless time is added to the operation.

3. Failure of the surgeon to avoid injury to the marginal vessels which supply essential blood to the reanastomosis site while he is closing the defect in the mesentery produced by removing the segment of intestine for ileal conduit.

4. Twisting of the conduit mesentery. The blood supply to the ileal segment must be carefully protected for if it is impaired by twisting, trauma, or tearing of the mesentery, an occlusion may develop and construction of a new conduit become necessary.

5. Failure to assure that peristaltic action of the ileal segment is directed toward the stoma.

6. Failure to anchor the butt of the conduit (Fig. 9.4) by suturing it to the posterior parietal peritoneum or to the fascia over the left psoas muscle threatens disruption of the ureteral conduit anastomosis by the weight of abdominal viscera with the patient erect.

7. Division of the ureters so low in the pelvis that excessive angulation occurs. The distal end of these ureters becomes devascularized, and an excessively long ureter draped over the pelvic brim becomes entrapped in dense scar tissue about the region of the common iliac artery.

8. Mistakes in identifying other structures as the ureter because of extensive fibrosis and disturbance of the normal appearance of tissues. The ovarian vein may be anastomosed to the conduit instead of the ureter.

9. Stripping away or retraction of the adventitia about the ureter should be avoided. Much of the blood supply to the ureter courses in the adventitia; it retracts easily and may be dissected from the ureter, and it should be maintained as an essential part of the vascular supply for the ureter.

10. Angulation of the ureter. Special attention is necessary to avoid acute angulation of the left ureter. This ureter, which may course through the mesial sigmoid or around its divided bases, should be mobilized to permit a slow curving course to the butt of the ileal segment. Likewise, on the right side, the ureter may be angulated as it exits from behind the peritoneum unless it is dissected free to above the level of the pelvic brim.

11. The technique for implantation of the ureter is critical. Excessive sutures will foul apposition of the full thickness of ureteral wall to the intestinal segment. If the entry hole in the intestinal segment is too large, too many sutures will be needed, overcrowding the end of the ureter. The implantation sites of the ureter in the ileal intestinal segment should be separated sufficiently so that mechanical problems are avoided and the blood supply is improved.

Colostomy

The level for division of the sigmoid colon for colostomy will vary individually because the mesentery must reach the abdominal wall freely. Adequate blood supply must be present to assure viability of the loop used for colostomy. Fortunately, the sigmoid colon has a favorable vascular supply which allows a choice of site for division. Consideration of the major arterial branches will assure vascularity to the stoma and facilitate hemostasis.

The stoma should not be created of intestine which has been badly injured by irradiation. Prior high dose irradiation to the sigmoid creates fibrosis of the bowel and shortens the mesentery, thus causing tension on the stoma. This, in turn, causes retraction below the surface of the abdominal wall. Neither should the bowel be divided too near the cancer for fear of inadequately excising the lesion. If secondary loops of the sigmoid become adherent to the central cancer mass in the pelvis, implantation can occur. Therefore, the bowel must be excised and a more proximal site chosen for the stoma.

Basic principles in establishing a colostomy are (1) the intestine must be drawn through the abdominal wall without tension; (2) the lateral gutter space must be obliterated to avoid trapping and volvulus of the small intestine; (3) the stoma must be in a favorable position for application of the irrigating apparatus; (4) the channel through the abdominal wall must be carefully selected to avoid herniation; (5) primary suture between the end of the colon and the skin favors a good healing and prevention of stricture; and (6) viability of the end must be evident.

Intestinal Anastomosis

Technical errors in the anastomosis of the

small intestine from which the ileal conduit was obtained may be followed by such serious consequences as intestinal obstruction or anastomosis, disruption, and leakage. Reapproximation of the two ends of the divided small intestine can be accomplished by a series of interrupted fine cotton or silk sutures in the seromuscular outer layer and a row of interrupted chromic catgut suturing the inside mucosa and muscular area. Good approximation will result if these sutures are placed at regular intervals in a neat row so that there is uniform tension. Excessively tight approximation caused by very tense knotting of the sutures sloughs through and loosens the attachment. Interrupted sutures are best since they have independent strength and the adjustment is better.

Inversion of an excessive amount of cuff of the bowel narrows the lumen at the site of the anastomosis, and since postoperative edema further reduces the already narrowed lumen, occlusion of the bowel with mechanical obstruction develops. With a long intestinal tube in place to keep the bowel deflated, the edema may resolve and the block open. At times, however, re-exploration and revision of the anastomosis may be necessary.

Postoperative Management

Many facets of postoperative care are controversial. Within a single institution there may be differences of opinion, and methods will vary in separate localities. Until experience establishes the best method or methods, this variation will continue. The suggestions given here are based on our own experiences.

Pelvic Pack

One of the more controversial facets of postoperative care is the proper care of the pelvic cavity. Some surgeons are reluctant to use packing in the cavity because of the danger of infection. The large coiled pelvic packs absorb and retain blood and lymph, become malodorous and irritating, and the exudates provide a rich medium for bacterial growth. We, however, have found that most of our patients have required a large, firm gauze pack, filling the lower pelvic cavity, to stop the multiple small sites of bleeding and also to support the

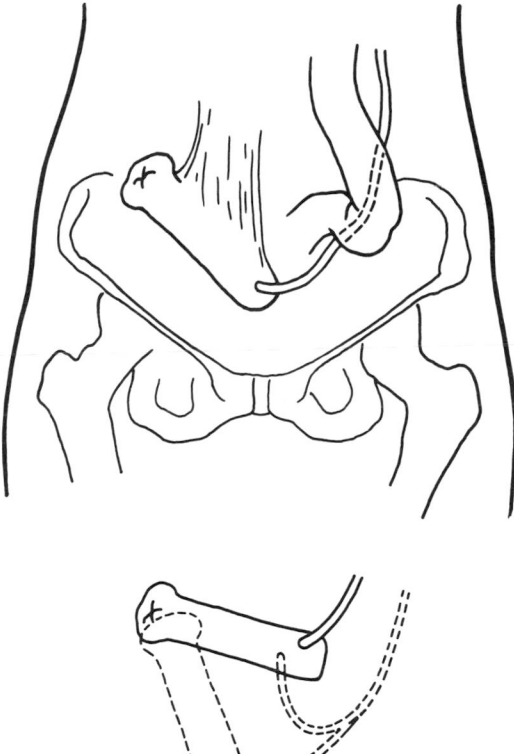

Fig. 9.4. The unsecured ileal conduit. Of those technical errors in construction of the ileal conduit, division of the ureter too low within the pelvic cavity and failure to anchor the base of the ileal segment are worthy of note.

A redundant portion of the ureter invites evulsion of the implantation by a force caused by the weight of dependent loops of intestine which drape across the ureter.

The unsupported base of the ileal segment may swing downward into the pelvic cavity. This strains the sutures of the ureteral conduit implantations. Also a dependent position for the conduit downward from the stoma may impede prompt conduction of urine from the ureters to the outside and contribute to urinary tract infections.

intestines above the open pelvic floor. The packs are removed when adequate time has passed to permit the sites of potential hemorrhage to be fully clotted and to allow the intestinal loops to react and become adherent to each other. They are then less likely to drop through the pelvic floor defect.

After the pack removal, the remaining pelvic spaces are still a source of septicemia. The contoured pelvic floor retains exudates in proportion to the degree of reconstruction of the floor at operation. Obviously, retention of this material is undesirable, but again the proper management is debatable. If the perineal body has been reconstructed, a noncollapsible tube drain should be placed to extend from the lowest level of the pelvic cavity to the outside. Pelvic cavity irrigations and topical applications of antibacterial agents have been used, but the merits of this practice are uncertain because it could prove harmful to some areas that are not infected and it might delay healing once the infection has been resolved. We are presently employing the mobilized omentum (Figs. 9.5 and 9.6) to serve the role of the pelvic pack whereby some gauze pack is still necessary but much less will serve and it can be removed sooner. More complete reconstruction of the perineum (Fig. 9.7) helps this effort to reduce the cavity and area of denuded tissues.

Postoperative Feeding

The urge to re-establish a positive nitrogen balance in the patient's metabolism by early oral intake can cause untimely feeding. Premature feeding of a patient with inactive intestine may precipitate problems of distension. A long intestinal (Miller-Abbott type) tube for the evacuation of bowel content should be put in place before the operation. This tube will prove useful because distention develops in spite of precautions.

The return of bowel function can be noted first in the peristaltic noises. When active bowel sounds and diminished return of fluid from the suction tube suggest that an oral intake may be tried, suction should be discontinued but the tube should be left in place. As oral intake proves tolerable, the tube may be cautiously extracted. Intussusception can be caused by hastily retracting the long intestinal tube.

Infection

Generally, infections are not avoidable after pelvic exenteration because contamination, resulting from invasion of the open pelvic wound, is inevitable either at some phase of the operation or postoperatively. Broad spectrum antibiotics, although in some ways objectionable, presently are given prophylactically. The antibiotics should be started in the preopera-

tive or intraoperative phase so that in the formation of blood clots and the development of the sequestrated exudate, the antibiotic will permeate the clot. Bacteria within an established hematoma are harbored from systemic medications; therefore, antibiotics in the blood that forms the clot should be effective.

Established infections are treated with more specific antibiotics. Alertness to the development of infection is important in the early postoperative phase because early diagnosis and prompt treatment may be life-saving. Therefore watchfulness for the common problems such as atelectasis, pneumonia, peritonitis, pyelitis, incision abscess, pelvic abscess, and phlebitis is an important part of postoperative care. A common error is neglecting atelectasis or failing to reaerate the lungs until consolidation with subsequent pneumonia develops. Peritonitis and intra-abdominal abscess can be elusive, however. When there is any sign of these conditions, localization and drainage should be instituted. Other and more serious complications are disruption of the bowel anastomosis with consequent fecal contamination, or breakdown in the ileal conduit construction with consequent peritonitis. Pyelitis is especially common since many of these patients have chronic bacteria before operation. Exenteration can change the subclinical urinary tract infection before operation into a febrile, threatening illness. Bacteremia and serious toxicity are reason for concern. Some patients have died from septic shock, persistent infection, or multiple abscess formation compounded by renal and liver infection.

There is considerable chance of wound infection during pelvic exenteration despite such preoperative cleansing, isolation while repairing the intestine, glove changes, etc., and irrigation lavage before closure. Some factors that contribute to this danger are prior injury by irradiation treatment, contamination during the operation to the open intestinal tract, the contamination of infected urine, or the infected vagina. Prevention of infection is preferrable, of course, but from a practical standpoint, it is difficult to prevent all exposure. Therefore, it is important that the incision be observed carefully for abscess formation so that these can be promptly opened for drainage.

The problem of infection in the denuded pelvic cavity has already been discussed. The

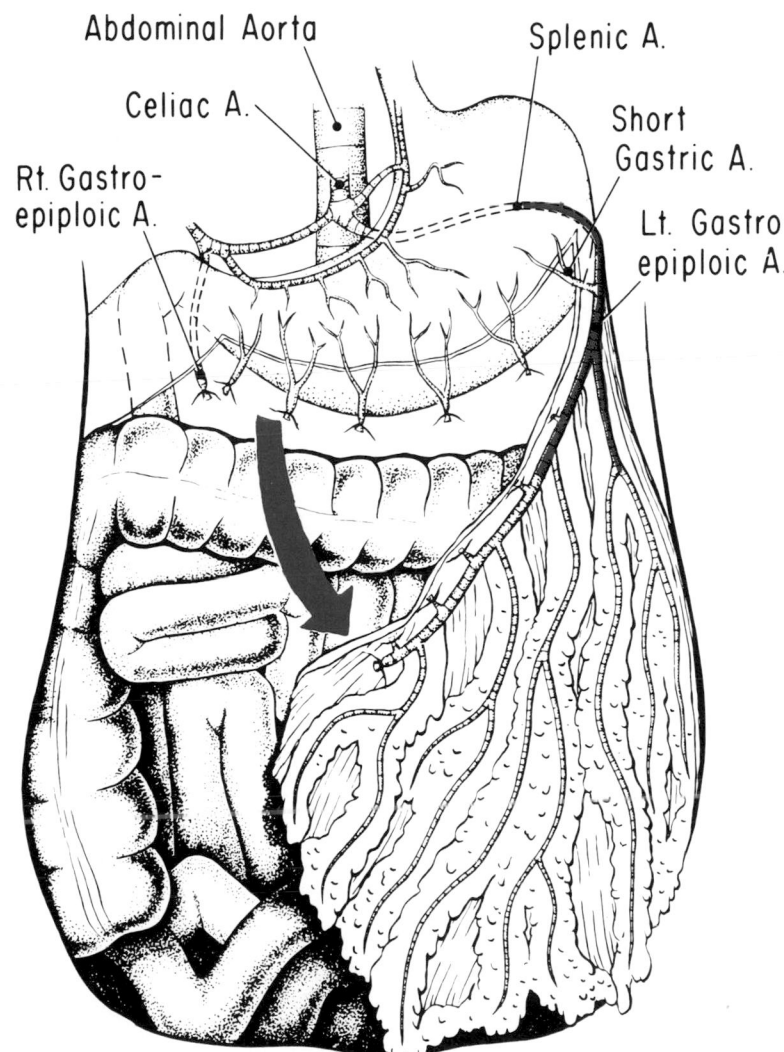

Abdominal Aorta

Celiac A.

Rt. Gastro-
epiploic A.

Splenic A.

Short
Gastric A.

Lt. Gastro-
epiploic A.

Fig. 9.5. Mobilization of the omentum. Dividing the attachment of the omentum from one side and its transfer to the denuded pelvic cavity after total exenteration is our current and best technique for dealing with this troublesome anatomic defect.

More often the arterial branch from the right gastric artery is severed to permit detaching the omentum from the greater curvature of the stomach and from the transverse colon. Progressively from the right to the left vascular connections to the stomach are severed, and the omentum is freed until the region of the splenic flexure region is near. The left gastric vascular supply to the omentum is preserved to maintain viability of the omentum.

The mobilized omentum can now be placed along the left lateral peritoneal gutter beyond to the descending colon and colostomy. The lower right part of the omentum will reach the pelvic floor. Here it is used to cover the denuded surfaces.

accumulation of blood clots, protein-rich lymph, and serum pools in the pelvic cavity provides a good culture medium for bacteria and consequent localized abscess formation. None of the treatment methods in present use is particularly effective.

Fluid and Electrolyte Balance

The criteria which determine proper management of fluid and electrolyte balance for other extended operations are generally applicable to patients who have undergone exenteration. These patients are especially susceptible to fluid and electrolyte imbalance for several reasons. (1) There is a need for prolonged intestinal tract suction, and oral feeding is unusually delayed. (2) Additional fluid is lost from the denuded pelvic cavity and the serum protein is diminished. (3) The urinary system is often crippled before the operation by the growth of cancer, and some loss in the compensatory powers of the system must be expected. (4) Because the operation involves a large area, several organ systems are modified, operating time is prolonged, and a large amount of fluid is lost.

The postoperative measures for any indications of abnormality are (1) careful measurement of the output of the gastric suction and urine, (2) regular weight checks for evidence of overloading and fluid retention, (3) a search of

Fig. 9.6. The omentum in position. The omentum serves as a floor and lining for the bare pelvic walls. Although sutures may be employed to attach it into desired position, there is no attempt to stretch the omentum across the pelvic outlet as a floor for support.

Our reference to this placement as an "omental carpet" is descriptive of its role. The fatty omentum consumes "dead space"—it brings a new source of vascularity to the pelvis and upon the omentum rest the intestines held away from the raw pelvic tissues where adhesions may produce obstruction of the bowel. The omentum protects the denuded pelvic wall from infection; exposed vascular channels are sealed; less serum and lymph exude; and, consequently, body proteins are conserved. Less fluid accumulates within the bowel of the pelvic cavity and pelvic abscesses are fewer.

The omental carpet corrects the objection of a pelvic lid constructed from an isolated segment of intestine for the pelvic space is better obliterated. Since employing the omental carpet, we have observed less severe postoperative sepsis originating within the pelvic cavity.

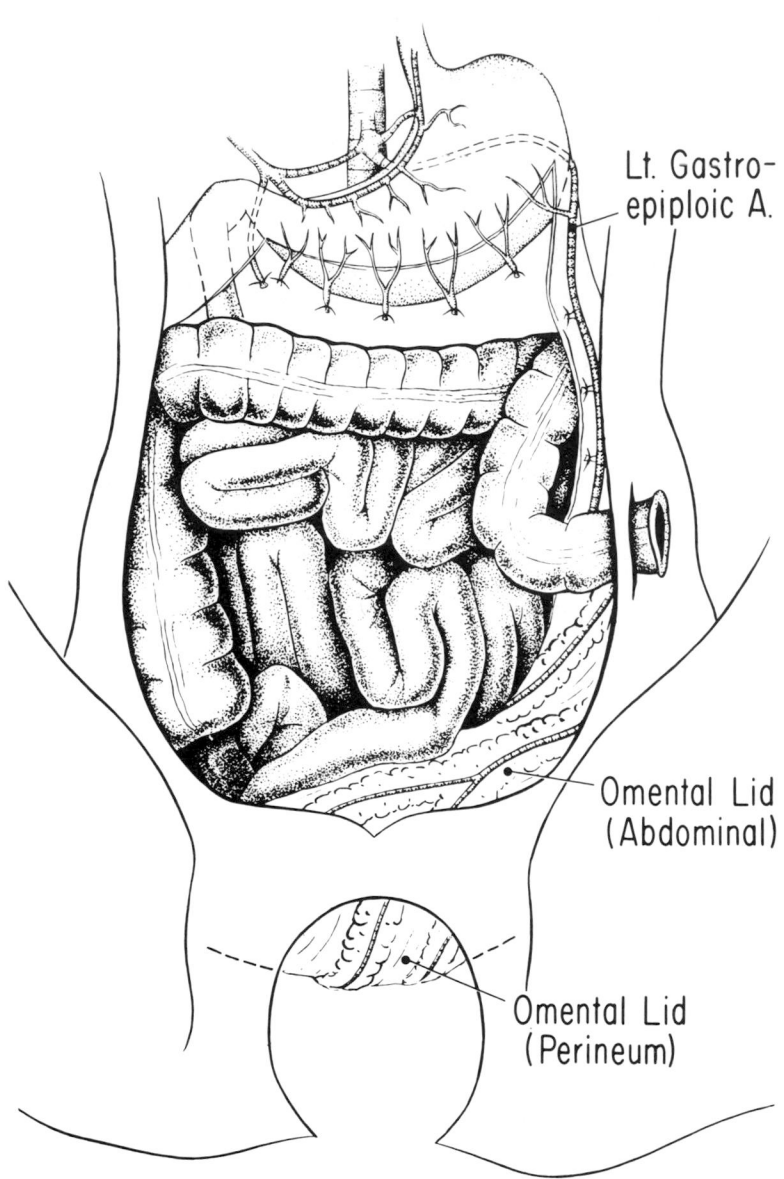

Lt. Gastro-epiploic A.

Omental Lid (Abdominal)

Omental Lid (Perineum)

the dependent regions of the body for evidence of edema, (4) regular auscultation of the chest for signs of decompensation, (5) examination of neck veins for overdistention, (6) frequent laboratory checks of the serum electrolyte levels, (7) notation of the respiratory characteristics and rate, (8) clinical evidence of dehydration and loss of skin turgor, and (9) carefully documented fluid intake and output.

Summary

The literature on pelvic exenteration shows that although this therapy has been established as beneficial to selected patients, there are still several sources of error and some questions still to be resolved. In patients with recurrent cancer or cancer too advanced for conventional treatment, this is the one remaining chance for cure.

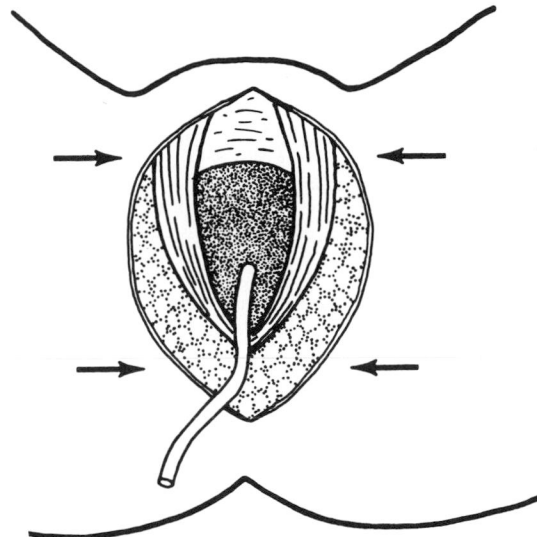

Fig. 9.7. Perineal closure following total pelvic exenteration. Reapproximation of incised margins of the levator muscles, subcutaneous fibrofatty tissues, and the perineal skin reduces serum loss and infection during the early part of the recovery phase. Also a reconstructed perineal defect lessens the risk of herniation during later months. Immediate and complete closure of the perineum will reduce the inevitable exudate from the denuded pelvic walls; however, they may collect and become infected unless provisions for evacuation are provided. A Saratoga-type sump-drain from the hollow of the sacrum through the buttocks will provide this drainage and allow more complete closure of this perineal defect.

If they are suitable for exenteration, then the chance should be taken because real benefits can be achieved. There are some hazards, however, which we must constantly strive to eliminate. In this chapter, we have listed some special problems which in our experience are particularly associated with pelvic exenteration. Perfection in all aspects of the procedure must be our goal if the operative mortality is to be minimal, the highest possible percentage of cures is obtained, and the rehabilitation of the patient is achieved.

Bibliography

1. Barber, H. R. K.: Results of surgical treatment of cancer of the cervix at the Memorial-James Ewing Hospitals, New York. In Advances in Obstetrics and Gynecology, edited by S. Marcus and C. Marcus, Vol. 1, p. 622. The Williams & Wilkins Co., Baltimore, 1967.

2. Barber, H. R. K., and Brunschwig, A.: Pelvic exenteration for extensive necrosis following radiation therapy for gynecologic cancer. Obstet. Gynecol. 25: 575, 1965.

3. Barber, H. R. K., and Brunschwig, A.: Pelvic exenteration for advanced and recurrent ovarian cancer. Surgery 58: 935, 1965.

4. Barber, H. R. K., and Brunschwig, A.: Results of the surgical treatment of recurrent cancer of the cervix. In New Concepts in Gynecological Oncology, edited by G. C. Lewis, Jr., W. B. Wentz, and R. M. Jaffe, p. 145. F. A., Davis Co., Philadelphia, 1966.

5. Barber, H. R. K., and Brunschwig, A.: Obstet. Gynecol. 28: 754, 1966.

6. Barber, H. R. K., and Brunschwig, A.: Excision of major blood vessels at the periphery of the pelvis in major surgery. Surgery 62: 426, 1967.

7. Barber, H. R. K., and Brunschwig, A.: Treatment of recurrent corpus cancer by anterior and total pelvic exenteration at the Memorial-James Ewing Hospitals, 1947 through 1962. Ann. Obstet. Gynecol. 4: 219, 1968.

8. Barber, H. R. K., Brunschwig, A., and Mangioni, C.: Advanced cancer of the vulva and vagina, treated by anterior and total pelvic exenteration 1947-1962 at the Memorial-James Ewing Hospitals. Cancer 22: 949, 1968.

9. Barber, H. R. K., Roberts, S., and Brunschwig, A.: Prognostic significance of the preoperative non-visualizing kidney in patients receiving pelvic exenteration. Cancer 16: 1674, 1963.

10. Bricker, E. M.: Symposium on clinical surgery; bladder substitution after pelvic evisceration. S. Clin. N. Am. 30: 1511, 1950.

11. Bricker, E. M.: Surgery 32: 372, 1952.

12. Bricker, E. M.: The technique of ileal segment bladder substitution. In Progress in Gynecology, edited by J. V. Meigs, Vol. III. Grune and Stratton, New York, 1957.

13. Bricker, E. M., Butcher, H. R., Jr., Lawler, W. H., Jr., and McAfee, C. A.: Surgical treatment of advanced and recurrent cancer of the pelvic viscera: an evaluation of ten years experience. Ann. Surg. 152: 388, 1960.

14. Bricker, E. M., Butcher, H. R., Jr., and McAfee, C. A.: Late results of bladder substitution with isolated ileal segments. Surg. Gynecol. Obstet. 99: 469, 1954.

15. Bricker, E. M., and Modlin, J.: Role of pelvic exenteration. Surgery 30: 76, 1951.

16. Brunschwig, A.: Complete excision of pelvic viscera for advanced carcinoma. Cancer 1: 177, 1948.

17. Brunschwig, A.: Total exenteration of the pelvic organs. In Surgical Treatment of Cancer of the Cervix, edited by J. V. Meigs, p. 307. Grune & Stratton, New York, 1954.

18. Brunschwig, A.: L'Exenteration pelvienne, p. 55. Masson et Cie, Paris, 1964.

19. Brunschwig, A.: What are the indications and results of pelvic exenteration? JAMA 194: 274, 1965.

20. Brunschwig, A.: Surgical treatment of carcinoma

of the cervix, recurrent after irradiation or combination of irradiation and surgery. Am. J. Roentgenol. Radium Ther. Nucl. Med. 99: 365, 1967.

21. Brunschwig, A., and Barber, H. R. K.: Extended pelvic exenteration for advanced cancer of the cervix. Long survivals following added resection of involved small bowel. Cancer 17: 1267, 1964.

22. Brunschwig, A., and Barber, H. R. K.: Pelvic exenteration combined with segments of bony pelvis. Surgery, in press.

23. Brunschwig, A., and Daniel, W. W.: Surgical treatment of cancer of cervix. Am. J. Obstet. Gynecol. 82: 60, 1961.

24. Brunschwig, A., and Pierce, V. K.: Partial and complete pelvic exenteration: Progress report based upon the first 100 operations. Cancer 3: 972, 1950.

25. Ingersoll, F. M., and Ulfelder, H.: Pelvic exenteration for carcinoma of the cervix. N. Engl. J. Med. 274: 648, 1966.

26. Ingersoll, F. M.: Pelvic exenteration for carcinoma of the cervix. Ob-Gyn. Digest 10: 49, 1968.

27. Ketcham, A. S., Bloch, J. H., Crawford, D. T., Liederman, J. E., and Smith, R. R.: The role of prophylactic antibiotic therapy in control of staphylococcal infections following cancer surgery. Surg. Gynecol. Obstet. 114: 345, 1962.

28. Ketcham, A. S., Lieberman, J. E., and West, J. T.: Antibiotic prophylaxis in cancer surgery and its value in staphylococcal carrier patients. Surg. Gynecol. Obstet. 117: 1, 1963.

29. Kiselow, M., Butcher, H. R., and Bricker, E. M.: Results of the radical surgical treatment of advanced pelvic cancer. Ann. Surg. 166: 428, 1967.

30. Mattingly, R. F.: Total pelvic exenteration. Clin. Obstet. Gynecol. 8: 705, 1965.

31. Parsons, L.: Total exenteration of the pelvic organs. In Surgical Treatment of Cancer of the Cervix, edited by J. V. Meigs, p. 322. Grune & Stratton, New York, 1954.

32. Parsons, L.: Pelvic exenteration. Clin. Obstet. Gynecol. 2: 1151, 1959.

33. Parsons, L.: Ann. NY Acad. Sci. 97: 830, 1962.

34. Parsons, L., and Bell, J. W.: Evaluation of pelvic exenteration operation. Cancer 3: 205, 1950.

35. Parsons, L., Cesare, F., and Friedell, G. H.: Primary surgical treatment of invasive cancer of the cervix. Surg. Gynecol. Obstet. 109: 279, 1959.

36. Parsons, L., Cesare, F., and Friedell, G.: Evaluation of lymphadenectomy in therapy of cervical cancer. Ann. Surg. 151: 961, 1960.

37. Parsons, L., and Friedell, G.: The evaluation of pelvic lymphadenectomy in the treatment of cervical cancer. In Progress in Gynecology, edited by J. Meigs and S. Sturgis, Vol. IV, p. 445. Grune & Stratton, New York, 1963.

38. Parsons, L., and Friedell, G. J.: Radical surgical treatment of cancer of cervix. Proc. Nat. Cancer Conf. 5: 241, 1964.

39. Rutledge, F.: The role of surgical resection in the management of cervical carcinoma. In Clinical Conference on Cancer, Anderson Hospital and Tumor Institute, 5th. 1960: Carcinoma of the Uterine Cervix, Endometrium and Ovary. (A Collection of papers . . .), pp. 149–173. Year Book Medical Publishers, Chicago, 1962.

40. Rutledge, F. N., and Burns, B. C., Jr.: Pelvic exenteration. Am. J. Obstet. Gynecol. 91: 692, 1965.

41. Symmonds, R. E., Pratt, J. H., and Welch, J. S.: Extended Wertheim operation for primary, recurrent or suspected recurrent carcinoma of cervix. Obstet. Gynecol. 24: 15, 1964.

42. Turnbull, R. B., and Weakley, F. L.: Atlas of Intestinal Stomas. The C. V. Mosby Co., St. Louis, 1967.

CHAPTER TEN

JOHN L. MOORE, JR.

GYNECOLOGIC ERRORS AND MEDICAL MALPRACTICE

The title of this textbook, *Gynecologic Surgery: Errors, Safeguards, and Salvage,* is provocative from the legal point of view. This chapter, commenting on legal questions concerning gynecologic error, will seek to demonstrate that use of the word "error" as in the title of this textbook differs entirely from the lay meaning of the word "error" which is frequently equated with "negligence" or "malpractice." Physicians will indeed be guilty of professional error if they do not understand at all times that there are at least three different relevant kinds of persons using the same or similar words but meaning quite different things and implying quite different conclusions. The physician must be able to understand his own language, the language of lawyers, and the language and understanding of patients.

The field of gynecologic surgery is well written up in the law reports—a fact probably realized by the gynecologist when he pays his malpractice insurance premium.

This chapter will start with some examples of misunderstanding of language between physicians and attorneys and between physicians and their patients. A discussion will follow concerning cases involving vesicovaginal fistulae, hemorrhage, or infection following various gynecologic surgical procedures. Reference will be made to the chapters on radical hysterectomy, fistulae, and other operative procedures. The particular cases will lead into a short discussion of the history of malpractice and predictions as to the future directions of malpractice in gynecologic surgery. The chapter ends with a more lengthy discussion of the currently very relevant question of "informed consent."

A classical 1921 Indiana case (1) illustrates graphically how physicians can misunderstand the legal meaning of words.

On April 26, 1920, Walter G. Luce was 48 years of age and in good health. He had never suffered from stomach or bowel trouble. He had worked almost every day for 25 years, weighed 160 pounds which was an appropriate weight for his height, and was employed as a shot-firer in a mine. On that day he was wounded in an explosion in the mine.

On admission to the hospital the admitting physician noted on the hospital record that Mr. Luce had grave wounds, including but not limited to, the following. He had a very severe scalp wound involving the pericranium. The scalp was lacerated and burned. The patient had numerous small lacerations and minor burns of the face, arms, forearms, and hands, and was bruised all over. Both ankles were fractured, the right ankle being a compound fracture. There was a fracture of the left tibia at the lower end and a comminuted fracture of the right leg involving the tibia and fibula. There was a possible fracture of the fourth cervical vertebra and much displacement of the fragments. The patient was in deep shock and his pulse could not be felt. The hospital records showed that by April 29, the patient's condition was very much improved. He was kept on a cot on his back, soup being his only nourishment, and he could take very little of that. The patient remained in a coma and was unconscious and delirious all the time.

On May 11, the patient began vomiting and was very ill. On May 12, he died. The deputy coroner and two other physicians performed an autopsy without the knowledge of the wife. Their report indicated they found an intestinal obstruction with no evidence of any abdominal injury to account for that obstruction. In their opinion, "he died from intestinal obstruction and from causes independent of the injuries received." The widow applied for workmen's compensation benefits, saying that the death was work-related. The Industrial Board, which by law was obligated to accept physicians' findings of medical fact, in effect overruled the three physicians and found that death was work-related and awarded compensation to the widow. On appeal the Indiana Appeals Court affirmed the action of the Industrial Board saying (2):

"Indeed, if it were not for the saving grace of what we call common sense, justice would be defeated in almost every case where opinion evidence is admitted. Moreover, it is sufficient if there be a causal connection between the injury and death. The injury need not be the sole cause."

One's initial reaction to the finding of the three physicians is to express incredulity that three could agree on such a ridiculous verdict. However, the matter is not that simple. Physicians are trained to look for the "immediate cause" of death for autopsy reports. Medically speaking, they were probably correct in saying that the immediate cause of death was "obstructed bowels." They do seem to have gone beyond this, however, in expressing an extraneous opinion that the cause of death was independent of the injuries received unless they were speaking only again of the "immediate cause." In the legal sense there can be no doubt that the "proximate cause" of death was injuries received in the work-related explosion in the mine. Had there been discussion by the three physicians with attorneys concerning the legal meaning of the term "proximate cause," the physicians easily could have rendered a medical verdict in their own terms and then translated it into legal language.

The above case, although it does not relate to gynecology, is an extreme example of the dangers to which physicians can be exposed if they do not understand how their own terminology can be misread by lay persons and attorneys.

What is the meaning of the word "error" in the title to this textbook? It is submitted that "error" is used in the sense of being an equivalent for "a deviation from the physician's ideal of perfect surgery." Remember the concept of Plato that for every idea there is in existence somewhere in the universe the perfect existence or expression of that idea or ideal. Gynecologic specialists writing in this textbook seek to find the ideal technique for each and every part of all of the procedures discussed in the various chapters. The writers of the various chapters seek to help the reader to perfect his

own techniques to the point where the ideal surgical result will be obtained. In that context a less than perfect result will involve the perforation or bruising of the bladder leading to a vesicovaginal fistula even though the hysterectomy was performed in a manner equal to the standard of skill of gynecologists in the community. The skilled surgeon need not concede that perforation or suturing or bruising of the bladder during the course of the performance of the hysterectomy is "error" equivalent to negligent malpractice. The physician should be free to refer to such an eventuality as a "risk of surgery," a "poor result," or an "error" in the platonic sense above mentioned. However, as will be shown by a discussion of subsequent cases, he will use the word "error" in the presence of his patients with some considerable risk to his pocketbook.

A 1953 decision of the California Appeals Court illustrates these points (3). Leakage of urine into the vagina was discovered 3 days after the performance of the total hysterectomy. The surgeon, upon complaint by the patient, made an examination and discovered a fistula in the plaintiff's bladder. Two operations followed with a final repair of the fistula. The patient testified at trial that the surgeon told her when discussing discovery of the fistula, "We all make mistakes." She also quoted the physician as saying that most probably the needle went through a portion of the bladder in sewing the incision between the bladder and the uterus and subsequently it broke out tearing a hole in the bladder. At the trial the physician denied that any such conversation occurred.

It is a little hard for this writer to believe that the patient could have come up with the quotes unless, in some way, the physician had given her an explanation of what might have happened. If he did say, "We all make mistakes," he undoubtedly was speaking in terms of deviations from the desired results of the ideal hysterectomy which is the concern of the chapters on that subject.

A later California case (4) sounds very similar. A vesicovaginal fistula developed 7 days after the performance of a hysterectomy. It was repaired by other surgeons. At trial the patient said that the defendant gynecologic surgeon, in explaining the fistula to her, showed her a chart and said, " 'I must have put a suture through the flap of the bladder there which caused the fistula' " (5).

In both cases the surgeon was totally exonerated, although in one of the cases the plaintiff was able to produce several physicians as expert witnesses in her behalf.

It is interesting to quote one paragraph from the opinion of the appellate court in the later case because the language speaks to the causes of fistulae very much along the lines of the safeguards against fistulae described by the surgeon in his chapter on radical hysterectomy:

"It is known that such fistulas result from devascularization and necrosis (cutting off of the blood supply and death of tissue) in the place where the fistula is formed; a number of factors can contribute to the devascularization and necrosis, and ordinarily it cannot be determined which of them were operative in a specific case. Among these factors are bruising of the bladder during the necessary separation of the uterus from the bladder, sutures or ligatures in the wall of the bladder to control bleeding caused in the separation, infection present in the cervix of the uterus and the vagina vault adjacent to the bladder, and the tissue reaction of the individual to surgery and suture materials. Tissue reaction may be affected by previously existent weakness of the area, impairment of the blood supply in the area, and prior X-ray treatment administered to any part of the patient's body" (6).

It is interesting that in the earlier California case, one of the plaintiff's medical expert witnesses stated that a fistula had never followed any of the approximately 300 hysterectomies he had performed in his career. Another gynecologic specialist testified that in his entire practice, he had observed approximately two dozen fistulae and that only in 0.1 to 0.2 of 1 percent of all hysterectomies does a fistula follow.

The majority of the judges considering the situation decided that the low incidence of fistulae following hysterectomies indicated that even if the performing surgeon sutured or bruised or perforated the bladder that, unless it could be affirmatively shown by expert testimony that he was guilty of negligence, the fact of the perforation, bruising, or suturing itself was not evidence of malpractice but was one of the side risks of having a hysterectomy. This finding seems to be borne out in a number of cases although one of the justices dissented from the decision saying:

"All the medical testimony showed that a fistula in the bladder caused by an hysterectomy operation was a very, very rare occurrence. One expert testified that in only one-tenth to two-tenths of one per cent did it happen. One testified that the incidence would be less than one per cent. One testified that a fistula had never happened in the approximately three hundred hysterectomy operations performed by him. It is not reasonable in view of this evidence for this court to say that such injury was an assumed risk, or one that would have ordinarily occurred" (7).

A more recent decision, in the Federal District Court in Virginia, seems to speak conclusively on the same subject:

"The record reflects that even the most competent board certified gynecologists will be confronted with inadvertent suturing of the bladder while performing like operations. Statistics indicate only a minimal percentage of such incidents, but it is nevertheless not uncommon and is a recognized hazard in the medical profession. As a vast majority of situations will not result in a fistula, or is otherwise repaired through a normal process, it is quite likely that the true percentage of inadvertent suturing is not reported. Because of the very nature of the operation and the requirement of working in a confined area, the surgeon doing the suturing is severely handicapped and medical science has not yet developed a procedure which will eliminate the calculated risk . . . . While plaintiff's counsel stresses the fact that witnesses referred to the suturing as a 'mistake,' this does not establish negligence as the duty owed is that degree of skill and diligence employed by the ordinary, prudent practitioner in his field and community, or in similar communities at the time" (8).

Several other cases of vesicovaginal fistula following hysterectomy can be summarized quickly. In a Connecticut case (9), the patient said that the defendant physician explained the fistula by saying that he had cut into her bladder during the operation. He referred her to another surgeon who repaired the fistula. The plaintiff was able to present no expert witness in her favor other than the defendant physician himself and judgment for the physician was affirmed.

Osburn v. Saltz, a Louisiana decision of 1964 (10), bears particular scrutiny because of its demonstration of how the patient's own anatomic anomalies may affect the surgeon, however skillful. The patient in this case had had previous surgery, and upon opening her abdomen for the performance of the hysterectomy, it was discovered that 90 per cent of the area was filled with adhesions. The difficult procedure was followed by a stormy and infectious recovery. The evidence in the records showed that the infection came from the colon. Seven days following surgery, the vesicovaginal fistula surfaced. The case is interesting because the report shows that the patient was handled exactly as is required in the chapter on fistulae. Conservative care until infection was cured was rigidly maintained in the face of strong insistence by the patient that surgery be performed sooner than thought wise by the surgeon. The repair was successful. The plaintiff at trial had two theories. The first was that the surgeon was guilty of negligent cutting of the bladder during surgery. The Court did not believe this testimony because expert testimony showed that either the surgeon would have known that he had cut the bladder during surgery and have repaired it or the fistula would have developed in 24 to 72 hours of surgery rather than 7 days later. The Court was therefore persuaded that the first theory had no evidence in support of it. The second theory was that the postoperative care by the physician was negligent so that he in effect allowed the infection to occur and the infection itself caused the fistula. The Court carefully reviewed the evidence and found that the physician had been careful in giving postoperative care. It was damaging to the plaintiff's case that well-intentioned relatives had given her baths in the hospital not prescribed or known by the physician or the hospital. The Court speculated that infection might have occurred because of such baths.

Three more cases, all involving fistulae following hysterectomies, were all won by the physicians. But note that in each case the patient relied on something she said the physician had said to her or in her presence: " 'Jim, here is your trouble. You've got a stitch in the kidney tube' " (11). " 'I cut too close . . .' " (to the bladder) (12). " 'I nipped her bladder' " (13).

To the attorney reading this chapter, this writer would advise that, based on reported decisions, he should not expect to prevail for a client who has suffered from a vesicovaginal fistula or a rectovaginal fistula following hysterectomy on the grounds of res ipsa loquitur or, indeed, because the physician has said something like, "I made a mistake," or "I cut the bladder." To the physician seeking to improve his techniques in the performance of procedures which might cause fistulae, this writer advises, after reading many reported cases, that naturally he should seek to perfect his techniques. Should a poor result eventuate, the result should be explained to the patient. Whether he performed the surgery or is making explanation after examination of a patient upon whom another surgeon has operated, he should carefully explain all of the different ways fistulae may develop. Some may be "caused" by the surgery, but the fact that a poor result has eventuated or there is a deviation from the surgical ideal should not be called by him "error" or "mistake" because he cannot be certain medically that it was anything other than a deviation from the surgical ideal and because if he reads the cases discussing this particular condition, he will realize that courts do not hold physicians to the same degree of care and skill to which the physicians writing the chapters of this textbook wish surgeons to achieve.

So that the surgeon contemplating performance of gynecologic surgery will not feel too much security, there follows a list of a few unfortunate results.

In a Washington case (14), a $25,000 judgment for the patient was affirmed and res ipsa loquitur was held to support a finding of negligence where the patient's arm was paralyzed following performance of hysterectomy on the patient in the Trendelenburg position.

In a New Mexico case (15), the physician was held possibly negligent in failing to discover a possible pregnancy prior to performing a hysterectomy.

In a Tennessee case (16), the patient's vagina closed following hysterectomy to the extent that marital relations were frustrated. After discharge from the hospital, the patient returned to the surgeon as required for postoperative followup. Until more than 6 months following the discharge and until the patient complained, the physician did not perform a manual examination on her. When he did perform a manual examination and discovered the closed vagina, he made a statement against his own interest that he could have avoided the result if he had examined her sooner as he should have done. The Court relied on the physician's statement as setting forth a prima facie case of negligence.

In a California case (17), the surgeon was held negligent for suturing the right ureter in two places during the performance of hysterectomy. The patient's right kidney had to be removed.

The surgeon reading the chapter on radical hysterectomy will find that in several places the author speaks of "error." For example, he says, in discussing when the physician should consider radical hysterectomy, "Misapplication of the operation is an error that should be credited against the surgeon." In another place, he says, "At this time, no error can be imposed by using either the open or closed procedure." His use of the word "error" in these contexts comes close to the legal definition of negligence, subject only to a discussion later in this chapter on the standard of practice in the particular location of the defending physician and whether the courts will impose on the defending physician only that degree of care and skill exercised in his own locality, or whether there may be a broader national standard.

The casual reader of the cases discussed so far in this chapter will certainly agree that careful discussion with the patient, whether the patient is discussing the situation with the surgeon who performed the procedure or with another physician, is certainly to be strongly recommended. In almost every one of the cases discussed, the patient at least thought she heard some confession against interest from the physician. Yet, to this date, the courts have been unwilling to impose liability on physicians for the appearance of fistulae following hysterectomies (18).

Malpractice cases against physicians have occurred since the beginnings of the practice of the profession. The general statement of law can be paraphrased as follows. The physician should bring to his practice the reasonable degree of care and skill possessed and exercised by others in the school or system of practice of medicine which he follows in the locality in which he practices or in similar localities. This standard can be broken into three parts: (1) the reasonable degree of care and skill possessed and exercised by others, (2) in the school or

system of practice which the physician follows, and (3) in the locality in which the defendant practices or in similar localities.

At the present time it appears that the first portion of the statement remains constant. The second portion of the standard has considerably less importance since the allopathic and homeopathic schools of medicine have been combined. There is considerable relevance at the present time in the second step with reference to osteopaths but the second portion of the standard has very little importance to make any differentiations among medical doctors at the present time.

However, the third portion of the standard may well be in a state of transition at the present time. The cases indicate that in the earliest days the courts moved to protect the rural physician who, in days of much harder transportation, could not be expected to have the same degree of care and skill as specialists located in metropolitan areas (19).

A decision in Massachusetts (20), while it dealt with the liability of a dentist, illustrates an important concept. In that case a dentist extracted three teeth from the patient's very infected gums. The dentist anesthetized with local novacaine around each tooth. He did not have the equipment or skill to use gas or deep-block novacaine. The court found that in Worcester, Massachusetts, the city in which the dentist practiced, in like situations of infected mouths, most dentists would ordinarily have used gas or deep-block novacaine. After the extractions the patient was ill and finally was hospitalized with osteomyelitis of the jaw bone. The defendant was held liable for malpractice. The court said the following:

"Nor is there anything in the findings inconsistent with the finding that the defendant's dentists should have advised the plaintiff to employ another dentist equipped to use a safer method of anesthetization rather than to have 'undertaken a less safe method.' Such may be the duty of a dentist who, for any reason, is unable personally to exercise the skill ordinarily exercised by dentists in the community." (21).

To bring the point of the Massachusetts decision home, one should ask the the following question. If a general surgeon or board-certified gynecologist does not have the skill to perform one of the specialized procedures discussed in this book, *e.g.*, pelvic exenteration, of some physicians in the same city, will he be held to be guilty of malpractice if he does not refer to the more experienced physician who does have the skill? To date the decisions of the court, aside from the decisions on informed consent to be discussed later in this chapter, would indicate that the answer will be determined by the practice in the community. Do general surgeons in the community as a matter of practice perform pelvic exenterations? Do board-certified obstetricians and gynecologists generally do pelvic exenterations? Of course, under most state licensing statutes, any person qualified as a medical doctor under the law may perform any recognized procedure. Under the by-laws of most hospital staffs, the performance of complicated, specialized surgery will be allowed only on proof of appropriate credentials of the surgeon. However, such by-laws, even in metropolitan centers, probably do not address themselves to quite the specialization implicit in those questions. They might indicate that the general surgeon, and certainly the general practitioner, would not be cleared to perform a pelvic exenteration although the board-certified obstetrician and gynecologist might be so cleared.

The prediction of this writer is that at some point in the future some more refinement in this area can be expected, and the case of the Massachusetts dentist should be remembered.

Beginning about 15 years ago the plaintiffs in malpractice actions against physicians began to take a different approach. Instead of looking at malpractice in the traditional sense of tort liability, *i.e.*, negligence law, the plaintiffs began to examine the contractual relationship between the patient and surgeon. From the beginning of time, if a physician were foolish enough to guarantee a result, the action against the physician would lie in contract, and the only question would be whether the result was obtained. The plaintiffs, for the last 15 years, have reasoned and argued to the courts that the entire relationship between the physician and patient is a contractual one. Underlying a contract must be a meeting of the mind on basic facts. Where one party to a contract is an expert about the subject of the contract and may take advantage of the other party to the contract, the courts will scrutinize the relationship as if the knowledgeable party were a trustee for the other party. Accordingly, plaintiffs have argued successfully before courts that physicians have strong obligations to disclose the nature of illness and the proposed treatment, the side risks, and the best source of treatment. Absent such information, there is no proper basis for the contract and some courts have ruled that, therefore, the physician is guilty of a nonconsensual touching of the patient. This amounts technically to "battery." Battery is classified as an intentional tort as distinguished from a negligent tort. If a person commits battery on another, he can be liable for damages to deter the wrongdoing even in the absence of proof of injury to the harmed party. The plaintiff who could break down the barrier of the contract and obtain a finding of battery against a physician therefore was not obligated to prove injury to his patient nor to use experts to prove the injury.

This line of cases has had something of a climax in the fall of 1972 with two important decisions, one in the federal appellate court in the District of Columbia (22), and the other in the Supreme Court of California (23). A review of the two cases in some detail is necessary to carry forward the discussion of malpractice and the requirements of informed consent. Both decisions are carefully considered and documented. It is likely that both being in agreement will have a heavy influence on other courts throughout the United States.

In *Canterbury v. Spence,* the District of Columbia decision, a 19-year-old male FBI employee suffered severe pain between his shoulder blades in December 1958. He consulted two general practitioners who could not help him but referred him to Dr. Spence, neurosurgeon. Dr. Spence found negative results on office examination. The X-ray was negative. He recommended a myelogram which was made on February 4, 1959, showing a "filling defect" in the region of the fourth thoracic vertebra. Dr. Spence recommended a laminectomy for a suspected ruptured disc. Apparently Mr. Canterbury did not raise any objection to the proposed operation nor did he probe into its exact nature, and Dr. Spence did not explain it to him. Dr. Spence did speak over the telephone to the mother but made no explanation to her other than that there was no greater risk involved in a laminectomy than in other surgery. The mother signed the consent after the performance of surgery.

The laminectomy was performed on February 11, 1959, and Dr. Spence found several anomalies. The spinal cord was swollen and unable to pulsate. There was an accumulation of large tortuous and dilated veins. There was a complete absence of epidural fat normally surrounding the spine.

The day following surgery the patient fell while attempting to void and while unattended. His bed had no rails up. He suffered paralysis and the physician immediately operated again to relieve pressure on the spine. The final result was partial paralysis and urinary incontinence.

At the trial the only expert witness was Dr. Spence called as an adverse witness. Dr. Spence testified that there was a 1 per cent chance of paralysis in laminectomy cases but that it was not good medical practice to inform the patient of that risk because it might adversely affect the patient's psychology and course of recovery. At the trial level the court directed verdicts for the physician and the hospital. The appellate court reversed and sent the matter back for trial.

The court started with a basic assumption: " '[E]very human being of adult years and sound mind has a right to determine what shall be done with his own body . . .' " (24).

The court, therefore, concluded that the physician must inform the patient of the proposed treatment, the risks, and alternative treatments. The court specifically stated that alternative treatments would include the referral to experts better qualified to perform particular procedures. The court pointed out that a physician is much more familiar with the facts confronting the patient than the patient can be himself. "To enable the patient to chart his course understandably, some familiarity with the therapeutic alternatives and their hazards becomes essential" (25). The physician has a duty to disclose dangers, the court saying that this is "surely a facet of due care" (26). Only a reasonable explanation to the patient, considering his level of education and sophistication, is allowable. The physician is neither required to give, nor exonerated by giving, a medical disposition or a short medical education. His obligation is to disclose more than he would disclose if he were trading with a person of equal education and sophistication in an arms-length transaction.

The court continued: "We now find, as a part of the physician's overall obligation to the patient, a similar duty of *reasonable* disclosure of the choices with respect to proposed therapy and the dangers inherently and potentially involved" (27).

The surgeon has an affirmative obligation to volunteer information and cannot simply answer questions posed by the patient. The affirmative duty to disclose is a part of the implied contract between the physician and his patient.

The court next found that a majority of courts ruling on the question up to the time of its decision had only found the kind of duty above described if it were also established by expert testimony that giving that kind of information and making such affirmative disclosures were the custom among similar medical doctors in the same community or similar communities. The Federal Court of Appeals for the District of Columbia agreed that a failure to disclose as much as was the medical practice in the particular community would give rise to liability, but it specifically declined to agree that there is no liability just because physicians in the same community do not make the kind of disclosure required. "Respect for the patient's right of self-determination on particular therapy demands a standard set by law for physicians rather than one which physicians may or may not impose upon themselves" (28).

The court then addressed itself to the question of how much disclosure should be given to the patient. The court specifically did not require "full" disclosure, not every risk no matter how small or remote. Again, the District of Columbia court said that most courts to date had referred to the medical practice in the community to determine how much disclosure, but the court stated that the law should set the amount of the disclosure, not the medical community. All risks potentially affecting the decision of the patient as to whether to have surgery must be unmasked.

The physician's liability for nondisclosure is to be based on foresight, not the 20/20 vision of hindsight. The reasonableness of disclosure will be measured by what the physician knew or should have known of the patient's needs to know in order to make an intelligent decision. The physician must make this determination, as a professional expert, based on his knowledge of the patient, the level of education and sophistication of the patient, and how the patient construes the information given him by the physician. The District of Columbia federal court gave some examples of where disclosure was required. These were: a 3 per cent chance of death, paralysis, or other injury (29); a 1 per cent chance of loss of hearing (30). It gave as examples from the legal literature of cases in which disclosure was not required the following: a 1/800,000 chance of aplastic anemia (31); a 1.5 per cent of chance of loss of eye (32); and a 1/250 to 1/500 chance of perforation of the esophagus (33).

The court went on to say that the dangers inherent in any operation, such as infection, need not be discussed with a person of average sophistication.

The court recognizes two exceptions to the foregoing rules. The first is the familiar exception for an unconscious patient where there is no relative conveniently nearby to consent and a true emergency requiring action exists. The court then recognized another exception where disclosure would cause psychologic harm or interfere with the course of recovery. The court hastened to say that this did not allow for nondisclosure just because the physician feared divulgence might prompt the patient to forego therapy the physician himself feels the patient really needs.

Even if the physician does not comply with all of the foregoing rules, before liability will attach, the unrevealed risk must eventuate and cause the patient harm. The necessary causal relationship between failure to divulge and damage to the patient must be based upon a factual finding that disclosure of a significant risk would have resulted in the patient's decision against having the treatment procedure. The court then examines what is the proper standard for determining whether the patient would have decided against the procedure if the risks had been disclosed. This is to be determined by what a prudent person in the same circumstances would have decided if he had known the risks and not by what the patient says on the stand after suffering the unfavorable result. Nonexpert, lay testimony may be taken by the court to determine whether a reasonable patient similarly circumstanced would have decided to have the therapy

knowing the risks. Presumably proof of the degree of risk would have to be made by experts, *i.e.*, whether a particular risk is a 1 or 10 per cent risk.

While the District of Columbia court pointed out that if the failure to disclose resulted in battery there was a 1-year statute of limitations against the plaintiff's claim and if it only resulted in negligence there was a 3-year statute of limitations, the court found it unnecessary to decide saying that in either event, the physician would have been negligent and, therefore, the patient's claim, filed between 1 and 3 years, was not barred by the statute of limitations. The court did not give insights into a differentiation between the two theories of action.

Such a differentiation is, however, found in the California decision in *Cobbs v. Grant* (34). The importance of the decision of the Supreme Court of California is emphasized by the fact that the Supreme Court sat en banc, meaning that it assembled the full court rather than sitting in separate panels. In that case the physician operated on the patient for a very small active duodenal ulcer. "The spleen injury, development of the gastric ulcer, gastrectomy and internal bleeding as a result of the premature absorption of a suture, were all links in a chain of low probability events inherent in the initial operation" (35). None of those unpleasant eventuating risks had been disclosed to the patient prior to the operation.

The California court indicated that there had been developing a line of cases to the effect that insufficient disclosure to the patient for him to give an informed consent automatically resulted in battery requiring no expert testimony. The California court declined to follow that line of reasoning except in the case of the physicians performing a wholly different operation from that to which consent had been given. If the physician performed the operation to which consent had been given but there had not been enough information for an informed consent to be given, the physician is only to be held to the standards of negligence in malpractice and, therefore, presumably expert testimony will have to be presented by the plaintiff to support his theory of action. The California court followed the decision of the District of Columbia in *Canterbury v. Spence*, saying that the amount of disclosure to be given to the patient is not to be determined by medical practice in the community but by law. It reaffirmed the idea that the adult patient in a nonemergency has a right of self-determination. In discussing the amount of disclosure, the court said:

"A mini-course in medical science is not required; the patient is concerned with the risk of death or bodily harm, and problems of recuperation. Second, there is no physician's duty to discuss the relatively minor risks inherent in common procedures, when it is common knowledge that such risks inherent in the procedure are of very low incidence" (36).

In a footnote to the quoted statement, the court pointed out, as one example which need not be disclosed, the side risks of vena puncture for a blood sample which include hematoma, dermatitis, cellulitis, abscess, osteomyelitis, septicemia, endocarditis, thrombophlebitis, pulmonary embolism, and death (37).

The California court also opined that it was only necessary for the physician to ask whether the patient had an adverse reaction to any antibiotics and that specific warning as to possible side effects from use of antibiotics is not necessary.

Finally, the California court cautioned:

". . . when there is a more complicated procedure . . . the jury should be instructed that when a given procedure inherently involves a known risk of death or serious bodily harm, a medical doctor has a duty to disclose to his patient the potential of death or serious harm, and to explain in lay terms the complications that might possibly occur. Beyond the foregoing minimal disclosure, a doctor must also reveal to his patient such additional information as a skilled practitioner of good standing would provide under similar circumstances" (38).

It is clear that, with respect to gynecologic surgical procedures discussed in this book, the surgeon must design his explanations to the patient or the patient's relatives with care. Further, he should, through the medical records if the explanation is in his office or the hospital records if the explanation is in the hospital, note carefully each instruction given and, if the physician decides not to disclose particular risks because of concern that the patient might have an adverse reaction, record the risks not disclosed and the reasons therefor. Incidentally, the other horn of the dilemma is occasioned by the cancerphobia case (39) in which a radiologist was held liable for dermatitis following X-ray treatment because the patient became neurotically fearful of cancer after being warned by the treating dermatologist to return for observation each 6 months.

The cases earlier described in this chapter indicate that physicians to date have not been held liable for vaginal fistulae following hysterectomy, these being considered to be risks variously appraised at from 0.1 of 1 per cent to 3 per cent of all cases. Yet if one carefully considers the decision of *Canterbury v. Spence* in which the court found the physician negligent in failing to disclose a 1 per cent chance of paralysis, should we raise the following questions? If a court finds that a physician, because of less training than a brother physician in the same community, has a 5 per cent possibility of untoward result of a fistula following hysterectomy where his brother has either none or a 0.1 of 1 per cent risk, does the more risky physician have an obligation to disclose that fact to the patient before the patient decides on surgery with the particular physician? If the more risky physician does not make the disclosure, does he become a guarantor that there will be no fistula following hysterectomy? If he is such a guarantor, it may be that the patient would not have to introduce expert testimony to prove the malpractice of the physician but only lay testimony as to what the patient should have heard before arriving at a decision for the surgery.

It seems to this writer that while the questions posed might make some sense in the context of the case of *Canterbury v. Spence*, it is highly unlikely that courts can ever be precise enough to say that one physician has a 5 per cent possibility of a poorer result and another has less than 1 per cent chance of a poor result. It is more probable that liability would only be imposed under this theory upon proof that the operating physician really was insufficiently trained to undertake the particular procedure. However, the degree of training for highly specialized surgery, especially in metropolitan areas, will undoubtedly be a question for consideration in future cases.

It is submitted that Mr. Canterbury, in *Canterbury v. Spence*, suffering as he was prior to his laminectomy, almost certainly would have elected surgery even if all side risks, including a 1 per cent chance of paralysis, were disclosed. It seems probable to this writer that when the matter is tried again by a jury that even lay persons will find this to be so if they can be made to understand the degree of pain suffered by a patient with a ruptured disc. Similarly, it seems that the patient in *Cobbs v. Grant* would elect surgery for a very painful active duodenal ulcer even if he had understood the side risks of internal bleeding and further operations. After all, if properly explained, he would know that he would probably have internal bleeding and a need for further surgery if he did not have the first surgery. It is a very different question, however, to ask whether Mr. Canterbury might have elected not to have the surgery with Dr. Spence if Dr. Spence really did not have as good training and record in the performance of laminectomies as another easily available surgeon. Therefore, the precise question of obligation to discuss referral to another more experienced physician may become one of the most critical elements of disclosure to a patient in order for the physician to have an informed consent to the procedure.

While a physician reading this chapter may well be able to design his discussions with the patient and the patient's spouse or relatives, he may welcome some attempt at organizing a procedure for laying out what to say in a particular case to a particular patient. The following paragraphs are organized in a way that seemed logical to this writer.

Kind of Procedure. A first distinction should be made between procedures essential to preserve life and those elective to improve health or the comfort of the patient or the reproductive or connubial function. With respect to the radical hysterectomy or the pelvic exenteration necessary because of the existence of a malignant tumor, less may need be said to the patient than with respect to elective procedures. For example, it would seem to this writer that the risk of general anesthesia need hardly be discussed with a patient facing nonelective life-saving surgery. On the other hand, the risk of general anesthesia might well be explained to the patient who had not previously undergone it but who is considering very elective surgery to relieve discomfort. Such a patient might well decide to proceed with more conservative treatment and to continue some discomfort rather than to run the risk of general anesthesia. It is inconceivable that, in the absence of clear contraindications for general anesthesia, any reasonable patient would decline surgery to remove a malignant tumor because of the risk of general anesthesia. Again, the patient facing pelvic exenteration hardly needs to have spelled out for her that she will not thereafter be able to bear children. Such an explanation should clearly be made with respect to less radical and elective surgery if there is a possibility of interfering with the reproductive function.

Nature of Patient. In line with the cases discussed, the education and sophistication of the patient are all important. Obviously, less need be said to a patient who is himself a physician than to a patient who is a lawyer, but less may need be said to the lawyer than would be proper to the plumber. If a decision not to disclose because of the possible adverse psychiatric damage is considered, it might be wise to have a psychiatric consultation to back up the decision not to disclose. Of course, a surgeon dealing with a hypertensive patient facing surgery could well harm the patient by suggesting a psychiatric consultation in his own interest.

Reproductive and Connubial Function. It is essential in all cases of elective surgery that the physician discuss with the patient and the patient's spouse, if any, the intended or possible effect of the surgery on the reproductive or connubial function. If there is a possibility, as a side risk of the surgery, that the reproductive function would be increased or decreased, that should also be discussed in all cases except those extreme ones such as pelvic exenteration as mentioned above.

Side Risks. Based on the cases discussed in this chapter, certain generalizations can be made. For the patient considering surgery in which vaginal fistulae may be a side effect, that possibility should always be discussed. It is suggested that the various possibilities for the occurrence of fistulae, including bruising in the close area of work and the danger of outside infection as well as the possible existence of anatomic anomalies which cannot be foreseen, all should be discussed. Apparently from the cases discussed in this chapter, it would be wise to mention as side risks any which have a possibility of occurrence of at least 1 per cent, although even more remote contingencies may need discussion if the side risk is extremely dangerous compared to the elective nature of the surgery.

No Guarantee. The physician should always be careful to indicate to the patient that no guarantee of results can be made. It is especially important if the intended effect of the operation is to increase or nullify the reproductive function. The physician, in his professional and almost paternal function of encouraging a patient who really needs surgery, must be careful not to brush aside the possibility that the intended result may not occur or the patient may well understand a guarantee that the physician did not intend to make. Remember that the court expects the physician to understand the patient to the degree of being able to know the patient's sophistication and education and an understanding of what the physician is saying as to be measured later against what a reasonable patient might decide to do in the circumstances.

Alternatives to Treatment. This may turn out to be the most critical area of the discussion with the patient. Is there a more conservative alternative to surgery? Is radiologic treatment possible instead of surgery? If so, what are the chances of cure and risks of not having the surgery? If the surgery is elective, what are the possible later consequences of not having surgery now and following a conservative course of treatment instead? The one alternative the surgeon must always consider is whether he should mention other physicians who may be more specialized in the performance of the particular procedure. What are the relative expenses to the patient in seeking such alternative physicians' treatment? Is the physician who has more experience practicing in the same community or must the patient travel at great trouble and expense to another location?

In summary, it appears that, despite some of the comfort offered the surgeon in this chapter, the future will bring more claims and malpractice exposure to the physician. The interesting question for speculation is whether the economics of rapidly rising malpractice premiums forcing higher fees will cause a reaction, as with automobile insurance, towards a "no-fault" insurance approach to professional malpractice. While no prediction can be made by this writer, it is his hope that such a result will be obtained.

It bears repeating that the surgeon should guard against quick statements sounding like a confession of professional self-fault or a finding of fault in another physician. As against himself these statements are probably admissible on the testimony of a patient as an "admission against interest." There is no substitute for a detailed, careful, and truthful but well planned explanation to the patient of the poor result.

Finally, the physician should not be overly concerned about his malpractice exposure. If a physician is well trained, hard-working, and not the touting or promoter prototype of an unethical professional, court and jury alike will differentiate very well between unprofessional negligence on the one hand and accident or error due to anatomic vagaries or poor tissue healing or failure of the patient to adhere to instructions, on the other.

References

1. *Miami Coal Co. v. Luce*, 76 Ind. App. 245, 131 N.E. 824 (1921).
2. *Id.*, at 76 Ind. App. 249, 131 N.E. 826.
3. *Dees v. Pace*, 118 Cal.App.2d 284, 257 P.2d 756 (Cal.App.1953).
4. *Silverson v. Weber*, 372 P.2d 97 (Cal.1962).
5. *Id.*, at 372 P.2d 98.
6. *Ibid.*
7. *Dees v. Pace*, 118 Cal.App.2d 284, 290-291, 257 P.2d 756, 759-760.
8. *Varga v. U.S.*, 314 F.Supp.671, 675 (E.D.Va. 1969), aff'd 422 F.2d 1333 (4th Cir.1970).
9. *Townsend v. Sullivan*, 149 Conn. 666, 183 A.2d 266 (1962).
10. 169 So.2d 687 (Ct.App.La.1964).
11. *Hart v. Steele*, 416 S.W.2d 927, 929 (Mo. 1967).
12. *Brear v. Sweet*, 155 Wash.474, 476, 284 P.803,804 (1930).
13. *Modrzyinski v. Lust*, 88 N.E.2d 76, 77 (Ohio App. 1949).
14. *Horner v. Northern Pacific Beneficial Association Hospitals, Inc.*, 62 Wash.2d 351, 382 P.2d 518 (1963).
15. *Burks v. Baumgartner*, 72 N.M. 123, 381 P.2d 57 (1963).
16. *Wooten v. Curry*, 362 S.W.2d 820 (Tenn.App. 1961).
17. *Tomei v. Henning*, 431 P.2d 633 (Cal.1967).
18. Other recent cases showing victories by the surgeon before juries or trial courts are *Huet v. Epstein*, and *Larson v. Genetti* reported in *The*

Citation, AMA Law Department, Vol. 25, No. 11, p. 165, September 15, 1972; *Dazet v. Bass*, 254 So.2d 183 (Miss.1971); *Tatro v. Lueken*, 212 Kan.606, 512 P.2d 529 (1973) (although the physician did not disclose the side risk of vesicovaginal fistula following hysterectomy).

19. e.g., *Josselyn v. Dearborn*, 143 Me.328, 62 A.2d 174 (1948) (proper for jury to consider what resources and skill osteopath in Lubec, Maine, had compared to physicians in Bangor; osteopath still held guilty of malpractice).

20. *Vigneault v. Dr. Hewson Dental Co.*, 300 Mass. 223, 15 N.E. 2d 185 (1938).

21. *Id.* at 300 Mass. 227-228, 15 N.E.2d 188.

22. *Canterbury v. Spence*, 464 F.2d 772 (D.C.Cir. 1972)., *cert. den.*, 409 U.S.1064.

23. *Cobbs v. Grant*, 502 P.2d 1 (Cal.1972).

24. *Canterbury v. Spence*, 464 F.2d 772, 780.

25. *Id.* at 781.

26. *Id.* at 782.

27. *Ibid.* Italics supplied.

28. *Id.* at 784.

29. *Bowers v. Talmage*, 159 So.2d 888 (Fla.App. 1963).

30. *Scott v. Wilson*, 396 S.W.2d 532 (Tex.Civ.App. 1965), aff'd 412 S.W.2d 299 (Tex.1967).

31. *Stottlemire v. Cawood*, 213 F.Supp. 897, 898 (D.D.C.), new trial denied, 215 F.Supp.266 (1963).

32. *Yeates v. Harms*, 193 Kan.320, 393 P.2d 982, 991 (1964).

33. *Starnes v. Taylor*, 272 N.C.386, 393, 158 S.E.2d 339, 344 (1968).

34. *Supra*, n.23.

35. 502 P.2d 1, 8.

36. *Id.* at 11.

37. *Id.* at 11, n.2. But *cf. Funke v. Fieldman*, 212 Kan.524, 512 P.2d 539 (1973) where the court, citing *Canterbury v. Spence*, fn. 22 *supra*, found that the defendant anesthesiologist could be held liable for failing to disclose the side risk of paralysis attendant to the use of spinal anesthesia instead of general anesthesia.

38. *Id.* at 11.

39. *Ferrara v. Galluchio*, 5 N.Y.2d 16, 152 N.E.2d 249 (1958).

INDEX

Abdomen
  closure, after hysterectomy, 25-26
  opening, incisions
    for adnexal surgery, 81
    general considerations, 8
    technique, 8-10
  surgical procedure, 8-11
Abcess
  pelvic
    following vaginal hysterectomy, 71-72
    in cul-de-sac, surgery, 88
    opened during laparotomy, 88
    postabortal, 89
    ruptured tubo-ovarian
      postoperative care, 91
      surgical treatment, 89, 90-91
    suburethral, incision and drainage, urethrovaginal fistula resulting from, 176
Adnexa
  disease: *see* Adnexal disease
  hemorrhage, diagnosis and treatment, 89-90
  removal during vaginal hysterectomy, 57
  surgery: *see* Adnexal surgery
  torsion of 89-90
  tumors, surgery, 82-85
Adnexal disease
  benign, surgery for, 78-113
  diagnosis, 78-79
  gynecologic emergencies due to, 89-91
  preoperative preparation, 79-80
Adnexal surgery, 78-113
  bowel involvement, 108-111
  common errors, 111-112
  for endometriosis, 85-87
  for residual pelvic inflammatory disease, 87-91
  incisions, 80-82
  indications, 78
  preparation in operating room, 80
  ureteral injury during, 91-108
Age, in pelvic exenteration, 279
Aldridge modification, of Goebell-Stoeckel-Frangenheim procedure, 131
  technique, 140-143
Ambulation, early
  following surgery for stress urinary incontinence, 149
  in prevention of thromboembolic complications, 39-40
Anesthesia
  in abdominal surgery, 7
  in vaginal hysterectomy, 47
Antibiotics, broad spectrum, use following tubal surgery for infertility, 239
Anticoagulants, postoperative, in prevention of thromboembolic complications, 39-41
Anuria, common errors in pelvic surgery, 112
Apareunia, following vaginal hysterectomy, 74
Appendix, removal during gynecologic surgery, 36

Bacteriuria, transient, following bladder manipulation during vaginal hysterectomy, 72
Ball and Hoffman modification, of Goebell-Frangenheim-Stoeckel procedure, 131

Barium
  enema, prior to pelvic exenteration, 281
  used in testing, evacuated preoperatively, 35
Bartholin gland
  removal, 245-246
  surgery, 244-247
    contraindicated during pregnancy, 246-247
Baylor balloon, for incompetent cervix, 228
Bladder
  at rest following injury, 33
  atonic, following radical hysterectomy, 271
  catheterized during abdominal surgery, 32
  detachment during radical hysterectomy, 267
  dissection in abdominal hysterectomy, safeguards, 16-17
  during abdominal surgery, 7-8
  exploration and manipulation after abdominal incision, 11
  infection, prior to abdominal surgery, 6
  injury
    at incision, 32
    by clamps in abdominal surgery, 32-33
    by sutures in abdominal surgery, 16
    complications if unrepaired, 34
    during adnexal surgery, 91-108
    fistulae caused by, 33, 34-35
    in abdominal surgery, 1, 31-35
    in dissection from cervix, 33
    management of complications in abdominal surgery, 31-35
    safeguards, 10
    to base, 33
    treatment of fistulae caused by, 34-35
    unrepaired, diagnosis of, 34
    warning signs, 31
  locating after abdominal incision, 31-32
  safeguards against incision of, 10
Bladder neck
  surgery, urethrovaginal fistula resulting from, 176
  transurethral resection of, condemnation of procedure, 186-188
Bladder wall, endometriosis of, treated by local excision, 87
Bleeding: *see also* Hemorrhage
  during abdominal surgery, 36-38
  during myomectomy, 215-218
  following surgery for stress urinary incontinence, 150
  following vaginal hysterectomy and repair, 68-71
  from abdominal incision, 9
  postoperative, management of, 37-38
  uterine, abnormal, indication for vaginal hysterectomy, 45
Blood loss, during surgery, 70-71
Blood replacement, during pelvic exenteration, 287
Blood volume, preoperative preparation in pelvic exenteration, 284
Bowels: *see also* Rectum
  adherent to fundus, in abdominal hysterectomy, 21
  common errors in surgery, 112
  injury
    during abdominal surgery, 35-36